TEXTBOOK OF ANATOMY

VOLUME 2

NEURAL, CARDIOVASCULAR, RESPIRATORY, DIGESTIVE, AND ENDOCRINE SYSTEMS

José Adán Amaya Duarte and
Kareling Alexandra Lopez Sandoval

ALLIED
HEALTH
PRESS

Textbook of Anatomy Volume 2

Neural, Cardiovascular, Respiratory, Digestive, and Endocrine Systems

Authors: **José Adán Amaya Duarte and Kareling Alexandra Lopez Sandoval**

Allied Health Press
4164 Lakeshore Road
Burlington ON L7L 1A4
Canada
www.alliedhealthpress.com
Email: orders@arclereducation.com

ISBN: 978-1-77956-771-0

ABOUT THE AUTHORS

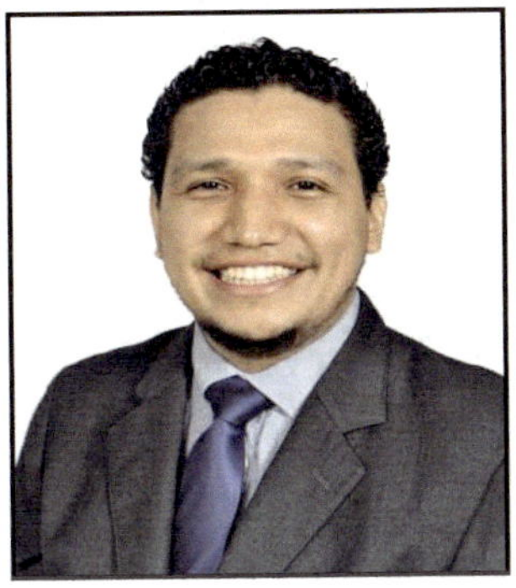

José Adán Amaya Duarte is a medical doctor, academic consultant, and entrepreneur with extensive experience in the industrial, educational, and public health sectors. He currently serves as General Manager (CEO) and co-founder of INVALA S.A., a manufacturing company in Nicaragua, where he has led operational and financial development since 2019.

With a medical degree from UNAN-León, where he also worked as a university professor and research assistant, his profile combines scientific rigor with advanced managerial skills. He also has worked as a medical academic content consultant on global platforms such as Upwork and as a technical advisor and instructional designer for the Pan American Health Organization (PAHO/WHO), participating in multiple virtual training projects, course design, and the updating of pedagogical health content.

In the academic field, he has served as an online tutor, academic coordinator, and designer of educational materials, including audiovisual media, for the Virtual Campus of Public Health. He has also conducted workshops and collaborated in international seminars on topics such as Biofabrication, anatomy, environmental toxicology, educational innovation, and human resource management.

Adán is fluent in English (advanced level) and has basic knowledge of German. In addition, he possesses strong skills in digital tools, ERP/CRM systems, data analysis (SPSS), audiovisual editing, and basic programming (AS3, Swift, Java). His multidisciplinary approach and leadership capacity position him as an influential figure at the intersection of medicine, virtual education, and business management.

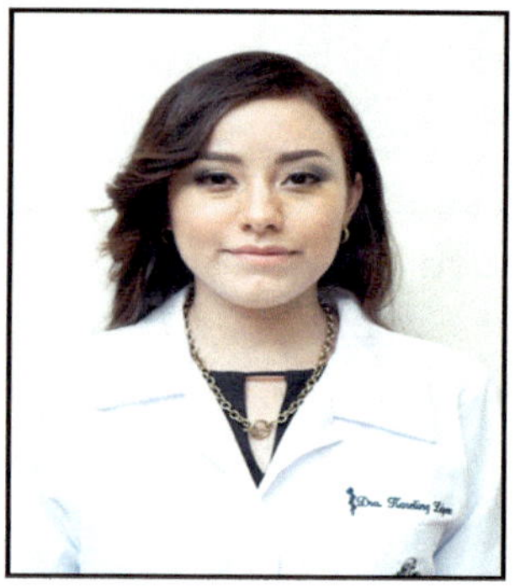

Kareling Alexandra López Sandoval is a medical doctor with experience in clinical care, healthcare operations supervision, and medical translation. She currently serves as Clinical Operations Supervisor at Oclinicals/GI Alliance, coordinating remote teams and maintaining direct communication with clinics in the United States to ensure high standards of patient care.

Graduated as a Doctor of Medicine and Surgery from the National Autonomous University of Nicaragua (UNAN-León), Kareling has worked across various medical areas, developing solid skills in patient assessment, diagnosis, and education. Her career includes roles in both hospital and remote settings, allowing her to adapt to diverse healthcare environments.

In the academic and scientific communication field, she has worked as a medical content reviewer for academic texts, medical article writer based on scientific evidence, and translator of medical documents (Spanish English) with technical accuracy. Her C2-level English proficiency has enabled her to collaborate on international projects, ensuring terminological precision and effective communication with global healthcare teams.

With a combination of clinical training, operational expertise, and medical communication skills, Kareling stands out for her commitment to quality, self-discipline, and continuous improvement in the healthcare sector.

Brief Table of Contents

Getting Started with This Book

Chapter Openers

A list of Chapter Outline is presented providing a brief Introduction to what will be covered in the chapter.

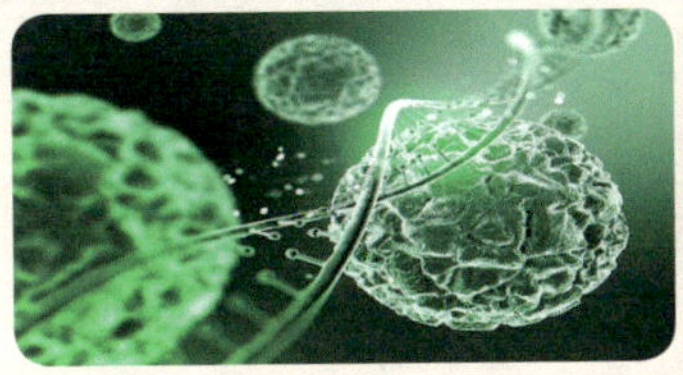

LEARNING OBJECTIVES

After studying this chapter, you will be able to:

1. Discuss the scientific method in biology;
2. Explain the cell theory;
3. Discuss the genetics and heredity;
4. Evolution and natural selection;
5. Focus on ecology and ecosystems;
6. Learn about human biology;
7. Evaluate the plant biology;
8. Explain the microbiology;
9. Focus on current trends in biology.

Introduction

Often referred to as the science of life, biology is a broad field of study aimed at comprehending the several kinds of life on Earth, from tiny creatures to sophisticated multicellular entities. Comprising several subfields, including molecular biology, ecology, and evolutionary biology, each of which advances our knowledge of living systems, this field clarifies the mechanisms controlling life events, including development, reproduction, and interaction with the surroundings, which is the central goal of biology. Moreover, biology fills in the void between the natural sciences and medicine by offering a necessary understanding of health, illness, and the interactions between organisms and their environments. Dealing with urgent global issues such as climate change, biodiversity loss, and new diseases depends on an awareness of these complex biological interactions, therefore highlighting the critical part biology plays in modern civilization. Fundamentally, biology explores and tests ideas about the living world using the scientific method. Through methodical observation and experimentation,

1.1. The Scientific Method in Biology

Learning Outcome

1. Describe the steps of the scientific method;
2. Focus on hypothesis formation;
3. Learn about experimental design.

Learning Outcomes

The beginning of each section of every chapter contains a set of Learning Outcomes that inform students of concepts they should understand. These outcomes help students understand what they should be able to do if they have mastered the material in that section.

Test Your Knowledge

Throughout each chapter, Test Your Knowledge cues you to note which topics have been covered and to self-test your understanding of the material presented.

Test Your Knowledge

1. Explain why correlation does not imply causation in scientific experiments.
2. How does the scientific method help reduce the influence of personal opinions in research?

Chapter Summary

The Summary Section appear at the end of each chapter and summarize main concepts covered throughout the chapter. These points provide key concepts in an engaging and meaningful way.

Summary

The investigation of biological principles highlights the importance of a comprehensive view of life by reflecting the intricate interactions that occur within living systems. The complexity of biology goes beyond individual species or systems, as this essay highlights; it also includes the interactions that mold ecosystems and affect biodiversity. Researchers can conduct in-depth analyses of metabolomic data using sophisticated technologies like MetaboAnalyst, which offer insights into the molecular mechanisms underlying these interactions. As demonstrated by the developments in MetaboAnalyst, for example, the integration of diverse omics data promotes a thorough understanding of metabolic pathways and helps identify important biological markers necessary for research on development and disease (Chong et al., 2018). Additionally, the phenomenon of ecological invasions is a key component of biological research and a vital field of study. The introduction of non-native species into unfamiliar habitats has significant ramifications and calls for multidisciplinary management strategies. Examining the origins and effects of these biological incursions, invasion science has become a crucial field that highlights the need to comprehend ecological dynamics and community interactions. As interest in biological invasions increases, new findings are emerging that put conventional ecological theories and practices to the test. The importance of incorporating various scientific viewpoints is shown by this developing discipline, which also highlights how invasive species shape ecosystems and advances our knowledge of ecological resilience (David et al., 2013). When taken as a whole, these discoveries from invasion science and metabolomics highlight the value of multidisciplinary biology research. Fostering cross-disciplinary collaboration and utilizing technological breakthroughs to improve our comprehension of intricate biological interactions are crucial as we look to the future of biological research. In addition to deepening our understanding of the complexities of life, this method lays the groundwork for tackling urgent environmental issues. Future studies can ensure the continued relevance of biology in a world that is constantly changing by acknowledging the interconnection of biological systems and opening the door to creative solutions that support sustainability and biodiversity conservation. We might imagine a thorough comprehension of life that serves both academia and society at large through ongoing investigation and integration of scientific knowledge.

Knowledge Assessment

The chapter includes material designed to review and reinforce each content. It includes Critical Thinking Questions to help test of your understanding of information presented in the chapter and Short answer Questions to review your understanding of the key concepts presented in the chapter.

Critical Thinking Questions

1. **Who is known as the "Father of Modern Biology"?**
   a. Aristotle
   b. Charles Darwin
   c. Gregor Mendel
   d. Louis Pasteur
2. **What is the basic unit of life?**
   a. Atom
   b. Molecule
   c. Cell
   d. Organism
3. **Which branch of biology studies the interaction of organisms with their environment?**
   a. Genetics
   b. Ecology
   c. Physiology
   d. Botany
4. **Which macromolecule is the main source of energy for living organisms?**
   a. Proteins
   b. Lipids
   c. Carbohydrates
   d. Nucleic acids
5. **DNA is primarily responsible for which function in living organisms?**
   a. Energy production
   b. Protein synthesis
   c. Storing genetic information
   d. Regulating body temperature

Short Answer Questions

1. What is biology, and why is it important to study biology?
2. What are the three main domains of life, and how are they different from one another?
3. Define homeostasis and give an example of how it works in living organisms.
4. What is the cell theory, and why is it fundamental to biology?
5. How do autotrophs and heterotrophs differ in the way they obtain energy?
6. What is the scientific method, and how is it applied in biological research?
7. Discuss how biology helps address global challenges such as climate change, disease, and food security.
8. Explain the levels of biological organization from the smallest unit to the largest. Provide examples at each level.
9. Describe the relationship between structure and function in biology, giving specific examples from cells or organs.
10. How has the discovery of genetics shaped our understanding of inheritance and variation among organisms?

Supplementary Materials

Key Terms: A list of key terms is given for quick reference

KEY TERMS FROM THIS CHAPTER

Annotation enrichment analysis	Biological structure	Cell
Cell theory	Cellular structure	Ecology
Ecosystems	Genetics	Human biology
Microbiology	Natural selection	Organism
Plant biology		

Further Resources: Recommendations for additional readings, websites, and multimedia resources.

References

1. Argelaguet, R., Velten, B., Arnol, D., Dietrich, S., Zenz, T., Marioni, J. C., Buettner, F., et al. (2018). Multi-omics factor analysis—A framework for unsupervised integration of multi-omics data sets. *Molecular Systems Biology, 14*. https://doi.org/10.15252/msb.20178124.
2. Bacher, S., Blackburn, T. M., Essl, F., & Genovesi, P. (2017). *Socio-Economic Impact Classification of Alien Taxa (SEICAT)*. https://core.ac.uk/download/286567949.pdf (accessed on 8th March 2025).
3. Barnett, R., Brace, S., Cucchi, T., & Dobney, K. (2013). *Divergent Evolutionary Processes Associated with Colonization of Offshore Islands*. https://core.ac.uk/download/20664364.pdf (accessed on 8th March 2025).

Detailed Table of Contents

CHAPTER 3

The Peripheral Nervous System 63

CHAPTER 4

Autonomic Nervous System 95

CHAPTER 5

The Cardiovascular System 131

CHAPTER 6

Blood Vessels and Circulation 165

CHAPTER 7

The Lymphatic System and Immunity 197

CHAPTER 10

The Urinary System 291

CHAPTER 11

The Reproductive System 325

CHAPTER 12

The Endocrine System 359

LIST OF FIGURES

PREFACE

Life-supporting functions extend far beyond the firm shape of the bone and contracting power of the muscles into a vast system of interlocking systems controlling everything from mind and emotion to fluid balance and immune defense. The body's nervous system, its matrix of synapses and neurons, is the command center—feeling the world for change, transmitting messages at light speed, and provoking responses that defend us and move us along. At the same time, the network of blood vessels delivers oxygen, nutrients, and hormones to all cells and removes waste products. In contrast, lymph vessels absorb excess fluid and filter out pathogens, performing immune surveillance. At the same time, endocrine glands secrete chemical messengers that regulate metabolism, growth, reproduction, and stress response. Exploration of interconnectivity among these systems teaches us about the body's remarkable capability for internal stability—tuning heart rate, blood pressure, hormone release, and nervous activity in real time as things change.

In *Textbook of Anatomy: Volume 2*, continuity is extended from the neural bases of sensation and control to the systems that convey nutrients, remove waste products, and trigger growth and reproduction. Each chapter is built on fundamental principles and contains elaborate schematics to aid in learning and remembering. Chapter 1 provides a general introduction to the nervous system, including its general divisions and organizational notions that are fundamental in scope. Chapter 2 deals with the central nervous system, explaining brain and spinal cord anatomy and sensation and control of movement aspects. Chapter 3 deals with the peripheral nervous system, explaining the cranial and spinal nerve patterns and the function of information transmission. Chapter 4 deals with the autonomic nervous system, demarcating sympathetic and parasympathetic pathways and their impact on organ function.

Chapter 5 is a summary of the anatomy of the heart, with descriptions of the chamber, valve, and conduction system tissues initiating the heartbeat. Chapter 6 discusses blood vessels and circulation, including arterial and venous circulation, and tissue microcirculation.

Chapter 7 addresses the immune and lymphatic system, which addresses the cellular immunity basis of immune protection, lymph transport, and lymphoid organs. Chapter 8 addresses the respiratory system, which includes gaseous exchange, respiratory surfaces, airways, and respiratory mechanisms.

Chapter 9 covers the digestive system, describing organs employed in processing nutrients from ingestion through to absorption. Chapter 10 covers the urinary system, kidney structure, urine formation, and fluid balance control. Chapter 11 covers the reproductive system, describing male and female structure, and gamete production mechanisms.

Chapter 12 covers the endocrine system, i.e., glands, hormone secretion, and feedback. Chapter 13 concludes with the special senses, namely the anatomy of vision, hearing, taste, smell, and balance receptors.

This text is directed to senior-level medical, nursing, and allied health students who are ready to combine structural information with clinical and physiological information. It will be of benefit to researchers who need a concise anatomy text. This brief chapter summary and quantity of information, combined with simple illustrations and an overview, make it a "must read" to become familiar with the highly interrelated systems that sustain human vitality and function.

NERVOUS SYSTEM: OVERVIEW

1

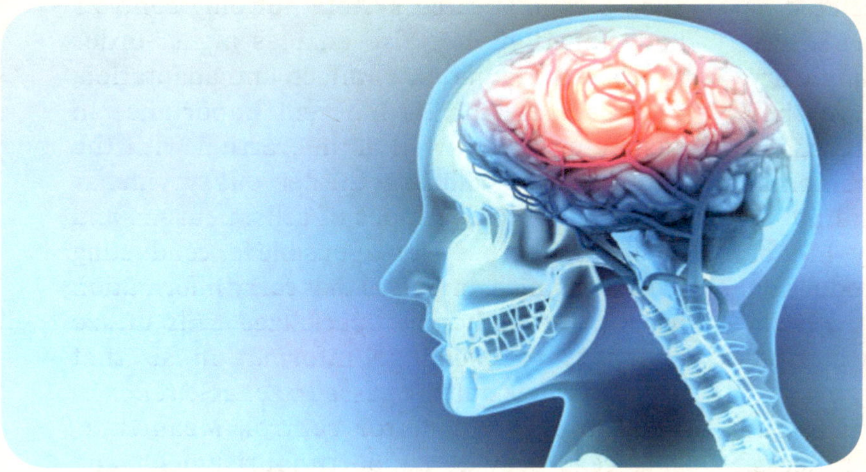

LEARNING OBJECTIVES

After studying this chapter, you will be able to:

1. Discuss the anatomical structure of the nervous system.
2. Discuss the overall function of the nervous system.
3. Make a distinction between the various neurons and their role.
4. Discuss how neurotransmitters are involved in neural communication.
5. Discuss usual nervous system diseases and their effects.
6. Discuss the connection between the nervous system and human behavior.

Introduction

The sophisticated and complex nervous system is the foundation for how living things function. In essence, the nervous system mediates the different physiological responses required for survival and adaptation by processing and transmitting information throughout the body. This system consists of two principal parts: the central nervous system (CNS) and the peripheral nervous system (PNS). The CNS, or brain and spinal cord, is the headquarters for transmitting sensory input and commanding motor outputs. The PNS is the link between the CNS and the limbs and organs, allowing communication between the brain and the entire body. Understanding the structure and function of these components is required to grasp the intricacy of neural processes, which will continue to be discussed throughout this chapter. In neuroscience, one of the most critical areas of study has been the mechanisms of neuronal functional diversity. Such diversity can be explained to a large extent by mechanisms such as alternative splicing, adding complexity to the function of the neuronal cells. Through the use of advanced text-mining techniques, researchers have begun creating databases that record instances of transcript diversity in a specific tissue, including the nervous system. These are invaluable aids to explaining the intricate splicing events that lead to neuron specialization. The LSAT database, for instance, allows scientists to study the implications of these alternative transcripts, thereby shedding more light on tissue-specific expression of genes and how this is related to neural behavior. Studying these processes serves to emphasize the accessibility and complexity inherent in the nervous system, further reinforcing its significance in biological research. Educational resources are also instrumental in creating an enhanced understanding of the nervous system's complexity by higher learning students. For example, the production of interactive multimedia tutorials on the brain and nervous system aims to make a topic that would otherwise be intimidating, easy to master. These tutorials not only instruct but engage students in an active learning process. The worth of innovative teaching techniques cannot be overemphasized, particularly in topics like neuroscience, where misconceptions can bar learning and retention. Employing a variety of methodologies, including multi-dimensions of visual and auditory assistance, instructors can enhance comprehension and facilitate a more in-depth examination of the nervous system's complexity. Therefore, integrating these innovations in education into curricula is necessary for the cultivation of well-educated prospective researchers and practitioners in neuroscience, as perceived from the current endeavors (Hall et al., 1995) and calls for innovation with respect to educational instruments (Lars et al., 2005).

Definition of the Nervous System

The nervous system is a tightly organized system of specialized cells that enables the body to communicate, thus allowing the organisms to respond suitably to their internal and external environment. It has two major divisions: the central nervous system (CNS) and the peripheral nervous system (PNS). The CNS, which consists of the brain and spinal cord, is the command center that processes sensory information and executes motor responses. In contrast to the CNS, the PNS comprises all neural connections beyond the CNS that connect the organs and tissues of the body to the central processor. Such a sophisticated system not only controls body functions but also enables higher-order processes, regulation of affect, and adaptation, thus emphasizing its inherent importance in sustaining life as well as interaction with the outside world. Cellularly, the nervous system has predominantly two types of cells: neurons and glial cells. Neurons are responsible for conducting electrochemical impulses that carry information around the body. The specialized cells utilize synapses to exchange information so that information is quickly passed to enable reflexes, sense input, and motor control. Meanwhile, glial cells provide support, nourishment, and protection to neurons and thus aid the operation and upkeep of the nervous system overall. The communication between the kinds of cells is also significant; some glial cells, for instance, can influence synaptic function and neuronal transmission, illustrating how their processes are interconnected. Understanding the cellular dynamics of the nervous system not only clarifies its mechanisms of function but also offers a basis for consideration of neurological disease and therapeutic intervention. One of the most critical aspects of the operation of the nervous system is that it is linked to consciousness and cognition. The interconnection between the brain's neural substrates and the abstract intellectual processes of thinking responds to the nature of this system. Recent neuroscience research suggests that consciousness does not arise as much from firing neurons as from the intricate dynamics of information processing in the brain, which connects various cognitive processes via some neural pathways. According to the informational model of consciousness, the nervous system is viewed as an information system that takes a central place in mediating experiences, internal states, and environmental interactions. Thus, knowledge regarding the mind-body problem indicates mental and physical neural processes interact, another aspect of emphasizing the nervous system's crucial role in building human experience and identity (Gaiseanu et al., 2019; Motofei et al., 2017).

Importance of the Nervous System in Human Physiology

The nervous system is a crucial component of human physiology, serving as the body's primary system of communication. This is achieved with its intricate structure, which is the CNS and the PNS. The CNS, the brain and spinal cord, consolidates sensory input and regulates responses, and the PNS connects the CNS to limbs and organs to facilitate motor and sensory functions. Homeostasis must be preserved, as physiological mechanisms such as heart rate, digestion, and temperature regulation are fine-tuned by neural input. Additionally, the nervous system's ability to adapt and reorganize itself depending on experiences through a process known as neuroplasticity emphasizes its critical role in learning, memory, and recovery from injury, thereby emphasizing the importance of its examination within physiological paradigms (Ainsworth et al., 2014). Moreover, the nervous system is extensively interconnected with other physiological systems such as the endocrine and immune systems. This coordination demonstrates the intricate process of physiological homeostasis, whereby diverse systems communicate with one another and interact to provide optimal functioning. For instance, the hypothalamus is a critical interconnection between the endocrine and nervous systems, regulating metabolic, stress, and growth hormone responses. In addition, recent evidence also indicates that the nervous system influences the immune system, and that emotional health as well as stress can have a significant influence on immune responses. This connectivity highlights the importance of an integrated perception of the nervous system, as disturbances in this network can lead to all types of medical conditions, from chronic illnesses to psychiatric illnesses, thereby demonstrating its crucial role in worldwide human health (Bich et al., 2019). Lastly, the role of the nervous system in human physiology extends beyond coordination and communication, as it also involves controlling adaptive behavioral responses to ensure survival. The system filters stimuli from the external world and delivers related actions via reflex arcs as well as higher-order thought processes. For instance, the fight-or-flight response, controlled by the autonomic nervous system, prepares the body for rapid response to an immediate threat by controlling heart rate, breathing, and mobilization of energy. Prolonged effects of stress on the nervous system can lead to maladaptive processes such as depression and anxiety, indicating how psychological functioning can be manifested physically. Thus, the nervous system has an important role, not only in respect to short-term physiological adjustment, but also in terms of shaping our conduct and emotional well-being, cementing its essential place in the complexity of human physiology (Ainsworth et al., 2014).

1.1. Anatomy of the Nervous System

Learning Outcome

1. Define the central nervous system (CNS) and the peripheral nervous system (PNS)
2. Discuss the major components and structures

The anatomy of the nervous system is a complex organization charged with coordinating the physiology of the body and traditionally divided into two large systems, namely the CNS and the PNS. The CNS, consisting of the brain and spinal cord, serves as the central command center, with the integration of sensory inputs and regulation of involuntary functions and higher mental processes. On the other hand, the PNS is a massive nerve network stretching from the spinal cord to the periphery of the body for two-way communication between the CNS and organs as well as tissues. It plays a crucial role in diagnosing and treating neurological conditions, which is why doctors and medical students need to know the structural associations that form the basis of the nervous system function. Also, ongoing innovation in education content, such as virtual reality (VR) software, significantly enhances the learning of nervous system anatomy. Innovations like human-innervated VR allow students to view and manipulate virtual 3D models of the human arm and observe the interaction between nerves and muscles. Not only does this virtual learning environment provide instant feedback, but it also allows visualization of the dynamic interaction of neural pathways with movement. By way of simulations, the students gain in-depth knowledge of innervation in nerves, overcoming book knowledge versus practical application. This kind of educational technology is pivotal in anatomy studies in modern times. It shows a proactive approach to more interactive learning methods in the field of medicine, as suggested in research on student motivation and spatial cognition in anatomy teaching (Lehman et al., 2023). In addition to human anatomy, comparative nervous system research in other organisms teaches us about evolutionary biology and neuroanatomy. As a case in point, the nervous system evolution of nervous system components is revealed through investigations of annelids such as species within the Family Nereididae. Detailed neuroanatomical analyses of *Neanthes arenaceodentata* yield considerable information about developmental morphology and interconnections of nervous systems. Understanding these evolutionary processes can clarify anomalies within previous research and advance the understanding of bilaterian nervous systems. This comparative analysis highlights the importance of studying different species since it can offer a bird's-eye view of the evolution of nervous systems, with instructive perspectives for the practice and study of medicine in neuroscience (Jacobs et al., 2010) (Figure 1.1).

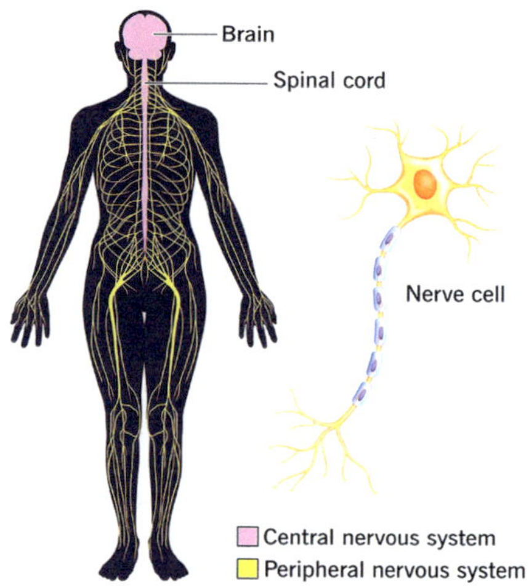

Figure 1.1. Your nervous system contains your brain, spinal cord and nerves.

Source: https://my.clevelandclinic.org/-/scassets/images/org/health/articles/21202-nervous-system.

1.1.1. Central Nervous System (CNS)

The CNS, or brain and spinal cord, is the primary processing center of the nervous system. Not only does it enable communication all over the body, but it also processes sensory data, enabling sophisticated behavior and response. Higher mental functions, emotions, and voluntary movements are the activities of the brain. In contrast, reflex movements and signal transmission from the brain to the peripheral nervous system and vice versa are the activities of the spinal cord. The organization of the CNS is mainly neuronal; neurons are the building blocks, specialized cells that transmit impulses within the system. Above all, the CNS is insulated and shielded by glial cells, which provide homeostasis, produce myelin, and provide the body support and protection to neurons. These intricacies bear witness to the intricacy of the CNS and its critical role in overall body operations, making it a focal point of neurological as well as psychological health. In understanding the central nervous system more, it is necessary to explore its structural composition. Approximately 50% of the brain's dry weight consists of lipids, the second-highest lipid content tissue after adipose tissue (Hornemann et al., 2021) (Figure 1.2).

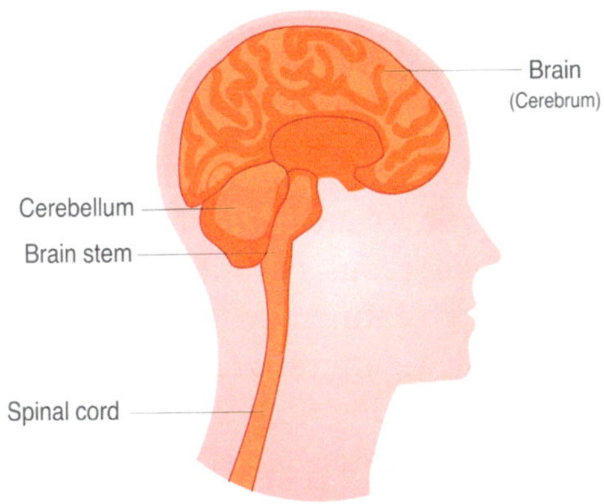

Figure 1.2. Central nervous system (CNS).

Source: https://mobilephysiotherapyclinic.net/wp-content/uploads/2023/11/central-nervous-system.webp.

While lipids have been well known for centuries for their roles in the structure of cells and storage of energy, their involvement in neurological diseases, particularly those concerning peripheral nerves, remains poorly comprehended. It is this void that inspires an examination of lipid metabolism in the CNS and its contribution to neurological health. In addition, the dynamic interaction among the various components of the cell, particularly the neuron and the glial cell, contributes to the complexity of this system. The CNS adapts to various stimuli through the phenomenon of neuroplasticity, the ability to recreate neural tracts, which is central to learning and recovery from trauma. Therefore, a discussion of both lipid functions and neuroplasticity gives real insight into CNS function and overall brain health. Microglial cells, an essential type of glial cell within the CNS, underscore the role of immune function in maintaining neural integrity and function. Non-muscle myosin II (II) is a motor protein expressed in numerous cell types, such as neurons and glial cells, and it facilitates key cellular processes such as vesicle transport, cell migration, and cytokine production (Pennella et al., 2021). NM II functions are particularly vital in microglia since microglia serve as the primary defenders of the CNS, responding to injury and disease through the production of pro-inflammatory mediators. However, excessive activation of microglia can lead to inflammatory responses that contribute to neurodegenerative conditions. Investigating NM IIs role in modulating these responses presents potential therapeutic avenues for treating CNS disorders. By understanding both the structural composition and the dynamic cellular interactions within the CNS, researchers can develop strategies for enhancing CNS resilience and functionality in the face of pathology.

1.1.2. Peripheral Nervous System (PNS)

PNS is a critical pathway connecting the CNS to the various organs and limb tissues of the body. Composed of ganglia and nerves peripheral to the CNS, the PNS transmits sensory input to the spinal cord and brain and also transmits motor commands from the CNS to muscles. Bidirectional communication is required for homeostasis as well as interaction with the external environment. Surprisingly, sensory axons of the PNS have lengths of up to three feet, indicative of the complexity and enormity of the system. However, the vulnerability of the PNS to external, hereditary, and metabolic forces requires more knowledge about its composition and functions, particularly how such elements can affect the overall health and functioning of nerves (Hornemann et al., 2021). In terms of cellular composition at the cellular level, the PNS is much different from the CNS, particularly about glial cells. The PNS has two principal forms of glia: Schwann cells and olfactory ensheathing cells (OECs) (Figure 1.3).

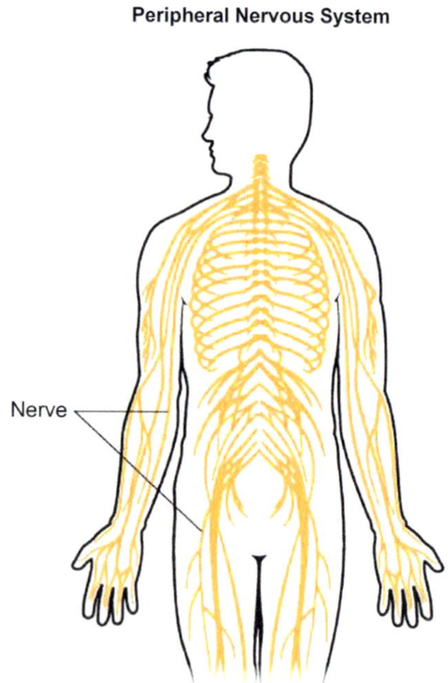

Figure 1.3. Peripheral nervous system (PNS).

Source: https://s3-us-west-2.amazonaws.com/courses-images-archive-read-only/wp-content/uploads/sites/902/2015/02/23224551/CNX_Psych_03_03_NervSystem.jpg.

Schwann cells are the core of peripheral nerve regeneration, which enhances the transmission of signals and particularly insulates the neurons' axons. Conversely, OECs are specific to the olfactory nerves and are responsible for ongoing neural regeneration during one's lifetime. Their shared and unique properties become evident on how these cells assist in nerve regeneration and repair. This cellular sophistication is essential; upon damage, PNS glial cells rapidly respond to remove debris and produce growth factors that promote regeneration, differentiating the PNS from the CNS for recovery potential (Barton et al., 2017). Understanding the regenerative ability of the PNS has tremendous therapeutic potential for the repair of nerve injury and neurological disease. With its higher regenerative potential than the CNS, research into PNS glial cells offers promising avenues for the treatment of both peripheral and central nervous system injuries. Transplantation of PNS glia can enhance regeneration by providing injured neurons with essential supporting niches. As research ever more clearly elucidates mechanisms involved in the regenerative processes, it presents new therapeutic avenues for repairing neural damage. These results hold the promise of revolutionizing treatment for many neurological diseases, with an increased focus placed on more research in this field to build further on the regenerative potential of the PNS (Barton et al., 2017).

1.1.3. Major Components and Structures

The nervous system is a complicated system composed of numerous parts working together to enable communication in the body. At its core are the CNS and the PNS. The CNS, comprised of the brain and spinal cord, is the master control center, where information is processed and responses coordinated. The brain is also segregated into different regions with specific functions such as processing sensory information, managing motor functions, and higher-level cognition. The spinal cord serves as a pathway for signal transmission between the brain and the rest of the body, as well as a means to regulate the reflex response. On the other hand, the PNS connects the CNS to limbs and organs to finalize a response mechanism. Dissimilarity of these two primary systems reflects the complexity of neural interaction necessary to sustain life and support adaptive behavior. Throughout the nervous system, certain structures play an important role in the organization and function of neuronal communication. Neurons represent the primitive units of the nervous system, with specialized cells utilized to propagate electrical impulses. These impulses carry information about synapses, in which neurotransmitters occupy the gap between adjacent neurons, conveying signals. Glial cells, other than neurons, provide support, providing necessary homeostasis, myelination, and protection. Such a relationship of glial cells to neurons is an illustration of the coordinated work that leads to successful signaling systems. Furthermore, such developments as the evolution of complex neural morphology in organisms like *Neanthes arenaceodentata* demonstrate the significance of these structures in evolution, which reveal information about both the structure of neural systems and the developmental processes, as evidenced by their acetylated α-tubulin labeling and confocal microscopy work (Jacobs et al., 2010). Spinal cord architecture demonstrates the intricate structural design required to defend neural structures and, nevertheless, allow for movement and reflexes. Encased within the vertebral column, the spinal cord consists of various segments, each corresponding to specific regions of the body. The organizational design allows for functional specialization and localized regulation of motor and sensory pathways. Although the spinal cord does provide some protection, it remains susceptible to trauma, which consequently can lead to primary injury that compromises its integrity. Following secondary injuries, secondary injury mechanisms can exacerbate damage and make recovery more challenging. It is critical to comprehend these two kinds of injuries to develop therapeutic strategies, as they highlight the complexity of not only the spinal cord but also the nervous system in general (Morin et al., 2018). This fact highlights the importance of continuing research on the significant elements and structures that comprise the nervous system towards potential treatment and rehabilitation improvements.

Test Your Knowledge

1. How does the peripheral nervous system (PNS) differ from the CNS?
2. Can you name two significant components of the nervous system and describe their roles?

1.2. Functions of the Nervous System

Learning Outcome

1. Define sensory input and processing
2. Discuss the motor output and coordination
3. Understand the homeostasis and regulation

The nervous system is the body's primary communication network, the transmission of information needed to survive and maintain function. Central to this communication is the neuron, the working unit that enables a range of activities, from the contraction of muscles to mental processes. Neurons communicate with each other and even glands and muscles by synaptic transmission, coordinating the responses and controlling most of the functions of the body. This intricate network allows for rapid response to stimuli such that organisms react efficiently to their environment. It is through understanding the neurophysiological processes behind these functions, including how neurotransmitters influence neuron discharge and signal conduction, that one comes to appreciate the intricacy of these functions of the nervous system in everyday life (Megaw et al., 2015). The nervous system also plays a critical role in maintaining homeostasis and body functions. The autonomic nervous system, as a subdivision of the peripheral nervous system, continuously regulates and adjusts the internal environment with little voluntary effort. It provides control over critical processes such as heart rate, digestion, and breathing rate, ensuring that vital parameters remain within optimal ranges. The two major branches are the sympathetic and parasympathetic systems, whose effects are contrary, thereby allowing delicate control of the physiological states. Through the regulation of these involuntary processes, the autonomic nervous system is a central facilitator between the brain and the body's systems, demonstrating the complexity and advanced nature of neural control for the sake of life and health. This regulatory aspect demonstrates the nervous system's greater significance above the mere reaction to stimuli (Megaw et al., 2015). Moreover, the recently emerging research on the roles of proteins, such as dystroglycan, illustrates the intricate interrelation between muscular and neurological functions. While classically focused on its involvement in muscular dystrophies, recent research demonstrates the participation of dystroglycans at cognition and neurological activities, such as brain development and synaptic plasticity. Its interaction with several proteins highlights the complexity of neuronal integrity and blood-brain barrier integrity, both offering a key window into how the nervous system functions in health and disease. By revealing such interactions and functions, scientists can better understand how neurodegenerative diseases might impact cognitive processes and overall neural function. This indicates the various roles of the nervous system in human health and the scope for targeted therapies in disorders affecting both muscle and neurological function (Figure 1.4).

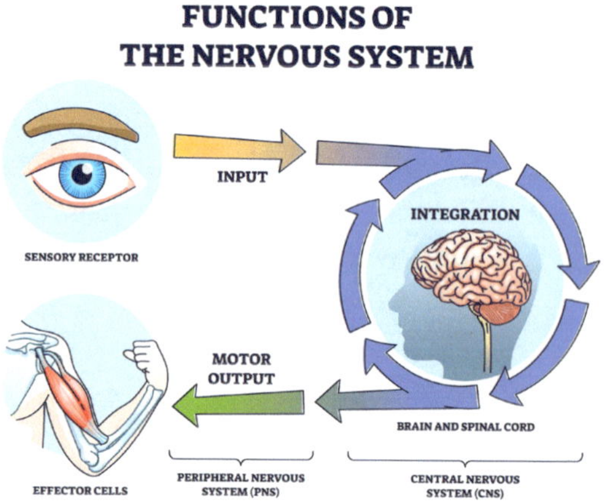

Figure 1.4. Functions of the nervous system.

Source: https://www.physio-pedia.com/images/thumb/f/f8/Functions_of_nervous_system.jpeg/400px-Functions_of_nervous_system.jpeg.

1.2.1. Sensory Input and Processing

The sensory input and processing are fundamental building blocks of the nervous system, assisting organisms in perceiving and interacting with the surrounding world. Sensory receptors distributed throughout the body are specialized to detect certain stimuli like light, sound, temperature, and chemical signals. Such receptors generate physical stimulation that is converted into neural responses, which are relayed to the central nervous system for processing. When the information reaches the brain, it is intricately integrated in a manner that permits perception of a unified sensory experience. This integration is essential for perceiving the environment and responding appropriately, highlighting the significant role sensory input plays in everyday functioning and existence. The relevance of personalized sensory processing lies particularly in special needs groups such as children with autism spectrum disorder (ASD) and cerebral palsy (CP). Empirical studies have established that personalized sensory environments are able to regulate levels of physiological arousal in these groups efficiently. For example, studies of multi-sensory environments (MSE) showed that children with ASD exhibited heterogeneous sensory responses to stimulation. Still, children with CP showed increased arousal levels when exposed to carefully designed sensory experiences. The results suggest that modifying sensory input according to specific needs can enhance therapy effectiveness and overall well-being, underscoring the importance of understanding sensory processing in diverse populations (Atari et al., 2014). Following up on the exploration of sensory input and processing mechanisms, information compression by multiple alignment, unification, and search (ICMAUS) offers insight into the neurobiology of perception. ICMAUS demonstrates that neural processes can effectively compress sensory information for effective retrieval and processing. This theoretical framework is an extension of traditional conceptions of neural assemblies, proposing that a neuron may belong to multiple assemblies, thus enhancing the capacity of the brain to create abstract representations and complex hierarchies. By understanding these higher-order processes, we gain a deeper insight into how the nervous system organizes sensory input into meaningful structures, enabling us to tailor our approach to foster learning and cognitive development, and to maximize therapeutic interventions across various fields (Wolff et al., 2003) (Figure 1.5).

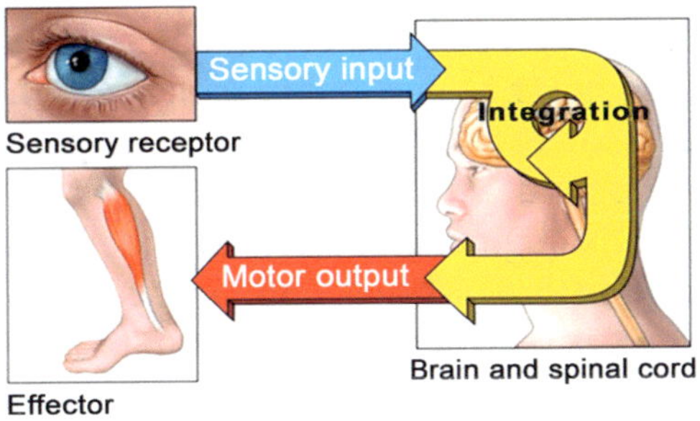

Figure 1.5. Sensory input and motor output processing.

Source: https://msgallagherlhs.weebly.com/nervous-system-function.html.

1.2.2. Motor Output and Coordination

Motor coordination and output are complex functions of the nervous system that allow interaction with the world. These are based on dynamic relationships among neural, muscular, and biomechanical systems from which effective movement emerges, both from the physiology of the body and the nature of the task to be executed. For instance, in the performance of a sophisticated motion such as object grasping, the neuromuscular system must translate neural commands into properly timed muscular activations that account for various loads and object textures. Such a complex interaction underlines the importance of understanding motion as a neuromechanical entity, where resultant behavior arises through neural inputs integrating with the mechanical demands of tasks (Santello et al., 2017). These results not only indicate the biological basis but also the importance of adaptive motor methods that allow subjects to conform their movements to various contextual situations. Coordination of motor output is deeply entangled with the mandates of distributed cognition, which makes it challenging to assume a centralized executive system with voluntary behavior. Research shows that motor behavior results from the interactive dynamics of multiple elementary cognitive processes, rather than a consequence of the command by a single control entity. It implies that each cognitive element performs semi-independent action, permitting selection of action through competition and coordination. Consequently, while coordinated motor coherence is crucial in task performance, it is an issue of concern about how separate cognitive pieces assemble to produce directed behavior (Christensen et al., 2006). This understanding of coordination indicates that there must be a top-down system that addresses conflict and prioritizes behavior, which suggests the evolutionary advantages of hierarchical cognitive organizations possessing executive function. Furthermore, the research into motor output and coordination has profound implications in robotics and rehabilitation domains. Insights developed from understanding how the human nervous system is capable of advanced motor control can be used to design next-generation prosthetics and rehabilitation systems. These technologies not only seek to mimic biological functions but also adapt through mechanisms that simulate the plasticity found in biological systems. By comparing the mechanisms of grasping in biology and robotics, researchers can identify the key differences and similarities that can lead to increased functional success in applications of rehabilitation (Santello et al., 2017). The investigation of motor output and coordination thus forms an essential component of our total knowledge of the nervous system and pushes the boundaries of both neurology research and applied biomedical engineering (Figure 1.6).

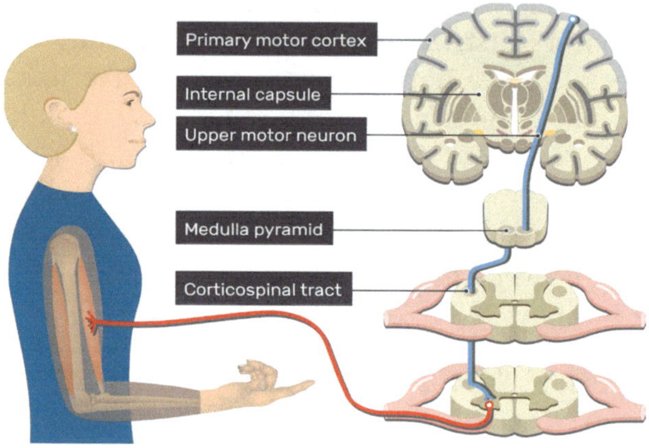

Figure 1.6. The pyramidal pathway is one of the main motor pathways in the spinal cord.

Source: https://www.getbodysmart.com/motor-system/pyramidal-tract-pathway/.

1.2.3. Homeostasis and Regulation

Homeostasis, the dynamic balance of the body, is a fundamental concept that highlights the tenuous interdependence of a number of bodily physiological systems, particularly the nervous system. This continuous activity is necessary to maintain the internal environment steady in the presence of changing environments and is controlled through finely balanced feedback systems. The role of the nervous system in facilitating homeostasis cannot be overemphasized, as it uses sensory inputs to perceive changes and orchestrate related responses. For instance, changes in blood pressure, temperature, and pH levels trigger related responses through neuronal pathways, keeping the body at the best range for functioning. This is sustained in stress responses, where repeated stress can disrupt homeostatic equilibrium. Recent research indicates that the modulators of the stress response, i.e., the corticotropin-releasing hormone family, play a role in chronic inflammation, which also undermines further homeostasis and disease evolution (Baritaki et al., 2019). Hormonal-nervous system interaction lies at the root of the maintenance of homeostasis, particularly of metabolism and energy control. Several peptide hormones secreted in the gut are significant in central nervous system processes and have a direct influence on energy homeostasis. A great example of this intricate relationship is glucagon-like peptide 2 (GLP-2) release after ingestion of food. As an anorexigenic factor, GLP-2 not only selectively stimulates the growth of the intestinal epithelial cells but also enhances nutrient absorption through various mechanisms, including increased intestinal blood flow and inhibition of gastric motility (Mule et al., 2011). This neuroendocrine conversation illustrates how hormones possess the ability to control brain function, thereby modulating hunger and satiety behaviors, enabling the regulation of energy balance and homeostasis. In addition, dysregulation of these control systems can cause profound disease, demonstrating the essential role of homeostasis in general health. Chronic stress, for example, shifts neuroendocrine activity with the potential to cause disease states like obesity and metabolic syndrome as the body attempts to stay in equilibrium. The interdependence of stress, hormone signaling, and neural function emphasizes the richness of homeostatic control. Continued research into the molecular basis of such interactions has potential for novel therapeutic directions in the therapy of stress disorders and metabolic diseases. As researchers learn more about how the nervous system maintains homeostasis through both neuronal and endocrine mechanisms, they are better equipped to individualize strategies toward personalized medicine and optimize health outcomes by specifically targeting the control networks (Baritaki et al., 2019).

Test Your Knowledge

1. How does the body coordinate motor output in response to stimuli?
2. How does the nervous system help maintain homeostasis and regulate body functions?

1.3. Types of Neurons

Learning Outcome

1. Identify and describe the roles of sensory neurons and motor neurons in transmitting sensory information
2. Understand the interneurons

The neuron grouping is a fundamental unit used to understand the complex design of the nervous system. The neurons may be grouped based on several traits like structure, function, and direction of impulse transmission. Primarily, the neurons have three main types: sensory neurons, motor neurons, and interneurons. Sensory neurons play a role in transmitting sensory information from the sensory receptors to the CNS. These cells are equipped with specialized terminals that perceive stimuli, such as light, sound, or touch, and convert these stimuli into electrochemical impulses for processing. Motor neurons, however, facilitate efferent communication by passing signals from the CNS to effectors like muscles and glands and thereby enable responses to sensory stimuli. Interneurons are the mediators of the CNS, accepting information and establishing relations between sensory and motor neurons, assisting with complex reflexes and higher-order cognitive processes. Still deeper in the morphology of the neuron, the structural categorization reveals its diverse functions. Neurons are categorized as unipolar, bipolar, or multipolar, each of which is constructed to perform specific tasks within the nervous system. Unipolar neurons, with one axon that bifurcates into two, are generally used in sensory pathways and effectively pass on the information from the periphery to the CNS. Bipolar neurons, with one axon and one dendrite, are less common but are crucial in passing sensory information, particularly in specialized locations such as the retina of the eye. Multipolar neurons, the most abundant of the three, possess multiple dendrites extending from one soma to facilitate extensive synaptic connections. These differences are critical in understanding the connectivity patterns observed in neural networks, as supported by studies that have probed synaptic structures and distance profiles across various organisms, including humans and rodents (Achacoso et al., 2009). Apart from mere categorizations, the functional variation of neurons also encompasses their role in complex signaling pathways. In addition, neurons are also heterogeneous in terms of qualities such as modulation by receptor interactions and in pain pathways. For instance, opioid receptor interactions with other receptors can modulate nociception significantly and, therefore, impact the pain response in the central nervous system (Agnati et al., 2013). This modulation is not only crucial to the explanation of pain mechanisms but also promises new therapeutic avenues for pain and neurological illness. Secondly, the capacity of neurons to achieve neuroplasticity, for example, reorganizations following damage or chronic stimulation, represents a test of their complex functional character. As the nervous system continues to be an area of ongoing investigation, the intricate mechanisms of neuron types will probably play a key role in continued advances in our comprehension of neuronal function and connectivity (Figure 1.7).

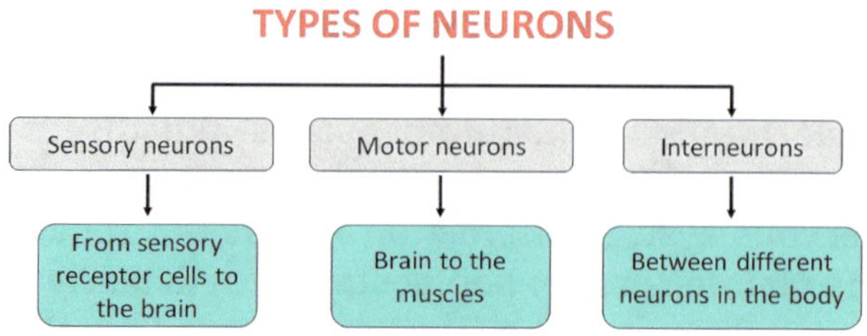

Figure 1.7. Types of neurons.

Source: https://cdn.teachoo.com/large/5303ab2f-7ebc-4e47-907f-bd1e860179e8/types-of-neurons---teachoo.jpg.

1.3.1. Sensory Neurons

Sensory neurons are significant constituents of the nervous system because they function as intrinsic information mediators between the external environment and the brain. Such specialized cells are capable of perceiving stimuli, i.e., light, sound, heat, and pressure, and transducing stimuli into electrical signals. Transduction is a critical function that allows sensations to be processed and interpreted by the central nervous system. Sensory neurons are classified based on the kind of stimulus they respond to, for example, photoreceptors that are responsive to light, mechanoreceptors that respond to touch and sound, and chemoreceptors that respond to chemical stimuli. These classifications demonstrate the flexibility and selectivity of sensory neurons to enable the organisms to respond to their environment and survive. The role of sensory neurons extends beyond detection. They are responsible for the initial sensory processing stage, whereby sensory input is sent to the spinal cord and ultimately to the brain for further analysis. Various nerve pathways facilitate this transfer, making it possible to incorporate sensory input with experience and prior knowledge. The functioning of these pathways not only influences everyday activities such as reflex action but also more advanced mental processes such as perception and decision-making.

Remarkably, sensory neurons' ability to adapt to constant stimuli—the process of sensory adaptation—reflects their dynamic nature. This phenomenon enables organisms to reject redundant sensory information and hence give more attention to novel stimuli, which is crucial for effective sensory perception. Furthermore, sensory neurons' capacity for regeneration, as exemplified by the PNS, reflects the complexity of neuronal recovery and repair. The PNS is more regenerative than the CNS, and this is very much a function of the activity of glial cells such as Schwann cells. They enable regeneration of the neurons by clearing away debris and providing important growth factors that are essential for repair following injury.

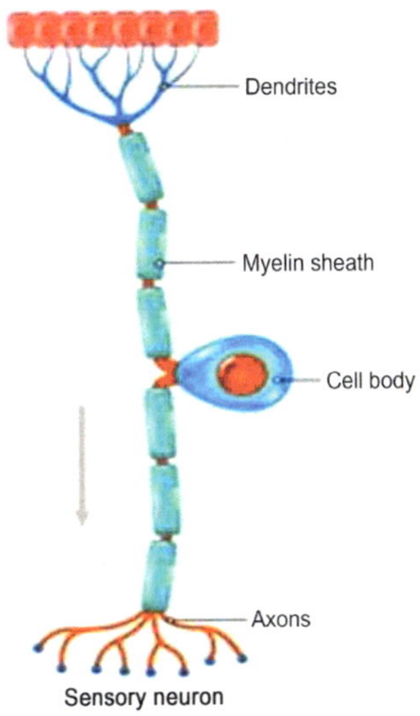

Figure 1.8. Sensory neurons.

Source: https://www.physio-pedia.com/images/thumb/0/04/Types_of_neurons.jpg/700px-Types_of_neurons.jpg.

A study of the difference in the response of PNS and CNS glia is necessary for the development of therapeutic strategies for the management of neural injuries and diseases. As new avenues of recovery remain to be explored, understanding the interaction between sensory neuron function, their capacity for regeneration, and the overall patterning of the nervous system remains an active area of evolving research with the potential to refine neurobiological and medical strategies that have the potential to introduce new treatments for sensory dysfunction (Bacik et al., 2016; Barton et al., 2017) (Figure 1.8).

1.3.2. Motor Neurons

Motor neurons are a critical component of the nervous system that serves as the necessary communication pathway between the CNS and muscles throughout the body. They originate in the spinal cord and brainstem, and their central function is to transmit signals that are responsible for causing voluntary contractions of muscles. By the conversion of electrical signals from neuronal activity into mechanical movements, motor neurons cause a variety of movements, from reflex to sophisticated voluntary motion. The process involves the release of neurotransmitters at the neuromuscular junction, which helps in the transmission between the nerve terminal and muscle fibers. Motor neuron functional continuity is fundamental not only for locomotion but also for posture and regulation of complex motor functions required for normal function and athletic performance. Motor neuron function complexity extends beyond mere muscle activation; it encompasses vital functions in muscle coordination and regulation of voluntary movement and muscle tone. The communication between the upper and lower motor neurons is essential, wherein upper motor neurons of the brain send impulses to lower motor neurons, which extend up to the muscles. Motor neuron diseases such as amyotrophic lateral sclerosis (ALS) can result in severe impairment and disability. As the health of the motor neurons deteriorates, patients exhibit weakness and wasting of the muscles, significantly impairing their quality of life. Understanding of the pathophysiology of such disorders is of utmost significance as it underscores the need to develop potent therapeutic interventions towards preserving motor neuron function and recovery following nerve trauma. Continued investigations have elucidated other cellular pathways underlying the maintenance of motor neuron function and survival. Interestingly, the non-muscle myosin II (II) is a critical component of the cytoskeletal machinery and plays a primary role in cellular processes integral to motor neuron survival, such as vesicle transport and contributing to the structural stability of neurons.

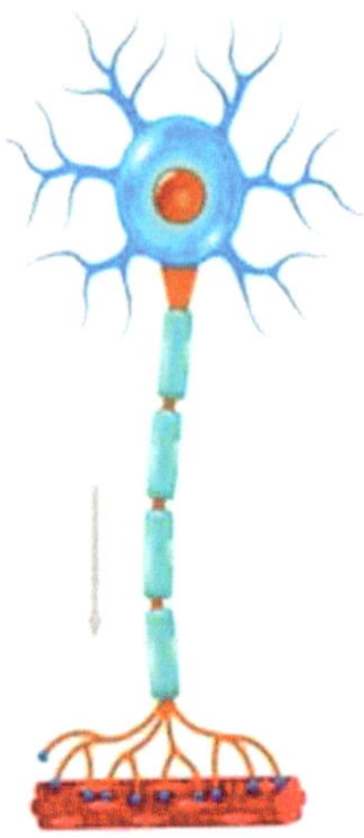

Figure 1.9. Motor neurons.

Source: https://www.physio-pedia.com/images/thumb/0/04/Types_of_neurons.jpg/700px-Types_of_neurons.jpg.

The implication of the involvement of NM IIs in various functions points to its importance in the nervous system, particularly in maintaining neuronal structure and reacting to cellular stress agents. Moreover, studies show that enhancing NM II activity will be capable of inducing mechanisms related to tissue repair and regeneration within the nervous system, and this presents new therapeutic opportunities for the treatment of neurodegenerative disorders and trauma. These findings on motor neurons' elaborate roles emphasize their central role in motor control and the nervous system's function as a whole, describing a highly complex dynamic of cellular mechanisms necessary for health and recovery (Barton et al., 2017; Pennella et al., 2021) (Figure 1.9).

1.3.3. Interneurons

Interneurons are a critical component of the nervous system, serving as integrative nodes that process and transmit information in neural circuits. Interneurons differ from sensory and motor neurons in that they are primarily found in the central nervous system and play a critical role in reflexes, sensory processing, and higher-order cognitive processing. Interneurons can change the activity of other neurons, thereby influencing the transmission of information along neural pathways. This modulation is important in state-dependent tasks, where interneurons assist with the organization and timing of neuronal discharge so that the response to stimuli is suitable to the context and effective. Their diverse morphologies and connections allow interneurons to form complex networks that modulate excitatory as well as inhibitory signals, with direct effects on global neural communication and function. This complex interaction emphasizes the importance of interneurons in maintaining balance to achieve optimal neurological function. Also, research on interneurons has opened new avenues to investigate how they participate in specific behaviors and neurological conditions. For instance, the ubiquitous distribution of interneuron types like class AIY across the nematode *C. elegans* illustrates how these neurons encode sensorial information to influence motor activities, namely the ability to navigate chemical gradients. Interneurons can flexibly track the variation of the environment with a subtle relationship between internal state and external stimulus. Information flow analysis has provided valuable information, which has demonstrated that interneurons such as AIY are strongly information-asymmetric in their synaptic forms and connectivity. This characteristic not only facilitates higher sensory processing but also forms a foundation for the prediction of behavioral outcomes, demonstrating the central roles of such neurons in transducing sensory input to motor output in complex animals (Beer et al., 2015). The significance of interneurons is not limited to basic motor control, as their dysregulation is increasingly linked with numerous neurological disorders. As a case in point, traumatic brain injury (TBI) disrupts the oscillatory rhythms that underlie cognitive processes, setting the stage for the potential role of altered interneuron function. Following TBI, injury can lead to enduring impairment of cognition and behavior and necessitate effective rehabilitative treatments. Electrical neuromodulation strategies have also emerged as effective treatments, aimed at restoring normal neural oscillations and cognitive functions that depend on the functioning of interneurons. Successful targeting of specific interneuron networks has delivered considerable enhancement of mental improvement, suggesting a central role of interneuron functionality in successful neurological recovery (Gurkoff et al., 2016). Hence, the understanding of interneurons not only clarifies essential neural functioning but also enhances therapeutic modalities for various neurological impairments (Figure 1.10).

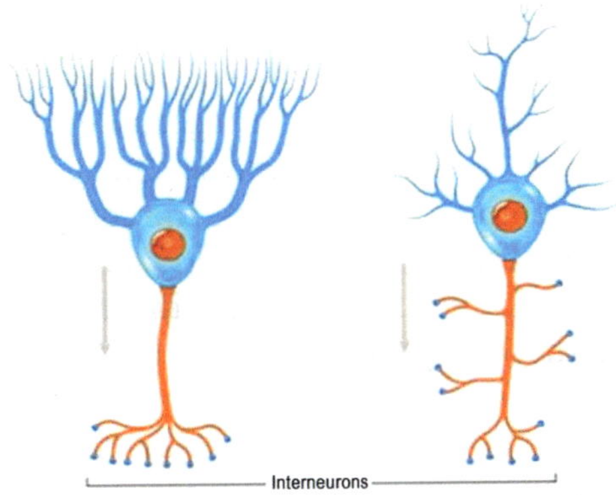

Figure 1.10. Interneurons.

Source: https://www.physio-pedia.com/images/thumb/0/04/Types_of_neurons.jpg/700px-Types_of_neurons.jpg.

Test Your Knowledge

1. How do motor neurons contribute to body movement?
2. What role do interneurons play in the nervous system?

1.4. Neurotransmitters and Signaling

Learning Outcome

1. Explain the role of neurotransmitters in communication
2. Identify the common neurotransmitters and their functions
3. Describe the mechanisms involved in synaptic transmission within the nervous system

The complex world of signal pathways and neurotransmitters is at the heart of understanding the nervous system's function and the intricate network of communication. Neurotransmitters, chemical messengers released by neurons, have the task of transmitting signals from synapses to target cells, thereby influencing various physiological and psychological processes. The ratio of excitatory to inhibitory neurotransmitters enables cognitive processes such as learning and memory to be applied proportionally. As an example, glutamate is the principal excitatory neurotransmitter, and gamma-aminobutyric acid (GABA) is the primary inhibitory neurotransmitter. This delicate balance is crucial for maintaining homeostasis in the nervous system, preventing disorders such as excitotoxicity or diminished neural function that result from failures in neurotransmitter signaling. Allosteric interactions of neurotransmitter receptors are a significant research field, particularly concerning pain mechanisms and their regulation. The study on receptor heteromers, such as the association between mu and delta opioid receptors, demonstrates the complexity of signaling mechanisms underlying pain and pain relief sensations. Not only do the heteromers change the receptors' function, but they also underlie the effects of morphine tolerance and dependence. The information thus gained through the study of such receptor interactions brings to the limelight the potential for targeted analgesics that might be able to suppress pain without the undesirable side effects of traditional opioids. The understanding of how such allosteric interactions work in specific signaling cascades may pave the way for new pain management strategies and therapeutic approaches with better therapeutic indices (Agnati et al., 2013). Moreover, the intersection of the immune system and neurotransmitters further testifies to the profound interrelatedness of body systems previously believed to exist in isolated realms. Recent research has now shed light on the involvement of cytokines, notably interleukin 15 (IL-15), in controlling synaptic transmission and influencing neurotransmitter concentrations, thereby revealing a neuroimmune signaling pathway. The CNS-immune dialogue is then used to illustrate how neuroinflammation may impact cognitive processes, and immune signaling affects neural growth and function. These data raise profound questions about the physiological role of inflammatory cytokines in health and disease, and the double-edged aspects of their roles as immunomodulators and neuromodulators. This increasing understanding serves to disentangle the processes of memory deficits and neuroinflammatory responses, and therefore could guide therapeutic strategies for neurodegenerative conditions (Carbonari et al., 2019).

1.4.1. Role of Neurotransmitters in Communication

The role of neurotransmitters in nerve-to-nervous communication is key to nervous system function. Neurotransmitters are chemical messengers that facilitate communication between neurons at synapses, the precise location where excitatory or inhibitory information is passed along. The molecules function by binding to specific receptors on the postsynaptic neuron, which triggers a range of physiological processes such as muscle contraction, emotional response, and mental processing. The dynamic interplay between neurotransmitters offers rapid and efficient communication, which is essential for the maintenance of homeostasis and adaptation to environmental changes. As an illustration, glutamate, the primary excitatory neurotransmitter, is used in synaptic plasticity. This process mediates learning and memory, thereby showing the intricate relationship between neurotransmitter activity and cognitive function (Gaiseanu et al., 2019). In addition to traditional neurotransmitters like dopamine and serotonin, the neuroimmune interactions illustrate how neurotransmitters participate in a long-range system dialogue. Researchers have determined that cytokines, traditionally provided with a function for immune reaction, are furthermore neuromodulators, recognizing an interactive pathway between the nervous and immune systems. This interaction alters neuronal transmission, influencing both mental health and immune reaction. For example, the cytokine interleukin-15 (IL-15) has been identified as a significant factor modulating neurotransmission and synaptic plasticity with an influence on cognitive functions like memory (Carbonari et al., 2019). These findings emphasize the multi-dimensional roles neurotransmitters and their related systems play in all-body communication and health, bridging the gap between psychological and physiological actions. Understanding the diverse functions of neurotransmitters also opens new therapeutic avenues to neurological and psychiatric disease. Depressive illness, for instance, anxious states, and schizophrenia have all been linked with disturbance in neurotransmitter systems such as serotonin, norepinephrine, and dopamine. Pharmacological treatments like SSRIs show the power of adjusting neurotransmitter levels to balance and reduce symptoms. Ongoing research on the signaling mechanisms and receptor dynamics in neurotransmitter activity continues to reveal potential new therapies. Interplay between neurotransmitters, immune responses, and neural health suggests that any advancement on this front could have profound impacts on therapeutic protocols for a broad spectrum of health conditions, which makes it a relevant area of investigation within the overall study of the nervous system (Gaiseanu et al., 2019) (Figure 1.11).

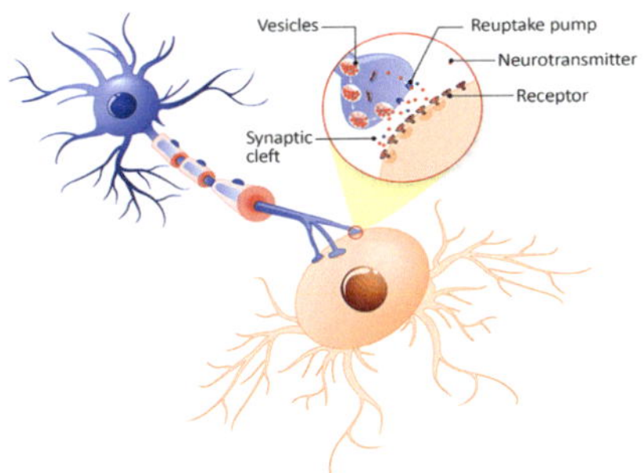

Figure 1.11. Neurotransmitters.

Source: https://qbi.uq.edu.au/brain/brain-functions/what-are-neurotransmitters.

1.4.2. Common Neurotransmitters and Their Functions

Understanding the common neurotransmitters and their various functions contributes to comprehending the intricacies of the nervous system. Neurotransmitters are chemical messengers passing signals between synapses, affecting a wide range of physiological functions. The primary neurotransmitters are dopamine, serotonin, acetylcholine, and gamma-aminobutyric acid (GABA). Dopamine operates within the brain's reward and pleasure centers, affecting motivation and mood. However, serotonin plays an essential role in mood control, appetite, and sleep patterns, and is generally linked to depression when deficient or excessive. Acetylcholine, the first neurotransmitter discovered, is involved in muscle contraction and memory, whereas GABA is the major inhibitory neurotransmitter, regulating the excitability of neurons throughout the nervous system. The intricate interaction and equilibrium of these neurotransmitters lay the foundation for many behavioral and physiological responses, demonstrating their significance in establishing homeostasis within the nervous system (Figure 1.12).

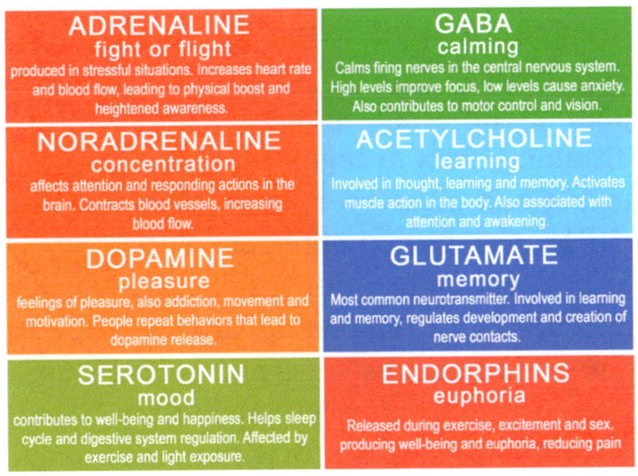

Figure 1.12. The key neurotransmitters.

Source: https://www.simplypsychology.org/neurotransmitter.html.

The various functions that dopamines have in human behavior are not just simple pleasure; it is critical to the regulation of motor control and reinforcement of rewarding behaviors. Dysregulation of it is associated with severe neurological disorders, such as Parkinson's disease, characterized by motor defects due to a deficiency of dopamine-producing neurons. Similarly, excessive dopamine has been implicated in neuropsychiatric diseases like schizophrenia, where the altered dopamine pathways can generate symptoms that include hallucinations and delusions. In addition, too, dopamine is at the heart of the brain's reward system, amplifying chemicals and activities' attractiveness and causing potential dependency. This points to the necessity of dopaminergic balance, reflecting the overall significance of neurotransmitter involvement in mental disease and behavioral economics (Haab et al., 2025). The impact of the immune system on neurotransmission also stands out, particularly concerning cytokines such as interleukin-15 (IL-15), which have proven to be of major importance in neuroimmune cross-talk. Long accepted as immunomodulators, cytokines are increasingly being recognized to possess neuromodulatory roles, modulating neurotransmitter release and synaptic plasticity (Carbonari et al., 2019). Recent findings indicate that cytokine signaling can shape neurotransmitter levels, positioning them in cognitive functions such as learning and memory. For instance, deficiency of IL-15 has been implicated with impaired spatial memory as well as altered levels of GABA, demonstrating an apparent intersection between immune response and neural function. This growing knowledge invites further research into the ways that immune signaling may impact neurological outcomes and reveal new avenues of therapeutic approaches for neuroinflammation and cognitive disorders. This interaction between neurotransmitters and the immune system illustrates the complicated web that governs brain function, and the value in employing a multidisciplinary perspective to studying neurobiology.

1.4.3. Mechanisms of Synaptic Transmission

Synaptic transmission processes are fundamental to the function of the nervous system in enabling neuronal communication and the conduction of impulses within the body. Electrical impulses from the presynaptic neuron at the synaptic junction trigger the discharge of neurotransmitters into the synaptic cleft, which is a critical step in this mode of transmission. These chemical messengers bind at particular postsynaptic membrane receptors, inducing changes in the postsynaptic neurons' membrane potential. This excites or inhibits the firing of the neurons and thus regulates the overall process of the synaptic interaction. This dynamic interaction is crucial to many cognitive functions like learning and memory storage, making it essential that synaptic mechanisms are comprehended within a complete discussion of the nervous system. Recent advances have made clear the immune system's role in modulating synaptic transmission, showing complex interactions between these two systems. The term " neuroimmune system " has emerged from the increasing evidence showing the collaboration between the nervous and immune systems. Cytokines, previously regarded as immunological regulators, are neuromodulators, influencing synaptic function and neural development. For example, interleukin 15 (IL-15) plays a pivotal role in synaptic transmission, where studies have indicated that its deficiency has been correlated with extreme fluctuation in the levels of neurotransmitters and memory storage. Such two-way communication between the immune and the nervous system not only enhances the literature on the mechanism of synaptic transmission but also suggests probable therapeutic approaches for the treatment of neurological disorders correlated with neuroinflammation and cognitive impairment (Carbonari et al., 2019). Functional architecture of synaptic transmission also needs to be considered from an informational point of view, highlighting the cellular-scale integration and processing of signals. Electrical impulses are binary units of information required for successful nervous system communication. The complex biochemistry of neurotransmitter interactions, in contrast, possesses a more complicated form of information dissemination, like the embodiment and disembodiment rules of information theory. This knowledge-based approach illuminates how neurons react to internal and external stimuli, conditioning responses that are essential to survival and adaptability. Knowledge of these processes pushes forward the study of cognitive functions and emotional states, contributing to debate regarding consciousness and the human condition (Gaiseanu et al., 2019).

Test Your Knowledge

1. What role do neurotransmitters play in neural communication?
2. What is the basic process of synaptic transmission between neurons?

1.5. Nervous System Disorders

Learning Outcome

1. Identify the common neurological disorders
2. Define causes and risk factors of neurological disorders
3. Explain the treatment and management options of neurological disorders

Nervous system disorders cover a wide range of diseases in the brain, spinal cord, and peripheral nerves, which have a significant social and personal impact. Generally, nervous system disorders can be classified as degenerative disorders, inflammatory disorders, developmental disorders, and traumatic injuries. Each class has its typical pathophysiologic mechanisms, supporting the need for respective therapeutic approaches. For example, degenerative conditions such as Alzheimer's and Parkinson's are defined by progressive neuronal dysfunction. In contrast, inflammatory conditions such as multiple sclerosis are characterized by immune-mediated injury to the myelin. This variability underscores the complexity of the nervous system itself and the need for an understanding of the particular etiology and presentation of each illness to allow effective intervention protocols. The recent advances in genomics have provided insight into the genetic etiology of a few of the nervous system diseases, revealing the essential role that non-coding RNAs play within neurodevelopment. Exome sequencing identified causative mutations in a large proportion of patients with intellectual disability in one such study, suggesting a genotype-phenotype correlation for many neurodevelopmental disorders. Notably, several long non-coding RNAs (lncRNAs) were implicated in processes such as synaptic transmission and neurogenesis. These findings indicate that the purported "junk" sections of the genome, long disregarded, play significant roles in brain development and brain function. By identifying lncRNAs implicated in central nervous system disorders, researchers have ushered in opportunities for discovery in the future that will determine their function in neuronal processes, which will further enlighten on complex illnesses such as autism spectrum disorder and intellectual disability (D'haene et al., 2016). The impact of environments on children with nervous system illnesses is being recognized more and more, particularly with regard to controlling anxiety. Studies comparing the effect of a multisensory environment (MSE) on children with autism spectrum disorder (ASD) showed heterogeneity in physiological arousal reactions, emphasizing the need for personalized treatment approaches. Sensory integration theory suggests that sensory stimulation tailored to an individual will reverse anxiety levels, which in children with conditions like cerebral palsy and ASD have a propensity to rise. Electrodermal measures indicated varying levels of arousal in participants, indicating differential sensory stimulation effects in children with different diagnoses. These results are legitimate reasons to use multisensory environments as therapy, providing leads toward various strategies for improving the quality of life of children with special health needs (Atari et al., 2014). Ultimately, understanding the relationship between the environment and neurological well-being is crucial for establishing effective interventions.

1.5.1. Common Neurological Disorders (e.g., Alzheimer's, Parkinson's)

The study of overall neurological disorders, particularly Alzheimer's disease (AD), and Parkinson's disease (PD) offers valuable facts about the nervous system's complexities. Alzheimer's is characterized most frequently by loss of memory, a decrease in cognitive function, and behavior change, typically represented as a state of disorientation or personality alteration. AD development is observed as a result of amyloid plaque and tau tangle formation, leading to eventual neuronal degeneration. As recent studies indicate, the dialogue between gut and neurological manifestations is growing in importance, uncovering the fact that gut dysbiosis is related to the onset and development of Alzheimer's. Understanding such an interaction can open the doors to novel therapeutic approaches concerning gastrointestinal health as a means to avoid neurodegeneration, underlining the need for interdisciplinary research combining neurology and gastrointestinal studies (Denman et al., 2023). In contrast to Alzheimer's, Parkinson's disease is primarily dominated by its motor features, for example, tremor, rigidity, and bradykinesia. PD is a neurodegenerative condition resulting from progressive loss of dopaminergic neurons in the substantia nigra region of the brain. Mounting evidence suggests PD may have connections with other conditions, particularly following infections such as SARS-CoV-2, which has stimulated scientific interest in potential connections between COVID-19 and PD. Post-viral onset of Parkinsonian symptomatology is similar to presentations of PD, possibly suggesting infection merely to unmask or speed up underlying neurodegenerative disease, providing a fertile ground for diagnosis and treatment. Investigating these connections will be crucial as populations will need to contend with the long-term health consequences of recent pandemics (Abbott et al., 2023).

Moreover, the social and psychological burden of living with these disorders adds further complexity. Alzheimer's and Parkinson's patients typically experience considerable challenges, both in motor and cognitive function as well as in emotional and mental state. This connection of the neurological state of these conditions and their psychosocial state emphasizes the necessity for an integrative method. The integration of cognitive therapies, medication, and social systems of support can enhance the quality of life of these patients. As studies continue, an understanding of how neurological illnesses affect overall health and social well-being continues to be important, emphasizing the need for integrated healthcare models specifically designed to suit the multiple needs of patients suffering from Alzheimer's, Parkinson's, and similar disorders (Figure 1.13).

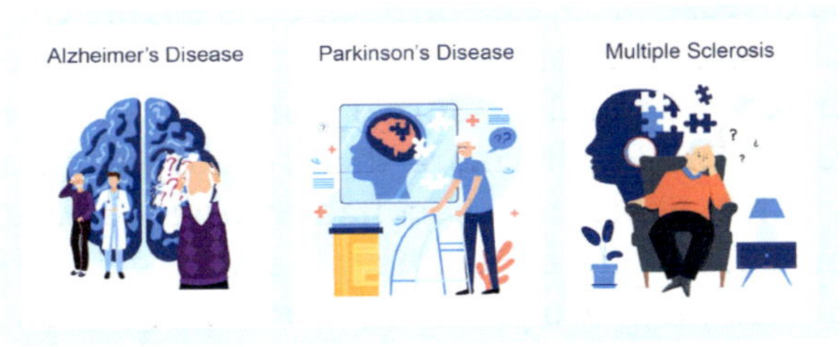

Figure 1.13. Common neurological disorders.

Source: https://lonestarneurology.net/wp-content/uploads/2024/09/2-What-Are-the-Most-Common-Neurological-Disorders.jpg.

1.5.2. Causes and Risk Factors

The intricate mechanism of the nervous system can be significantly affected by numerous reasons and risk factors, which in turn manifest as different neurological disorders. One such severe risk factor is hyperhomocysteinemia (hHCy), which is characterized by a raised blood concentration of homocysteine. It has been proven through various studies that hHCy is strongly associated with enhanced oxidative stress, which may result in neuronal injury and is associated with brain ischemia. The mechanisms underlying this association involve complex interactions between signaling pathways within the brain, but specifically those involved in mitogen-activated protein kinases (MAPKs). Understanding how these factors interact may lie at the forefront of therapeutic intervention strategies for ischemic diseaseand therefore highlight the need for , thereby highlighting the need for a detailed understanding of risk factors surrounding neurological health (Beňová et al., 2016). Another significant aspect of risk factor study is the influence of environmental factors and lifestyle on neurological health. For instance, individuals with intellectual disability are exposed to unique health inequalities that lead to premature death caused by avoidable diseases. Evidence from a Confidential Inquiry also shows that 37% of deaths for people with intellectual disability were graded as avoidable through improved healthcare, and this is a stark contrast compared to the rate of the general population at 13% (Blair et al., 2013). Underlying determinants of factors like poor care provision, inadequately developed advanced care planning, and poor levels of living also contribute to these variations. Hence, addressing these systemic vulnerabilities is crucial in risk reduction and facilitation of health gains in such a vulnerable population. Furthermore, genetic inclinations are also critical in the causation of the onset of such neurological diseases. Inherited characteristics can make an individual susceptible to conditions such as Alzheimer's disease, Parkinson's disease, and multiple sclerosis. Genetic differences have the potential to affect various biological pathways, such as inflammatory reactions and neurotransmitter activity, all of which are crucial for proper neuronal well-being. This genetic context, together with environmental risk factors such as improper diet, sedentary lifestyle, or exposure to neurotoxins, exists in a complex arena where prevention and treatment at an early stage can be helpful. These causes and risk factors are thus to be thoroughly examined to ensure effective measures of prevention and therapeutic intervention in the framework of neurological health (Figure 1.14).

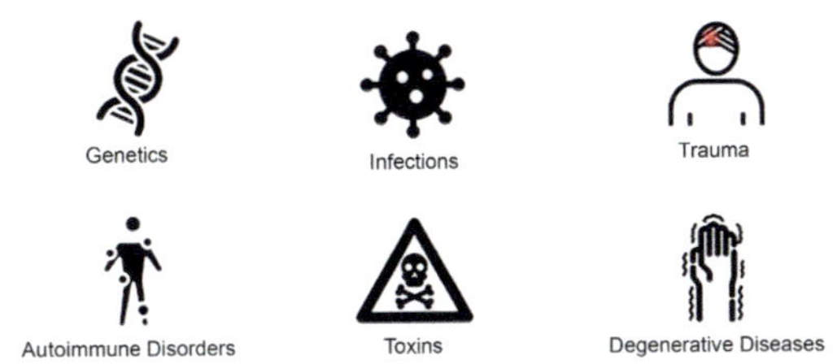

Figure 1.14. Causes of neurological disorders.

Source: https://cdn-jcbbn.nitrocdn.com/ZzJTQPFExwgabqaRdCGLAPQIlofRPyyW/assets/images/optimized/rev-5ae967d/psrihospital.com/wp-content/uploads/2023/10/PSRI-Blog-banner-1-1.jpg.

1.5.3. Treatment and Management Options

Management and care of nervous system diseases need holistic care that considers the intrinsic nature of the condition, the background of the patient, and overall health. Various modalities are applied in the treatment of brain metastases, which are common in cancer patients with advanced disease. Whole-brain radiation therapy is a conventional technique that treats not just symptoms but also avoids neurologically induced death and intellectual impairment. In addition, other therapies such as stereotactic radiosurgery, neurosurgery, and chemotherapy are usually combined with the treatment to enhance patient response. However, with the resulting CNS toxicity risk, investigation remains ongoing into other such therapies, such as radiosensitizers, that could reduce these toxicities but enhance efficacy in the treatment of brain metastases (Baschnagel et al., 2008). In the context of inherited nervous system diseases such as Von Hippel-Lindau syndrome (VHL), management is not just a case of simple instant intervention. VHL patients typically require multidisciplinary management due to the multidimensional aspect of the tumors responsible for the disease. Regular genetic screening and surveillance through advanced imaging technologies are critical in monitoring the disease progression. Such tests enable early diagnosis of tumors and prompt treatment, either through removal by surgery or through other treatments. Furthermore, the demand presented by VHL necessitates collaboration between specialists like oncologists, genetic advisors, and primary care physicians to deliver patients with holistic care that treats their physical as well as psychological health (Amanuel et al., 2017). A second critical component of treatment and management strategies is the integration of neuropsychological testing and biomarker research to quantify CNS toxicity from various treatments. As therapy continues to develop, it is crucial to identify what cognitive impairment can arise so that long-term patient care can be optimized. Neuropsychological testing has the potential to be highly informative regarding the impact of treatments on cognitive function and allows for tailored interventions that optimize patients' quality of life. In addition, biomarker search is promising in the identification of high-risk patients and in the prediction of outcomes of treatment, thereby maximizing management strategy in neurosciences. As scientists continue to discover the correlations between treatment modalities and CNS action, individualized medicine in neurological therapy may present the key to improved therapeutic outcomes for patients with nervous system diseases (Baschnagel et al., 2008).

Test Your Knowledge

1. What are some common causes or risk factors associated with neurological disorders?
2. What are two treatment or management options for neurological disorders?

1.6. The Nervous System and Behavior

Learning Outcome

1. Define the influence of the nervous system on emotions
2. Describe the role of the nervous system in cognitive functions
3. Identify the impact on social interactions

The complex relationship between the nervous system and behavior is at the core of understanding how organisms respond to their surroundings. The nervous system, consisting of the central and peripheral systems, constitutes a highly developed system for the processing of sensory input and the coordination of responses. Behavior, on the other hand, can be considered to be the manifestation of neuron function, influencing everything from reflex behavior to decision-making. For instance, neurotransmitters regulate moods and emotional responses, illustrating the biological underpinnings of behaviors such as aggression, social behavior, and anxiety. An understanding of these connections is central to fields such as psychology and neuroscience, where researchers attempt to account for patterns of behavior through the framework of neurological functioning. New research has investigated the influence of extrinsic factors on the nervous system and how environmental stimulus affects behavior. Examples include research that has illustrated how stressors powerfully influence neural circuits and neurotransmitter function, leading to a change in behavior. An investigation had considered the application of a work-stress management intervention and its subsequent influence on blood pressure and emotional health in hypertensive employees. These findings highlight the elaborate feedback cycle between environmental stress, physiological reaction, and resultant behavior, and suggest that targeted interventions can yield increased well-being and cognitive functioning under stress. This is indicative of the flexibility of the nervous system and its capacity to modulate behavior when subjected to changing demands. Additionally, unconventional research approaches have started to investigate the long-term impacts of non-biological inputs on the nervous system, especially in Russia. Studies into high-penetrating emissions and their potential biological effects may reveal additional layers of sophistication in the ways that living organisms are shaped by their worlds. This research supports the argument that the nervous system reacts not only to internal stimulation but to external, even non-traditional, stimulation. As scientists venture into these new frontiers, the potential for discovering new interactions between the nervous system and behavior grows, with the hope of a greater understanding of the biological determinants of human and animal behavior in a variety of contexts and stimuli (Tomasino et al., 2003; Kernbach et al., 2013).

1.6.1. Influence of the Nervous System on Emotions

The intricate relationship of the nervous system with the emotions is the very betokenment of human complexity. Emotions not only arise in response to external stimuli but are also deeply embedded in the physiological functioning of the body, which is primarily governed by the nervous system. The brain processes sensory data, balancing it, which leads to emotional responses experienced as joy, sorrow, fear, or anger. Neurotransmitters such as serotonin and dopamine are at the forefront of mood modulation and emotional states, with direct nervous system control over the expression and feeling of emotions. Furthermore, the autonomic nervous system, divided into the sympathetic and parasympathetic divisions, aids in the modulation of physiological responses that possess a link with emotions and thus shows the intertwined nature of body responses and emotional states. Research in affective neuroscience illuminates the neurophysiological correlates of emotional expression and the idea that body and brain work together to reflect the affective state of a person. Physiological measures, such as heart rate and skin conductance, are indicators of emotional arousal. Studies have shown that both body and brain responses can convey a person's emotional status in subtle ways. Additionally, while affect recognition from physiological signals is highly challenging, evidence shows consistent patterns between specific emotional responses and identifiable physiological states. Elaboration of the patterns offers significant information on how biological mechanisms are the foundation for human emotions and therefore contribute to enhanced understanding of emotional well-being and possible treatments for emotional disorders (Mühl et al., 2009). The influence of emotion on behavior and decision-making can be traced back to several information systems mediated by the nervous system.

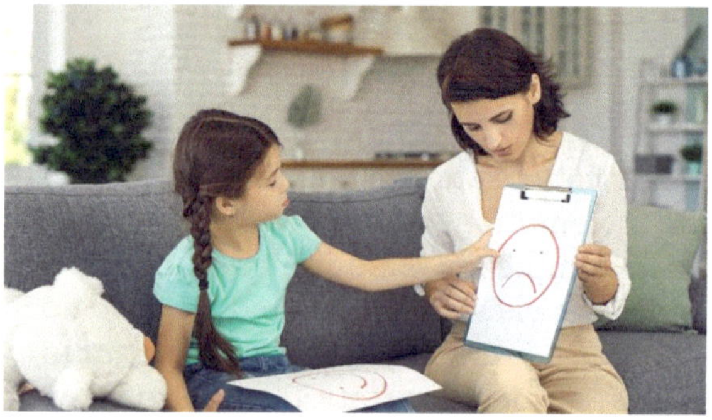

Figure 1.15. Nervous system influences our emotions.

Source: https://cdn.neurofit.app/learn/images/emotions_autonomic_nervous_system/16x9-mobile.jpg.

These systems retain different aspects of human emotional experience and cognition, which suggests that individuals behave in a context of YES/NO decisions based on their emotional state. Emotional pain and certain affective states are, in certain situations, causal conditions for behavior that determines the direction of a person's life course and outcomes, and the significance of emotional regulation. Positive engagement results in healthier adaptation and decision-making style, while negative emotion creates maladaptive behavior resulting in chronic anxiety or stress. It is necessary to understand these dynamics both for individual health as well as for integrated educational and parenting practices promoting emotional health and resilience for future generations (Gaiseanu et al., 2018) (Figure 1.15).

1.6.2. Role in Cognitive Functions

The nervous system is also responsible for playing a significant role in numerous mental functions, including memory, attention, and decision-making. It facilitates these processes by complex networks of neurons and synaptic links, which are vital for information exchange and communication between the brain and body. For instance, memory formation is controlled by the hippocampus, which is a region of the brain that illustrates the power of neural connectivity and plasticity in mental processes. Disturbances in these neural networks have the potential to lead to severe cognitive impairment, highlighting the importance of intact nervous system function. Emerging research suggests the participation of proteins such as dystroglycan in brain development and synapse formation, with implications that disturbances in these processes not only threaten muscular integrity but also lead to cognitive impairment, testifying to a sophisticated relationship between physical health and cognition (Samwald, 2007). Recent research has also highlighted the importance of neuroplasticity-the ability of the brain to modify and adapt through the formation of new neural pathways- as a major factor influencing cognitive ability. Higher levels of neuroplasticity are linked with various factors, such as sleep, learning, and physical activities like yoga. Yoga practice has been shown to profoundly influence the nervous system's flexibility, thereby contributing to cognitive enhancement. Yoga exercises of restraint in breathing and awareness can facilitate the regulation of emotions, ensuring good stress management and mental resilience. Such adaptability is paramount to the mind's functionality as it provides for improved processing and also reaction to adversity within the environment. Through its facilitation of enhanced neuronal plasticity, yoga represents actual application methods of enhancing intellectual functions in the context of nervous system resilience (Biesok et al., 2024). The nexus between the nervous system and cognitive processes can also be observed in stress and anxiety, which are commonly known to pose adverse effects on intellectual acuity and decision-making capabilities. Chronic stress, on the other hand, can impair neural circuits involved in learning and memory, and robust methods will be needed to reverse these processes. Techniques like mindfulness meditation, grounded in principles not significantly different from those of yoga, hold promise in developing cognitive resilience. By creating a more balanced autonomic nervous system response, these procedures can induce alterations in mood regulation and cognitive functioning. As research continues to shed light on the interplay between lifestyle factors and cognitive health, this type of information is most welcome in the formulation of unified strategies that directly address the needs of the nervous system but promote cognitive function. Thus, it is critical to identify the role of intrinsic and extrinsic factors in maintaining cognitive health and overall well-being.

1.6.3. Impact on Social Interactions

The intricate interaction between the nervous system and social behavior is deeply embedded in the way individuals interact and develop interpersonal relationships. The nervous system not only regulates physiological responses but also guides emotional responses and interpersonal relationships. For instance, an individual's level of arousal, established by the autonomic nervous system, may influence the quality of the way an individual converses and sympathizes with other individuals. When levels of physiological arousal are too high or too low, a person's ability to communicate effectively is disrupted. This dynamic is particularly pertinent in a discussion of racial and cultural difference because implicit biases alter communication patterns and impact relational outcomes. Such processes explain the complex entwinement of physiological state and social action, and therefore have implications for maximizing interpersonal relationships in a range of contexts. Moreover, the influence of attachment styles on social relationships is rooted in the functioning of the nervous system. Attachment theory holds that early interpersonal relationships with caregivers shape patterns of behavior that get translated into adult relationships. These attachment patterns influence emotional regulation, producing either secure or insecure relationships among individuals. The physiological responses linked to attachment can also control stress levels, which in turn may affect health outcomes and social interactions. This connection highlights the need for the integration of psychology and physiology in a bid to appreciate the complexity of human interaction. Secure attachment, for instance, encourages openness in communication, while insecure attachment can make a person vulnerable to anxiety or avoidance, thus complicating social interaction. Discussing such nuances deepens our understanding of interpersonal connection and fills gaps that are likely to be there in social interaction. The two-edged nature of the nervous system's contribution to the building of trust and communication is also pointed out by its influence on interpersonal satisfaction and confidence, particularly in health care. Mistrust and dissatisfaction can develop from miscommunication or presumed bias, as illustrated with physicians and patients. Research has indicated that physician implicit racial bias has negative implications for patient trust and satisfaction, leading to underutilization of healthcare services among already vulnerable communities (Fetters et al., 2018). Such interactions underscore the value of good communication in establishing trust and adherence. As healthcare providers pay attention to their communication habits and work towards reducing bias, they strengthen not only the individual patient experience but also the social environment of healthcare communication as a whole. Thus, examining the convergence of communication, trust, and physiological response is an articulation of the fluid interplay between individual relationships and system infrastructure for enhancing positive health outcomes and social consciousness.

Test Your Knowledge

1. What role does the nervous system play in cognitive functions like memory and decision-making?
2. In what ways does the nervous system impact social interactions?

SUMMARY

The projection of the nervous system reveals that this intricate network is the foundation of human function. The ability to process and respond to stimulation is a hallmark of not just survival but also advanced decision-making and emotional regulation. Each component, from neurons to synapses, has a critical role in transferring information that governs our interaction with the environment. The understanding of these processes focuses on the nervous system's role in normal physiological conditions as well as the onset of a vast array of neurological disorders. This synthesis of knowledge then augments the paradigms of treatment towards the goal of enhancing neural health and resilience, which points to further research and application in clinical settings. In addition, the latest developments in the field also reveal the core, mutually integrated functions of the nervous system beyond traditional boundaries of neurobiology. For instance, genomic studies reveal the vital functions of long non-coding RNAs (lncRNAs) in neurodevelopment and intellectual processes, suggesting that the genetic foundation of intellect and behavior is far more complex than previously imagined. Identification of lncRNAs that play a role in synaptic transmission and neural system development is opening avenues for new therapeutic strategies, and specifically in intellectual disability disorders. As it becomes increasingly clear from evidence, such findings need to be integrated into educational practice as well as clinical work to understand how genetic inputs are a factor in neural function and welfare. In total, the end of our examination of the nervous system reveals not only the elementary components of its organization and its operation but also the cumulative advance of knowledge within this field. The integration between biological, psychological, and environmental factors provides a universal underlying theme in developing an integrated comprehension of the nervous system's contribution to human life. The knowledge reached through both past and present research sets a firm foundation to address neurological health concerns. Moreover, as the body of knowledge expands with research on the implications of free will and decision-making frameworks, as was exemplified with regard to personal trajectories and centers of cognition (Gaiseanu et al., 2018), it is clear that a multi-dimensional approach will be crucial in advancing knowledge and understanding of the nervous system. These findings help support the development of a cooperative endeavor across fields to optimize interventions for the promotion of nervous system health and function (D'haene et al., 2016).

A foray into the nervous system reveals its intricate organization and diverse functions. The central point, the nervous system branches out into two key components: the CNS and the PNS. The CNS, comprised of the brain and spinal cord, processes information and integrates actions, acting as the control center of the body. On the other hand, the PNS contains all the neural tracts that carry information beyond the CNS, making it possible for the brain to communicate with the body's extremities. The difference is fundamental to organisms' adjustment to their surroundings, response to stimuli, and obtaining homeostasis with intricate neural networks. New developments in anesthesia, like the concept of Receptor-focused Magnetic Resonance anesthesia, illustrate the ongoing progress in medical practice related to the PNS. This new method proposes the application of electromagnetic models of medicinal preparations for the administration of anesthetic action with none of the poisonous side effects associated with conventional drug delivery. Through the application of advanced high-resolution magnetic resonance imaging technology to identify receptor sites, this method may enhance accuracy in anesthesia delivery and transform surgical interventions and patient treatment. Such advances not only signify technological integration in medicine but also a greater understanding of the nervous system's diverse functions and how they can be manipulated for therapeutic purposes (Golyanishchev et al., 2016). Further, studies of nerve morphology in some taxonomic groups, e.g., Family Nereididae, add to general knowledge about nervous systems within species. Neuroanatomical studies of **Neanthes arenaceodentata** uncover the incredible intricacy of neural development even at post-embryonic stages. Sophisticated imaging techniques have enabled scientists to record the early formation of essential structures like the brain and segmental nerves. The findings oppose previous assumptions about nerve structure and development in annelids, uncovering evolutionary adaptations and variability potential within related groups. Thus, these results are significant because they bring to light the intricate evolutionary background that has shaped the annelid nervous system and its context within the bilaterian evolutionary framework (Jacobs et al., 2010).

KEY TERMS FROM THIS CHAPTER

- Central Nervous System
- Brain
- Neurons
- Synapse
- Myelin Sheath
- Autonomic Nervous System
- Motor Neurons
- Neurotransmitters
- Peripheral Nervous System
- Spinal Cord
- Neuroglia
- Nerve Impulse
- Reflex Arc
- Somatic Nervous System
- Interneurons

CRITICAL THINKING QUESTIONS

1. **Which of the following is the primary function of the nervous system?**
   a. Production of hormones
   b. Transport of nutrients
   c. Coordination of body activities
   d. Absorption of oxygen
2. **The two main parts of the central nervous system (CNS) are:**
   a. Brain and spinal cord
   b. Nerves and ganglia
   c. Brain and nerves
   d. Spinal cord and sensory organs
3. **Which type of neuron carries impulses from the body to the central nervous system?**
   a. Motor neuron
   b. Sensory neuron
   c. Interneuron
   d. Connector neuron
4. **The peripheral nervous system (PNS) consists of:**
   a. Brain and spinal cord
   b. Spinal cord only
   c. Nerves and ganglia outside the CNS
   d. Sensory organs only
5. **Which part of the nervous system is responsible for involuntary actions like heartbeat and digestion?**
   a. Somatic nervous system
   b. Central nervous system
   c. Autonomic nervous system
   d. Sensory nervous system

Short Answer Questions

1. What are thc main components of the central and peripheral nervous systems?
2. List two primary functions of the nervous system.
3. What are the three main types of neurons and their roles?
4. What is the role of neurotransmitters in neural communication?
5. Name two common disorders of the nervous system.
6. How can damage to the nervous system affect behavior?
7. What is the difference between the sympathetic and parasympathetic nervous systems?

Answer to Critical Thinking Questions

1. (c); 2. (a); 3. (b); 4. (c); 5. (c)

REFERENCES

1. Iacono, S., Schirò, G., Davì, C., Mastrilli, S., Abbott, M., Guajana, F., Arnao, V., Aridon, P., Ragonese, P., Gagliardo, C., Colomba, C., Scichilone, N., & D'Amelio, M. (2023). COVID-19 and neurological disorders: what might connect Parkinson's disease to SARS-CoV-2 infection. *Frontiers in Neurology, 14*. https://doi.org/10.3389/fneur.2023.1172416

2. Achacoso, A., Amirikian, B., van Ooyen, A., Baruch, I., Binzegger, T., Borisyuk, R., et al. (2009). A simple rule for axon outgrowth and synaptic competition generates realistic connection lengths and filling fractions. http://arxiv.org/abs/0906.0685 (accessed on 14th June 2025).

3. Agnati, L. F., Borroto-Escuela, D. O., Fuxe, K., et al. (2013). On the G-protein-coupled receptor heteromers and their allosteric receptor-receptor interactions in the central nervous system: Focus on their role in pain modulation. https://core.ac.uk/download/55762900.pdf (accessed on 14th June 2025).

4. Ainsworth, B. E., Avitsur, R., Baumeister, R. F., Beedie, C., Biomarker Definitions Working Group, Bolger, N., et al. (2014). The attachment system and physiology in adulthood: Normative processes, individual differences, and implications for health. https://core.ac.uk/download/294625964.pdf (accessed on 14th June 2025).

5. Atari, R. (2014). *Rawan Atari–The Influence of Multi-Sensory Environment on Physiological Response in Children with Autism Spectrum Disorders and Children with Special Health Care Needs.* https://core.ac.uk/download/67757154.pdf (accessed on 14th June 2025).

6. Bacik, K. A., Barahona, M., Beguerisse-Díaz, M., et al. (2016). Flow-based network analysis of the *Caenorhabditis elegans* connectome. https://core.ac.uk/download/77017459.pdf (accessed on 14th June 2025).

7. Baritaki, S., Chatzaki, E., de Bree, E., et al. (2019). Chronic stress, inflammation, and colon cancer: A CRH system-driven molecular crosstalk. https://core.ac.uk/download/323076588.pdf (accessed on 14th June 2025).

8. Barton, M. J., Clarke, M., Ekberg, J., et al. (2017). The glia response after peripheral nerve injury: A comparison between Schwann cells and olfactory ensheathing cells and their uses for neural regenerative therapies. https://core.ac.uk/download/196605084.pdf (accessed on 14th June 2025).

9. Baschnagel, A., Camphausen, K., & Wolters, P. L. (2008). Neuropsychological testing and biomarkers in the management of brain metastases. https://core.ac.uk/download/pdf/8195806.pdf (accessed on 14th June 2025).

10. Beer, R. D., Izquierdo, E. J., & Williams, P. L. (2015). Information flow through a model of the *C. elegans* klinotaxis circuit. http://arxiv.org/abs/1502.04262 (accessed on 14th June 2025).

11. Beňová, A., Kalenská, D., Kaplán, P., et al. (2016). Forebrain ischemic stroke and the phenomenon of ischemic tolerance: Is homocysteine foe or friend? https://core.ac.uk/download/322427793.pdf (accessed on 14th June 2025).

12. Bich, L., Moreau, J. F., & Pradeu, T. (2019). Understanding multicellularity: The functional organization of the intercellular space. https://core.ac.uk/download/228134961.pdf (accessed on 14th June 2025).

13. Biesok, M., Lewoniuk, N., Macherski, M., et al. (2024). Analysis of the effects of regular yoga on the adaptive capacity of the nervous system. https://core.ac.uk/download/620863318.

pdf (accessed on 14th June 2025).

14. Blair, P. S., Fleming, P. J., Heslop, P., et al. (2013). The confidential inquiry into premature deaths of people with intellectual disabilities in the UK: A population-based study. https://core.ac.uk/download/29026952.pdf (accessed on 14th June 2025).
15. Carbonari, L. (2019). *IL-15/IL-15Rα signaling and synaptic transmission: A crosstalk between the immune and the nervous system?* https://core.ac.uk/download/188833274.pdf (accessed on 14th June 2025).
16. Christensen, W. (2006). The evolutionary origins of volition. https://core.ac.uk/download/pdf/87234.pdf (accessed on 14th June 2025).
17. D'haene, E., De Meyer, T., Jacobs, E., et al. (2016). Identification of long non-coding RNAs involved in neuronal development and intellectual disability. https://core.ac.uk/download/84041574.pdf (accessed on 14th June 2025).
18. Denman, C. R., Jo, J., & Park, S. M. (2023). Gut-brain axis: Gut dysbiosis and psychiatric disorders in Alzheimer's and Parkinson's disease. https://core.ac.uk/download/622101581.pdf (accessed on 14th June 2025).
19. Fetters, M. D., Hagiwara, N., Lafata, J. E., et al. (2018). Study protocol for investigating physician communication behaviors that link physician implicit racial bias and patient outcomes in Black patients with type 2 diabetes using an exploratory sequential mixed methods design. https://core.ac.uk/download/232207266.pdf (accessed on 14th June 2025).
20. Gaiseanu, F. (2018). Destiny or free will decision? A life overview from the perspective of an informational modeling of consciousness. Part II: Attitude and decision criteria, free will and destiny. https://core.ac.uk/download/186331556.pdf (accessed on 14th June 2025).
21. Gaiseanu, F. (2019). Informational mode of the brain operation and consciousness as an informational related system. https://core.ac.uk/download/210995796.pdf (accessed on 14th June 2025).
22. Gaiseanu, F. (2019). The informational model of consciousness: Mechanisms of embodiment/disembodiment of information. https://core.ac.uk/download/287611919.pdf (accessed on 14th June 2025).
23. Golyanishchev, M. (2016). Hypothesis of Rfmra development–the receptor-focused magnetic and resonant anesthesia. https://core.ac.uk/download/301580510.pdf (accessed on 14th June 2025).
24. Gurkoff, G. G., Izadi, A., Lee, D. J., et al. (2016). Making waves in the brain: What are oscillations, and why modulating them makes sense for brain injury. https://core.ac.uk/download/323070739.pdf (accessed on 14th June 2025).
25. Haab, T. C., & Roe, B. E. (2025). Using biomedical technologies to inform economic modeling: Challenges and opportunities for improving analysis of environmental policies. https://core.ac.uk/download/pdf/7130413.pdf (accessed on 14th June 2025).
26. Hall, M., & Robinson, D. (1995). The multimedia brain. https://core.ac.uk/download/9630635.pdf (accessed on 14th June 2025).
27. Hornemann, T. (2021). Mini review: Lipids in peripheral nerve disorders. https://www.zora.uzh.ch/id/eprint/205258/1/1-s2.0-S0304394020307254-main.pdf (accessed on 14th June 2025).

28. Jacobs, D. K., Valencia, J. E., & Winchell, C. J. (2010). Confocal analysis of nervous system architecture in direct-developing juveniles of *Neanthes arenaceodentata* (Annelida, Nereididae). https://core.ac.uk/download/4886525.pdf (accessed on 14th June 2025).
29. Jensen, L. J., Shah, P. K., Bork, P., Bourne, P., & Boué, S. (2005). Extraction of transcript diversity from scientific literature. https://core.ac.uk/download/pdf/3711515.pdf (accessed on 14th June 2025).
30. Kebede, A. A., Owusu-Dapaah, H., Bhullar, J. S., Lather, J., Kaushik, M., & Varshney, N. (2017). A review of Von Hippel-Lindau syndrome. https://core.ac.uk/download/206431858.pdf (accessed on 14th June 2025).
31. Kernbach, S. (2013). Unconventional research in USSR and Russia: Short overview. http://arxiv.org/abs/1312.1148 (accessed on 14th June 2025).
32. Lehman, C. D. (2023). *Human InNervate VR*. https://core.ac.uk/download/596995564.pdf (accessed on 14th June 2025).
33. Megaw, P. (2015). *Neurophysiology for Allied Health Students, Book 1: The Basics*. https://core.ac.uk/download/303779636.pdf (accessed on 14th June 2025).
34. Morin, D. (2018). Spinal cord trauma: An overview of normal structure and function, primary and secondary mechanisms of injury, and emerging treatment modalities. https://core.ac.uk/download/158970372.pdf (accessed on 14th June 2025).
35. Motofei, I. G., & Rowland, D. L. (2017). Psycho-physiologic emergentist; Four minds in a body. https://core.ac.uk/download/144553869.pdf (accessed on 14th June 2025).
36. Mühl, C. (2009). Neurophysiological assessment of affective experience. https://core.ac.uk/download/pdf/11473076.pdf (accessed on 14th June 2025).
37. Mule, F. (2011). The glucagon-like peptide-2. https://core.ac.uk/download/46602309.pdf (accessed on 14th June 2025).
38. Pennella, A., Porro, C., Panaro, M. A., & Trotta, T. (2021). Functional role of non-muscle myosin II in microglia: An updated review. https://core.ac.uk/download/541260282.pdf (accessed on 14th June 2025).
39. Samwald, M. (2007). Review: Dystroglycan in the nervous system. https://core.ac.uk/download/pdf/287398.pdf (accessed on 14th June 2025).
40. Santello, M., & Valero-Cuevas, F. J. (2017). On neuromechanical approaches for the study of biological grasp and manipulation. http://arxiv.org/abs/1710.08557 (accessed on 14th June 2025).
41. Tomasino, D., Atkinson, M., & McCraty, R. (2003). Impact of a workplace stress reduction program on blood pressure and emotional health in hypertensive employees. https://core.ac.uk/download/71342520.pdf (accessed on 14th June 2025).
42. Wolff, J. G. (2003). Neural mechanisms for information compression by multiple alignment, unification and search. https://core.ac.uk/download/pdf/85392.pdf (accessed on 14th June 2025).

THE CENTRAL NERVOUS SYSTEM

2

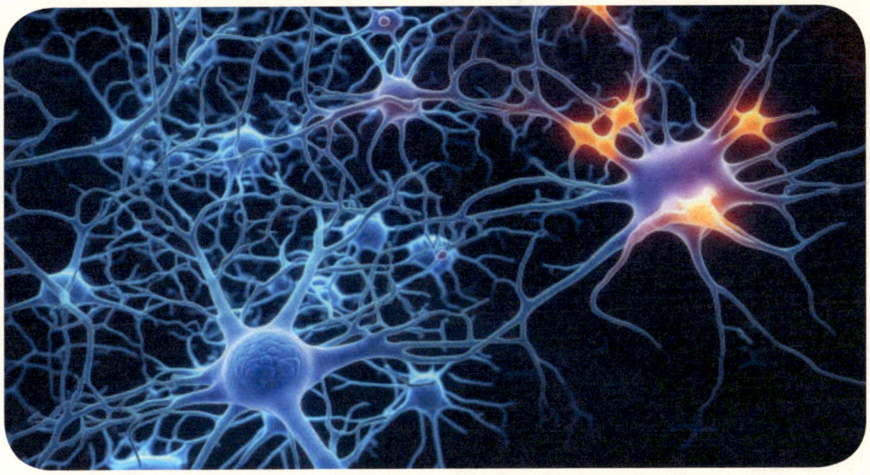

LEARNING OBJECTIVES

After studying this chapter, you will be able to:

1. Identify and describe the central nervous system anatomical structures
2. Outline the chief functions of the central nervous system
3. Describe the roles played by neurons and the process of neurotransmission in the central nervous system
4. Recognize common central nervous system disorders and their implications
5. Describe the role of the central nervous system in regulating behavior

Introduction

The central nervous system (CNS) is the command center of the body, coordinating a vast number of activities crucial for survival and environmental adaptation. It consists of the brain and spinal cord, processing sense data, integrating responses, and maintaining control over body functions. At its core is the neurobiological support system offering cognition, emotion, and motor control. This intricate system not merely supports primitive reflexes but also ensures higher-order conduct and cerebral function. The discovery of the CNS function is greater than what is known by anatomical structure; it is what is known by cellular process and molecular mechanisms that direct its function. An exploration of such processes is of utmost importance because they are the foundation for neuroscience and medical research and ultimately therapeutic intervention for neurological disease and prognosis for mental illness. Current studies emphasize the interconnectedness of stress, inflammation, and the CNS and thus have wide-ranging implications for general health. As the study has shown, neuroendocrine mechanisms can be turned on by chronic stress and modulate inflammation and contribute to disease development, including cancer. CNS-body inflammatory process interaction is particularly noteworthy with the action of corticotropin-releasing hormone (CRH) and its receptors. As a result of actions in the various body systems, these neuropeptides have complex regulatory circuitry governing results in health. Evaluation of such a relationship is crucial in understanding the CNS reaction to stress and homeostatic regulation. From such an understanding of molecular interactions, scientists can acquire novel information on mechanisms for the design of personalized medicine strategies aimed at chronic inflammation and associated diseases that can lead to more effective therapeutic outcomes.

Organization of the CNS is a mirror of its evolutionary history as a response to the need for information processing in the optimum manner under the constraint of environmental demands. The Informational Model of Consciousness is a model for the study of the structure and function of CNSs. Information acquisition and processing, in this system, are at the core of the brain activities and are thus specialized centers for decision-making, emotional processes, and genetic inheritance. The anterior cingulate cortex, the most important of these regions of interest, is involved in affective signal modulation and facilitation of adaptive behavior. Thus, understanding hierarchical integration of information in the CNS elucidates dynamic interaction between cognition, emotion, and bodily response to human adaptation and survival mechanisms. Continued studies can reveal more sophisticated processes controlling these functions to advance neuroscience and psychological well-being by explaining the utmost significance of the CNS to human existence.

Definition of the Central Nervous System

CNS is a central organ of the body, for instance, the brain and the spinal cord, that oversees action and the passing of sensory impulses within the body. In operation, CNS is where sensory input is stored, manages the body's operations, and is the site of conscious thinking and feeling. Control of voluntary and involuntary behavior is essential in obtaining homeostasis and the organism's capacity to adapt to environmental stimuli. It is manifested in the formation of neural circuitry that integrates varied sensory information in a bid to support sagacious responses. Being an information system, it acts upon distinctive items that stand for consciousness, and distinct interrelating is expressed in the result of explicated intellectual behavior and activities, which are stimulated by the postulate that consciousness is a result of such operational activity of the CNS, as proposed by recent studies giving significant weightage to information at its core (Gaiseanu et al., 2019). The brain, therefore, as the foremost organ of the CNS, is structured hierarchically so that it can process information in a complex manner to influence both elementary survival responses as well as more complex cognitive processes. According to the Informational Model of Consciousness, this theory suggests that different regions in the brain, such as the Info-Emotional Center and the Center of Decision and Command, are responsible for specific but complementary roles in a person's structures of feeling and action. The functioning of these areas also places into context an active interaction that not only detects external information but also unifies this with internal states and points to the importance of neuro-connectivity in global brain function. The dynamic functioning of the anterior cingulate cortex, to name but one example, with its role to weigh up emotional input and decision-making operations, only further hinders the CNS as regards handling human experience and survival mechanisms (Gaiseanu et al., 2020) (Figure 2.1).

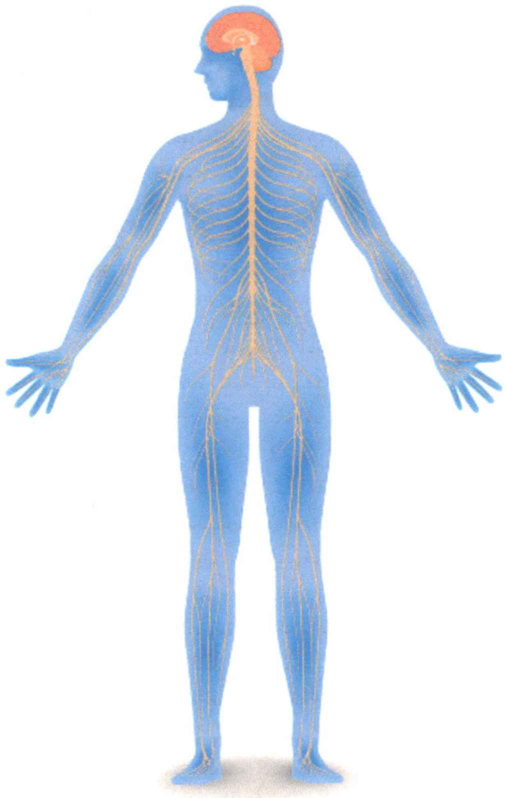

Figure 2.1. Diagram of the human nervous system, illustrating the central and peripheral components, including the brain, spinal cord, and peripheral nerves.

Source: https://external-content.duckduckgo.com/iu/?u=https%3A%2F%2Fqbi.uq.edu.au%2Ffiles%2F27993%2Fcentral-nervous-system-QBI.jpg&f=1&nofb=1&ipt=cf676b0b0f30e08464925ff2cd8777a7481602444081aed7d18b955698d1866e.

Besides, the spinal cord also acts as the main route of information flowing from the brain to and from the rest of the body, through the sensory and motor tracts. Intactness of the spinal cord cannot be overstressed since it directly impacts reflex arcs and automatism of responses needed for reflex reactions to immediate danger. Spinal cord injury has long-range effects, e.g., paralysis or loss of sensation, to emphasize the CNS's function and role in health. The CNS's capacity to process is the plasticity of the CNS, which creates epigenetic outcomes that permit the organism to adjust to environmental pressures. This knowledge builds upon our current understanding of how the CNS participates not only in short-term survival but also in long-term evolutionary success (Gaiseanu et al., 2020).

Importance of the Central Nervous System in Human Physiology

The CNS performs the role of governing and managing human physiology as the central processor and controller of sensory data and motor responses. Under the influence of the environment, the CNS allows for proper responses, which are essential for survival. The complex system manages autonomic functions such as heart rate, breathing, and digestion to ensure homeostasis—a balancing of body processes. Also, having the capacity to learn and adapt through experience is important. Neuroplasticity enables the realignment of neuronal tracts in response to new stimulation, effectively reforming behavior and facilitating recovery from trauma. Thus, the CNS not only facilitates basic physiological processes but is also responsible for advanced ones, such as cognition and emotion regulation, that are indispensable for full health and well-being. In understanding the role of the Central Nervous System, care must be exercised regarding how it intersects with psychological elements that influence physiological well-being. There is evidence recorded of the interdependence of emotional well-being and physiological response; stress, for instance, can elicit a series of reactions based on the CNS. It can be understood through knowledge of the function of attachment styles, for example, why affective relationships influence physiological processes for stress. It has been documented in the literature that attachment theory can account for individual differences in stress response and ensuing health consequences. Therefore, the CNS is not only a conduit for body response but also plays an integral part in emotional processing and sociality, highlighting its multifaceted role in psychological and physiological well-being mechanisms (Ainsworth et al., 2014). Moreover, long-term stress brought about by inefficient emotional regulation carries immense influence on physiological functioning through the CNS. Chronic stress has been found to disrupt homeostasis and lead to an array of diseases, from cardiovascular to metabolic disease. A significant gap is observed between paradigms of care that focus on either psychological or physical components of health, while neglecting the interdependence within human physiology. By this bridging, a more integrated conceptualization of health is achieved, whereby the CNS is a mediator of mental as well as physical conditions. Management of such complexity requires an interdisciplinary approach, which promotes interprofessional collaboration among health professionals, hence improving the efficacy of intervention tactics to stress diseases (Estrine et al., 2006). Lastly, the Central Nervous System's role of controlling the mind and body also underscores its importance in human physiology.

2.1. Anatomy of the Central Nervous System

Learning Outcome

1. Understand the major components: brain and spinal cord
2. Discuss the protective structures: meninges and cerebrospinal fluid
3. Explain the functional regions of the brain

The CNS's anatomy is very well suited to provide for the many functions that come with maintaining homeostasis and sensing. At its core is the brain and spinal cord that are enveloped in protective bony structures—the skull and vertebral column, respectively. The brain is further broken down into segments that comprise the cerebrum, cerebellum, and brainstem, each of which possesses unique cognitive and physiological functions. The cerebrum, for instance, processes the higher-order activities of reasoning, emotion, and sensory interpretation, while the cerebellum is central to motor coordination. Segmentation in this case assists in the specialized processing of several neural functions, a critical evolutionary step to enhance the sensitivity of organisms to external and internal stimuli. The CNS anatomy includes glial cells that perform vital supporting tasks to the neurons. These glial cells also provide homeostasis and myelination, as well as aid in immune function in the CNS. Astrocytes, oligodendrocytes, and microglia are some of the most recognized glial cells that serve specific functions essential to neural function and health. Oligodendrocytes, for instance, play a significant role in the process of myelination, which raises the speed of conduction of electrical impulses along axons, thereby facilitating effective communication between neurons. Moreover, glial cells facilitate the repair of damaged tissues, as they can divide and form a supportive background upon injury. The information regarding the synergy between neurons and glial cells contributes to CNS anatomy information and application in neurological health. Recent techniques continuously evolve our understanding of CNS anatomy, particularly due to advancements in imaging and modeling techniques. New imaging modalities such as computer tomography (CT) and magnetic resonance imaging (MRI) allow detailed three-dimensional reconstructions of the CNS that can image soft tissues and neurovascular structures. They are not only but also crucial in studies and in the clinic, e.g., surgical planning and rehabilitation. With practical segmentation algorithms, scientists can construct models of anatomy that tell us about biomechanics and neurological disease. In addition, the models enable simulations to be created that enhance the outcome of surgery in minimally invasive surgical operations using real-time anatomical data on surgical methods, attesting to the dynamic character of CNS research among academics and in the clinic (Audenaert et al., 2010) (Figure 2.2).

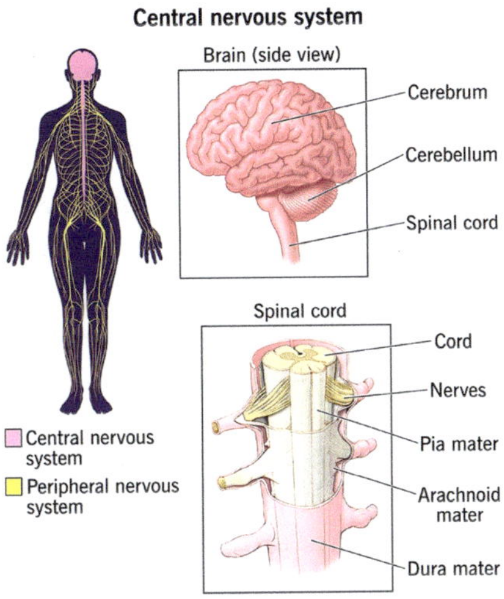

Figure 2.2. Your central nervous system is made up of your brain and spinal cord. It connects to your peripheral nervous system.

Source: https://my.clevelandclinic.org/-/scassets/images/org/health/articles/central-nervous-system.

2.1.1. Major Components: Brain and Spinal Cord

The brain is the control center of the central nervous system (CNS), integrating a vast array of functions required for homeostasis and supporting complex behavior. It consists of several types of characteristic areas, with each containing a specific function. The brain processes sensory information, regulates motor function, and is linked with intellectual functions such as memory and emotion. The brainstem, cerebellum, and cerebral cortex are among the structures that make it function so intricately. In addition, the brain holds not only neurons, but also glial cells, and these have key roles in sustaining neuronal health and communication. Since it continues to evolve, understanding how the dynamic interplay between such cell types functions has become increasingly critical, particularly in characterizing therapeutic strategies for neurological disease. Such complex intermingling of glial and neuronal cells, as with astrocytes, serves to demonstrate the synergistic character of brain function, wherein dysfunction in such interaction is responsible for CNS pathologies. The spinal cord is an essential channel of information exchange between the peripheral nervous system and the brain for reflexes and voluntary movement. It has segments corresponding to spinal nerves that supply innervation to specific regions of the body, making it particularly valuable. The grey and white matter structure in the spinal cord facilitates its role in sensory processing and the execution of motor commands. Rising tracts transmit sensory impulses to the brain and falling tracts transmit motor commands to muscles (Figure 2.3).

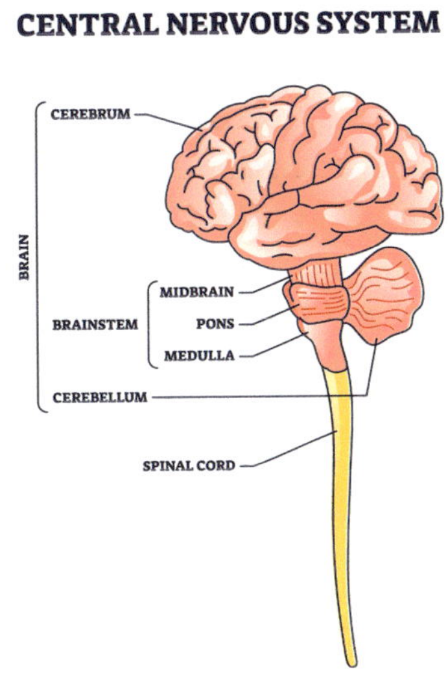

Figure 2.3. The CNS consists of two parts: the brain and the spinal cord.

Source: https://www.physio-pedia.com/Introduction_to_Neuroanatomy.

In addition, injuries to the spinal cord have the potential to disastrously interfere with these pathways with devastating effects, such as paralysis. Research is ongoing on neuroregenerative therapy for the restoration of function in spinal cord injury. New methods involve combining neurorehabilitative techniques with innovative technologies to replace destroyed spinal pathways, offering new hope for the return of function through synergistic interactions between brain-machine interface technology and neuroplasticity protocols. Recent studies also established the central role of glial cells, specifically astrocytes, in the well-being and functioning of the spinal cord and brain. Not just do astrocytes offer direct metabolic support to neurons, but they are also implicated in complex networks of signaling that regulate synaptic transmission and facilitate myelination. Upon CNS injury, these cells can express several different phenotypes, some of which are inhibitory to recovery but others stimulating it (Barnett et al., 2016). These two roles need to be understood to create therapy that is engineered to optimize repair processes with fewer inhibitory reactions. Further, the cell-to-cell communication between astrocytes and other cells, such as oligodendrocytes and neurons, teaches us about the cellular support required for effective regeneration after injury. With further research, utilizing the potential of astrocytes and their supportive roles could be a revolutionary treatment to aid recovery after CNS injury, eventually filling in gaps from nervous system damage and disease (Edgerton et al., 2016).

2.1.2. Protective Structures: Meninges and Cerebrospinal Fluid

The CNS is protected by protective structures, i.e., the meninges, which play a role in the protection of neural tissue. The meninges create three layers of coverings: dura mater, arachnoid mater, and pia mater. These membranes all act as protection from potential damage and infection, but at the same time provide support and stability for the brain and spinal cord. The most peripheral dura mater is thick and hard and serves as the first line of defense. Below it lies the arachnoid mater, a web-like covering over the brain. The pia mater then envelops the CNS tightly, permitting the exchange of nutrients. Through the creation of them as a physical barrier and medium for nutrient exchange, the meninges are crucial to the well-being and operation of the CNS overall. Cerebrospinal fluid (CSF) is a protective CNS component, located in the subarachnoid space between the meninges. CSF is a clear, colorless body fluid that fills several essential functions, including cushioning the brain and spinal cord against injury, buoyancy, and removal of products of metabolism. CSF is a shock absorber as well, which significantly reduces the potential of injury due to impacts. It is also essential in maintaining homeostasis in the environment of neurons through regulation by pressure and electrolytes. CSF production and circulation are associated with the structure of meninges since it is secreted in the choroid plexus and circulates through ventricles and re-enters the blood circulation (Figure 2.4).

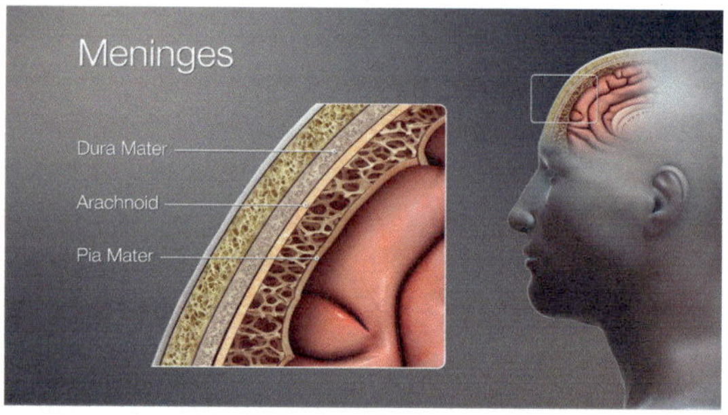

Figure 2.4. Depicting meninges around the brain.

Source: https://upload.wikimedia.org/wikipedia/commons/1/13/3D_Medical_Illustration_Meninges_Details.jpg.

Thus, the dynamic nature of CSF ensures the protective function of the meninges and cooperates with the global stability of the CNS. Meningeal interaction with CSF and immune response is essential in the protective function of the CNS. New research highlights the roles of the immune cells, like mast cells and microglia, which interact in the meninges and thereby facilitate protective immunity against assumed pathogens. These immune cells stand ready to respond rapidly against inflammatory stimuli, as systemic inflammation may trigger neuroinflammatory processes that disrupt the function of the brain. The meninges create an interface modulating leukocyte migration into the CNS in a way that the CNS is immune-privileged but is otherwise competent to defend itself whenever the occasion arises. This marvelous equilibrium highlights both the immunological and physical function of the meninges and CSF in maintaining the health and integrity of the CNS, affirming that such protective systems are greater than mere barriers but are directly involved in the intricate ballet of immune defense and neuroprotection (Alhouayek et al., 2017; Attwell et al., 2022) (Figure 2.5).

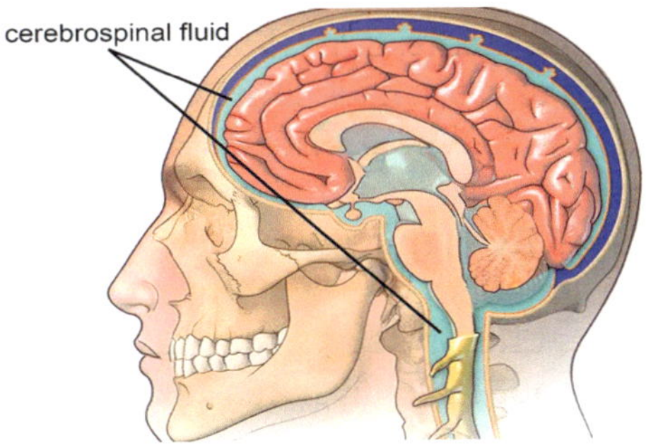

Figure 2.5. Cerebrospinal fluid.

Source: https://img.lb.wbmdstatic.com/vim/live/webmd/consumer_assets/site_images/article_thumbnails/BigBead/cerebrospinal_fluid_bigbead/1800x1200_webmd_rf_cerebrospinal_fluid_bigbead.jpg?resize=750px:*&output-quality=75.

2.1.3. Functional Regions of the Brain

One has to become acquainted with the brain's functional areas to get to know the complex areas of the central nervous system (CNS). The human brain, as a general concept, is divided into several areas that have distinct functions, such as the cerebrum, cerebellum, and brainstem. The cerebrum, the largest and most significant part of the brain, is divided into the right and left hemispheres, each comprising four lobes: frontal, parietal, temporal, and occipital.

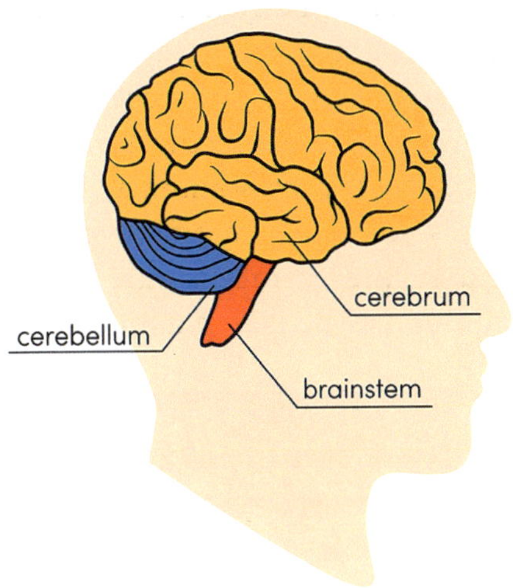

Figure 2.6. The brain can be divided into the cerebrum, brainstem and cerebellum.

Source: https://www.hopkinsmedicine.org/-/media/images/health/1_-conditions/brain/brain-main-parts.png.

The lobes control a vast array of functions, from reasoning and problem-solving in the frontal lobe to vision processing in the occipital lobe. The interactive dynamic of these areas enables the CNS to analyze sensory input, perform motor functions, and oversee emotional responses, thereby illustrating the integrated and complicated nature of brain function in the grand scheme of human anatomy. Coordination of sensory and motor functions is another key brain function, best illustrated by areas such as the pre-central and post-central gyri. The pre-central gyrus is involved in the planning and execution of voluntary movement. It houses the primary motor cortex, which serves to send signals to the various muscles of the body. The post-central gyrus is involved in the processing of somatosensory information so that touch, pain, and temperature can be felt (Figure 2.6).

Pathology of these regions is linked to severe motor dysfunction and sensory impairments, which highlights the importance of these regions for daily life. Above all, studies on subjects of spinal cord injury have shown decreased functional connectivity of such areas, showing how harm can not only reduce the capability for movements but actually reorganize the brain's adaptive properties to harm, and further establish the necessity for more studies on neural plasticity (Budde et al., 2016). Secondly, studies have broadened our knowledge about lesser-studied regions and their possible functions in the CNS. For instance, neuropeptides such as the adipokinetic hormone/corazonin-related peptide (ACP) exhibit hormonal and neurological function overlap. ACP and its receptor are found in brain regions, indicating neuromodulatory function that potentially influences stress response, energy mobilization, and cognition. This finding opens up new avenues of research into how neuropeptides might affect brain function and direct overall health and behavior. By recognizing the role of both established systems and new neuropeptide systems, a more accurate picture of brain function within the CNS can be built, ultimately contributing to better ways of treating neurological disease and our capacity as a whole to understand human behavior (Wahedi et al., 2018).

Test Your Knowledge

1. How do the meninges and cerebrospinal fluid protect the brain and spinal cord?
2. Can you name one functional region of the brain and its primary role?

2.2. Functions of the Central Nervous System

Learning Outcome

1. Explain the processing of sensory information
2. Discuss the coordination of motor functions
3. Understand the regulation of homeostasis

The CNS has numerous functions essential to organismal existence, which are based on its role of maintaining organismal homeostasis as well as negotiating with the environment. The CNS is responsible for consolidating the sensory input of the peripheral nervous system, i.e., visual, auditory, and tactile. Consolidation facilitates the generation of responses to stimuli, thus playing a significant role in survival. Secondly, the CNS controls voluntary motor function to control muscle activity in fine motor performance. Such coordination of sensory and motor response dictates the CNS's role as a channel for responses that reflect not only physiological needs but also behaviorally conditioned responses, propelling organismal adaptability to varied environmental demands. Its control functions about emotional and cognitive functions are among the most significant roles played by the CNS. The brain, the body's focal organ of the CNS, plays a strong role in influencing mood, making decisions, and interacting socially. Neurotransmitters such as dopamine and serotonin, through being produced and controlled within the CNS, directly influence emotional reactions as well as mental sharpness. Besides, the brain's intricate webs of neurons enable the complexity of thinking processes such as reasoning and solving problems. Such processes are vital to high-level functions, distinguishing humans from most other animals. As a result, comprehension of the methods by which CNSs participate in cognitive processes significantly adds to our understanding of psychological illness and neurological diseases, which may interrupt regular brain operation and, therefore, behavior. Recent observations have brought into focus the fundamental role of glial cells, especially astrocytes, in CNS functioning, along with their conventional support cell function. Astrocytes contribute to CNS homeostasis by providing trophic support to neurons and participating in neurotransmitter recycling, a function essential to synaptic efficacy. Astrocyte function also encompasses blood-brain barrier functioning and immune responses to maintain the neural environment favorable for normal brain function. Furthermore, astrocyte dysfunction has also been known to be an etiologic agent for numerous neurologic disorders, suggesting their probable contribution to disease pathogenesis. Awareness of the specific contribution of astrocytes and other glia not only enriches CNS function comprehension but also offers promising avenues for therapeutic intervention in neurodegenerative disease, where neuron-glia integrity is vital (Efthymiou et al., 2014; Lakatos et al., 2016).

2.2.1. Processing Sensory Information

The intricate process of central nervous system sensory information processing is an elementary attribute of organism-environment interaction. Segregation and integration of multimodal data are central to sensory processing so that organisms respond appropriately to a variety of stimuli. Sensory pathways are typically segregated, and sensory types of data follow different paths of neural transmission. This modularity is essential for initial sensory processing, where the other modalities are handled independently in a manner that is consistent with signal transmission. But the brain's capacity to converge these streams of information is what enables later higher-order cognition, allowing for perception, awareness, and more reflective responding to the outside world. This segregation-integration duality is one of the features of the neural elements governing the processing of the senses. It highlights the intricacy of the operation of the central nervous system in encoding and interpreting sensory inputs (Zhou et al., 2010). Furthermore, sensory processing may be elaborated by the cooperative action of adjacent neurons. Experiments with electrosensory systems reveal that overlapping receptive field cells possess high correlations in their activity, which enhances informational encoding. Stimulation of such types of systems produces coincident spikes among the neurons. It substantially enhances the combined ability to detect specific stimulus features, such as upstrokes and downstrokes of voltage changes (Gabbiani et al., 2002) (Figure 2.7).

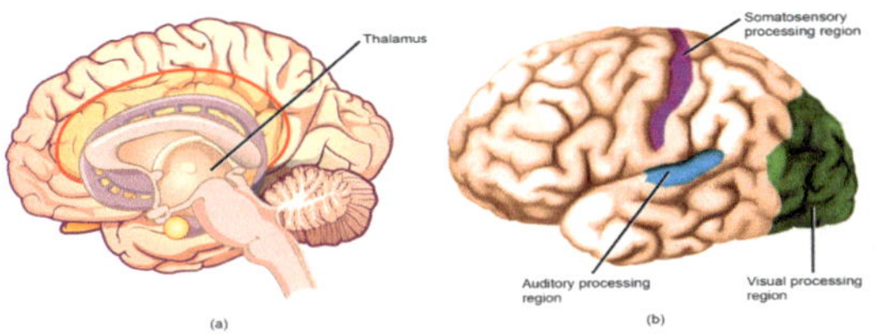

Figure 2.7. In humans, except olfaction, all sensory signals are routed from the (a) thalamus to (b) final processing regions in the cortex of the brain. (Credit b: modification of work by Polina Tishina) Scientific Method Connection.

Source: https://opentextbc.ca/biology/chapter/17-1-sensory-processes/.

This phenomenon points to the significance of population activity in neurons and that information integration occurs over several levels of processing. Hence, as sensory input rises through the neural hierarchy, it gets transformed in such a way that the convergent output of groups of neurons results in progressively greater complex understanding of the stimuli. This contributes to better feature extraction as well as the operation of the entire sensory system. Lastly, dynamic interaction between segregation and integration within the central nervous system allows not just primitive perception of sensation, but also intricate cognitive processes. The presence of nodes within cortical networks is necessary for multisensory information control and integration, which allows for a more global and contextually richer interpretation of stimuli. These hubs play a crucial role in creating connections between distant sensory modalities and, hence, in enabling an integrated percept. In addition, the ability of the brain to integrate redundant and complementary sensory information is also the foundation of higher-order processes like decision-making and motor planning. Through inspection of the central nervous system handling of sensory information, cognition, and behavior functions are grasped on a more fundamental level, and respect is achieved for the complicated system of interacting processes, through which understanding about the interface between sensory information and conscious experience is gained (Zhou et al., 2010).

2.2.2. Coordination of Motor Functions

Motor coordination is a complex process relying primarily on the sophisticated network of the CNS. The CNS integrates sensory information with motor signals to create smooth, coordinated movement. Coordination is acquired through multiple loops of the nerve impulses between various regions of the brain, including the motor cortex, cerebellum, and basal ganglia. In the spinal cord, neurons play an essential role in transmitting signals for reflex and voluntary movement. Dorsal hindbrain and spinal cord neurons, as per the literature, are crucial to receiving, processing, and transmitting sensory perception and also in integrating sensory-motor output (Birchmeier et al., 2017). This highlights the role of neuronal networks in handling sensory input across modalities and, therefore, performing coordinated motor functions. The cerebellum also helps coordinate motor function accuracy and timing, as well as movement adjustment.

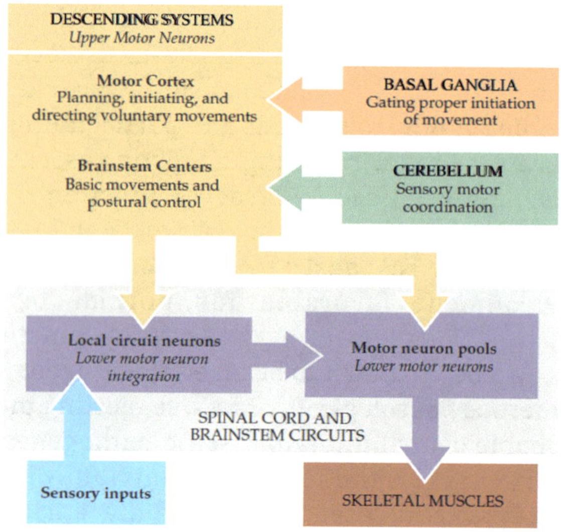

Figure 2.8. Organization of motor control in the central nervous system.

Source: https://www.researchgate.net/figure/Organization-of-motor-control-in-the-central-nervous-system-At-the-lowest-level-sensory_fig9_328134715.

It receives continuous sensory feedback on position, balance, and movement and sustains muscle coordination and postural control. Sensory information integration with motor commands prevents errors and changes movements in real time, so action is smooth and effective. The cerebellum is not independent, however, in its operation; instead, it operates with aid from the motor cortex and other brain areas. Such cooperative processes strengthen the arguments of distributed cognition against a single chief executive control system. Instead, they suggest that motor control arises from the competitive and cooperative interplay of many relatively simple cognitive systems (Christensen et al., 2006) (Figure 2.8).

This is important in the understanding of how different neural pathways give rise to motor coordination. Motor function coordination can also be viewed from the adaptability perspective, leading to survival. With organisms engaging in more complex functions that require more precise motor function, the CNS has found means of ensuring efficiency and flexibility in movement. This evolutionary perspective presumes that selective pressures favor the structure of an increased-level control system to integrate well sensory input and motor output. Integration of many cognitive systems not only favors complex motor behavior but also makes sense of the possible conflict that arises when action is being carried out. A comprehension of how all the CNS comes together to organize motor functions is thus of utmost importance in the formulation of therapeutic measures in motor control disorders. By studying the subtle harmony between interaction and competition amongst neural networks, scientists are better able to understand and maybe even enhance recovery mechanisms for motor function.

2.2.3. Regulation of Homeostasis

Homeostasis is an inherent quality of biological systems whose purpose is to keep internal conditions constant regardless of external changes. In the CNS, regulation of homeostasis is of paramount concern, and it enables maximum efficiency of neuronal processes. The role of calcium ions (Ca^{2+}) is at the heart of this delicate equilibrium; intracellular Ca^{2+} content is kept under strict regulation by a complex system including the plasma membrane, mitochondria, and endoplasmic reticulum. When all these systems function as they should, they prevent excitotoxicity, an event that results in neuronal injury and cell death due to an influx of excess Ca^{2+}. The complex interaction of these elements highlights the value of accurate regulation in the maintenance of neuronal integrity, also demonstrating how alterations can lead to neurodegenerative diseases and other cognitive impairments and, in so doing, emphasize the crucial role played by homeostatic mechanisms in the CNS (D\\u27Orsi et al., 2017). In addition, outside of calcium regulation, the gut-brain axis has also become a key contributor to homeostatic processes that affect the CNS. This complex web of communication links the gut and the brain, engaging a multitude of signals that impact neurotransmitter production and immune modulation. Microbiota, a polymicrobial community that colonizes the gut, is key to this interaction, affecting the body's metabolic pathway and overall homeostasis. Dysbiosis, or disturbance of this microbiota, has also been linked to various neuropsychiatric conditions such as depression and anxiety, as evidence of the profound impact that gastrointestinal health has on psychological welfare. Thus, it is not only crucial for metabolic health but for overall emotional and cognitive functioning in the CNS as well (Czerska et al., 2025). Homeostasis regulation within the CNS is closely associated with bioenergetics and apoptotic pathways, which are essential for the health and survival of the cell. The Bcl-2 family of proteins plays an important role in this context, influencing cell death as well as maintenance of calcium homeostasis. The proteins regulate mitochondrial function, which is essential for ATP production and the supply of energy to the neurons. When homeostatic regulation goes awry, either because of increased levels of Ca^{2+} or by failure of Bcl-2 proteins, neurons are threatened with degeneration and death. This link comes into action most significantly under circumstances like neurodegenerative diseases, when loss of control by the cell can have disastrous consequences. Thus, understanding the complexities of homeostatic regulation in the CNS not only sheds light on normal physiological functions but also underscores potential therapeutic targets for intervention in various neurological disorders (D\u27Orsi et al., 2017).

Test Your Knowledge

1. Which part of the brain is primarily responsible for processing sensory information?
2. How does the nervous system coordinate motor functions in the body?

2.3. Neurons and Neurotransmission

Learning Outcome

1. Understand the structure and types of neurons
2. Discuss the mechanism of neurotransmission
3. Describe the role of neurotransmitters in communication

The fundamental constituents of the CNS are the neurons, specialized cells that are skilled at transmitting information by way of electrical and chemical signals. Neurons communicate with one another through synapses, where neurotransmitters, the chemical messengers, are emitted from one neuron to bind to receptors on a second neuron. The process of neurotransmission is complex; it begins with the reception of an action potential, which triggers the entry of calcium ions and the consequential release of neurotransmitters into the synaptic cleft. This very complex dance of signals allows for fast and precise communication, required for voluntary as well as involuntary functions. Interestingly, the balance among neurotransmitters can exert powerful influences on physiology, which underscores the importance of demarcating neuron interaction within the broad context of the CNS. Of particular interest is the feature of cotransmission, wherein two or more transmitters are released concurrently from a single neuron. This aspect adds complexity to synaptic transmission, since different combinations of transmitters may have other effects. For example, ATP is a cotransmitter along with classical neurotransmitters such as acetylcholine in the bladder and noradrenaline in sympathetic nerves, and therefore plays a significant role in regulating synaptic responses. Not only does the presence of cotransmitters diversify the signal, but it also provides fine regulation of various physiological processes, such as movement, sensation, and autonomic functions. Understanding cotransmission expands our understanding of the way that neural networks may be functionally variable and adapt to meet physiological demands (Burnstock et al., 2025). However, the subtle balance of neurotransmission is subject to being disrupted by neurotoxic chemicals, which pose a danger to the integrity of the CNS. These chemicals, whether naturally occurring or synthesized, can act on neural cells or metabolic events essential to the efficient functioning of neurons. Neurotoxicity could be of different forms, leading to acute or chronic deficits depending on the character of exposures and duration. The symptoms could instantly occur or develop gradually, complicating diagnosis and treatment. The impact also persists long after exposure has been terminated, which necessitates ongoing research in the field. An understanding of neurotransmitter-neuron-neurotoxic agent interactions will guide treatments and preventive measures for maintaining neural health in the case of exposure (Brust et al., 2014).

2.3.1. Structure and Types of Neurons

It is necessary to learn the morphology and classification of neurons in order to grasp the complexity of the CNS. Neurons, being the fundamental units of neural interaction, are divided into three basic parts: the soma (cell body), dendrites, and axon. The soma holds the nucleus and organelles for cellular functions, while dendrites are the areas where signals are received from other neurons and synaptic interaction takes place. The axon, typically covered by myelin, transfers electrical signals long distances to engage with target cells. The intricate morphology is specialized for the specific functions of neurons, categorizing them into various types like sensory, motor, and interneurons. Each type has a role in information processing and reflex action and underscores the vital role played by neurons in the overall function of the CNS. Variety among neurons is also apparent in their morphological and functional classifications. Motor neurons, for instance, extend from the CNS to effectors to facilitate motion and body response. Sensory neurons are geared to detect stimuli in the environment and transmit sensory information to the CNS for processing. Interneurons act as bridges, with significant functions being realized in reflex arcs and complex neural circuits to enhance processing abilities. In addition, structural variations, such as the presence or absence of myelin sheaths, have an impact on the velocity and efficacy of signal conduction. The structural differences are particularly noteworthy when considering the developmental trajectory of neurons; as research shows, the ability of neurons to regenerate when damaged differs considerably by their type and level of maturity (Blackmore et al., 2016) (Figure 2.9).

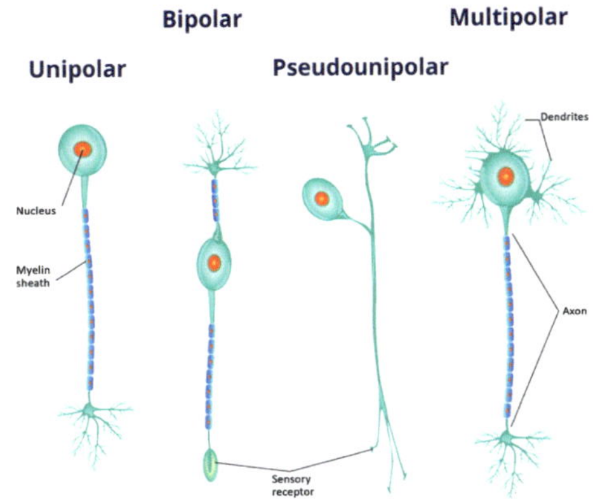

Figure 2.9. Types of neurons based on structure.

Source: https://interactivebiology.com/wp-content/uploads/2021/09/Types-of-Neurons.png.

Other more recent studies have also described more intricate relationships between neuron types and biochemical properties. Some subsets of neurons, for example, have distinctive glycosphingolipid expressions, the roles of which are cell recognition and signaling in the CNS. Research into Gb3 distribution has seen its expression in numerous populations of neurons, including those of the cerebral cortex and olfactory bulbs, and it illustrates how structural variations influence function (Abbott et al., 2010). This variation highlights the interdependence of neuronal structures and functions within the CNS, and the prospect for novel therapeutic options to arise from a better understanding of these interdependencies. As we delve into the complexity of neuronal structure, it becomes increasingly clear that their diversity underlies the neural functional complexities and overall cognitive processes (Figure 2.10).

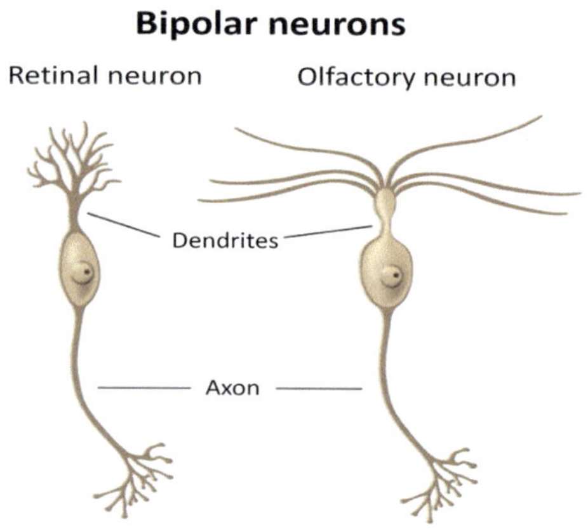

Figure 2.10. Illustration of bipolar neurons, showing the structural differences between retinal and olfactory neurons, each with distinct dendrites and a single axon.

Source: https://interactivebiology.com/3247/the-neuron-external-structure-and-classification/.

2.3.2. Mechanism of Neurotransmission

Neurotransmission is the functional process through which neurons communicate with one another and is the core of CNS function. Neurotransmission entails the release of neurotransmitters from the presynaptic neuron into the synaptic cleft, where they bind to receptors on the postsynaptic neuron. This binding initiates a cascade of biochemical events that either end in an excitatory or inhibitory response, which decides the transmission of the neural signal. The timing and concentration of neurotransmitters are precise, as they determine the amplitude and the length of the synaptic response. The delicate balance achieved by neurotransmitter discharge, receptor sensitivity, and resultant cellular is essential to normal brain functioning and is the basis for activities such as learning, memory, and mood regulation. New research has also shown purinergic signaling, in which ATP and other purines are used as neurotransmitters in both the peripheral and central nervous systems, to be vital. This discovery, now salient since the 1970s, positions ATP as a vital cotransmitter, collaborating with conventional neurotransmitters such as acetylcholine and dopamine. The identification of P1 and P2 receptor families has testified to the diversity of roles of purinergic signaling in neurophysiology. Experiments attest that ATP plays not just a role in synaptic transmission but influences long-term neuronal health through trophic signaling—modifying cell proliferation, differentiation, and overall neural homeostasis. Moreover, new findings in purinergic pathways emphasize the significance of such mechanisms in neurological disease and suggest that changes in purinergic cotransmission can be implicated in various CNS pathologies causing neuropathic pain and neurodegeneration, as in studies that have examined purinergic neuropathology (Burnstock et al., 2009) (Figure 2.11).

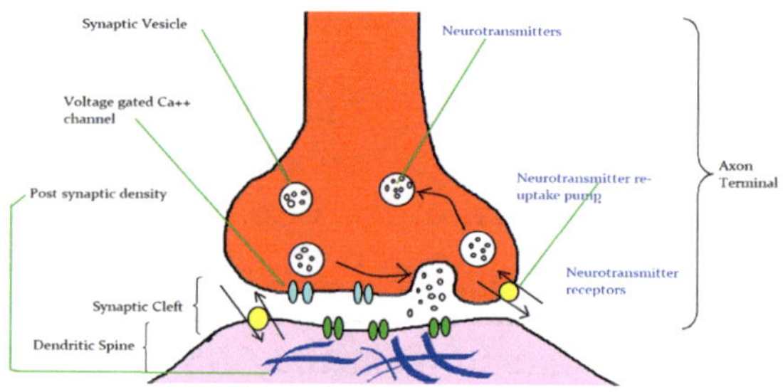

Figure 2.11. The mechanism of action of neurotransmitters.

Source: https://www.researchgate.net/figure/The-mechanism-of-action-of-neurotransmitters_fig5_368062783.

In addition to purinergic signaling, chemokines have also been shown to be potent regulators of neurotransmission within the CNS. For instance, the chemokine CXCL16 has been reported to potentiate both excitatory and inhibitory synaptic transmission, thus having an active role in the modulation of synaptic contacts. Noteworthy is the interaction of CXCL16 with astrocytes, showing dynamic glial-neuronal communication, which emphasizes the role of the neuroinflammatory environment in dictating the neuron's response. Modulation of synaptic transmission is not the role of individual neurotransmitters but a complex interaction of various signaling pathways and cellular receptors, such as adenosine receptors. These findings underscore the multivalent nature of neurotransmission and its susceptibility to alteration in pathological conditions, which suggests potential therapeutic options for neurodegenerative diseases in which chemokine function would be utilized to reverse synaptic transmission and confer neuroprotection (Castro et al., 2016).

2.3.3. Role of Neurotransmitters in Communication

The role of neurotransmitters in CNS communication is fundamental to the functioning of normal neuronal networks. Neurotransmitters are charged messengers that facilitate synaptic transmission so that neurons can communicate and coordinate many physiological events. Neurotransmitters such as dopamine, serotonin, and norepinephrine strongly influence mood, motivation, and cognition. Their release from presynaptic neurons interacts with specific receptors on postsynaptic neurons, triggering a cascade of events that control neuronal excitability and plasticity. This biochemistry organizes everything from reflexes to complex behaviors, emphasizing the importance of neurotransmitter signaling in maintaining homeostasis and mediating responses to environmental inputs. In addition to their more familiar roles in synaptic transmission, neurotransmitters also play roles in the modulation of other critical systems, including immune responses. For instance, the adenosine system is a neuromodulation pathway that is representative of this integrative function. As described in the literature, adenosine-neuron surface receptor interaction has profound consequences for the regulation of neurotransmitter release and the reactivity of the neuron to various stimuli. Disruption by alcohol of adenosine-carrying nucleoside transporters is representative of how exogenous agents influence neurotransmitter systems to impact central functions and behavioral outcomes. This complex interplay between neurotransmitters, modifiers, and behavioral responses accentuates the multidimensional nature of CNS communication (Figure 2.12).

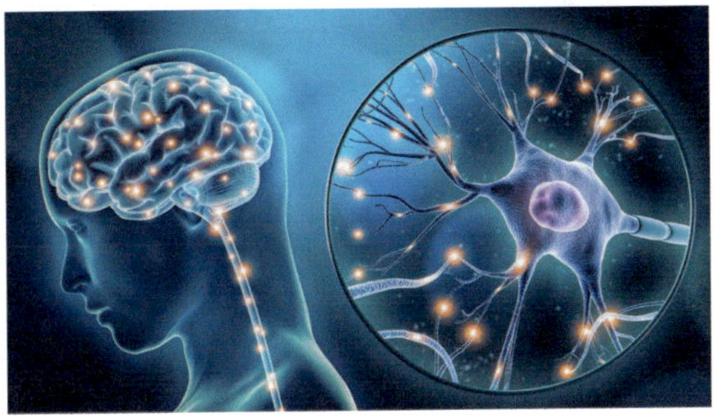

Figure 2.12. Neural activity in the brain and spinal cord with a magnified view of a signaling neuron.

Source: https://bhoperehab.com/wp-content/uploads/2024/02/drugs-nervous-system-scaled.jpeg.

Further, the connection between neurotransmitters and CNS pathological diseases proves the inherent importance of neurotransmitter malfunction. Obesity and cardiovascular diseases have warped neural communication patterns, which affect overall health. Research indicates that the central neural pathways governing peripheral nervous system activity can exacerbate these disorders, correlating neurotransmitter signaling with metabolic deficiency. The spleen's novel role as a hub of neural-immune interactions illuminates how neurotransmitters may modulate responses not only within the CNS but also throughout the rest of the body. In research carried out in recent years, being aware of these interactions further informs the identification of potential therapeutic targets for managing metabolic and cardiovascular disease conditions related to neurotransmitter dysregulation (Carnevale et al., 2017).

Test Your Knowledge

1. What are the three main types of neurons, and what are their functions?
2. How do neurotransmitters help in communication within the nervous system?

2.4. Central Nervous System Disorders

Learning Outcome

1. Identify the common disorders: Alzheimer's and Parkinson's disease
2. Identify the impact of trauma on the central nervous system
3. Explain the neurodegenerative diseases and their effects

The complexities of CNS illness encompass a wide array of conditions that carry a profound impact on neurological function and well-being. One case in point is Multiple Sclerosis (MS), a chronic disease in which the myelin sheath enveloping nerve fibers breaks down. MS manifests through a myriad of heterogeneous symptoms like fatigue, sensory impairment, and cognitive impairment that have profound impacts on an individual's capability to carry out daily functioning. Studies have illustrated the multifaceted effect of MS on its caregivers and patients, as it documents the dual load of the disease symptoms and the caregiver stress, illustrating an endemic demand for comprehensive care support services in managing such conditions (Bernabeu et al., 2010). In addition, the etiology of many CNS disorders is likely to extend beyond genetic predisposition to encompass environmental precipitants and exacerbators of these conditions. Maternal immune activation during gestation is a particular point of interest, since existing research indicates potential long-term impacts on the offspring's health. These immune responses lead to the development of neurodevelopmental diseases, meaning the effects of CNS diseases can typically begin even before birth, influencing an individual throughout their life (Groenink et al., 2024). This paradigm shift towards understanding CNS disorders emphasizes the importance of immediate intervention and follow-up, as the detection and management of these factors can revolutionize health outcomes. Further, treatment of CNS disorders must involve multidisciplinary interventions encompassing medical treatment, psychological counseling, and rehabilitation therapy. Effective management strategies are crucial in enhancing the quality of life in individuals with CNS disorders. The range of treatment methods encompasses, in most instances, pharmacotherapeutic interventions aimed at minimizing symptoms or modifying disease trajectory. Further, psychological counseling for associated mood disorders may have an integral function in assisting patients and their families in managing the emotional impact of the diseases. A comprehensive understanding of the interaction between psychosocial and biological components must be possessed when organizing therapeutic interventions for patients with CNS diseases. And as research continues to evolve in the field, future studies will undoubtedly bring more light to other avenues of innovation in treatment methods.

2.4.1. Common Disorders: Alzheimer's and Parkinson's Disease

The prevalence of neurodegenerative diseases, particularly AD and PD, points to serious problems with the central nervous system. AD is predominantly characterized by deterioration of the mind and loss of memory due to amyloid plaque deposits and neurofibrillary tangles in the brain. The disruption causes neurons to progressively degrade, ultimately ending with elementary brain functions being impaired. Conversely, PD is marked by motor impairment due to the loss of dopamine within the substantia nigra, causing tremors, rigidity, and bradykinesia.

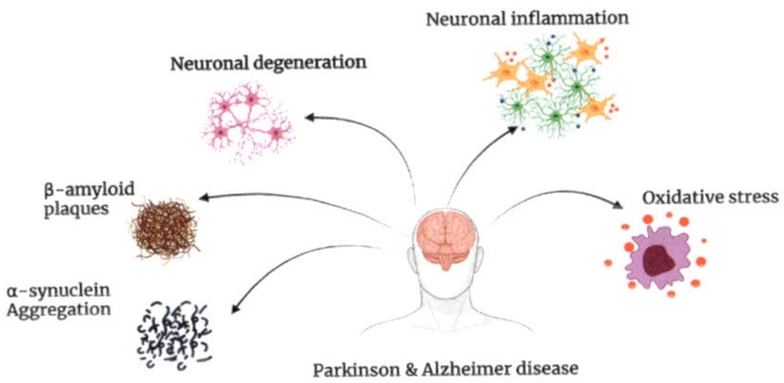

Figure 2.13. Pathogenesis of Alzheimer's' disease and Parkinson's' disease.

Source: https://www.researchgate.net/figure/Pathogenesis-of-Alzheimers-disease-and-Parkinsons-disease-AD-and-PD-share-common_fig1_368902613.

Both indicate the vulnerability of the central nervous system as it disrupts normal physiological processes, emphasizing a critical area of research towards developing proper interventions and treatments to enhance the quality of life of the targeted population. The relative pathological processes of AD and PD are instructive regarding neurodegenerative processes that can inform treatment strategies. Misfolded and aggregated protein is responsible for cell injury and death in both disorders. The pathogenesis of these cytotoxic proteins not only manifests in specific clinical presentation but also has broader implications for neural form and function, according to research. An understanding of the intricacies of protein aggregation and the mechanisms involved is vital to grasping the etiology and pathogenesis of such diseases (Figure 2.13).

Specifically, the research of potential treatments, such as pathologic protein targeting, is increasingly important as the world's population ages and these diseases become more common, highlighting the urgency of the necessity for scientific research (Mack et al., 2018). Further, cerebrovascular contribution to AD and PD is increasingly seen as a component of neurodegeneration. Emerging evidence suggests that compromised blood-brain barrier (BBB) function is most probably the central mechanism involved in AD and vascular dementia (VaD) pathophysiology. Dysfunctional BBB leads to increased permeability, which allows toxic plasma components to penetrate the brain, exacerbating neuroinflammation and neuronal damage (Acharya et al., 2015). This shared vascular involvement presents a novel perspective, situating AD and VaD on an age continuum of vascular disease that could bridge gaps in the understanding of these multifactorial illnesses. By pointing out cerebrovascular disease and its connection to the development of neurocognitive disorders, further research has the promise to identify fundamental connections that will enable diagnostic and therapeutic advances with improved accuracy.

2.4.2. Impact of Trauma on the Central Nervous System

The impact of trauma upon the CNS is a rich area of study, particularly concerning how traumatic events alter neurobiological processes and emotional regulation. Trauma, most often defined as an inescapable stressful event, overwhelms existing coping abilities, leading to a variety of psychological and physical responses. Bessel van der Kolk, the leading trauma expert, theorizes that trauma is not merely a memory of past occurrences; rather, it sidetracks the present by becoming ensconced in the neural architecture. The change can manifest itself in a range of symptoms such as mood changes, insomnia, and anxiety, describing how deeply trauma influences the CNS. Understanding the specific ways in which trauma builds the brain is crucial not just for treatment practice but also to knowing the long-term effects of such experiences on a person's mental state and cognitive processes (et al., 2021). Furthermore, the relationship between trauma and the CNS extends into the realm of neuroplasticity—the brain's capacity to reorganize itself by the formation of new neural circuits.

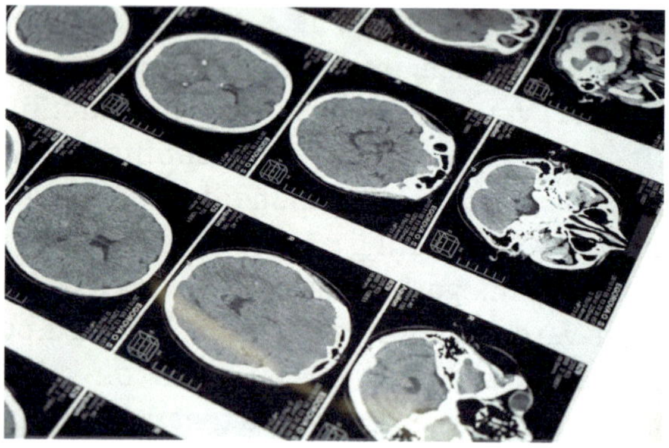

Figure 2.14. Trauma can leave invisible scars on our brains, but some long-term effects can have an observable impact.

Source: https://www.primaltrust.org/the-effects-of-trauma-on-the-brain/.

This elasticity has two sides: it suggests that traumatic events leave permanent marks on the structure and function of the brain, even while it also permits healing and adaptability. To illustrate, individuals who have suffered unimaginable trauma, e.g., physical abuse or combat exposure, may find that their neural modes are fixed to hyper-vigilance or affect dysregulation. Research has also shown that trauma may lead to changes in areas such as the amygdala, which handles emotion processing, and the hippocampus, which affects learning and memory. This neurobiological foundation suggests the necessity of specialized interventions to enable individuals to work through traumatic experiences and normalize the CNS (et al., 2021) (Figure 2.14).

In some cases, such as following combat operations, the mechanisms by which trauma acts upon the CNS can be even more complex. Research into mild to moderate traumatic brain injury (mTBI) indicates that pressure waves from explosive devices can produce severe nervous system damage even if the presentation may not appear severe on initial inspection. Evidence exists that these types of pressure waves can interact with the thoracic cavity and consequently impact the health of the brain in new mechanisms. This observation highlights the complex nature of the effect of trauma on the CNS, demonstrating that trauma can occur not just due to psychological pathology but also due to physical impacts that decimate brain function. Knowing how these processes operate can inform preventive strategies and treatment protocols, particularly in groups that are exposed to extreme physical and emotional stress, and identify the need for further research.

2.4.3. Neurodegenerative Diseases and Their Effects

Neurodegenerative diseases represent a serious and multifaceted threat to the central nervous system in the form of progressive degeneration of neurons in terms of structure and function. Diseases such as Alzheimer's disease, Parkinson's disease, and multiple sclerosis depict the diversity of disease conditions that can disrupt normal neural functioning to produce severe cognitive and motor dysfunction. These diseases not only affect the neurological functions required for daily performance, but also have considerable impacts on the psychological well-being of the patients and their relatives. The pathophysiology of such illnesses typically entails complex interactions between genetic predisposition, environmental influences, and deranged cellular processes that result in pathological neurotransmission and ultimate neuronal loss. This cascade of events highlights the importance of a greater understanding of neurodegenerative processes in the development of more effective therapeutic strategies, particularly those at the root cause of these disabling disorders. Existing research illustrates the pivotal role that neuroprotective drugs have in modulating the effects of neurodegenerative disorders. One such avenue under investigation is that of the Klotho protein, which is now a potential target for therapies. Klotho proteins are involved in several cellular processes, such as maintenance of oxidative stress and mitochondrial function, which are of significance in the preservation of neuronal health. Abnormality of Klotho signaling pathways has been implicated in a variety of central nervous system disorders, and mounting evidence indicates involvement in neurodegenerative disorders where myelin integrity is compromised. Encouragingly, these therapies that boost Klotho expression and activity are expected to cause remyelination and restore pathologically lost critical functions in conditions like multiple sclerosis, and this is a thrilling area for future research in neurotherapeutics. New treatment approaches are needed, especially considering the limitations of current treatments that focus primarily on symptomatic alleviation rather than disease modification (Chen et al., 2020) (Figure 2.15).

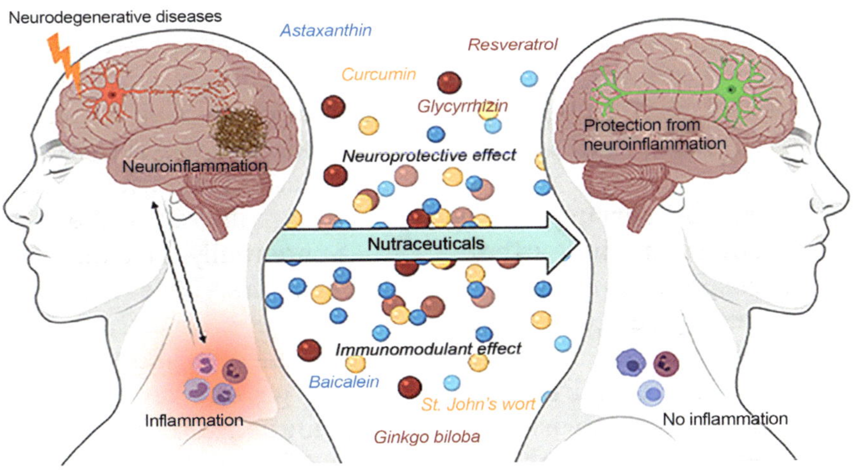

Figure 2.15. Neurodegenerative diseases.

Source: https://taylorandfrancis.com/wp-content/uploads/2023/02/image-Neurodegenerative-Diseases-768x436.jpg.

Investigation of the viral etiology of other neurodegenerative diseases has also extended our knowledge of their complex nature. Fresh evidence has implicated viral infection in disease causation, for example, in multiple sclerosis, and has posited a potential interaction between host immune mechanisms and specific viral pathogens. Experimental animal models of Theiler's murine encephalomyelitis virus (TMEV) and mouse hepatitis virus (MHV) infections have played a crucial role in the acquisition of knowledge regarding host-pathogen interactions and ensuing effects on neuronal function and integrity. These findings emphasize the necessity for an interdisciplinary framework in understanding neurodegenerative disease, including virology, immunology, and neurology, to uncover possible therapeutic directions based on viral mechanisms. By elucidating the role of infectious agents in neuroinflammatory processes, researchers can develop new prophylactic and therapeutic modalities aimed at limiting the impact of these disabling neurological illnesses (Buchmeier et al., 1999).

Test Your Knowledge

1. What are the main symptoms of Alzheimer's and Parkinson's diseases?
2. What are neurodegenerative diseases, and how do they impact brain function over time?

2.5. The Role of the Central Nervous System in Behavior

Learning Outcome

1. Define influence on emotions and mood
2. Analyze the relationship between the central nervous system and cognitive functions
3. Discuss the behavioral responses to environmental stimuli

The CNS regulates behavior, serving as the primary site where environmental stimuli are interpreted and responded to. CNS is made up of the brain and spinal cord, which collectively govern complex operations such as perception, emotion, and motor control. All these processes rely on intricate neural networks that communicate through electrical and chemical signals. Through the integration of sensory information, the CNS enables individuals to make decisions and take actions that are necessary for adaptation and survival. In addition, the CNS performs the function of shaping behavior as a function of experience, which shows its role in learning and memory. This adaptability points to the capacity of the CNS to mold not only the behavior of an individual but also social behavior, as learned behavior in one set of circumstances can be applied to new sets of circumstances in the future. Additionally, the interactions of biochemicals within the CNS significantly influence behavior. Neurotransmitters such as serotonin and dopamine control psychological states, including mood and drive. For instance, dysbalances in these neurotransmitters would result in behavioral aberrations of mental health disorders, once again pointing towards the interconnection between CNS function and behavior. Genetic research, that is, genes like DISC1, associated with severe psychiatric illness, once more illustrates the biological foundations that potentially have an influence on behavior. Experiments have revealed that the DISC1 gene plays a crucial role in synaptic function within the CNS and show that predispositions at the genetic level can make a significant contribution to behavioral outcomes in a vast array of circumstances (Brandon et al., 2017). It becomes possible to make better sense of how molecular changes translate into tangible changes in behavior. In addition, the CNS not only reacts to sudden environmental stimuli but also plays an integral part in long-term behavioral adaptations. Neuroplasticity—the ability of the brain to reorganize itself by creating new neural connections—is a factor in modifying behavior through experience and learning. For instance, during recovery from remyelination, axon integrity is required in order to regulate successful behavior because it is highlighted in molecular protein Ptprz research that ensures oligodendrocyte survival, critical for remyelination processes (Castro et al., 2012). This provides a direct indication of how CNS health relates to being able to change behaviors effectively. As our understanding of the CNS deepens, it becomes increasingly clear that its complex structure is not merely a facilitator of behavior but a dynamic system that actively shapes the very framework of individual and social behavior patterns.

2.5.1. Influence on Emotions and Mood

The complex interaction between the CNS and emotional control suggests the substantial impact of bodily processes on affective states. According to this model, the brain not only functions as an interpreter of stimuli from outside but also as an emotional response generator. The autonomic nervous system (ANS), sympathetic and parasympathetic pathways, plays a role in such modulation. For instance, during stressful times, an apparent sympathetic dominance increase can lead to heightened anxiety and negative affect and undermine well-being. Conversely, states involving positive emotions note an increase in parasympathetic dominance, which enhances restorative processes. This dynamic relationship determines how states of the body influence emotional expression, demonstrating emotional experience to be inextricably linked with both neural functions and bodily physiology (Crawford et al., 2015). Emotional states influencing cognitive processing are another key mechanism through which emotions shape human experience. Research demonstrates that older adults possess a particular attentional bias for positive information, especially when faced with aversive stimuli. This phenomenon, referred to as the positivity effect, is an adaptive emotion-regulation strategy for distress minimization. In particular, under conditions of emotion regulation required, like stressor exposure, older adults are biased to engage more strongly with positive information but struggle to disengage from negative information. This implies that patterns of changes in levels of mood contribute not only to emotional well-being but also to attentional engagement and disengagement tactics. Thus, the CNS's ability to orchestrate such cognitive processes underscores the importance of mood regulation as an organizer of emotional and mental health (Raedt et al., 2017) (Figure 2.16).

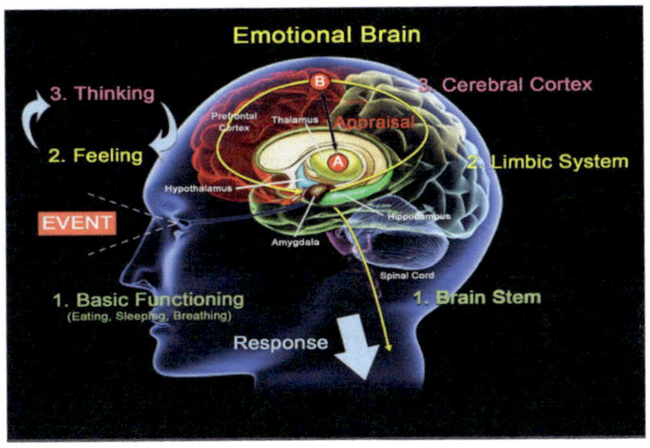

Figure 2.16. Four major brain regions are: the brain stem, cerebellum, neocortex (cerebrum) and limbic system.

Source: https://karengosling.com/understand-your-emotional-brain/.

Also, comments on the complex feedback processes between the brainstem and limbic system indicate the interaction of physiological activity on emotional states. Cardiorespiratory coherence (CRC) is a concept that may be employed to explain the interaction of emotional expression with physiological regulation. When positive emotional states occur, CRC rises, initiating a state of well-being and optimal emotional function. On the other hand, negative states often coincide with reduced levels of CRC, suppressing emotional regulation and contributing to stress-related issues. All such evidence indicates the promise of techniques like meditation and pranayama for the promotion of emotional well-being through physiological coherence. Thus, understanding these underlying mechanisms within the CNS facilitates a better grasp of the complicated processes of emotions and how these impact mood, paving the way for specific interventions in mood disorders (Crawford et al., 2015).

2.5.2. Connection Between the Central Nervous System and Cognition

The intricate dynamic between the CNS and mental functioning forms the foundation of human cognition, emotion, and behavior. The CNS, or brain and spinal cord, is responsible for the processing and integration of sensory information and for the execution of motor functions. The system works as a living network such that various neuronal structures and brain regions can communicate and facilitate complex processes like perception, reasoning, and decision-making. Neurons reorganize their connections according to experience through neuroplasticity, significantly influencing cognitive processes. An understanding of this harmony between the physical architecture of the CNS and higher-level cognitive processes is central to exploring the underlying processes at the root of behavior, learning, and the formation of memory. In addition, the development of frameworks such as the Information Compression by Multiple Alignment, Unification, and Search (ICMAUS) gives insight into how neural processes model cognitive processes. The ICMAUS model describes how to describe abstract higher-level cognitive processes, such as problem-solving and language processing, in terms of distinctive patterns of neural activity corresponding to many information alignments. This theoretical innovation denotes a move away from the classical notion of neuronal assemblies to an appreciation that cells are members of special assemblies based on the functional role they take. Such knowledge ties the neurobiological underpinnings of cognition to actualized purposes in artificial intelligence and language perception, which supports the degree of expertise required within the study of cognition's origin in the CNS (Wolff et al., 2003). Further research into CNS involvement in cognition also includes implications for learning by dynamic neural events. Research has discovered that learning is not merely a passive accumulation of information but a persistent process intertwined with the reorganization of neural networks. ICMAUS broadens the initial principles of Hebbian learning, subject to the qualification that any neuron can belong to any set of assemblies, permitting more detailed encoding of higher-level abstractions. Cognitive flexibility and the ability to form complex hierarchies of information are facilitated by this flexibility. By fractally organizing information in such neuron patterns, the CNS not only accommodates the storage of learned information but also supports cognitive processes such as reasoning and problem-solving, thereby clarifying the intimate association of the CNS with the world of cognition (Machamer et al., 2002).

2.5.3. Behavioral Responses to Environmental Stimuli

The interaction between organisms and the environment is intensely mediated by the CNS, which translates sensory input and evokes corresponding behavioral outcomes. The neurons in the CNS, particularly those that act upon environmental stimuli, are the ones responsible for these interactive dynamics. For instance, in the domain of nociception—nervous system reaction to harmful stimuli—specialized cells known as nociceptors are activated by bodily harm or threat and transmit signals of pain to induce defensive behaviors. This is demonstrated by the work with patients who have mutations in specific genes, such as KCNH8 and ITSN2, that impact their pain sensitivity as well as their environmental temperature-related behavior. Through the recognition of these genetic factors and their implications on sensory processing, we are given insight into the processes behind behavioral adaptation to environmental changes as mediated by the CNS (Bullock et al., 2018) (Figure 2.17).

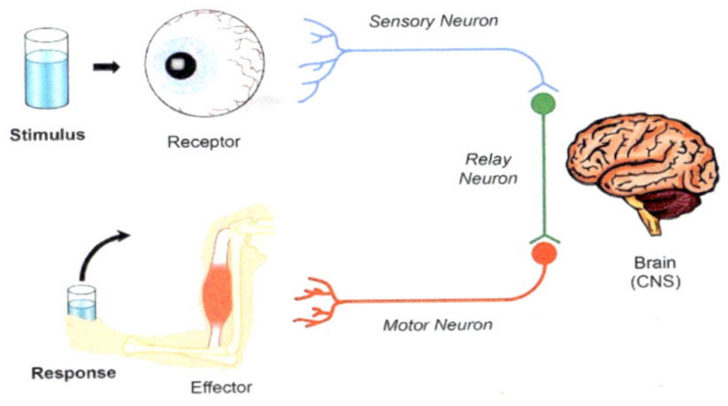

Figure 2.17. The stimulus-response pathway.

Source: https://old-ib.bioninja.com.au/standard-level/topic-6-human-physiology/65-neurons-and-synapses/stimulus-response.html.

Environmental stimuli also cause sophisticated behavioral reactions that can differ substantially from person to person because of genetic, anatomical, and physiological variations within the CNS. Stress is a major contributor to these behavioral reactions, especially about visceral sensitivity and pain perception. In experimental models, varying stressors can cause the response of animals to distress to change, as those with differing genetic backgrounds show varying sensitivities and adaptation mechanisms. For instance, modulation of visceral pain by the brain-gut axis illustrates the impact psychological stressors have on physical pain sensitivity and response. Investigation of such physiological responses to stress could give rise to the therapeutic targets that reverse stress-evoked changes in sensory perception. With a better understanding of these mechanisms, it is possible to progress in manufacturing targeted treatments for pain disorders of stressful or environmental origin (Larauche et al., 2011). Furthermore, the behavioral responses to environmental stimuli are not just significant when trying to understand sensitivity and pain but also in increasing the general quality of life. The CNS integrates the processing of sensory input, memory, and motor output to allow organisms to survive and adapt in their environments. For example, changes in environmental temperatures trigger different behavioral responses, as shown by the distinct temperature preferences of the KCNH8 and ITSN2 mutant mouse models. In those studies, observed temperature sensitivity changes not only mimic certain human diseases but also indicate a changeable nature of behavioral responses controlled by genetic regulation and neural adaptation. While scientists delve deeper into the neurobiology and genetics of such reactions, it is clear that the CNS is at the epicenter of not only adaptation mechanisms but also potential interventions that promote increased resilience to environmental stress (Larauche et al., 2011; Bullock et al., 2018).

Test Your Knowledge

1. What is the connection between the central nervous system and cognitive functions like thinking and memory?
2. How does the nervous system generate behavioral responses to environmental stimuli?

SUMMARY

In looking at the multifaceted role of the central nervous system, it is clear that its influence reaches well beyond simple neural processing. What emerges from numerous studies is how beneficial interventions can improve the quality of life for those who endure internal and central nervous system disorders. For instance, research has established that respiratory muscle training (RMT) substantially improves pulmonary function, exercise capacity, and general sense of well-being in patients with the disorder. This shows that targeted interventions can promote adaptation or recovery in patients, further emphasizing the necessity of developing evidence-based treatment programs for not just relief of symptoms but also functional improvement and quality of life (Baldan et al., 2022). Besides, advances in therapeutic technology, such as functional electrical stimulation and ankle foot orthoses, have provided new avenues for the restoration of mobility in patients with central nervous system disorders. The two interventions are comparably effective at enhancing walking speed, stressing the potential for adaptive technologies to aid in rehabilitation. However, note should be taken of current limitations of the evidence base, which fail to fully explain how such improvements manifest in everyday clinical environments or what the underlying mechanisms are. Future research must address these gaps with studies that involve numerous central nervous system diagnoses and examine precise outcomes that reflect the specificity of rehabilitative requirements (Hollands et al., 2017). The central nervous system remains a highly relevant area of study, particularly in understanding how disruptions in its processes can impact overall health. As our comprehension deepens, the development of specialized interventions that treat the unique needs of central nervous system disorder patients will be crucial. Effective therapeutic approaches such as RMT and adaptive technologies illustrate the potential for modern medicine to enhance patient care. But further investigation into the subtlety of these treatments is required to establish their value in everyday life for patients. Such efforts will ultimately lead to a more compassionate and better-informed approach to the treatment of central nervous system disorders, promoting resilience and improved quality of life for patients.

The research on the central nervous system (CNS) is extensive, with major subjects being its developmental stages and mechanisms. The significant rise in neurodevelopmental disorders is a major characteristic that necessitates prompt identification and treatment. Although growth charts, traditionally used by pediatricians to monitor growth, do not identify neurodevelopmental issues beforehand. Linear model and standard growth assumptions can hide important patterns of deviation. Emerging methods introduce velocity-based growth charts that incorporate dynamic motor performance change and thus enhance the identification of early developmental delay indicators. Emerging interventions hold promise to revolutionize early interventions and results for risk populations (Brincker et al., 2016). A second emphasis is the role of model systems for unraveling the intricacy of CNS development. Research with zebrafish has provided valuable insights into the cell-cell interactions accountable for neural patterning and morphogenesis. Gastrulation observations reveal reproducible neurectodermal cell spatial arrangements that are reminiscent of future brain morphology. These organizational processes, especially at decisive stages of development, allow investigators to track the differentiation pathways to building the largest brain regions, such as forebrain, midbrain, and hindbrain. The meticulous reorganization of blastoderm cells accentuates the intrinsic order of development, which suggests patterning interactions start much earlier than has long been considered (Fraser et al., 1995). This data not only illuminates our understanding of typical neurological development but also serves to explain abnormalities found in genetic mutation. Finally, the cross-disciplinary nature of CNS research emphasizes the persuasive value of interdisciplinary cooperation between genetics, neurobiology, and pediatrics. As outlined in recent reports, blending information from enhanced analytical strategies and model organism research unlocks the potential for improved diagnostic technologies and therapeutic strategies. The ability to spot early developmental issues using superior growth markers, along with accurate fate mapping and model systems, provides a sound basis for elucidating CNS disorders. This combined strategy ultimately aims at the creation of proactive interventions that will minimize developmental risk and enhance involved individuals' quality of life, thereby justifying the continued research in neurodevelopment (Brincker et al., 2016; Fraser et al., 1995).

KEY TERMS FROM THIS CHAPTER

- Sympathetic Division
- Sensory Neurons
- Cerebral Cortex
- Midbrain
- Medulla Oblongata
- Ventricles
- Meninges
- White Matter
- Parasympathetic Division
- Cerebrum
- Thalamus
- Pons
- Cerebellum
- Cerebrospinal Fluid
- Gray Matter
- Basal Ganglia

CRITICAL THINKING QUESTIONS

1. **What structures make up the central nervous system?**
   a. Brain and spinal cord
   b. Brain and nerves
   c. Spinal cord and sensory organs
   d. Nerves and ganglia
2. **Which part of the brain is responsible for coordinating voluntary muscle movements and maintaining balance?**
   a. Cerebrum
   b. Brainstem
   c. Cerebellum
   d. Medulla oblongata
3. **The largest part of the brain, responsible for higher brain functions like thinking and memory, is the:**
   a. Brainstem
   b. Cerebellum
   c. Cerebrum
   d. Hypothalamus
4. **Which part of the CNS acts as a communication highway between the brain and the rest of the body?**
   a. Cerebellum
   b. Spinal cord
   c. Brainstem
   d. Thalamus
5. **The medulla oblongata, which controls vital functions like breathing and heart rate, is part of the:**
   a. Cerebellum
   b. Midbrain
   c. Brainstem
   d. Cerebrum

Short Answer Questions

1. What are the main anatomical parts of the central nervous system?
2. What are two key functions of the central nervous system?
3. What is the basic structure of a neuron, and how does it transmit signals?
4. What role do neurotransmitters play in central nervous system communication?
5. Name two common disorders that affect the central nervous system.
6. How does the central nervous system influence human behavior?
7. What is the function of the brainstem within the central nervous system?

Answer to Critical Thinking Questions

1. (a); 2. (c); 3. (c); 4. (b); 5. (c)

REFERENCES

1. Obata, F., & Obrig, T. (2010). Distribution of GB3 immunoreactivity in the mouse central nervous system. *Toxins, 2*(8), 1997–2006. https://doi.org/10.3390/toxins2081997
2. Acharya, N., Goldwaser, E., & Nagele, R. (2015). Cerebrovascular and blood-brain barrier compromise: A mechanistic link between vascular disease and Alzheimer's disease subtypes of neurocognitive disorders. https://core.ac.uk/download/214464755.pdf (accessed on 14th June 2025).
3. Ainsworth, B. E., Avitsur, R., Baumeister, R. F., Beedie, C., Biomarker Definitions Working Group, Bolger, N., et al. (2014). The attachment system and physiology in adulthood: Normative processes, individual differences, and implications for health. https://core.ac.uk/download/294625964.pdf (accessed on 14th June 2025).
4. Alhouayek, M., Amor, S., Appel, S. H., Bankston, A. N., Biber, K., Biran, V., et al. (2017). Neuroinflammation, mast cells, and glia: Dangerous liaisons. https://core.ac.uk/download/129593018.pdf (accessed on 14th June 2025).
5. Courtney, A., & Courtney, M. (2008). A thoracic mechanism of mild traumatic brain injury due to blast pressure waves. https://core.ac.uk/download/pdf/287975.pdf (accessed on 14th June 2025).
6. Attwell, D., Barkaway, A., & Korte, N. (2022). Immune-vascular mural cell interactions: Consequences for immune cell trafficking, cerebral blood flow, and the blood-brain barrier. https://core.ac.uk/download/519723104.pdf (accessed on 14th June 2025).
7. Audenaert, E., Mahieu, P., Pattyn, C., et al. (2010). Soft tissue structure modelling for use in orthopedic applications and musculoskeletal biomechanics. https://core.ac.uk/download/55761253.pdf (accessed on 14th June 2025).
8. Baldan, F., Cacciante, L., Federico, S., Pregnolato, G., Rutkowska, A., Rutkowski, S., & Turolla, A. (2022). The use of respiratory muscle training in patients with pulmonary dysfunction, internal diseases or central nervous system disorders: A systematic review with meta-analysis. https://core.ac.uk/download/554066152.pdf (accessed on 14th June 2025).
9. Baritaki, S., Chatzaki, E., de Bree, E., et al. (2019). Chronic stress, inflammation, and colon cancer: A CRH system-driven molecular crosstalk. https://core.ac.uk/download/323076588.pdf (accessed on 14th June 2025).
10. Barnett, S. C., Hosseinzadeh, S., Kiray, H., et al. (2016). The multifaceted role of astrocytes in regulating myelination. https://core.ac.uk/download/42370602.pdf (accessed on 14th June 2025).
11. Beckers, P. (2025). *Nemertean Nervous System: A Comparative Analysis.* https://core.ac.uk/download/pdf/304639045.pdf (accessed on 14th June 2025).
12. Bernabeu, M., Hernandez-San-Miguel, J., Marnetoft, S. U., et al. (2010). Rehabilitation for multiple sclerosis in adults (I); impairment and impact on functioning and quality of life: An overview. https://riunet.upv.es/bitstream/10251/103163/3/Part%201%20VANCOUVER%20FINAL%20v2%2019.6.12.pdf (accessed on 14th June 2025).
13. Birchmeier, C., Hernandez-Miranda, L. R., & Müller, T. (2017). The dorsal spinal cord and hindbrain: From developmental mechanisms to functional circuits. https://core.ac.uk/download/300325565.pdf (accessed on 14th June 2025).

14. Blackmore, M. G., Coley, D. M., Simpson, M. T., et al. (2016). Epigenetic profiling reveals a developmental decrease in promoter accessibility during cortical maturation *in vivo*. https://core.ac.uk/download/213085162.pdf (accessed on 14th June 2025).

15. Brandon, N. J., Brown, J. T., Kurihara, M., et al. (2017). Disrupted in schizophrenia 1 and synaptic function in the mammalian central nervous system. https://core.ac.uk/download/79655619.pdf (accessed on 14th June 2025).

16. Brincker, M., Mistry, S., Smith, B., et al. (2016). Neonatal diagnostics: Toward dynamic growth charts of neuromotor control. https://core.ac.uk/download/287581414.pdf (accessed on 14th June 2025).

17. Brust, P., Creeley, C., Feldman, R., Grandjean, P., Herken, H., Panzica, G., et al. (2014). Neurotoxicity. https://core.ac.uk/download/286729125.pdf (accessed on 14th June 2025).

18. Buchmeier, M. J., & Lane, T. E. (1999). Viral-induced neurodegenerative disease. https://core.ac.uk/download/323075723.pdf (accessed on 14th June 2025).

19. Budde, M. D., Kalinosky, B., Kaushal, M., et al. (2016). Alterations in cortical sensorimotor connectivity following complete cervical spinal cord injury: A prospective resting-state fMRI study. https://core.ac.uk/download/213083667.pdf (accessed on 14th June 2025).

20. Bullock, D. (2018). Evaluation of behavior in transgenic mouse models to understand human congenital pain conditions. https://open.bu.edu/bitstream/2144/31217/5/Bullock_bu_0017N_13665.pdf (accessed on 14th June 2025).

21. Burnstock, G. (2009). Purinergic signaling: Past, present and future. https://core.ac.uk/download/1670991.pdf (accessed on 14th June 2025).

22. Burnstock, G. (2025). Purinergic cotransmission. https://core.ac.uk/download/pdf/8443838.pdf (accessed on 14th June 2025).

23. Carnevale, D., Lembo, G., Lori, A., et al. (2017). The spleen: A hub connecting nervous and immune systems in cardiovascular and metabolic diseases. https://core.ac.uk/download/98347401.pdf (accessed on 14th June 2025).

24. Castro, G. M. de, Ferrari, C. C., Franklin, R. J. M., et al. (2012). Accelerated axonal loss following acute CNS demyelination in mice lacking protein tyrosine phosphatase receptor type Z. https://core.ac.uk/download/37738730.pdf (accessed on 14th June 2025).

25. Zhou, C., Zamora-López, G., & Kurths, J. (2010). Cortical hubs form a module for multisensory integration on top of the hierarchy of cortical networks. https://core.ac.uk/download/pdf/8402616.pdf (accessed on 14th June 2025).

26. Chen, X., Faller, D. V., Glavas, I. P., et al. (2020). Klotho pathways, myelination disorders, neurodegenerative diseases, and epigenetic drugs. https://core.ac.uk/download/322973341.pdf (accessed on 14th June 2025).

27. Christensen, W. (2006). The evolutionary origins of volition. https://core.ac.uk/download/pdf/87234.pdf (accessed on 14th June 2025).

28. Crawford, M. W., & Jerath, R. (2015). How does the body affect the mind? Role of cardiorespiratory coherence in the spectrum of emotions. https://core.ac.uk/download/131207333.pdf (accessed on 14th June 2025).

29. Czerska, M. A., Furtak, K., Kamińska-Omasta, K., et al. (2025). Gut microbiota and its impact

on brain function and mental health. https://core.ac.uk/download/646079917.pdf (accessed on 14th June 2025).

30. D'Orsi, B., Mateyka, J., & Prehn, J. H. M. (2017). Control of mitochondrial physiology and cell death by the Bcl-2 family proteins Bax and Bok. https://core.ac.uk/download/83917578.pdf (accessed on 14th June 2025).

31. De Raedt, R., Demeyer, I., & Sanchez Lopez, A. (2017). Older adults' attentional deployment: Differential gaze patterns for different negative mood states. https://core.ac.uk/download/84045283.pdf (accessed on 14th June 2025).

32. Di Castro, M. A., Limatola, C., Maggi, L., et al. (2016). The chemokine CXCL16 modulates neurotransmitter release in hippocampal CA1 area. https://core.ac.uk/download/54538364.pdf (accessed on 14th June 2025).

33. Diamond, I., Dohrman, D., & Gordon, A. (1997). The role of the neuromodulator adenosine in alcohol's actions. https://core.ac.uk/download/323079180.pdf (accessed on 14th June 2025).

34. Edgerton, V. R., Krucoff, M. O., Rahimpour, S., et al. (2016). Enhancing nervous system recovery through neurobiologics, neural interface training, and neurorehabilitation. https://core.ac.uk/download/323078214.pdf (accessed on 14th June 2025).

35. Efthymiou, A. G., Heman-Ackah, S., Malik, N., et al. (2014). Comparison of the gene expression profiles of human fetal cortical astrocytes with pluripotent stem cell derived neural stem cells identifies human astrocyte markers and signaling pathways and transcription factors active in human astrocytes. https://core.ac.uk/download/38067677.pdf (accessed on 14th June 2025).

36. Gargi, M. M., et al. (2021). Pangs of trauma in *Anita: End of a beginning and a life apart*. https://core.ac.uk/download/621412820.pdf (accessed on 14th June 2025).

37. Fraser, S. E., & Woo, K. (1995). Order and coherence in the fate map of the *zebrafish* nervous system. https://core.ac.uk/download/4879704.pdf (accessed on 14th June 2025).

38. Gabbiani, F., Koch, C., Krahe, R., et al. (2002). Stimulus encoding and feature extraction by multiple sensory neurons. https://core.ac.uk/download/17182330.pdf (accessed on 14th June 2025).

39. Gaiseanu, F. (2019). The informational model of consciousness: Mechanisms of embodiment/disembodiment of information. https://core.ac.uk/download/287611919.pdf (accessed on 14th June 2025).

40. Gaiseanu, F. (2020). Information-based hierarchical brain organization/evolution from the perspective of the informational model of consciousness. https://core.ac.uk/download/322492692.pdf (accessed on 14th June 2025).

41. Groenink, L., Hofsink, N., & Plösch, T. (2024). The fetal programming effect of maternal immune activation (MIA) on the offspring's immune system. https://core.ac.uk/download/620188758.pdf (accessed on 14th June 2025).

42. Hollands, K. L., Kenney, L. P., Onmanee, P., et al. (2017). Functional electrical stimulation and ankle foot orthoses provide equivalent therapeutic effects on foot drop: A meta-analysis providing direction for future research. https://core.ac.uk/download/110588624.pdf (accessed on 14th June 2025).

43. Estrine, J., & DeLisle, L. (2006). Stress: Putting the brain back into medicine. https://core.ac.uk/download/71356692.pdf (accessed on 14th June 2025).
44. Lakatos, A., Patani, R., & Tyzack, G. (2016). Human stem cell-derived astrocytes: Specification and relevance for neurological disorders. https://core.ac.uk/download/288347706.pdf (accessed on 14th June 2025).
45. Larauche, M., Mulak, A., & Taché, Y. (2011). Stress-related alterations of visceral sensation: Animal models for irritable bowel syndrome study. https://core.ac.uk/download/323080393.pdf (accessed on 14th June 2025).
46. Machamer, P., Quartz, S., Scarantino, A., et al. (2002). Session 5: Development, neuroscience and evolutionary psychology. https://core.ac.uk/download/11920468.pdf (accessed on 14th June 2025).
47. Mack, J. (2018). Protein aggregates and polyglutamine tracts in neurodegenerative disease. https://core.ac.uk/download/213462874.pdf (accessed on 14th June 2025).
48. Wahedi, A. (2018). Characterization of the adipokinetic hormone/corazonin-related peptide signaling system in the mosquito, *Aedes aegypti*. https://core.ac.uk/download/161989738.pdf (accessed on 14th June 2025).
49. Wolff, J. G. (2003). Neural mechanisms for information compression by multiple alignment, unification and search. https://core.ac.uk/download/pdf/85392.pdf (accessed on 14th June 2025).

THE PERIPHERAL NERVOUS SYSTEM

3

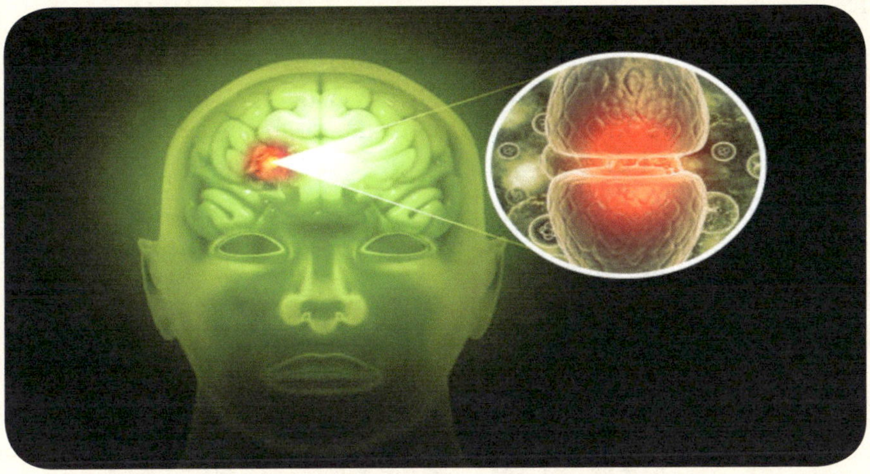

LEARNING OBJECTIVES

After studying this chapter, you will be able to:

1. Explain the anatomy of the peripheral nervous system
2. Describe the roles of the peripheral nervous system
3. Identify the different types of nerves in the peripheral nervous system
4. Identify frequent disorders of the peripheral nervous system
5. Explain diagnostic techniques employed to establish peripheral nervous system disorders

Introduction

The peripheral nervous system (PNS) has the key responsibility of transmitting information between the central nervous system (CNS) and the rest of the body. Made up of nerves and ganglia, the PNS runs from head to toe in the body and is responsible for sensory as well as motor functions. The two principal components—the somatic and autonomic nervous systems—regulate voluntary and involuntary movements, respectively. Understanding the PNS is essential because it enables communication between the brain and the world, which in turn enables complex behaviors such as reflexes and organized movements. Moreover, with its participation in numerous physiological processes, derangements of the PNS can lead to a broad range of medical conditions, hence making it necessary to study this system. Thus, a careful exploration of the PNS can lead to a greater realization of health and disease on a general basis and lay the foundation for advances in neurological medicine. Recent research has shed light on the complex interconnection of the PNS with other body systems, such as the endocannabinoid system (ECS), which is a key player in the function of the gastrointestinal (GI) tract. The ECS is also a significant signaling pathway involved in the regulation of GI motility, secretion, and sensitivity.

Endocannabinoids are involved in intestinal inflammation and mucosal barrier permeability and therefore may modulate functional and organic GI disorders. Genetic studies have documented significant associations between cannabinoid receptor gene polymorphisms and diseases like irritable bowel syndrome (IBS) and inflammatory bowel disease, uncovering the intricate relationship between the PNS and various physiological responses. With this understanding, researchers unveil promise for new therapies, demonstrating evidence of the worth in studying peripheral mechanisms in achieving complete health outcomes. The evolutionary features of the PNS and its varied structures also deserve consideration. Changes in peripheral nerve structures among different taxa tell us much about the evolutionary changes that have been undertaken over time. For example, the cephalic sensory organs in the Opisthobranchia exhibit striking morphological variation, leading to examinations of their homologous relationship. Scientists attempt to reconstruct the evolutionary history of these structures using neuroanatomical methods with the ultimate aim of informing us about the adaptation of peripheral systems to environmental pressures. This question not only raises our understanding of the PNS but also provides avenues for exploring comparative anatomy and evolutionary biology. Thus, a detailed description of the PNS from different viewpoints—functional, clinical, and evolutionary—adds richness to our knowledge as a whole concerning its function in health and disease.

Definition of the Peripheral Nervous System (PNS)

Knowledge of the PNS requires examination of its structure and function, which forms the core basis of distinguishing it from the CNS. The PNS comprises all the neural elements outside the brain and spinal cord, including sensory and motor neurons that carry information to and from the central nervous system. Structurally, it can be divided into the somatic and autonomic nervous systems. The somatic nervous system is responsible for voluntary muscle movements and the conduction of sensory information. In contrast, the autonomic nervous system controls the involuntary functions, such as heart rate and digestion.

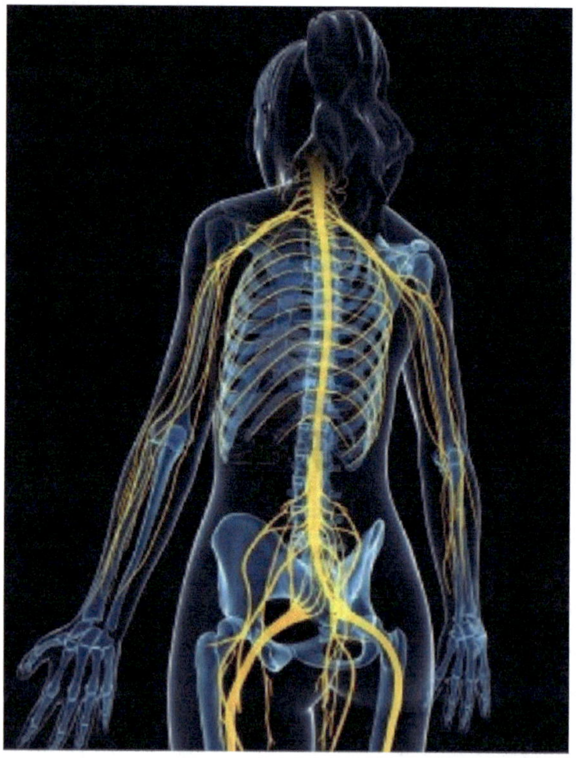

Figure 3.1. Posterior view of the human nervous system showing spinal cord and peripheral nerve pathways.

Source: https://barefootstrongblog.com/wp-content/uploads/2014/09/nervous-system.jpg?w=144.

This dual function of the PNS makes it a central part of both sensory experience and motor response, and its importance in connecting the brain with the body's many physiological activities cannot be underestimated. The PNS is also implicated in many clinical conditions, where its dysfunctions lead to a wide range of diseases. One of these conditions is for peripheral nerve transmission disorders, which lead to neuropathies resulting in muscular weakness, pain, or loss of sensation. It has also been implicated, according to recent research, with a variety of systemic health diseases, including mental illness. It has been found that peripheral interactions with the autonomic nervous system can potentially influence emotional control and cognitive function. Advances in understanding these interactions may also help identify potential interventions, as proposed by initial studies into how variations in peripheral nervous function could impact disorders such as autism (Brincker et al., 2017) (Figure 3.1).

Such findings underscore the importance of recognizing the PNS's extensive impact on overall health and functioning. Furthermore, the implications of the PNS cross new therapeutic approaches, particularly considering its interplay with the gut-brain axis. New evidence shows that peripheral systems' health is tightly linked to the microbiota and how it influences neurocognitive processes. Dysbiosis, or imbalance in gut microbiota, has also been associated with psychological and neurological illness, illustrating a complex relationship between gut health and peripheral nervous system health. For example, probiotic supplementation has been shown to improve neurocognitive function while lowering peripheral immunological activation levels in individuals who have compromised health, including HIV (Bianchi et al., 2017). This underlines the potential for the use of non-pharmacological interventions in PNS dysfunction-related conditions, thereby promoting a total holistic initiative towards well-being. Here, the PNS not only enhances key body functions but also serves as a bridge between various physiological systems, reiterating its core role within both clinical and routine situations.

3.1. Anatomy of the Peripheral Nervous System

Learning Outcome

1. Understand the components of the PNS
2. Discuss the classification of nerves: cranial and spinal
3. Describe the role of ganglia in the PNS

The peripheral nervous system (PNS) is a vast network that connects the central nervous system (CNS) to limbs, organs, and other parts of the body. It consists of nerves and ganglia outside the brain and spinal cord, facilitating communication between the CNS and the rest of the body. This system has two large subdivisions: the somatic nervous system, which manages voluntary actions through skeletal muscle, and the autonomic nervous system, which manages involuntary activities such as heart rate and digestion. The neuroanatomy of the PNS comprises sensory receptors, which gather information from the external environment, and motor neurons, which carry commands from the CNS to effectors. Understanding this multifaceted set is crucial in understanding how messages are being conveyed and how many body functions are being processed, highlighting the PNS's role in overall physiology (Figure 3.2).

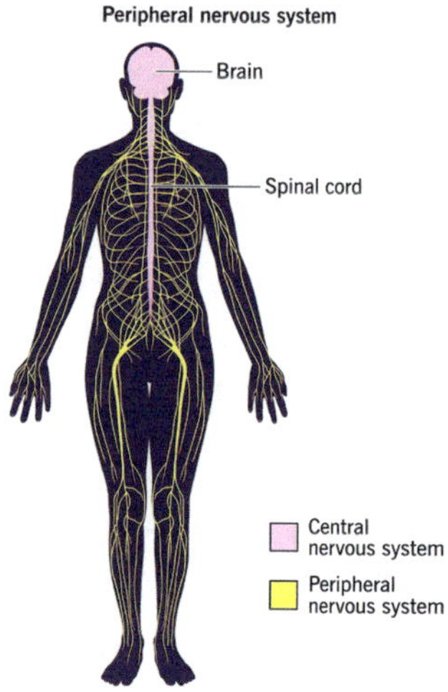

Figure 3.2. The peripheral nervous system branches outward from the spinal cord and brain to reach every part of your body.

Source: https://my.clevelandclinic.org/-/scassets/images/org/health/articles/23123-peripheral-nervous-system.

The anatomy of the PNS is also very diverse, particularly in glial cell composition, the significance of which is related to function and healing. The peripheral glia, i.e., Schwann cells and satellite cells, are very different from central nervous system glia. The Schwann cells, for instance, play an essential role in myelinating peripheral nerves, enhancing signal conduction speed. They also possess excellent regenerative abilities, acting rapidly to repair nerve injury by removing cell debris and encouraging axonal growth; this contrasts considerably with the poor regenerative ability of CNS glia. It is through research that PNS glia are seen not only to be involved in the recovery from injury, but also in supportive functions in maintaining normal neuronal function at all points throughout life, emphasizing dynamic structure-function relationships in peripheral neural anatomy (Barton et al., 2017). Delving deeper into certain genera, for example, members of Nereididae, provides more insight into the evolutionary processes of the PNS. For instance, studies have proven that the neuroanatomy of organisms like *Neanthes arenaceodentata* develops complex structures early in life, a hypothesis suggesting a highly advanced development pattern. Bigger central nervous systems and segmental nerves in such organisms are an adaptive advantage for ecological niches. In addition, these morphological traits could be a marker of evolutionary processes with advantages in a variety of physiological functions, including sensory processing and movement coordination. By examining peripheral neuroanatomy in various species, researchers can understand the evolutionary developmental biology of the PNS and develop a basic foundation essential for further research on neural anatomy and repair mechanisms within taxon groups (Jacobs et al., 2010).

3.1.1. Components of the PNS

The peripheral nervous system (PNS) comprises essential components that play a vital role in maintaining the central nervous system (CNS) in contact with the rest of the body. The PNS can be divided structurally into sensory and motor pathways, which contain various types of neurons that are responsible for sending messages. Sensory neurons transmit afferent impulses from sensory receptors located throughout the body to the CNS for the perception of external stimuli such as touch, temperature, and pain. Motor neurons transmit efferent commands from the CNS to effectors such as muscles and glands to enable responses to sensory stimuli. Understanding of such pathways is essential to comprehensively appreciate the overall functioning of the PNS because it highlights the intricate relationships that blend sensory inputs and motor outputs harmoniously. In addition, the PNS is characterized by the presence of supporting cells known as glial cells, which provide crucial support and maintenance for neural functions. Among these, the Schwann cells are critical for myelination, which enhances the transmission of signals in nerves by increasing their speed and efficiency. Myelination of the PNS is contingent on the expression of prominent myelin proteins such as Peripheral Myelin Protein 22 (PMP22). Effective myelination is vital for normal peripheral nerve function because it affects the conduction velocity of signals and the integrity of the nerves. A PMP22 overexpression mutation, for example, leads to Charcot-Marie-Tooth disease (CMT), which shows the significance of myelin stability. The coordinated roles of central transcription factors like Egr2 and Sox10, and others, are significant in regulating PMP22 expression, highlighting the delicate balance among cellular and genetic processes involved in the formation of peripheral nerves (Chang et al., 2011) (Figure 3.3).

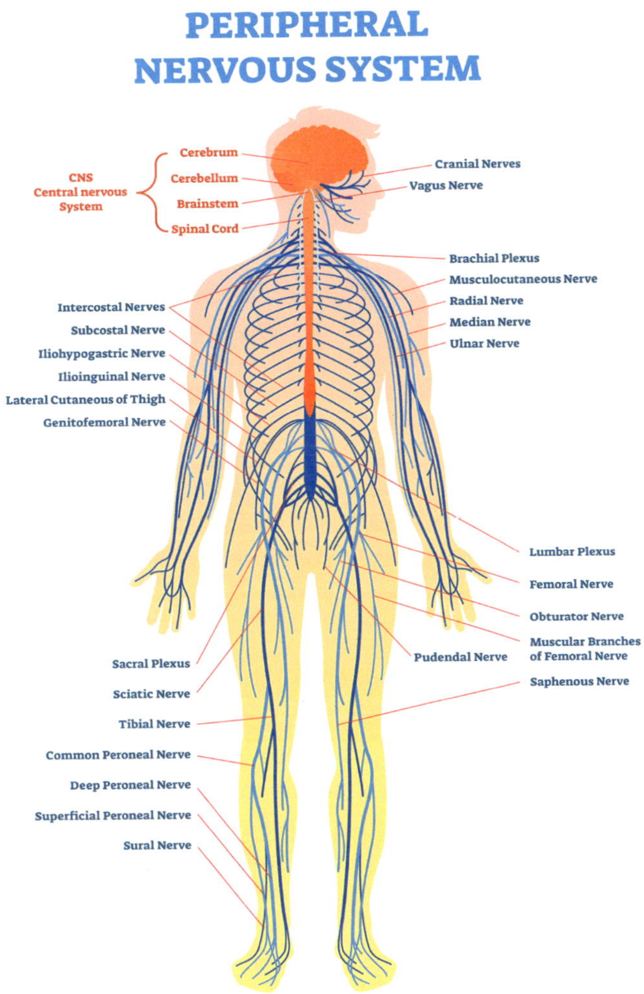

Figure 3.3. Components of peripheral nervous system (PNS).

Source: https://external-content.duckduckgo.com/iu/?u=https%3A%2F%2Fcmtrf.org%2Fwp-content%2Fuploads%2F2019%2F10%2FPeripheral-Nervous-System-1-651x1024.jpg&f=1&nofb=1&ipt=54c7d827a22b363e207d86263facdd8954256b3db8fcd4dc8c49e26ab674fd15.

Besides the Schwann cells, the PNS contains other types of neurons that all play distinct roles based on their location and function. The occurrence of cyclins such as cyclin E during cell cycles in the neurons illustrates how complex transcriptional regulation is within the peripheral nerve cells. A high-resolution analysis of Drosophila cyclin E reveals that its expression is regulated by multiple cis-regulatory elements that respond to tissue-specific and developmental cues. This suggests that standard cell cycle regulators do not exclusively regulate the expression of cyclin E; rather, it is the output of a intricate network of regulatory mechanisms that respond to various physiological conditions in various areas of the PNS (Jones et al., 2000). Such appreciation of the molecular mechanism of PNS components highlights the importance of appreciating both cellular and genetic factors responsible for its functioning and well-being (Figure 3.4).

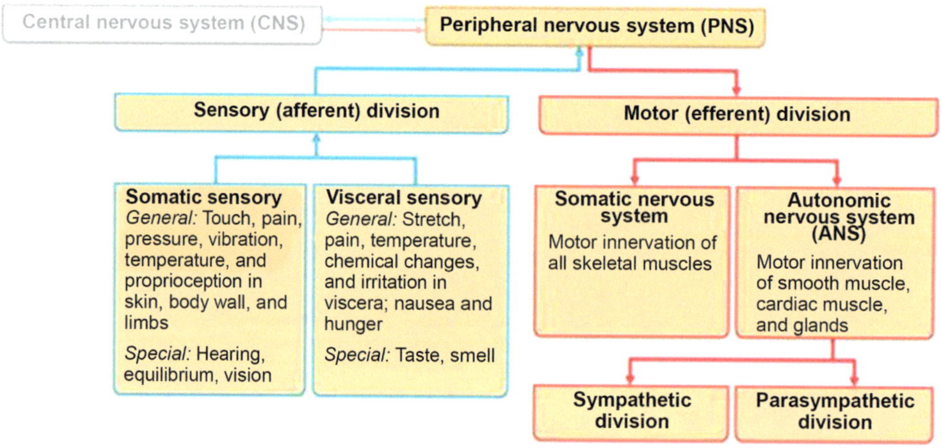

Figure 3.4. Functional organization of the PNS.

Source: https://external-content.duckduckgo.com/iu/?u=http%3A%2F%2Fantranik.org%2Fwp-content%2Fuploads%2F2011%2F11%2Ffunctional-organization-of-peripheral-nervous-system.jpg&f=1&nofb=1&ipt=e2e888d9d30a5b2c0a2e6caa6c8067962714a5db6ba5299fddcbc74aafe18628.

3.1.2. Classification of Nerves: Cranial and Spinal

The peripheral nervous system is further divided into two categories, namely cranial nerves and spinal nerves. Cranial nerves have a direct connection to the brain and are primarily sensory and motor functions of the head, neck, and internal organs. There are twelve pairs of cranial nerves with specific functions, from eye movement to transmitting sensory input from the face. On the other hand, spinal nerves emanate from the spinal cord with thirty-one pairs of spinal nerves that are tasked with transmitting sensory and motor impulses between the body and itself. They further break down into cervical, thoracic, lumbar, sacral, and coccygeal, each serving distinct areas of the anatomy. This division aids in the elaboration and structure of the peripheral nervous system, which is crucial in maintaining a harmonious body function. Cranial and spinal nerves also possess specific structural and functional characteristics that differentiate them from one another. Cranial nerves tend to go around the spinal cord and directly originate from the forebrain or brainstem, making their responses quick, particularly in the reflex movements of the facial region (Figure 3.5).

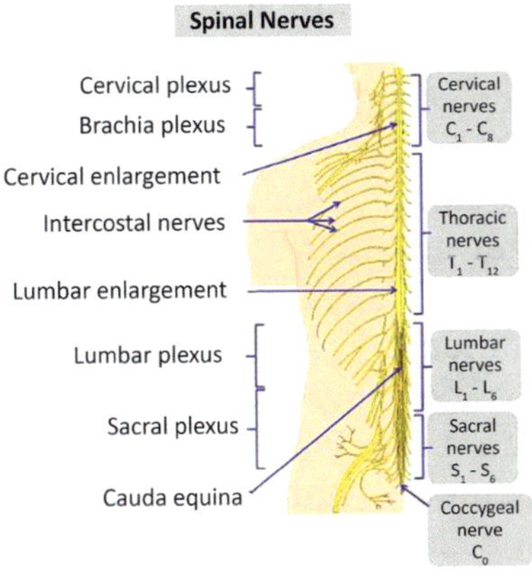

Figure 3.5. Spinal nerves.

Source: https://www.teachoo.com/17638/3522/How-many-spinal-and-cranial-nerves-are-present-in-the-human-body-/category/Teachoo-Questions/.

For instance, the optic nerve (Cranial Nerve II) transmits visual data directly from the retina to the brain without intervention by the spine. Spinal nerves are formed by the union of dorsal (sensory) and ventral (motor) roots, which allows for two-way transmission of data—both sensation and motor feedback. This bilateral role is essential for activities as varied as sensory perception to movement under voluntary control, thus emphasizing the intricate coordination present within the peripheral nervous system, including that observed in conditions like schwannomatosis affecting nerve function and regrowth (Chin et al., 2019). The clinical relevance of understanding the classification of nerves extends beyond simple anatomical context; they are essential in diagnosing and treating neurological disorders of various severities. Research on cranial and spinal nerve functions has unraveled conditions such as dog histiocytic sarcoma, which can manifest with inflammatory presentations on the central nervous system (Crowe et al., 2020). While the work here is principally established on animal models, it points out the biological and pathological importance of nerve classification. A thorough understanding of these classifications aids in symptom identification and therapy choices for nerve illnesses in humans as well. Therefore, the classification not only increases our knowledge of the peripheral nervous system but also encourages innovations in clinical practices and therapies for nerve injuries or disorders (Figure 3.6).

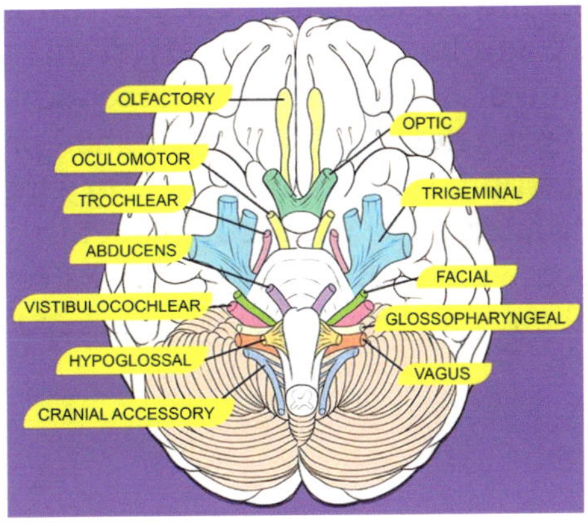

Figure 3.6. Cranial nerves.

Source: https://cdn1.byjus.com/wp-content/uploads/2018/11/biology/2018/04/24082909/Cranial-Nerves2-1.jpg.

3.1.3. Role of Ganglia in the PNS

Ganglia are central locations within the PNS that are responsible for allowing communication from the CNS to other body functions. These collections of neuron cell bodies that have sensory or autonomic function are located throughout the body in strategic positions. Sensory ganglia, such as dorsal root ganglia, house the cell bodies of primary sensory neurons that carry information from peripheral receptors to the CNS. This relay is of extreme importance in the processing of sensory information, including touch and pain. The organizational pattern of ganglia not only facilitates neuronal signal effectiveness but also functional integrity within the PNS, where ganglia serve a vital function in reflex arcs and autonomic response processing, a primary network in guaranteeing homeostasis and sensory perception. In addition, ganglia within the PNS are highly variable in structure and function, tailored to their specific role in the nervous system. Sympathetic ganglia, for instance, are involved in the body's fight-or-flight responses, sending signals that prepare the organism to respond with a rapid response. Sympathetic ganglia secrete neurotransmitters that act upon a variety of target organs, regulating such activities as heartbeat and digestion. Parasympathetic ganglia, located closer to target organs, support "rest and digest" behavior, which includes energy-saving activities. The disparity in neuron structure and types in these ganglia is indicative of the complex nature of PNS functions, where local integration of sensory input and autonomic output is responsible for much of the physiological response in real time. Recent research underscores the nuanced role of ganglia, particularly regarding regulatory functions involving neuropeptides and growth factors. For instance, studies show the expression of KISS1 and its receptor KISS1R in the sympathetic ganglion cells, suggesting involvement in the regulation of peripheral chemoreception and autonomic function (Caro et al., 2011). Moreover, the roles of peripheral ganglion-contained primary sensory neurons, such as dorsal root ganglia, reveal their function of transmitting sensory modalities and pain to the CNS, showing the increased focus on their interaction with growth factors like neurturin (Wang et al., 2011). Together, these findings underscore the vital role of ganglia within the PNS, revealing their intricate functions and providing hints about possible therapeutic prospects for a variety of neurological disorders (Figure 3.7).

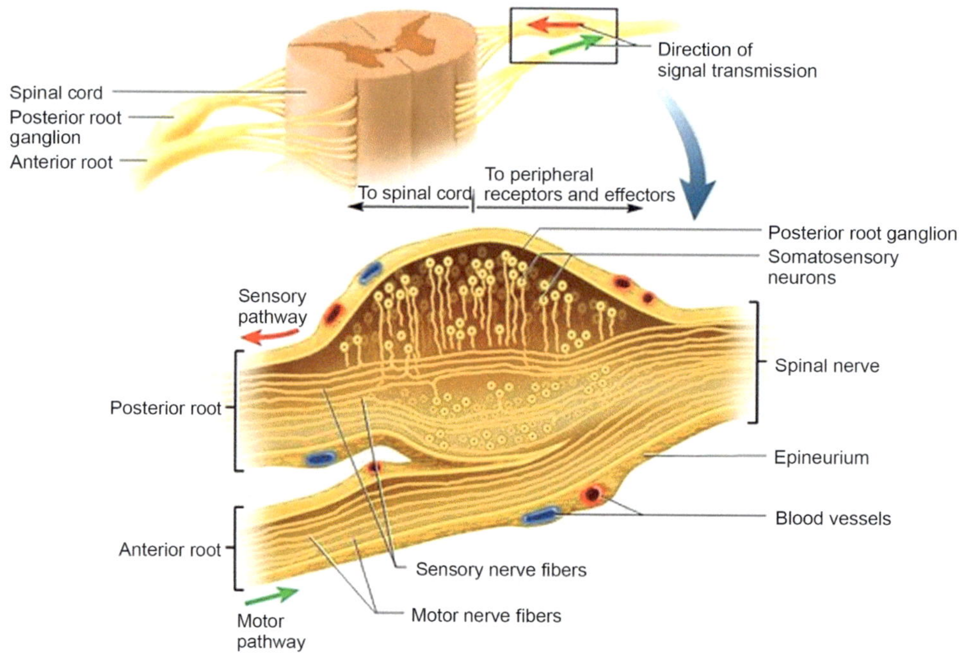

Figure 3.7. Anatomy of ganglions in the PNS.

Source: https://qph.cf2.quoracdn.net/main-qimg-58ed660c01921ef670e741282cdf4b33-lq.

Test Your Knowledge

1. What are the main components of the peripheral nervous system (PNS)?
2. How are nerves in the PNS classified into cranial and spinal nerves?

3.2. Functions of the Peripheral Nervous System

Learning Outcome

1. Explain the sensory functions and sensory receptors
2. Understand the motor functions and muscle control
3. Define autonomic functions and involuntary responses

Functions of the PNS are critical in facilitating communication between the CNS and body so that both sensory and motor processes can function. The PNS consists of two central units: the somatic nervous system for voluntary control of muscle movement, and the autonomic nervous system for involuntary physiological function. Under the autonomic system, there are additional subdivisions between the sympathetic and parasympathetic systems, wherein the body can react with ease to anything from an emergency to routine upkeep of homeostasis. This highly regulated system not only aids in complex movement and response but also provides reflex action that occurs without thinking, showcasing the PNS's role in spurring responsiveness and flexibility to the environment as a whole. In addition, the peripheral nervous system also plays a significant role in regulating some of the physiological functions via modulation of neurotransmitters and other signal molecules. A good example is the corticosterone effect on neuronal physiology, showing how peripheral hormones impact neurotransmitter systems, particularly by inhibiting transport processes that clear monoamines from synaptic compartments. This rapid, GR-independent action is to underscore the intricate interactions of the endocrine substances with the peripheral nervous system, ultimately influencing behavior and physiology. These interactions emphasize the necessity of integrating hormonal function with the PNS's ancient roles, thereby providing a more enlightened perspective on how these two systems interact to balance vital functions within the organism and adapt to altered conditions, as illustrated in the study on OCT3-mediated monoamine transport (Gasser et al., 2018).

Furthermore, the function of the PNS can be augmented by identifying multiple pathways of signaling that considerably enhance heart rate and other autonomic functions. Studies aimed at inhibitory heterotrimeric G proteins demonstrate the complex mechanisms through which the PNS controls cardiac function, symbolized by that of specific G protein-coupled receptors in modulating heart rate. The function of RGS proteins to increase the GTPase activity of such proteins further confirms the intricacy of communication in neurons of the PNS, demonstrating how it can finely tune body functions based on internal and external stimuli. These observations are essential for an understanding of how peripheral signals get translated into system-wide physiological changes, showcasing the PNS's vital function in not only voluntary motor control but also fundamental autonomic regulation, hence its broad applicability in homeostasis maintenance and overall well-being (Ang et al., 2012).

3.2.1. Sensory Functions and Sensory Receptors

The sensory role of the PNS forms the foundation of how organisms' sense and respond to the world. Sensory receptors, the receptor structures that are specialized to receive various stimuli, play a crucial role in this function. The receptors may be classified into several types based on their modalities, including mechanoreceptors that respond to touch, thermoreceptors that react to temperature, and photoreceptors that respond to light. All receptor types transform specific environmental changes into neural signals that are carried to the CNS for interpretation.

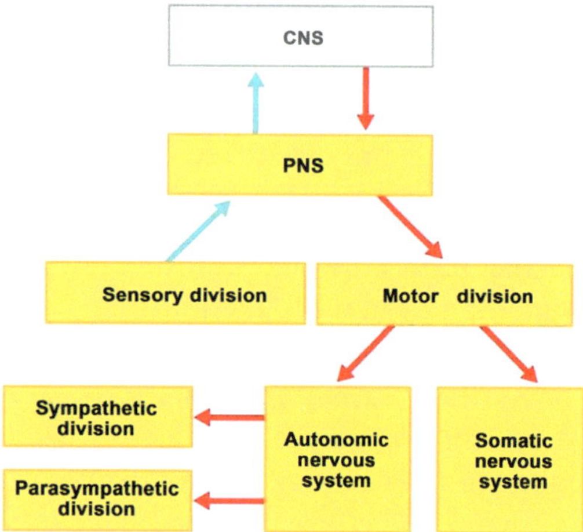

Figure 3.8. Function of the PNS.

Source: https://external-content.duckduckgo.com/iu/?u=https%3A%2F%2Fimage1.slideserve.com%2F2432186%2Fpns-in-the-nervous-system-l.jpg&f=1&nofb=1&ipt=54d063ce8b6f3a6eb8efb407cdf8379eebfabbc65f2c98a5199ec9ab4198f9a4.

The conversion of external stimuli into electrical signals ensures that sensations such as pain, pleasure, and temperature are properly relayed to the brain, allowing effective responses. An understanding of the variety of sensory receptors and their pathways makes us aware of how complex and efficient the PNS is. One such example illustrating the interplay between peripheral function and sensory receptors is the activities of single glial cells, i.e., the Schwann cells, of the PNS (Figure 3.8).

Besides providing structural support, the cells also facilitate the regeneration of sensory nerves upon injury, and therefore, sensory functions are very well preserved. After injury, Schwann cells release growth factors required in neural repair as well as guide regrowing axons to the target tissue. This regenerative capacity, according to research, presents a stark contrast to the poor capacity for regeneration of the CNS. The ability of the PNS to recover from damage emphasizes the need to maintain healthy sensory pathways because sensory receptors rely on intact nerve health to work correctly. Such information about PNS glial functions significantly advances therapeutics for inducing sensory regeneration and recovery. Expression of some receptor subunits, such as the α7 nicotinic acetylcholine receptors (nAChRs), adds yet another level of understanding to sensory functions within the PNS. The receptors are expressed during embryonic development early in tissues, suggesting their organizing function in the development of the nervous system. Within the PNS, the presence of α7 nAChRs in organizations such as the dorsal root ganglia suggests their sensory transmission function. Furthermore, prenatal nicotine exposure has also been discovered to affect the expression of these receptors, and such may have lasting implications for sensory functions and processing. The significance of such findings cannot be overemphasized, as it underscores the necessity to investigate receptor dynamics not only concerning sensory function but also in the context of neural health. This research brings to the fore the intricate interaction between developmental biology and sensory receptors in the case of the PNS, and how they participate in physiology as well as potential pathologies.

3.2.2. Motor Functions and Muscle Control

Motor function and muscle control are central aspects of human motion and are intensely rooted in the complex interplay between the peripheral and central nervous systems. The spinal cord is centrally located in the control of these functions, particularly in voluntary movements such as walking. It facilitates motor control and maintenance of posture through input from the motor cortex and the periphery, including muscle spindles.

The ability of the spinal cord to blend higher-order cognitive processes and sensory feedback data allows for fine-tuning of muscle contractions when moving with a high level of complexity. Dynamic control highlights the importance of spinal cord operation in enabling proper and smooth motor activities, demonstrating how crucial the peripheral nervous system is in conducting intentional behaviors and in responding to external stimuli in real-time (340 et al., 2023). Primitive reflex theory and motor primitives provide further understanding of motor function maturation. Primitive reflexes, or spontaneous, automatic responses of movement to specific stimuli, are the first level of motor control in early development.

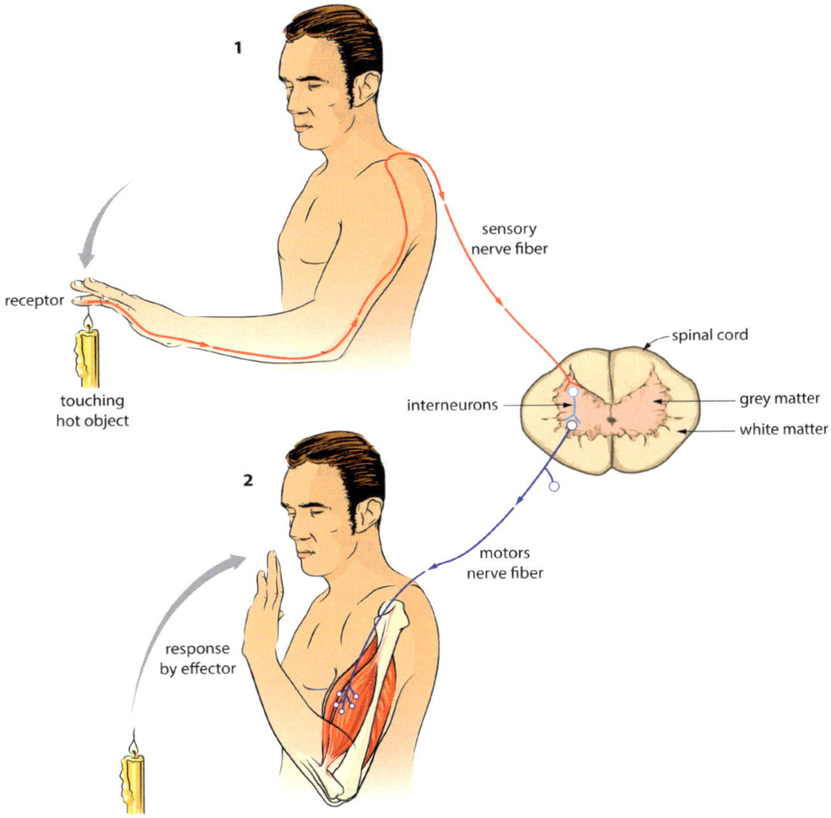

Figure 3.9. The brain works with the peripheral nervous system and continually responds to changes in muscle contraction.

Source: https://www.acquiredbraininjury-education.scot.nhs.uk/wp-content/uploads/360969659-Reflex.jpg.

Motor primitives are hierarchical sets of voluntary motor patterns that remain invariant throughout the life of an individual. Both motor primitives and primitive reflexes are intrinsically associated with the spinal cord's structure and function, which generate these reflexive movements. It is through an understanding of the relationship between such factors that the richness and variability of motor control, as well as of human movement, are realized, ultimately elucidating how the peripheral nervous system functions in harmony with the higher cortical areas to optimize and carry out motor tasks (Konczak et al., 2005) (Figure 3.9).

Furthermore, modulation of spinal cord function by higher central nervous system structures accentuates the intricacy of control of the motor system. Cognitive processes, specifically those of voluntary motor behavior, significantly contribute to spinal cord function, according to studies of the H-reflexes of muscle response. According to these studies, regions such as the parietal association cortex and the prefrontal cortex are implicated in the control of spinal disinhibition to permit sophisticated motor activities. The interaction of cognitive function and spinal cord processing exhibits a feedback system in which sensory input, motor planning, and reflexive output converge. Not only does this cooperation allow for finer motor function, but it also points to the robust capabilities of the peripheral nervous system in undertaking simple reflexive movements as well as more complex, goal-oriented movement (340 et al., 2023).

3.2.3. Autonomic Functions and Involuntary Responses

The autonomic activities governed by the peripheral nervous system play a crucial role in maintaining homeostasis and also in managing involuntary physiological responses. This branch of the nervous system operates predominantly beneath the level of awareness, managing functions such as heart rate, digestion, and respiratory rhythm. These mechanisms are essential to the body's adaptation to altering internal and external milieus, exhibiting the autonomic nervous system's inherent ability to balance itself. Heart rate variability—a process mediated by the respiratory cycle—is a prime example of this interaction between respiration and cardiac function. The alteration of heart rhythms through inhalation and exhalation, as detailed in studies of respiratory rhythms, illustrates how respiratory mechanics control other autonomic activities, and therefore how interdependent these systems are in regulating body states (Barnes et al., 2014). Furthermore, involuntary responses are not merely primitive reflexes but also highly evolved physiological compensations that can impact affective and cognitive states. Studies have established the mechanisms by which individuals, particularly those with autism, deal with social and environmental hardship using both central and peripheral autonomic processes. Disjunction between social cognition and behavior can frequently reflect more integral physiological adaptation than mere cognition loss. This information indicates that the driving biological forces governing autonomic processes significantly contribute to the nature of behaviors traditionally viewed as abnormal. By examining movement variability and its relation to systemic neurophysiology, researchers have endeavored to map how such imperceptible involuntary responses can inform the general knowledge of cognitive and emotional development across broad populations (Brincker et al., 2017). In addition to its role in moderating fundamental bodily functions, the autonomic nervous system also has a significant role as a facilitator of stress reactions. In times of emotional or physical stress, the sympathetic branch of the autonomic nervous system is activated, resulting in a cascade of involuntary actions, including increased heart rate and blood pressure. Concurrent activation of the parasympathetic system provides for restoration and relaxation and underscores the delicate balance required for overall health. States of panic or anxiety attacks can cut short this balance, demonstrating the significance of autonomic dysregulation to daily functioning. Studying these involuntary acts not only enhances our understanding of the complexity of the peripheral nervous system but also opens doors to healing against ailments of ill health. It is hence of paramount importance in clinical and educational settings to identify the interaction between autonomic functions and involuntary response (Barnes et al., 2014).

Test Your Knowledge

1. How do motor functions contribute to muscle control?
2. What are autonomic functions, and how do they regulate involuntary responses?

3.3. Types of Nerves in the Peripheral Nervous System

Learning Outcome

1. Define afferent nerves and sensory information
2. Discuss the efferent nerves and motor commands
3. Explain the mixed nerves and their dual functions

The PNS consists of a vast array of different types of nerves that facilitate communication between the CNS and the remainder of the body. Primarily, these include sensory, motor, or mixed nerves. Sensory nerves are responsible for transmitting sensory input from the various regions of the body to the CNS. They send vital information regarding touch, temperature, pain, and proprioception to allow the organism to react properly to its surroundings. Motor nerves, in contrast, carry impulses from the CNS to effectors such as muscles and glands to enable actions ranging from simple reflexes to sophisticated voluntary movements. Mixed nerves contain both sensory and motor fibers to allow feedback and command functions to be performed in parallel, thus serving significant conduits for functional organization of the PNS. In addition to the basic sensory and motor categorizations, peripheral nerves can also be categorized based on their myelination. Myelinated nerves, encased within a fatty sheath known as the myelin sheath, enable quicker conduction of impulses through saltatory conduction. This mechanism significantly enhances the speed with which nerve impulses travel down the axon, facilitating rapid movement in voluntary and reflex movements. In contrast, unmyelinated nerves conduct impulses at slower speeds, which may be necessary for those actions that are not as urgent. Notably, various types of nerve fibers, such as A, B, and C fibers, exhibit this variation of myelination. Fibers are heavily myelinated and transmit sharp, smart pain sensation, whereas C fibers lack myelination and transmit dull, thudding pain sensation, thus influencing pain perception. Understanding the diverse categorization of nerves within the PNS is also connected with their anatomical and functional roles in specific systems. For example, sensory neurons in the dorsal root ganglia are central to the afferent pathways by which sensory input is transmitted. At the same time, autonomic nerves are involved in the involuntary control of body functions like digestion and heart rate. Recent research has also shown that specific nerves are differentially sensitive to treatments like photodynamic therapy, wherein specific populations of nerves are spared from damage while others are targeted. Research suggests that the effectiveness of treatments may rest upon the particular morphology and functional characteristics of peripheral nerves, emphasizing the need for a clear comprehension of such nerve types and their relevance to health and disease (MacRobert et al., 2007; Jacobs et al., 2010) (Figure 3.10).

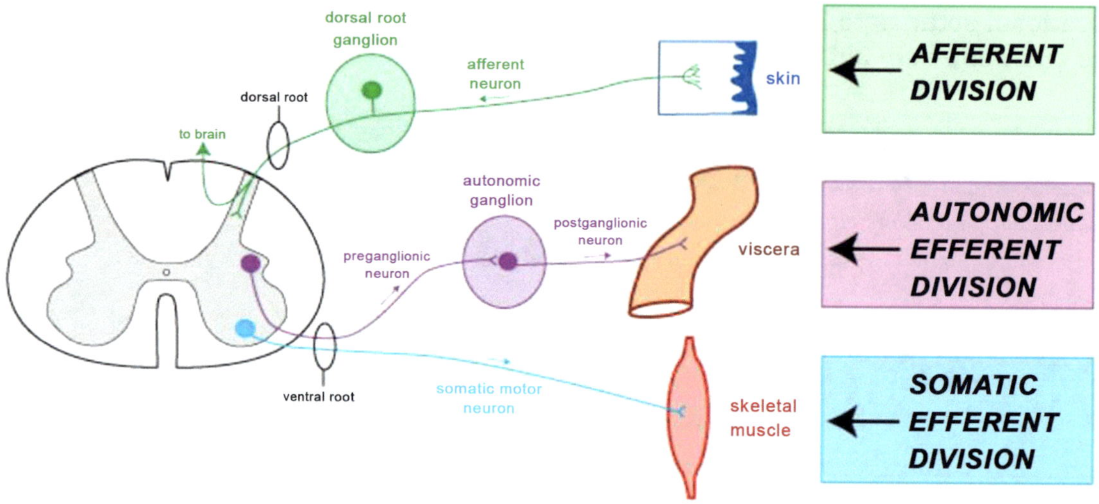

Figure 3.10. Types of nerves in the peripheral nervous system.

Source: https://courses.washington.edu/pbio375/PNS-org/SC-schematic.png.

3.3.1. Afferent Nerves and Sensory Information

Afferent nerves play a pivotal role in conveying sensory information by prioritizing as the most critical pathway along which external stimuli are passed to the central nervous system. Afferent nerves are responsible for the transmission of sensory modalities such as touch, temperature, pain, and proprioception from throughout the body. Because they are the first point of contact for environmental stimuli, afferent fibers originate from particular receptors in dermal, muscular, and visceral tissues. Information picked up on these routes is crucial to the body's ability to respond appropriately to environmental change, ensuring survival through the ability to react immediately to potential dangers or condition shifts. The complex interplay between afferent nerves and central processing areas is essential to the processing of sensory data. Sensory information is not only conveyed but also integrated with autonomic function to influence physiological response throughout the body. For instance, it has been found that processing of brief somatosensory stimulation can alter radically as a function of phase in the cardiac cycle, showing that sensory perception is influenced by physiological states like heart rate and blood pressure. Afferent pathways carry diverse sensory information to structures such as the amygdala and insula, illustrating dynamic interplay between autonomic control, sensory information, emotional response, and physiological state (Critchley et al., 2009) (Figure 3.11).

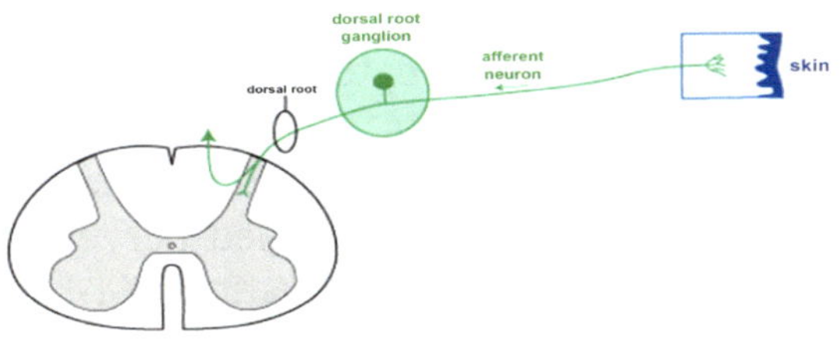

Figure 3.11. Afferent neurons have a unique structure that differs from most other neurons.

Source: https://upload.wikimedia.org/wikipedia/commons/thumb/e/ea/Afferent_and_efferent_neurons_en.svg/1024px-Afferent_and_efferent_neurons_en.svg.png.

Hence, this afferent activity plays a critical role in homeostasis and acts adequately to internal and external stimuli. In addition, the diversity of afferent nerves, like those specialized in mechanoreception, illustrates sensory pathway specialization in the peripheral nervous system. For example, in the spiny eel, dedicated lateral-line nerves have been shown to connect mechanosensory information from new peripheral sources to the cerebellum in different regions (Hofmann et al., 1991). This is proof that afferent projections are not uniformly distributed but are tailored to the sensory requirements of the organism and the trends in the environment. The convergence of these signals allows for subtle responses to complex stimuli, illustrating the sophistication of the peripheral nervous system to provide sense perception and motor response for maintenance and interaction with the world.

3.3.2. Efferent Nerves and Motor Commands

The PNS plays a crucial role in transmitting motor commands from the central nervous system to muscles, mainly through efferent nerves. Efferent nerves convey impulses that result in voluntary and involuntary movements, which are crucial for body functions like walking and reflex actions. They are classified into autonomic and somatic nerves; somatic efferent nerves supply skeletal muscles with the ability to make voluntary movement, while autonomic efferent nerves control involuntary functions such as heart rate and digestion. This dichotomy highlights the PNS's twofold capability, making it possible for both conscious control and autonomous regulation, thereby enabling the organism to respond appropriately to internal and external stimuli. Research has shown that the use of therapeutic interventions following spinal cord injury has the possibility of significantly enhancing motor function through targeted use of the efferent nerves. Functional electrical stimulation (FES) is one possible technique for restoring movement in paralyzed individuals suffering from spinal injury. By administering controlled electrical currents into the injured nerves, FES can cause muscle contractions and enable activities once thought not possible for spinal injury patients. In addition to triggering the attempt to help with locomotion, the procedure enhances the quality of life of the patients through the restoration of some degree of mobility and independence, thus showing the significant interaction between technological innovation and neural function (Hunt et al., 2002). Furthermore, novel methods of directly controlling prosthetic devices through efferent neurons have been made possible by technology developments in brain interfaces, which has important implications for amputee rehabilitation plans. Intrafascicular electrodes, which talk to peripheral nerves, provide a low-invasive method for reading motor instructions to prostheses. Intrafascicular electrodes can translate volition into action in prosthetic limbs with enhanced dexterity and function by reading the neural signals attendant to movements of intent. Early trials have been encouraging, with the potential of such systems to restore fine motor function. The applications are beyond mere functionality, since they can greatly improve the quality of life of individuals who are required to rely on prosthetic limbs, and are under the spotlight in future medical technology research (Carpaneto et al., 2010).

3.3.3. Mixed Nerves and Their Dual Functions

Mixed nerve theory lies at the heart of understanding the neural functionality of the PNS, as mixed nerves contain both motor and sensory fibers. This binary arrangement allows mixed nerves to play a vital role in transferring a wide variety of signals from the brain to the body. Sensory fibers are responsible for sending information from the peripheral receptors—i.e., pain, temperature, and proprioceptive receptors—to the CNS. Motor fibers, conversely, transmit signals from the CNS to the muscles to trigger voluntary and involuntary movements. Mixed nerves thus play a key role in integrating sensory feed and motor function, essentially enabling organisms to respond quickly and efficiently to their surroundings. The dual function of mixed nerves demonstrates the complexity and sophistication of the PNS. The sciatic nerve, for instance, one of the largest mixed nerves in the body, not only innervates the muscles of the leg but also conducts sensory information from the lower extremities to the brain. This lends credence to the concept that the PNS is more than a pipe, but rather an integral participant in homeostasis via feedback mechanisms. Disturbance of these hybrid nerves, either through disease or trauma, can lead to severe impairments in sensory function and motor activity, highlighting their role in everyday, ordinary physiological processes. It is essential to know this dual role to design therapeutic interventions for numerous neuropathic illnesses that can occur after nerve damage. Furthermore, recent studies have illuminated our understanding of the pathophysiological functions of mixed nerves. For instance, the modulation of some cytokines involved in nerve damage has been shown to influence pain hypersensitivity, highlighting a biological communication process by mixed nerves after trauma. In particular, the activation of T-helper cells with algesic cytokine IL-17A expression after peripheral nerve injury shows the intricate relationship between the mixed nerves and the immune system that may complicate neuropathic pain. This association emphasizes the dual role of mixed nerves, not just as conduits for conduction but as components of the body's constitution in reacting to injury, highlighting the importance of such structures in both physiological and pathological states (Angert et al., 2015). Moreover, technical improvements in neurophysiological monitoring have provided optimism for improving results in mixed nerve procedures (Doan et al., 2016) (Figure 3.12).

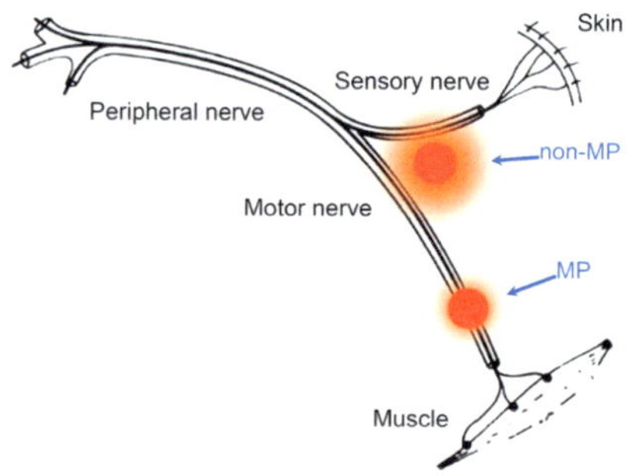

Figure 3.12. Schematic representation of a mixed peripheral nerve and two stimulation sites.

Source: https://www.researchgate.net/figure/Schematic-representation-of-a-mixed-peripheral-nerve-and-two-stimulation-sites-When-the_fig1_260380215.

Test Your Knowledge

1. What role do efferent nerves play in the nervous system?
2. What are mixed nerves, and why are they important for nervous system function?

3.4. Common Disorders of the Peripheral Nervous System

Learning Outcome

1. Explain the causes and characteristics of peripheral neuropathy
2. Describe Guillain-Barré syndrome and its effects on the nervous system
3. Identify the symptoms and clinical features of carpal tunnel syndrome

PNS is distributed through a wide variety of disorders with profound effects on sensory and motor functions. The most common disorders are peripheral neuropathies, which are often due to diabetes, infections, and toxic exposure. These cause variable degrees of symptoms like pain, numbness, and weakness, thus severely impairing the quality of life in a person. Individual presentations can differ with the type of nerves involved; e.g., damage to sensory nerves typically provokes paresthesia and alteration in sensation, while motor nerve impairment can present as muscle weakness or wasting. Thus, a thorough neurological examination is essential to establish the character and severity of these conditions. Because of the complex interaction between the PNS and other neurological systems, early and accurate diagnosis is crucial to prevent progression and optimize patient outcomes (LeCouteur et al., 1999). Another frequent category of disorders that affect the PNS is entrapment syndromes such as carpal tunnel syndrome and ulnar nerve entrapment. These syndromes result from compression or inflammation of nerves at specific anatomical sites, causing pain limited to the region, sensory loss, and motor weakness. An example is carpal tunnel syndrome, which consists of compressive impingement of the median nerve where it traverses through the carpal tunnel to cause numbness and tingling of the first three fingers. Recognition of the causative pathophysiology underlying these syndromes is critical not only to diagnosis but also to successful management. Treatment can span from conservative interventions, including immobilization and physical therapy, to surgical options that ensure alleviation of pressure over compressed nerves (Falla et al., 2014). Therefore, treatment programs must consider both the functional and physical consequences of nerve entrapment syndromes. Finally, the impact of traumatic injury on the PNS is a crucial element of peripheral nerve conditions. Acute and chronic types of injuries, such as lacerations and fractures, and repetitive strain injury, can produce severe nerve damage. This could be in the form of neuropraxia, axonotmesis, or neurotmesis, each defining the severity of nerve injury and referencing outcomes in terms of recovery. Additionally, following such trauma, patients may be left with neuropathic pain, a complex and often hard-to-treat condition. The multidimensional character of pain of peripheral nerve injury necessitates a sophisticated understanding of pain neurophysiology, so effective intervention goes beyond anatomic damage. With more study, a clearer picture of the nociception-motor relationship will be needed to continue to develop treatment strategies for people with peripheral nervous system disorders (LeCouteur et al., 1999; Falla et al., 2014).

3.4.1. Peripheral Neuropathy and Its Causes

Education on peripheral neuropathy is about finding the multitude of causes that lead to it. Peripheral neuropathy occurs when the peripheral nerves are injured, and this leads to a number of symptoms that can range from pain, weakness, and numbness. Diabetes mellitus is one of the major causes of the disorder, whereby long-standing high levels of blood sugar can lead to nerve damage over time. Additionally, autoimmune diseases, such as lupus or rheumatoid arthritis, can induce inflammatory responses that injure peripheral nerves. Viral infections, including herpes zoster, have also been seen to possess the potential to induce neuropathy. All such causes possess unique mechanisms through which they impact the peripheral nervous system, indicative of the multiplicity of a range of health conditions along with nerve function. Furthermore, certain drugs and toxins have a significant effect on the occurrence of peripheral neuropathy. For example, chemotherapy agents used in the management of cancers, such as those used in acute lymphoblastic leukemia, have been associated with severe toxic effects on peripheral nerves, which lead to clinical presentations of neuropathy in patients. The intensity of the side effects is generally variable based on the specific treatment protocols implemented (Attarbashti et al., 2016) (Figure 3.13).

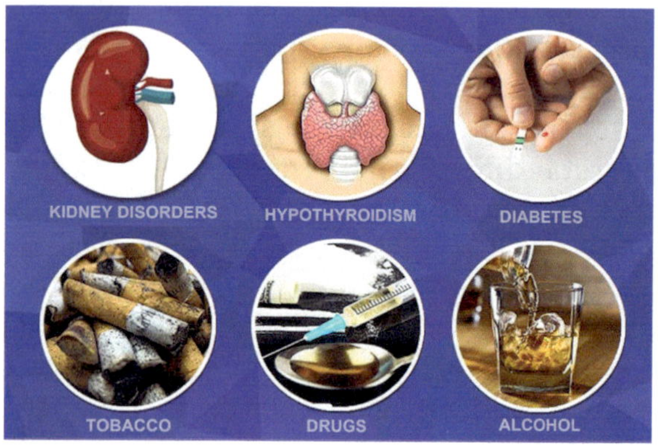

Figure 3.13. Causes of peripheral neuropathy.

Source: https://cdn1.byjus.com/wp-content/uploads/2018/11/biology/2018/04/12044631/Causes-of-peripheral-neuropathy.jpg.

Moreover, contact with heavy metals, e.g., lead or mercury, can lead to toxic neuropathy, which can be particularly dangerous because such poisons are silent in the sense that they do not automatically lead to symptoms. Hence, therapy of peripheral neuropathy must not only address the symptom but also identify and manage exposure to the causative agents, thus placing significant emphasis upon integral healthcare practices. One of the newer fields of investigation in peripheral neuropathy studies is how mitochondrial dysfunction, particularly in Schwann cells, contributes to maintaining nerve integrity. Dysfunctional mitochondria have been implicated in new studies to cause extensive demyelination to result in varying neuropathy conditions. Specifically, the mitochondrial protein Prohibitin 1 is recognized as a key player in this process; without it, Schwann cells exhibit persistent activation of demyelination-related pathways (Nunes et al., 2021). This points towards the importance of cellular health in accounting for peripheral neuropathy since abnormalities at the mitochondrial level have distant-reaching implications throughout the peripheral nervous system. Generally, a multifactorial cause combining metabolic, environmental, and genetic factors along with mitochondrial integrity is required in the attainment of a holistic perspective regarding peripheral neuropathy and its diverse etiologies.

3.4.2. Guillain-Barré Syndrome (GBS) and Its Effects

GBS is a perfect illustration of how autoimmune conditions affect the peripheral nervous system (PNS) negatively. The disease is acute inflammatory demyelinating polyradiculoneuropathy and most often comes after viral or bacterial infection, specifically with *Campylobacter jejuni.* The immune process triggered during infections tends to demolish the myelin sheath surrounding peripheral nerves. This demyelination is then followed by a variety of neurological impairments, from muscle weakness and paralysis, which is the most frequent etiology of acute flaccid paralysis. The heterogeneous presentation of the symptoms and rapid development of GBS emphasize its devastating impact on patients, resulting in many cases in long-term rehabilitation and therapy for the recovery of motor function and autonomy (Pésinho et al., 2019). Besides the immediate physical sequelae, GBS encompasses a vast spectrum of complications that have the potential to significantly impair one's quality of life. Respiratory insufficiency is frequently observed, characterized by the involvement of nerves that control crucial respiratory muscles. Autonomic dysfunction is another critical factor that can manifest as alteration of blood pressure and heart rate, further destabilizing the control of this complex syndrome. Cognitive and affective outcomes also occur in the course of the disease, with the majority of patients suffering from anxiety and depression because of their physical impairment and doubt of recovery. Additionally, unpredictability of GBS often necessitates a treatment protocol with multiple disciplines, including neurologists, physical therapists, and psychologists, underpinning holistic care for effective recovery (N/A, 2016) (Figure 3.14).

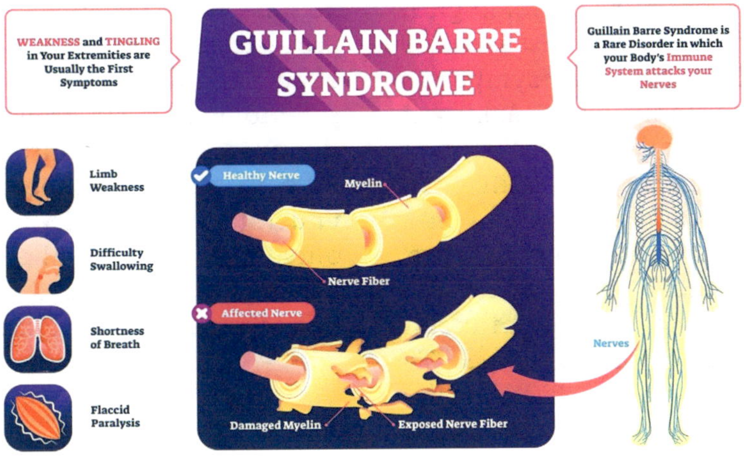

Figure 3.14. Guillain-Barré syndrome.

Source: https://propelphysiotherapy.com/wp-content/uploads/2020/08/guillain-barre-syndrome-treatment-propel-physiotherapy.jpg.

The pathophysiologic basis of GBS remains an area of ongoing research, where an urgent need exists for a better understanding of the immunological triggers and mechanisms. The process through which genetic predisposition combined with environmental factors serves as a stimulus for the activation of these autoimmune processes is yet to be well elucidated. Current research on GBS is aimed at identifying specific biomarkers that can enable early diagnosis as well as tailoring individual therapy according to individualized immunological characteristics. In addition, research on novel treatments such as immunotherapies is a mirror of the active measures being taken to mitigate against the incapacitating effects of GBS. As evidence accumulation continues in this field, there is hope for improved treatments that can ultimately improve prognosis and quality of life in affected patients (Pésinho et al., 2019).

3.4.3. Carpal Tunnel Syndrome and Its Symptoms

Carpal tunnel syndrome (CTS) is a common disorder due to median nerve compression within the carpal tunnel at the wrist. Characterized by a symptom pattern of numbness, tingling, and weakness in the hand, CTS illustrates a vital interface between peripheral nerve disease and functional disability.

Worsening of symptoms with activity such as gripping or repetitive wrist flexion, for instance, typing or use of hand tools, are often the presenting complaint of the patient. Nocturnal symptoms are also frequent and disrupt sleep, leading to secondary associated conditions such as fatigue and mood disturbances. This symptom complex is indicative not only of the neurological basis of CTS but also of the broader impact on the quality of life of patients, thereby imposing the need for effective management strategies that are sensitive to both the physiological and psychological effects of this disease. The presentation of CTS in terms of symptoms occurs variably among individuals, making it challenging to diagnose and treat. Recent studies have introduced a pain phenotype classification model for CTS, which categorizes them into nociceptive, neuropathic, and nociplastic types. This is significant because it may alter the approach to treatment and the type of result that can be anticipated. As stated, while CTS is fundamentally a neuropathic disorder, the occurrence of nociplastic pain components in a subset of patients suggests that holistic treatment modalities may become essential. For instance, the prevalence of overlapping symptoms would indicate that treatments according to the conventional treatments of the carpal tunnel may not be effective for cases involving nociplastic mechanisms, and therefore, there is a need to apply a more sophisticated understanding of the unique symptom profile of each patient (Arendt-Nielsen et al., 2023).

New treatments have explored therapy beyond conventional corticosteroid injections, offering potential avenues towards improvement of CTS symptoms. For example, a randomized controlled trial is currently assessing the efficacy of locally administered progesterone as second-line treatment versus cortisone, and its neuroprotective effects (Ginanneschi et al., 2010). Preliminary results indicate that while corticosteroids provide quick symptom relief, in the long term, they are not particularly helpful, with relapse being common. However, progesterone's more widespread neuroprotective effect might provide lasting improvement of symptoms in some groups. Study of such new therapies in the context of the peripheral nervous system is important to advancing our understanding of CTS and improving patient outcomes, as it highlights the commonality between structural and biochemical processes in nerve disorders (Figure 3.15).

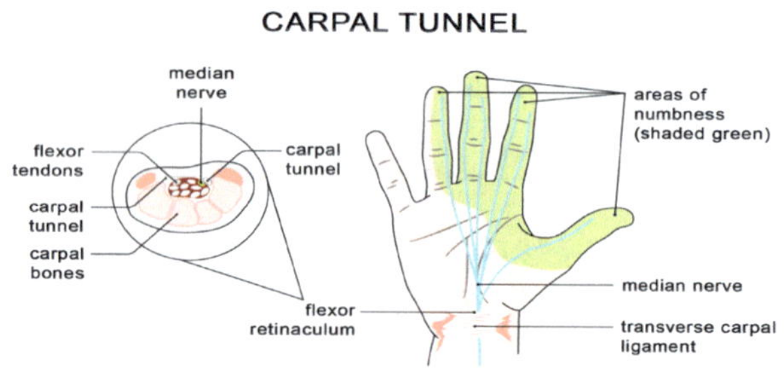

Figure 3.15. Carpal tunnel syndrome.

Source: https://www.medicalnewstoday.com/articles/184337.

Test Your Knowledge

1. What is peripheral neuropathy, and what are some common causes?
2. How does Guillain-Barré syndrome affect the nervous system?

3.5. Diagnostic Techniques for PNS Disorders

Learning Outcome

1. Understand the use of electromyography (EMG) in diagnosing peripheral nervous system (PNS) disorders
2. Explain the principles and applications of nerve conduction studies
3. Describe the role of imaging techniques, including MRI, in evaluating PNS disorders

The diagnostic techniques employed in the diagnosis of PNS disorders are crucial for precise estimation and treatment planning. These tests usually begin with a thorough clinical evaluation of motor, sensory, and reflex function. Neurologists employ various techniques such as EMG and nerve conduction studies (NCS) to assess the electrical activity of muscles and the speed of electrical signals within nerves. EMG can identify neuromuscular junction abnormalities, while NCS provides data on nerve function. Clinicians can diagnose specific PNS dysfunctions by relating clinical findings to physiological data obtained from the tests. The utility of the methods also extends beyond diagnosis in that they can be used to track the course of the disease and drug response longitudinally, improving patient management. Current imaging modalities tend to augment traditional forms of diagnosis, particularly when the signs and symptoms present in an abnormal manner. Imaging modalities such as magnetic resonance imaging (MRI) and computed tomography (CT) scanning can provide valuable visual data regarding the structural integrity of nerve roots and adjacent tissue. A case point involves imaging assisting in the diagnosis of pathologies like cervical radiculopathy or tumors involving the PNS. The case of a military man who was diagnosed with multiple sclerosis after inconclusive X-rays shows the importance of whole imaging in making a diagnosis when initial results are still unclear (Stafrace et al., 2015). By making anatomical lesions that underlie abnormalities visible, imaging facilitates differential diagnoses and leads to more specific therapeutic approaches. Combining imaging data with physiological assessment thus provides a holistic view of PNS disorders. In addition to traditional methods, emerging diagnostic approaches are in sight that address physiological variability in movement patterns, or micro-movements. In light of recent research, testing of those subtle differences can reveal evidence of systemic responses behind PNS disorders, especially disorders such as autism spectrum disorders that may involve both peripheral and central nervous system mechanisms (Brincker et al., 2017). This focus on variability of movement is a new approach to conceptualizing the dynamic interactions in sensorimotor systems, advancing the understanding of motor control and regulation. Through the use of advanced data collection and statistical analysis, medical practitioners can better quantify personal conditions and enhance diagnostic accuracy. Lastly, the application of numerous diagnostic techniques, from conventional to advanced research, holds great promise for improved identification and management of peripheral nervous system disorders.

3.5.1. Electromyography (EMG)

EMG is an essential diagnostic tool applied in the evaluation of the peripheral nervous system. EMG gives details about muscle function and neurologic integrity through the recording of electrical muscle activity. EMG is helpful in the diagnosis of conditions that affect nerve and muscle function, including neuropathies, myopathies, and neuromuscular junction disorders. The method involves the placement of electrodes on the skin or the penetration of the muscle by needle electrodes to measure electrical activity at rest and during contraction. Data obtained from EMG provides valuable information about the health of peripheral nerves along with the innervated muscle, allowing clinicians to decide the presence of pathology with effectiveness. Thus, EMG not only aids in diagnosis but also acts as a complementary aid in the process of treatment planning and monitoring the course of various neuromuscular disorders. One of the most critical applications of EMG is observed in its use during surgery in the form of intraoperative monitoring. Intraoperative EMG offers assessment of the functional integrity of nerves while operating on the spinal cord and peripheral nerves, which plays a crucial role in reducing post-surgical complication risk. As suggested by a study conducted at Aga Khan University Hospital, EMG was employed in spinal scoliosis correction operations, acoustic neuroma excision, and peripheral nerve repairs, among others. The monitoring technique provided immediate feedback regarding the nerve function, lowering the risk of iatrogenic damage. The study recorded that there were no worthwhile neurological deficits after surgery in the patients, highlighting the efficacy of EMG in preserving nerve function during complicated surgeries (Ali et al., 2016) (Figure 3.16).

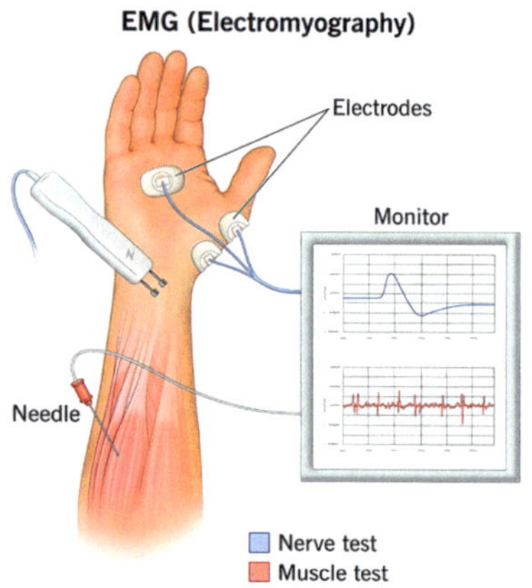

Figure 3.16. Electromyography (EMG) is a diagnostic test.

Source: https://my.clevelandclinic.org/-/scassets/images/org/health/articles/4825-electromyography.

As a practice standard, intraoperative EMG is the pinnacle of the importance of intraoperative neurophysiological monitoring to optimize the surgical outcome. Further, EMG research continues unabated as technology further advances, and its use and accuracy become increasingly more costly. Technology has enabled the development of high-density electrode arrays and improved signal processing algorithms to enhance the capability and performance of EMG recordings. Enhanced EMG methods are now available to offer greater spatial resolution so that it is feasible to identify neuromuscular transmission defects accurately with greater localizing ability. Increased use of EMG results in other neurophysiological tests such as nerve conduction studies and imaging is demonstrated in research to develop a comprehensive diagnosis of peripheral nervous system disorders. This integrative approach not only allows for definitive diagnoses, but it also facilitates an improved understanding of the pathophysiological mechanisms underlying. Consensus nomenclature reports issued by organizations with a neuromuscular health specialty signal the necessity for common practices and terms in the discipline further expanding the potential for improved clinical applications (Abramov et al., 2016).

3.5.2. Nerve Conduction Studies (NCS)

NCS are important diagnostic procedures used to evaluate the functional integrity of peripheral nerves. Through the determination of conduction velocity and amplitude of electrical impulses conducted along nerves, the tests provide valuable information regarding conditions of the peripheral nervous system. The technique in general involves stimulation of a nerve at one location and evaluation of the response elsewhere so that both myelinated and unmyelinated fibers can be evaluated. Anomalies of conduction velocity may point to a variety of neuropathies, and these may result from injury, metabolic disorder, or genetic defect. For instance, slowed conduction velocity can be observed in demyelination, while decreased amplitude could suggest axonal damage. These variations are essential in correct diagnosis and management of peripheral neuropathies so that correct therapeutic regimens can be adopted depending on etiology. In the case of neurological disease, understanding the role of NCS is all the more critical. As an example, in diseases such as Rett syndrome, peripheral nerve function as a result of a genetic mutation can be assessed based on comprehensive nerve conduction studies. Research has shown that although the central nervous system is significantly engaged in Rett syndrome, there are also subtle peripheral nerve morphology and function changes, specifically in myelinated fibers. These, as they occur through alterations in diameter and densities of mitochondria, demonstrate the intricacy of peripheral nerve pathology in disease conditions characterized primarily by central nervous system dysfunction. As discussed in studies in Mecp2+/- mice, while conduction characteristics of peripheral nerves could be normal, global structural alterations could provide some insight into the phenotypic manifestations, thereby highlighting the importance of NCS in the comprehensive evaluation of the central and peripheral nervous systems. NCS could also identify disease states not immediately linked with neuropathies, e.g., recurrent laryngeal neuropathy in equines. This condition damages the function of the recurrent laryngeal nerve, leading to stridor and intolerance to exercise. The pathophysiology of the condition has been controversial as to whether it is caused by distal axonopathy or primary myelinopathy. With the application of nerve conduction studies, researchers can elucidate electrophysiological deficits that define this disorder, which can be helpful in precise classification as well as understanding of its pathophysiology. The ability to accurately assess conduction properties in disparate contexts finally allows clinicians and researchers to make intelligent treatment choices and directions for future investigation. NCS is thus a rudimentary examination in further elucidating the peripheral nervous system and its intricate disorders, illuminating the way toward more effective interventions (Figure 3.17).

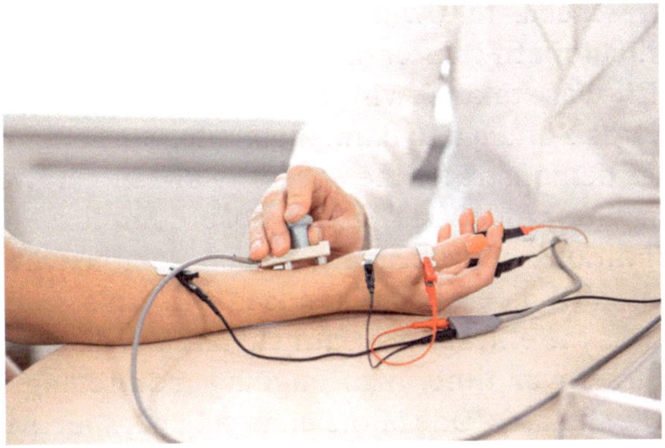

Figure 3.17. Electromyography (EMG) procedure being performed to assess muscle and nerve function.

Source: https://www.spineinfo.com/wp-content/uploads/2023/06/EMG-scaled.jpg.

3.5.3. Imaging Techniques Such as MRI

The use of advanced imaging technologies like MRI greatly improves the investigation of the PNS. MRI is a non-invasive imaging diagnostic tool that provides high-definition images of soft tissues, making it highly effective for imaging neurological structures. MRI does not use ionizing radiation like other imaging modalities, making it safer for patients who need to have repeated images taken. Specifically, in the circumstances of the patient's PNS, MRI can be employed to detect lesions, nerve entrapments, and other pathologies not detectable with standard X-rays. According to numerous case reports, visualization of the intricate array of peripheral nerves allows clinicians to design targeted treatment strategies, ultimately improving outcomes of neurological disorders in patients.

The MRI value in diagnosis is not merely visualization but rather an essential feature in the identification of atypical presentations of neurological disorders. A case in point is an initial diagnosis that fails the test, or patients that do not respond to standard treatment, where high-technology imaging takes precedence. A soldier is a prime example who reported persistent paresthesia following a diagnosis of cervical radiculopathy. After non-definitive X-rays, an MRI was taken, which diagnosed multiple sclerosis and led to immediate intervention. The case demonstrates the necessity of using newer imaging modalities to diagnose complex PNS conditions appropriately. It also demonstrates that MRI not only diagnoses but also helps assess the efficacy of treatment and the disease's course over time, with ongoing monitoring of patient status. One of the emerging perspectives is the merger of traditional medicine practices with modern imaging techniques to further our understanding of patient care. For example, acupuncture, an integral component of traditional Chinese medicine (TCM), is being increasingly studied through modern neuroscientific lenses. Recent research using functional MRI (fMRI) has demonstrated specific neural patterns triggered through acupuncture at specific acupoints and possibly relating to peripheral nerve systems. This coming together of ancient heritage and cutting-edge imaging makes possible an extended model of human health, bridging the gaps between classical anatomical knowledge and contemporary neuroanatomy. With increasing knowledge about these correspondences, new insights into the dynamics between acupuncture and the PNS can potentially illuminate new pathways for therapeutic intervention, and thereby improve clinical care and patient outcomes through a multidisciplinary healing process.

Test Your Knowledge

1. How is electromyography (EMG) used to diagnose peripheral nervous system (PNS) disorders?
2. Why are imaging techniques like MRI important in evaluating nervous system disorders?

SUMMARY

In assembling the complex details regarding the PNS, one sees that the system is an essential facilitator of communication between the central nervous system and the rest of the body. As all the components and functions inherent in the PNS were being discussed, it has become clear that the anatomical as well as physiological characteristics of this system are both requisite for homeostasis and coordination of a vast array of body functions. The complex processes of PNSs' sensory input processing and motor output control underscore their significance in everyday function, underscoring the need for ongoing research and understanding in this critical area of neuroscience. Molecular influences, such as Semaphorin3A, on guiding the development of neurons in the PNS cannot be overstated. Experiments have indicated that Semaphorin3A serves as a chemorepellent signal to guide axon trajectories in development during embryonic stages, and this plays a significant role in the correct specification of neural circuits. Surprisingly, knockout mouse experiments with Semaphorin3A revealed complex patterns of corrective processes that appear to compensate for early developmental abnormalities within the PNS by later stages, validating the dynamic nature of neural development and the inherent capacity to adjust within the nervous system. These results emphasize the complex interaction between the genetic factors and environmental factors in the creation of the functional integrity of the PNS, and they further enrich our understanding about peripheral neuropathies. Lastly, research about the PNS and its associated diseases emphasizes the critical function played by this system in neural function and overall well-being. For instance, research on genetic diseases, such as Sandhoff disease, has shown the predominant influence of enzymatic defects on the integrity of the nervous system. The absence of meaningful functional impairment of peripheral nerves, despite the presence of structural adversity, suggests compensatory mechanisms in action and better insight into myelin structure and function. With more research, such findings will not only enlighten us on the mechanistic mechanisms of several neurological disorders but also guide potential therapeutic interventions that can restore or enhance peripheral nervous system function, paving the way for novel treatments and better patient management (Berezikov et al., 2000; Federico et al., 2007).

The PNS is a vital communication channel between the central nervous system and the body that enables voluntary and involuntary action. It contains sensory neurons that transmit information from the outside world to the brain, as well as motor neurons, which transmit signals that enable the movement of muscles. Further, the PNS is also responsible for regulating body functions by its autonomic divisions, which regulate essential processes such as heart rate, digestion, and respiratory rate. When treating many neurological disorders, an understanding of the PNS is necessary because abnormal peripheral nerve signaling can generate disabling symptoms and influence overall well-being. This has highlighted the necessity of ongoing research investigating the interaction between the peripheral and central nervous systems, particularly how peripheral excitation can significantly influence central nervous functions. Recent studies have illustrated the interwoven relationship between peripheral immune responses and CNS functions. For instance, it has been shown that peripheral immune stimulation—i.e., inflammation—has the potential to influence brain activity and behavior significantly. Experiments involving a model of psoriasis-like cutaneous inflammation have identified that inflammatory chemokines and immune cell invasion can modulate animal behavior and neurogenesis. These findings indicate that peripheral immune dynamics are not merely local, but instead suggest that cytokines and leukocyte activity can transmit significant modifications in CNS function. These findings are opposed to traditional assumptions that view the CNS as very insulated from peripheral immune effects, emphasizing the need for such insight in the development of effective therapy strategies in conditions involving both the immune and neurological dysfunctions, highlighted in the literature. Additionally, advances in procedures, such as those used in research on human gait dynamics, have further enlightened the role of the PNS in motor coordination as well as general physiology. A significant contrast between ankle dynamics in healthy individuals and diabetic patients means that feedback from the feet is essential in enabling optimal movement functions. However, the findings also suggest knee movement to be comparatively unaffected, meaning that there is a complex relationship between some aspects of the PNS and neural control of walking. These results serve to emphasize the importance of technology and pattern recognition in extracting useful data from movement studies and expanding our knowledge of how the signals from the periphery are incorporated into the overall neuromuscular control systems. Gaining information from these kinds of studies not only expands our understanding of the PNS's vital roles but also provides the basis upon which future studies can be conducted into the design of specific interventions for those experiencing peripheral nerve impairments.

KEY TERMS FROM THIS CHAPTER

- Cranial Nerves
- Sensory Division
- Somatic Nervous System
- Ganglia
- Dorsal Root
- Mixed Nerves
- Neuromuscular Junction
- Endocannabinoid system
- Spinal Nerves
- Motor Division
- Sympathetic Nervous System
- Plexus
- Ventral Root
- Sensory Receptors
- Peripheral Nerve Fibers
- Gastrointestinal (GI)

CRITICAL THINKING QUESTIONS

1. **What does the peripheral nervous system mainly consist of?**
   a. Brain and spinal cord
   b. Nerves and ganglia outside the CNS
   c. Sensory organs only
   d. The cerebrum and cerebellum
2. **Which division of the peripheral nervous system controls voluntary movements?**
   a. Autonomic nervous system
   b. Somatic nervous system
   c. Sympathetic nervous system
   d. Parasympathetic nervous system
3. **The autonomic nervous system regulates:**
   a. Skeletal muscle movement
   b. Conscious sensory input
   c. Involuntary functions like heart rate and digestion
   d. Voluntary speech production
4. **The part of the autonomic nervous system that prepares the body for "fight or flight" is called:**
   a. Parasympathetic nervous system
   b. Sympathetic nervous system
   c. Somatic nervous system
   d. Central nervous system
5. **Sensory neurons in the peripheral nervous system carry signals:**
   a. From the CNS to muscles
   b. From muscles to the CNS
   c. From sensory organs to the CNS
   d. Between interneurons only

Short Answer Questions

1. What are the main anatomical components of the peripheral nervous system?
2. What are the primary functions of the peripheral nervous system?
3. Name the different types of nerves found in the peripheral nervous system.
4. What is the difference between sensory and motor nerves in the PNS?
5. List two common disorders that affect the peripheral nervous system.
6. Which diagnostic techniques are commonly used to evaluate peripheral nervous system disorders?
7. How does the autonomic nervous system fit within the peripheral nervous system?

Answer to Critical Thinking Questions

1. (b); 2. (b); 3. (c); 4. (b); 5. (c)

REFERENCES

1. Bo, K., Frawley, H. C., Haylen, B. T., Abramov, Y., Almeida, F. G., Berghmans, B., Bortolini, M., Dumoulin, C., Gomes, M., McClurg, D., Meijlink, J., Shelly, E., Trabuco, E., Walker, C., & Wells, A. (2016). An International Urogynecological Association (IUGA)/International Continence Society (ICS) joint report on the terminology for the conservative and nonpharmacological management of female pelvic floor dysfunction. *Neurourology and Urodynamics*, *36*(2), 221–244. https://doi.org/10.1002/nau.23107
2. Ali, L., Tahira, B., Iqrar, A., et al. (2016). Utility of intraoperative neurophysiological monitoring (IONM) in various surgeries at a tertiary care hospital in Karachi, Pakistan. https://core.ac.uk/download/47264786.pdf (accessed on 14th June 2025).
3. Alingh Prins, A., Scheurink, A., Steffens, A. B., Steffens, A. B., Steffens, A. B., Steffens, A. B., Steffens, A. B., et al. (1996). Overfeeding, autonomic regulation and metabolic consequences. https://core.ac.uk/download/pdf/12942087.pdf (accessed on 14th June 2025).
4. Ang, R., Opel, A., & Tinker, A. (2012). The role of inhibitory G proteins and regulators of G protein signaling in the *in vivo* control of heart rate and predisposition to cardiac arrhythmias. https://core.ac.uk/download/30697484.pdf (accessed on 14th June 2025).
5. Angert, M., Chernov, A. V., Dolkas, J., et al. (2015). The alternatively spliced fibronectin CS1 isoform regulates IL-17A levels and mechanical allodynia after peripheral nerve injury. https://core.ac.uk/download/323064557.pdf (accessed on 14th June 2025).
6. Arenas, A., Babloyantz, A., Bezerianos, A., Brovelli, A., Goldberger, A., Pikovsky, A., Tarca, A., et al. (2010). Rhythmic dynamics and synchronization via dimensionality reduction: Application to human gait. https://core.ac.uk/download/45296.pdf (accessed on 14th June 2025).
7. Arendt-Nielsen, L., Basson, A., de-la-Llave-Rincón, A. I., et al. (2023). Carpal tunnel syndrome: Neuropathic pain associated or not with a nociplastic condition. https://core.ac.uk/download/580117506.pdf (accessed on 14th June 2025).
8. Attarbaschi, A., Barzilai, S., Escherich, G., et al. (2016). Consensus definitions of 14 severe acute toxic effects for childhood lymphoblastic leukemia treatment: A Delphi consensus. https://core.ac.uk/download/42370388.pdf (accessed on 14th June 2025).
9. Bahey, N. G., Bailey, M. E. S., Cobb, S. R., et al. (2017). Reduced axonal diameter of peripheral nerve fibers in a mouse model of Rett syndrome. https://core.ac.uk/download/84148418.pdf (accessed on 14th June 2025).
10. Balaban, Z., & Kurt, G. (2023). Neurotransmitters of autonomic nervous system. https://core.ac.uk/download/588401315.pdf (accessed on 14th June 2025).
11. Barnes, V. A., Cearley, S. M., Junca, S., et al. (2017). The dynamic role of breathing and cellular membrane potentials in the experience of consciousness. https://core.ac.uk/download/131210584.pdf (accessed on 14th June 2025).
12. Barnes, V. A., Crawford, M. W., Harden, K., et al. (2014). Widespread depolarization during expiration: A source of respiratory drive? https://core.ac.uk/download/131210052.pdf (accessed on 14th June 2025).
13. Barton, M. J., Clarke, M., Ekberg, J., et al. (2017). The glia response after peripheral nerve injury: A comparison between Schwann cells and olfactory ensheathing cells and their uses

for neural regenerative therapies. https://core.ac.uk/download/196605084.pdf (accessed on 14th June 2025).

14. Berezikov, E., Bischoff, R., de Boer, R. A., et al. (2000). The development and subsequent elimination of aberrant peripheral axon projections in *Semaphorin3A* null mutant mice. https://core.ac.uk/download/pdf/82176684.pdf (accessed on 14th June 2025).
15. Bianchi, L., Cavallari, E. N., Ceccarelli, G., et al. (2017). Improvement of neuropsychological performances and reduction of immune-activation markers after probiotic supplementation and change of lifestyle in an HIV positive male: Targeting the microbiota to act on gut-brain axis. https://core.ac.uk/download/141694703.pdf (accessed on 14th June 2025).
16. Boivin, A., Constant, A., Walter, A., Bachstetter, A. D., McColl, A., Winner, B., Fife, B. T., et al. (2016). TLR7-mediated skin inflammation remotely triggers chemokine expression and leukocyte accumulation in the brain. https://core.ac.uk/download/42371113.pdf (accessed on 14th June 2025).
17. Brincker, M., & Torres, E. (2017). Why study movement variability in autism? https://core.ac.uk/download/131210732.pdf (accessed on 14th June 2025).
18. Broide, R. S., Chen, Y., Leslie, F. M., et al. (2019). Distribution of α7 nicotinic acetylcholine receptor subunit mRNA in the developing mouse. https://core.ac.uk/download/323075429.pdf (accessed on 14th June 2025).
19. Brust, P., Creeley, C., Feldman, R., Grandjean, P., Herken, H., Panzica, G., et al. (2014). Neurotoxicity. https://core.ac.uk/download/286729125.pdf (accessed on 14th June 2025).
20. Buchman, V. L., Millership, S., Ninkina, N., et al. (2013). γ-synuclein is a novel player in the control of body lipid metabolism. https://core.ac.uk/download/42130506.pdf (accessed on 14th June 2025).
21. Carpaneto, J., Citi, L., Dario, P., et al. (2010). Decoding information from neural signals recorded using intraneural electrodes: Toward the development of a neurocontrolled hand prosthesis. https://core.ac.uk/download/9995711.pdf (accessed on 14th June 2025).
22. Chang, L. W., Jones, E. A., Krueger, C., et al. (2011). Regulation of the PMP22 gene through an intronic enhancer. https://core.ac.uk/download/70382013.pdf (accessed on 14th June 2025).
23. Chin, C. T., Jacques, L., Lee, A. T., et al. (2019). Schwannomatosis of the spinal accessory nerve: A case report. https://core.ac.uk/download/323075253.pdf (accessed on 14th June 2025).
24. Critchley, H. D., Gray, M. A., Harrison, N. A., et al. (2009). Following one's heart: Cardiac rhythms gate central initiation of sympathetic reflexes. https://core.ac.uk/download/2710256.pdf (accessed on 14th June 2025).
25. Crowe, C. M., Dickinson, P. J., Giuffrida, M., et al. (2020). Clinicopathological characteristics of histiocytic sarcoma affecting the central nervous system in dogs. https://core.ac.uk/download/323069047.pdf (accessed on 14th June 2025).
26. D'Alessandro, A., Esposito, G., Gigli, S., et al. (2018). Endocannabinoid-related compounds in gastrointestinal diseases. https://core.ac.uk/download/127586499.pdf (accessed on 14th June 2025).
27. De Caro, R., Fenu, G., Macchi, V., et al. (2011). *KISS1* and *KISS1R* expression in the human and rat carotid body and superior cervical ganglion. https://core.ac.uk/download/11692080.pdf (accessed on 14th June 2025).

28. Della-Flora Nunes, G., Feltri, M. L., He, B., et al. (2021). Activation of mTORC1 and c-Jun by Prohibitin1 loss in Schwann cells may link mitochondrial dysfunction to demyelination. https://core.ac.uk/download/490700174.pdf (accessed on 14th June 2025).
29. Doan, A. T., Evans, J. J., Kenning, T. J., et al. (2016). Intraoperative neurophysiological monitoring for endoscopic endonasal approaches to the skull base: A technical guide. https://core.ac.uk/download/83050037.pdf (accessed on 14th June 2025).
30. Dorsher, P. (2009). The neuroanatomic basis of the acupuncture principal meridians. https://core.ac.uk/download/pdf/288827.pdf (accessed on 14th June 2025).
31. Draper, A. C. E., & Piercy, R. J. (2018). Pathological classification of equine recurrent laryngeal neuropathy. https://core.ac.uk/download/157583314.pdf (accessed on 14th June 2025).
32. Falla, D., Lluch, E., Meeus, M., et al. (2014). Influence of shoulder pain on muscle function: Implications for the assessment and therapy of shoulder disorders. https://core.ac.uk/download/55799562.pdf (accessed on 14th June 2025).
33. Federici, A., Zenzola, A., Xu, A., Akay, M., Aldroubi, A., Simone, F., Gonnella, G., et al. (2005). Response of autonomic nervous system to body positions: Fourier and wavelet analysis. http://arxiv.org/abs/physics/0310125 (accessed on 14th June 2025).
34. Federico, A., Taylor, C., Denny, C. A., Kirschner, D. A., Hauser, E. C., Kaye, E. M., Norflus, F., et al. (2007). Peripheral nervous system manifestations in a Sandhoff disease mouse model: Nerve conduction, myelin structure, lipid analysis. https://core.ac.uk/download/pdf/7696008.pdf (accessed on 14th June 2025).
35. Gasser, P. J., & Lowry, C. A. (2018). Organic cation transporter 3: A cellular mechanism underlying rapid, non-genomic glucocorticoid regulation of monoaminergic neurotransmission, physiology, and behavior. https://core.ac.uk/download/213087190.pdf (accessed on 14th June 2025).
36. Giannini, A. M., Haggard, P., Leemhuis, E., et al. (2019). The homuncular jigsaw: Investigations of phantom limb and body awareness following brachial plexus block or avulsion. https://core.ac.uk/download/188832051.pdf (accessed on 14th June 2025).
37. Ginanneschi, F., Mazzocchio, R., Milani, P., et al. (2010). Progesterone–new therapy in mild carpal tunnel syndrome? Study design of a randomized clinical trial for local therapy. https://core.ac.uk/download/pdf/8411226.pdf (accessed on 14th June 2025).
38. Häming, D. (2012). Evolution and development of the sympathetic nervous system. https://core.ac.uk/download/12011354.pdf (accessed on 14th June 2025).
39. Hofmann, M. H., Meyer, D. L., & Wullimann, M. F. (1991). The valvula cerebelli of the spiny eel, *Macrognathus aculeatus*, receives primary lateral-line afferents from the rostrum of the upper jaw. https://core.ac.uk/download/12164204.pdf (accessed on 14th June 2025).
40. Hunt, K. J., & McLean, A. N. (2002). Exciting innovations for the spinally injured. https://core.ac.uk/download/1633337.pdf (accessed on 14th June 2025).
41. Jacobs, D. K., Valencia, J. E., & Winchell, C. J. (2010). Confocal analysis of nervous system architecture in direct-developing juveniles of *Neanthes arenaceodentata* (Annelida, Nereididae). https://core.ac.uk/download/4886525.pdf (accessed on 14th June 2025).
42. Jones, L., Richardson, H., & Saint, R. (2000). Tissue-specific regulation of cyclin E transcription during *Drosophila melanogaster* embryogenesis. https://core.ac.uk/download/12750286.pdf (accessed on 14th June 2025).

43. Konczak, J. (2005). On the notion of motor primitives in humans and robots. https://core.ac.uk/download/pdf/86573.pdf (accessed on 14th June 2025).
44. LeCouteur, R. A., & Vernau, K. M. (1999). Feline vestibular disorders. Part II: Diagnostic approach and differential diagnosis. https://core.ac.uk/download/323068734.pdf (accessed on 14th June 2025).
45. MacRobert, A. J., Phillips, J. B., & Wright, K. E. (2007). Intracellular localization of mTHPC and effect of photodynamic therapy in cells of the mammalian peripheral nervous system. https://core.ac.uk/download/81856.pdf (accessed on 14th June 2025).
46. Micallef Stafrace, K., & Psaila, M. (2015). An unexpected cause of palmar paranesthesia in a soldier: A case report. https://core.ac.uk/download/46603556.pdf (accessed on 14th June 2025).
47. N/A. (2016). GBS100: Celebrating a century of progress in Guillain-Barré Syndrome. https://core.ac.uk/download/74362846.pdf (accessed on 14th June 2025).
48. Pésinho, I. V. (2019). Multiple sclerosis vs. Guillain-Barré syndrome: Differences in two autoimmune disorders with a common target in two different regions. https://core.ac.uk/download/322655387.pdf (accessed on 14th June 2025).
49. Staubach, S. (2008). *Evolution Der Cephalic Sensory Organs Interhall Der Opisthobranchia*. https://core.ac.uk/download/14505921.pdf (accessed on 14th June 2025).
50. Wang, T. (2011). Neurturin's role in sensory neuron plasticity. https://core.ac.uk/download/12208716.pdf (accessed on 14th June 2025).

AUTONOMIC NERVOUS SYSTEM

4

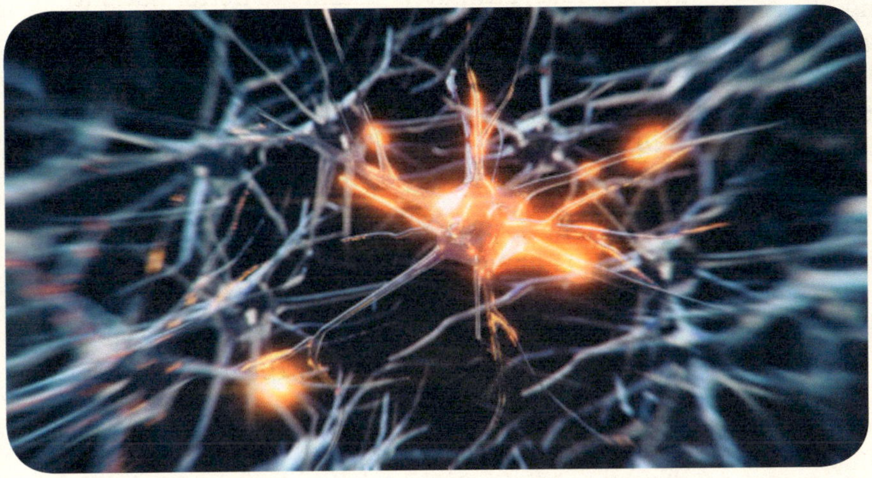

LEARNING OBJECTIVES

After studying this chapter, you will be able to:

1. Discuss the structures of the autonomic nervous system
2. Describe the functions of the autonomic nervous system
3. Discuss the neurotransmitters of the autonomic nervous system
4. Emphasize the autonomic nervous system and health
5. Study diagnostic resources for autonomic jumpy system diagnosis
6. Assess the treatment and management of autonomic disorders

Introduction

The autonomic nervous system (ANS) plays a critical role in the maintenance of homeostasis in the human body, for the most part working subconsciously. It regulates involuntary bodily functions such as heart rate, blood pressure, respiration, digestion, and sexual arousal. The ANS is neatly lumped into three categories: the sympathetic, parasympathetic, and enteric nervous systems. Each of these divisions works in conjunction with the others to manage physiological response, from the fight-or-flight response initiated by the sympathetic system to the rest-and-digest functions mediated by the parasympathetic system. Not only is learning about the sophistication of the ANS valuable for comprehending elementary human physiology, but also for examining the interconnectedness of mind and body health, as this system has a direct correlation to stress and emotional well-being. Recent research highlights a significant link between practices like yoga and the improvement of the adaptability of the ANSs, revealing its potential benefits in addressing mental illness and reducing stress. Naming an example, regular yoga practice has the potential to improve neural resilience and adaptive capacity in the case of the ANS and create new avenues for the treatment of mental illness. Research has illustrated that yoga can considerably affect the nervous system's adaptive capacity, promoting better physical and psychological health. As the literature presents, yoga methods, especially respiratory maneuvers, have been associated with decreases in cortisol levels, a hormone indicating stress, thus increasing autonomic function and emotional regulation (Biesok et al., 2024). This implies that lifestyle treatments focused on the ANS may bring significant benefits to overall health. In addition, note should be taken of the implications of autonomic dysfunction in comparison to other chronic diseases.

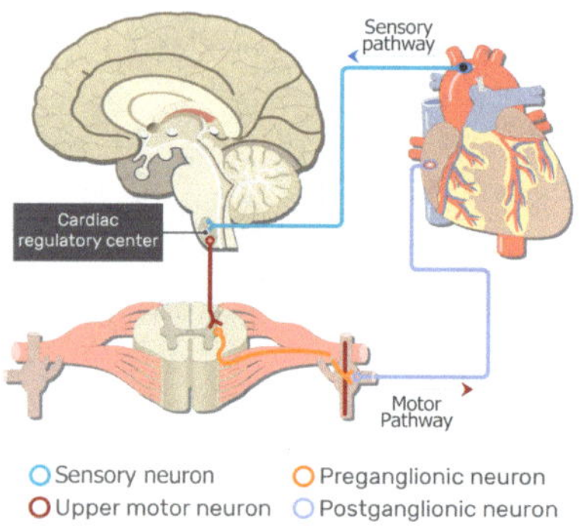

Figure 4.1. Sample-autonomic-nervous-system-pathways.

Source: https://www.getbodysmart.com/wp-content/uploads/2017/10/Sample-Autonomic-Nervous-System-Pathways-Labeled-1024x1024.png.

Fibromyalgia, for example, which affects about 2% of the population, reflects the synergistic relationship of the autonomic nervous system with pain mechanisms that define chronicity. The disease is characterized by an array of symptoms ranging from fatigue, headaches, to sleep disorders, which make treatment regimens challenging (Dorsher, 2008). A neuroendocrinologic model of fibromyalgia places particular value on knowing the pathophysiology of interdependencies between body and mind in the treatment of the disorder. Through continued exploration of the capabilities of the ANS in these conditions, clinical practitioners can design holistic approaches that not only alleviate symptomatology but also work to the direct autonomic processes at their core, ultimately leading to better patient management and resilience to states of chronic disease (Figure 4.1).

Definition of the Autonomic Nervous System

The ANS is a primary homeostatic regulatory system that regulates a large variety of involuntary physiological events. It functions without conscious control to regulate basic functions like the rate of heartbeat, breathing rate, digestion, and blood pressure. The very intricate system is roughly divided into three primary systems: the sympathetic nervous system, the parasympathetic nervous system, and the enteric nervous system. Every component has a unique contribution to body regulation, such as the sympathetic system's activation of the fight or flight response for stressful states and the parasympathetic system's dominance in resting states, allowing recovery and energy conservation. Therefore, the ANS not only maintains an equilibrated internal environment but also allows the body to respond adaptively to both internal and external stimuli, thereby clarifying its central function within human physiology. The definition of the autonomic nervous system goes beyond visceral function regulation; it is an interaction between neural and hormonal responses that adapts to the various needs of the body. The complicated structure of the ANS is a typical case of distributed cognition, where multiple sensors and neural pathways collaborate to realize homeostasis without one supreme executive system commanding every movement. This decentralized organizational structure encourages a rethinking of volition and decision-making in physiological contexts. Since Christensen et al. (2006) contend, the lack of a unified integrated control center means that regulation of internal states emerges from the dynamic interactions between more basic cognitive systems rather than from some central volitional agency. The implications of this perspective extend to the research into diseases and disorders involving these neural interactions that are in disarray, producing dysfunctional autonomic function. In addition, the relationship between the ANS and higher mental processes makes this nervous system central to psychological and neurological debates, primarily the mind-body problem. (Motofei et al., 2017) considers that the difference between somatic brain processes and abstract psychological processes provides an avenue for exploration of the interrelationship between autonomic functions and cognitive experience in terms of reasoning and judgment. As far as various autonomic responses bear influence on emotional states and decisional processes, the formation of an understanding of the ANS should encompass both its physiologic contributions and its psychological importance. This dual anxiety at once enriches the definition of the autonomic nervous system. It propels future research to understand how these complex interactions shape our mental lives and overall well-being. So, the ANS begs a nuanced answer that recognizes its foundational significance in both body and mind.

Importance in Human Physiology

The ANS plays a very crucial role in maintaining homeostasis in the human body, which is vital for survival. It regulates involuntary bodily functions like heart rate, digestion, and respiratory rate. With its two divisions, i.e., the sympathetic and parasympathetic nervous systems, the ANS provides a dynamic equilibrium that is essential during stress states as well as during relaxation. The sympathetic branch prepares the body for "fight or flight" responses, triggering processes such as increased heart rate and increased alertness. The parasympathetic branch, conversely, promotes "rest and digest" processes, facilitating recovery and energy conservation. Through the process of balancing these opposing functions, the autonomic nervous system directly contributes to physiological processes, maintaining health, illustrating the sophisticated interaction between body systems necessary for human physiology. Moreover, the significance of the autonomic nervous system transcends the complexity of heart rate regulation and cardiovascular functioning. Recent findings have unveiled the inhibitory heterotrimeric G protein's role in the regulation of heart rate through ion channel function, thus emphasizing the biochemical basis of cardiac regulation. Through the regulation of heartbeat frequency, the ANS exerts an immediate influence on the circulation, oxygenation, and metabolic processes in the body. This interaction is of special significance in the case of exercise, stress, and relaxation, when the response of the heart needs to be fast and by the body's changing demands. Awareness of the processes through which the ANS controls the heart rate and cardiovascular health in general gives us vital information about ailments like arrhythmias and hypertension, further underlining the system's significance within the context of human physiology (Ang et al., 2012). Further, the ANS is at the heart of the delicate interplay between neurophysiology and higher body function. The relationship between visceral systems and neurophysiology underscores the importance of such autonomic control in physical as well as mental health. For instance, control over visceral organs is not only a physiological function but also exerts influences on psychological status and exhibits psychosomatic correlations. Autonomic nervous system disorders have various mechanisms of action leading to diverse symptoms, including anxiety, gastrointestinal disorders, and blood pressure fluctuations. Investigating these relationships is helpful in improving our understanding of physiological science and for the creation of new therapies. Through research in the fields of physiological cybernetics and artificial intelligence-assisted health monitoring, scientists can gain deeper insight into the regulatory function of the Autonomic Nervous System in health and disease and highlight its crucial importance in human physiology (Lange, 2025) (Figure 4.2).

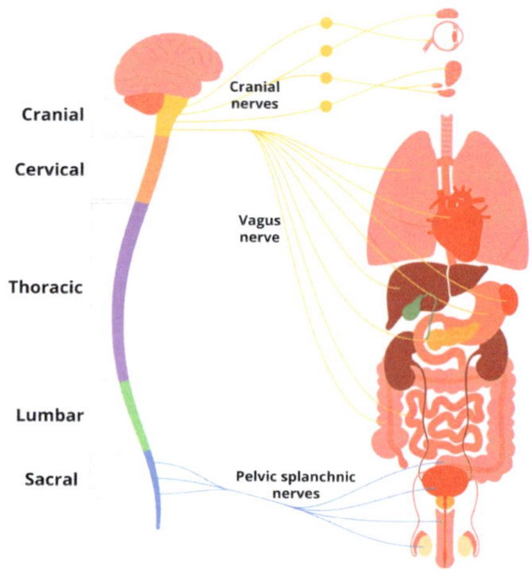

Figure 4.2. Structure-of-the-parasympathetic-system.

Source: https://teachmeanatomy.info/wp-content/uploads/Structure-of-the-Parasympathetic-System-949x1024.png.

4.1. Components of the Autonomic Nervous System

Learning Outcome

1. Describe the sympathetic nervous system
2. Focus on the parasympathetic nervous system
3. Learn about the enteric nervous system

Autonomic nervous system (ANS) is a complex and vital aspect of human physiology, which regulates involuntary action to bring homeostasis. ANS is usually divided into three functional systems, namely the sympathetic, parasympathetic, and enteric nervous systems. The sympathetic nervous system prepares the body for fight or flight when there is stress, such as an increased rate of heartbeat, dilated pupils, and secretion of adrenaline. Conversely, the parasympathetic nervous system is in charge of rest and digest processes, for inducing relaxation and recuperation by reducing heart rate and augmenting digestive processes. The enteric nervous system, or second brain, regulates gastrointestinal function independently but also interacts with the other two systems, illustrating the intricate balance needed for maintaining health and reacting to environmental change dynamically. Investigating the role of heart rate variability (HRV) is an educational way in which to view the activity of the autonomic nervous system. HRV reflects the balance between autonomic sympathetic and parasympathetic inputs and is prognostic for the understanding of a person's cardiovascular health. HRV modifications have also been found to be present in conditions such as chronic cerebral ischemia and angina pectoris, and these serve to illustrate how autonomic regulatory disturbance can be manifested clinically. Such as, diminution of parasympathetic activity, as would be expected in patients who are unwell with such conditions as chronic cerebral ischemia, might manifest as augmentation of the low-frequency spectral components of heart rate variability. These findings indicate that it is necessary to measure autonomic function through HRV analysis to identify risk and tailor therapy for cardiovascular patients (Inhula et al., 2018). Further research into the divergence of physiological reactions elicited by the autonomic nervous system as the body is altered between positions further reaffirms its critical role in maintaining cardiovascular homeostasis. Research employing methods such as wavelet transformations has shown that different body positions yield differing responses in blood pressure and heart rate variability, showing how the ANS compensates to maintain balance. Specifically, such trials involving comparison between supine and head-down tilt postures have revealed enormous differences between low-frequency and very low-frequency blood pressure and heart rate components, pointing to a dynamic pattern that reflects responding to changing external and internal demands. The ability of the ANS to regulate cardiovascular parameters adaptively in response to posture change emphasizes its key role in controlling the body's capability to respond maximally to environmental stimuli to ensure optimal functioning under the various states of physical activity (Federici et al., 2005) (Figure 4.3).

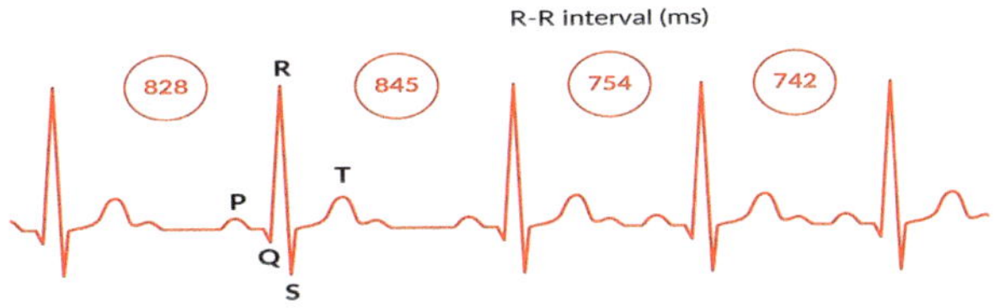

Figure 4.3. Heart rate variability (HRV).

Source: https://www.firstbeat.com/wp-content/uploads/2018/04/heart-rate-variability-firstbeat.jpg.

4.1.1. Sympathetic Nervous System

The sympathetic nervous system (SNS), a significant component of the autonomic nervous system, is primarily responsible for the fight or flight function of the body so that rapid physiological modifications can be achieved under stress or danger. This intricate system functions by virtue of an interweaving of pathways that originate in the thoracic and lumbar regions of the spinal cord. When stimulated, the SNS secretes catecholamines, including adrenaline and norepinephrine, which stimulate increased heart rate, high blood pressure, and mobilization of energy. The body is thus preadapted to respond at once in order to survive under conditions of threat. The SNS operates not only in states of acute stress but also plays a significant role in regulating body functions under normative states, i.e., digestion and thermoregulation, demonstrating its dual role in emergency and homeostatic processes. Under psychological and physiological well-being, the sympathetic nervous system can have beneficial and detrimental effects. Continuous stimulation of the SNS, most often triggered by chronic stress or anxiety, can lead to a variety of health issues, including cardiovascular disease, metabolic syndromes, and psychiatric illness. For instance, constant hyperactivity of the SNS can generate continuous high blood pressure and tachycardia with serious consequences. In addition, the hyperactivity is able to influence the autonomic balance by disturbing the balance with the parasympathetic nervous system (PNS), which is associated with rest and digestion. Understanding the health implications of sympathetic activation guides the development of interventions in stress management as well as overall treatment approaches that are directed towards psychological as well as somatic symptoms of stress-related disorders (Li et al., 2025). Besides, recent research recognizes the synergy between the sympathetic nervous system and various therapeutic approaches, including the use of psychedelics. Evidence demonstrated that certain psychedelics have the ability to influence autonomic processes by regulating SNS activity, offering interesting insight into cardiovascular well-being and stress reaction (Li et al., 2023). This relationship emphasizes the need for a better understanding of the SNS both in the context of traditional physiological considerations but also in exploring new psychiatric treatments. Explanation of how substances can act upon the SNS permits researchers to develop targeted therapies that capitalize upon the intrinsic relationships between states of physiology and states of mind. These developments will ultimately contribute to new types of health care, emphasizing the integrated nature of the autonomic nervous system and its role in presenting a unified image of human health (Figure 4.4).

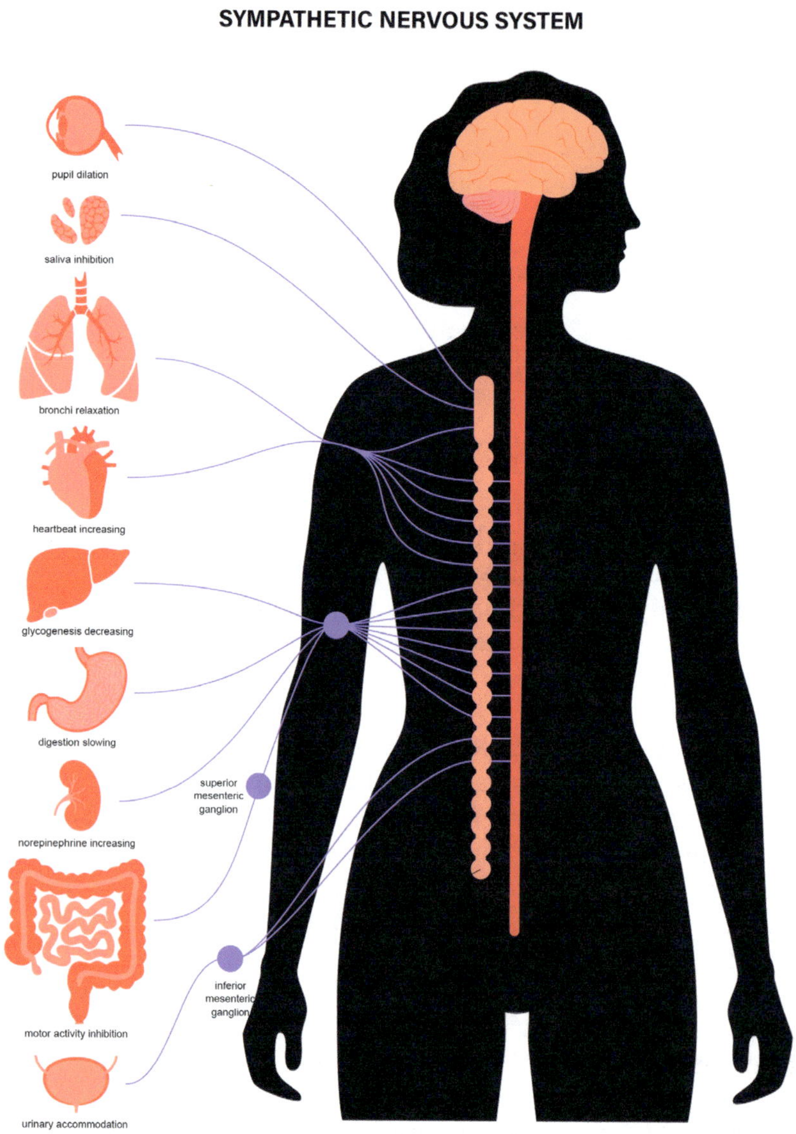

Figure 4.4. Sympathetic-nervous-system.

Source: https://www.simplypsychology.org/wp-content/uploads/Sympathetic-Nervous-System.jpeg.

4.1.2. Parasympathetic Nervous System

The PNS plays a significant role in the overall scheme of the ANS and is primarily responsible for inducing a state of rest and digest. This branch of the ANS conserves energy by initiating relaxation and assisting in the functions of digestion when the body has experienced stress. The PNS accomplishes this through neurochemical communication, using acetylcholine as its primary neurotransmitter, which acts upon many target organs. Through its action to slow heart rate, enhance intestinal and gland function, and relax sphincter muscles, the PNS reverses the aroused state induced by its counterpart, the SNS. This fine balance between sympathetic and parasympathetic divisions is required for maintenance of homeostasis, thereby highlighting the importance of the PNS in general health and well-being. Research has suggested that impaired function of the PNS may lead to severe health issues, particularly in obese and metabolic disorder patients. When 100 volunteers were studied, it was observed that parasympathetic activity was extremely low among obese patients, as reflected by a very impaired standing to lying ratio, a significant autonomic dysfunction measure (Grewal et al., 2011). This loss of parasympathetic control can predispose the individual to a range of cardiovascular complications, since the body is unable to control its resting function and adequately respond to environmental stimuli. As such, understanding the mechanisms of the PNS is not just crucial in the mitigation of current health issues but also in the formulation of prevention methods to safeguard cardiovascular well-being. Furthermore, the effect of chronic stress on the PNS complicates the interpretation of the interactions between body health and mental well-being. Stress activates the SNS, usually leading to a predominance of sympathetic responses that can inhibit parasympathetic function after a duration of time. Such an imbalance may contribute to the pathogenesis of most stress disorders, which explains why means of improving the PNS function are applied in the clinical environment. These practices, such as mindfulness, relaxation, and regulated breathing, have been seen to stimulate PNS function and thus reverse the harmful consequences of chronic stress. This is founded on an understanding that health interventions must tackle both the psychological and physiological dimensions, bridging the rift between different healthcare therapies in pursuing to comprehend the blending of body and mind (Estrine et al., 2006) (Figure 4.5).

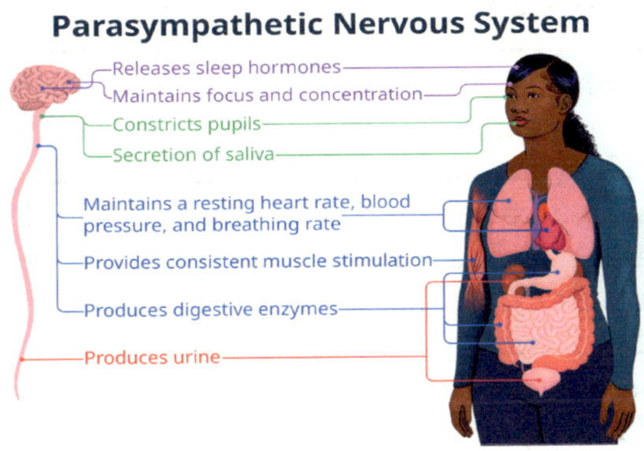

Figure 4.5. Parasympathetic nervous system.

Source: https://www.verywellhealth.com/thmb/H7h3nagrjjGQqcMjxcd4NkqJ__g=/1500x0/filters:no_upscale():max_bytes(150000):strip_icc()/ParasympatheticNervousSystemPSNS-v1-8992348880a4400aa46680b8113b4433.png.

4.1.3. Enteric Nervous System

The enteric nervous system (ENS), or the "second brain," is a central part of the ANS responsible for regulating gastrointestinal function apart from the CNS. Made up of approximately 100 million neurons, this sophisticated network of neural components strategically resides in the walls of the gastrointestinal tract. It is tasked with regulating such processes as peristalsis, blood flow, and secretory processes. Because it is conventionally considered to be a subservient aspect of the ANS, the ENS has been recognized to have independent functions, exhibiting high sophistication and functional independence placing it well within the running as a likely contender for serious participation in the general regulation of the body, bridging gastrointestinal well-being with overall physiological and psychological health (Steinhart et al., 2001). As research into the ENS expands, its contribution to disease and health is increasingly elucidated. The cross-talk between the ENS and the CNS highlights the bidirectional communication between these two systems and provides windows for further advanced understanding of gut-brain axis function. Valuable information has been gleaned regarding the function of enteric neurotransmitters like serotonin and ATP, which play pivotal roles in gut motility and sensation. Above all, the function of purinergic signaling has come to be understood, where ATP acts as a cotransmitter in the peripheral and central nervous systems. This is not just true in gastrointestinal disease but even in conditions such as anxiety and depression because the neurochemical microenvironment of the ENSs can have profound effects on emotional and cognitive function (Burnstock et al., 2009). Thus, demystifying the complex interactions between ENS function and psychological well-being remains a relevant research focus. The examination of the possible functions of the ENS in the various pathological conditions is also compounded by its involvement in the autonomic control processes. Irritable bowel syndrome and inflammatory bowel disease are examples of functional gastrointestinal illnesses that can arise from dysregulation of the enteric circuits, highlighting the critical connection between the ENS and general health. Research has come to focus more on the role of neuron-glial interactions of the ENS and their relation to neuropathologies, with indications that alterations in this network can be associated with alterations in gut flora or inflammation. Clarification of how the ENS reacts to stressors or damage offers therapeutic potential, emphasizing its integrative role within the ANS. The ENS not only affects gastrointestinal health but also plays a central role in the integrated network of systems that support homeostasis in the entire body (Steinhart et al., 2001).

Test Your Knowledge

1. What are the two main divisions of the autonomic nervous system?
2. Which division of the ANS is responsible for the 'fight or flight' response?

4.2. Functions of the Autonomic Nervous System

Learning Outcome

1. Explain the regulation of involuntary bodily functions
2. Define the role in stress response
3. Learn about the impact on homeostasis

The ANS is tasked with regulating involuntary physiological activity, which enables elementary functions to be performed unconsciously. ANS is primarily composed of two systems: the sympathetic and parasympathetic nervous systems, which are in charge of varied responses to internal and external stimuli. The sympathetic nervous system is also referred to as the fight or flight system and is tasked with inducing a body response when there is a need for stress. For instance, the system increases blood pressure, dilates airways, and shunts blood supply to essential organs and thereby prepares the body for activity. Conversely, the parasympathetic system, or rest and digest system, facilitates recuperation and relaxation. It assists in digestion, slows heart rate, and conserves energy, illustrating a balancing interplay required for homeostasis. This regard for function underscores the ANS's pivotal role in body equilibrium. Apart from homeostasis, the ANS is also intricately involved in stress and emotional modulation through its physiological actions. Stimulation of the sympathetic nervous system with stress can cause physiological alterations that affect health; for example, prolonged stimulation of the sympathetic nervous system can lead to increased blood pressure and elevated cortisol levels, which could have effects on long-term health. The parasympathetic nervous system, on the other hand, can undo stress effects through recovery and relaxation and thus enhance general well-being. Recent research has also been conducted on whether variation in responding to stress, in turn influenced by attachment styles, will also affect physiological outcomes. For instance, individuals with secure attachment styles may react to stress with adaptive physiological responses, while insecurely attached individuals may express heightened reactivity. Identifying these dynamics also underscores the importance of the ANS not just in physical health but in emotional and psychological resilience (Ainsworth et al., 2014). Additionally, the ANS is networked with other physiological systems, a sign of the complexity and interrelatedness of bodily functions. Inhibitory heterotrimeric G proteins, for instance, play a critical role in the heart by governing heart rate through the action of G protein-coupled receptors. Such proteins can decelerate the heart rate following numerous stimuli, reflecting the ANS's effectiveness in managing cardiovascular health. The breaking of this pathway has been shown to create deleterious cardiovascular outcomes, making it essential to understand the network of regulators that influence heart functioning (Ang et al., 2012). In short, the functions of the ANS are more complex than mere control over automatic reactions; they involve connection with emotional and cognitive processes, highlighting the system's pivotal contribution to general well-being and resilience in the wake of life's numerous adversities (Figure 4.6).

Functions of ANS	
Sympathetic	Parasympathetic
► Heart	► Heart
► ↑ heart rate	► ↓ heart rate
► ↑ force of contraction	► ↓force of contraction
► Blood vessels	► Blood vessels
► *Constriction*	► No effect
► Lungs	► Lungs
► Bronchodilation	► Bronchoconstriction
► GIT	► GIT
► ↓ motility	► ↑ motility
► Sphincter contraction	► Sphincter relaxation
► Decreased secretions	► Increased secretions

Figure 4.6. Functions of autonomic nervous system.

Source: https://howmed.net/wp-content/uploads/2010/09/functions-of-autonomic-nervous-system.bmp.

4.2.1. Regulation of Involuntary Bodily Functions

Control of involuntary bodily functions is precisely managed by the ANS, whose workings operate primarily below the conscious level. The system is composed of two large branches: the sympathetic and parasympathetic nervous systems. The sympathetic division is responsible primarily for the body's fight or flight response, producing instantaneous physiological changes upon stress by increasing heart rate, dilating airways, and redirecting blood supply to essential organs. Unlike the sympathetic branch, the parasympathetic branch is involved in rest and digest functions that drive body processes such as digestion and storing energy. There is a balance required between the two branches to attain homeostasis, wherein the body can adapt to varying amounts of physical as well as environmental pressure and also accommodate necessary involuntary functions such as breathing and cardiac regulation. Recognition of the biomechanical processes of autonomic function illustrates the complexity of physiological regulation, particularly with the mechanism of respiration. Not only does breathing deliver life through gas exchange, but, through modulation of cardiac rhythms and blood pressure, it also significantly influences cardiovascular health. For instance, changes in heart rate with inhalation and exhalation can lead to changes in autonomic tone as well as overall cardiovascular health. Research indicates that respiration is a modulator of cellular membrane potential, with inspiration relating to widespread minor hyperpolarization and expiration relating to depolarization. This delicate interaction identifies respiratory drive as a potential therapeutic target for conditions like anxiety and hypertension, citing the importance of investigating such automatic functions to uncover both physiological mechanisms and broader clinical utility (Barnes et al., 2014). The ANS regulation is more complex than mere automatic function since it displays the interlinked intertwining of neural, hormonal, and environmental effects. Dysregulation of the ANS may adopt variable clinical presentations, particularly in individuals with autism spectrum disorder, in which aberrant autonomic function might be an index of associated generalized physiological challenges. Research suggests that the person with autism may face difficulties with both peripheral and central nervous system functioning, which may be responsible for creating the heterogeneity of their behaviors and coping mechanisms. Determination of such multi-level factors is crucial for creating efficient evaluations and interventions. Knowledge of the role of micro-movements and their relation to autonomic responses can shed light on cognitive development and regulation mechanisms (Brincker et al., 2017). Therefore, the study of automatic functions demonstrates a rich interface among basic biological processes and their complex implications for health and behavior (Figure 4.7).

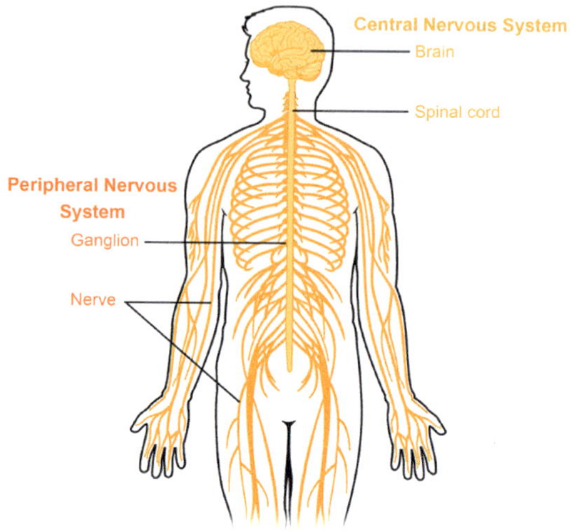

Figure 4.7. Peripheral nervous system functions.

Source: https://qbi.uq.edu.au/files/38434/Nervous_System.jpg.

4.2.2. Role in Stress Response

The ANS is at the center of the physiological stress response, controlling several basic body functions. Comprising two broad branches—the sympathetic and parasympathetic systems—the ANS regulates the body's involuntary reactions to internal and external stimuli that occur with stress. The sympathetic branch is activated primarily in a state of stress, and this creates physiological reactions such as a heightened rate of heartbeats, a rise in blood pressure, and increased alertness, all of which prepare the body for a fight or flight scenario. The parasympathetic branch, on the other hand, controls relaxation and recuperation, facilitating restoration to homeostasis. The delicate balance between these two branches is not only crucial for immediate stress responses but also for long-term effects on health. Sustained sympathetic system activation can lead to chronic states of stress, quite aptly illustrating the ANS's critical role in maintaining overall well-being. Research points to the interplay between stress responses and brain function regulated by the ANS. Under stressful conditions, the brain activates various neural circuits, which subsequently trigger hormonal responses largely linked with the ANS. This is most evident in the regulation of the hypothalamic-pituitary-adrenal (HPA) axis, which governs the secretion of cortisol, a key stress hormone. Elevated levels of cortisol can affect numerous body systems, usually resulting in mood disorders, cardiovascular illness, and impaired immune function. Furthermore, coordination of heart and respiratory functions, particularly during meditation, is a testament to the ANS's role in modulating stress response (Barnes et al., 2014).

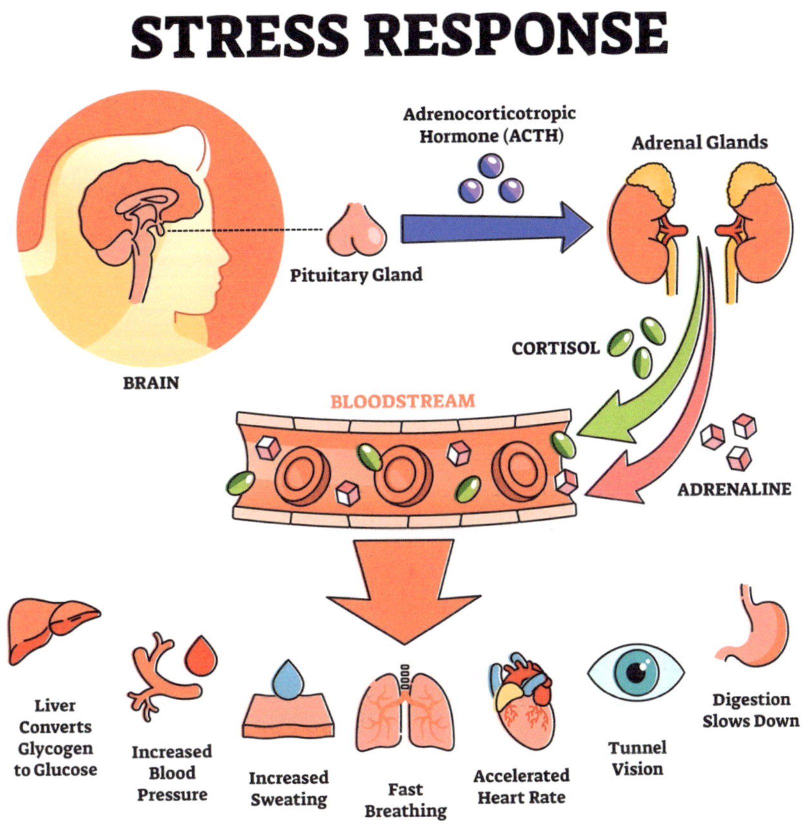

Figure 4.8. Stress response.

Source: https://www.simplypsychology.org/wp-content/uploads/hpa-stress-response.jpeg.

Recognition of these dynamics provides the foundation for further research into specially targeted intervention that utilizes the restorative capacity of the ANS in reducing the harmful consequences of stress. In the clinical management of the ANS implications, it is necessary to identify the double tracks of health intervention: those focused on neurological functions and those that focus on bodily health. Conventional paradigms in medicine prefer the head-up approach, emphasizing brain-centered interventions and ignoring complex messaging between the brain and the body (Estrine et al., 2006). However, with an integrated frame of mind that appreciates bidirectional communication between the central nervous system and the ANS, therapeutic protocols for disease of stress can be optimized. Techniques such as meditation, relaxation, and biofeedback are the best practices that can easily stimulate the parasympathetic system to alleviate stress effects. With a complete understanding of ANS's role in responding to stress, medical experts can better address the overall needs of individuals experiencing stress-related problems (Figure 4.8).

4.2.3. Impact on Homeostasis

Homeostasis, or the body's capacity for maintaining stable internal conditions, is largely regulated by the ANS. The ANS controls involuntary functions of the body, including heart rate, digestion, and breathing rate, which are essential for maintaining homeostasis in the presence of changing external environments. Employing stressors, the fight or flight response is engaged by the sympathetic branch of the ANS, leading to such physiological responses as increased heart rate and blood pressure. Although these adaptations prepare the body to act, they cause homeostatic disruptions if the stress lasts (Barnes et al., 2014). Chronic stimulation of the sympathetic nervous system can ultimately result in such diseases as hypertension and metabolic disease, illustrating the necessity for adaptive processes that restore equilibrium to the body. Conversely, the parasympathetic branch of the ANS plays an essential role in recovery and restoration of homeostasis. Relaxation behaviors such as meditation have been reported to activate parasympathetic activity, which has been found to synchronize cardiorespiratory rhythms. This synchronization helps to modulate neuronal function along the autonomic pathways and may lead to favorable physiological changes, for instance, reduced amygdala activity associated with stress responses. Induction of calm through stimulation of the parasympathetic nervous system not only enables emotional control but also ensures homeostatic stability through balancing sympathetic activation. Becoming parasympathetically dominant is crucial in the maintenance of overall health and functioning, encapsulating the delicate balance that the ANS must achieve (Barnes et al., 2014). Moreover, new therapeutic methods, such as INH, illustrate the plasticity of the ANSs to engage in homeostasis in varied clinical situations. Indeed, research shows that INH is effective in enhancing autonomic function, particularly in cerebral palsy and epilepsy patients, by facilitating sympathetic-parasympathetic equilibrium. This maximizes cardiovascular function and lung capacities, thereby stimulating homeostasis repair. The efficacy of INH underscores the importance of developing the ANS for general health, particularly in groups that have encountered varying extrinsic stressors, such as those subjected to contaminated environments. By stimulating higher vegetative centers, INH constitutes a practical intervention to help achieve homeostasis and re-establish biological balance, illustrating the flexibility of the ANS in responding to different challenges.

Test Your Knowledge

1. How does the autonomic nervous system regulate heart rate and blood pressure?
2. What role does the parasympathetic division play in digestion?

4.3. Neurotransmitters in the Autonomic Nervous System

Learning Outcome

1. Explain the acetylcholine and norepinephrine
2. Describe the neuropeptides and hormones

The ANS is vital in regulating involuntary physiological responses, such as heart rate, digestion, and respiratory rate, through the action of several neurotransmitters. Of significance are acetylcholine, norepinephrine, and epinephrine, which provide for communication between peripheral organs and the central nervous system. Acetylcholine, primarily active in the parasympathetic branch, ensures a state of rest, while norepinephrine and epinephrine, associated with the sympathetic branch, prepare the organism for stress and conditions of emergency. The neurotransmitters also influence the emotional and cognitive functions, besides the visceral functions. It is critical to recognize the individual functions of these chemical messengers for the creation of targeted treatments of psychological disorders, since dysregulation in neurotransmitter activity within the ANS has been correlated with anxiety disorders and mood instability. In unraveling the complex interrelation between emotions and the autonomic nervous system, it is revealed that neurotransmitters not only mediate physiological change but also modulate emotional experience. Under stress situations, high norepinephrine leads to high sympathetic activity that creates hyperarousal states. Under favorable emotional conditions, on the other hand, a higher concentration of acetylcholine tends to stimulate the parasympathetic system to create feelings of relaxation and calmness. Research emphasizes the significance of cardiorespiratory coherence (CRC) in understanding emotional state, where negative emotions lower CRC, suggesting a shift towards sympathetic dominance, and positive emotions elevate it, suggesting parasympathetic dominance. This interactive process that it would be possible to control neurotransmitter function through cognitive and behavioral techniques, which may offer evidence-based practical techniques in treating mood and anxiety disorders, as elucidated through various therapeutic modalities. Several recent studies suggest that integrative methods, such as meditation and controlled breathing exercises, may prove to be practical add-ons or substitutes for pharmacotherapy in controlling emotional dysregulation related to neurotransmitter imbalance. Through the regulation of autonomic nervous system activity, these techniques can improve homeostasis and check sympathetic dominance induced by stress. Specifically, clinicians report that exercises in breath control and meditation complement CRC, possibly via brainstem and limbic system mechanisms linking feedback from emotional and physiological states. Such effects, being beneficial, form the basis for new treatment approaches focusing on the management of neurotransmitters in the ANS rather than reliance on drugs. Hence, a greater knowledge of how neurotransmitters influence both the physiological and affective response is essential for proceeding with therapeutic intervention for stress, anxiety, and related disorders, as highlighted in current research (Barnes et al., 2015; Crawford et al., 2015).

4.3.1. Acetylcholine

Acetylcholine (ACh) is a key neurotransmitter within the ANS, regulating a wide range of physiological activities. Found as a key component in both the sympathetic and parasympathetic branches, ACh influences numerous processes, including cardiac rhythm, digestion, and glandular secretion. Release of ACh at synapses between target organs and neurons binds to cholinergic receptors, enabling nervous system communication. Significantly, its role transcends mere transmission; ACh also plays a significant role in modulating synaptic action, and thus the effectiveness of neural communication. Its dual role underscores its importance in ensuring homeostasis throughout an organism, showing its utility in addressing environmental stimuli as much as internal balance. Moreover, the specifics of AChs mechanism underscore its sophistication as a functionary of the ANS. The neurotransmitter elicits its actions primarily through two forms of receptors: nicotinic and muscarinic receptors. Fast synaptic transmission, particularly at neuromuscular junctions and autonomic ganglia, is due to ionotropic nicotinic receptors. Metabotropic muscarinic receptors are primarily involved in slower, longer-term signaling, and this results in a variety of physiological effects in organs such as the heart, lungs, and gastrointestinal tract. This variation in receptor allows for fine control of body function, varying responses to meet the needs of the specific situation. It also positions ACh as a central mediator in processes such as bronchoconstriction, slowing heart rate, and gastrointestinal motility, further highlighting its pivotal position in ANS function. While acetylcholine is essential to proper autonomic function, its deregulation can result in significant health issues. For instance, ACh level imbalances are the cause of a range of neurodegenerative conditions, including Alzheimer's disease, with cholinergic neuron loss. In addition, hyperactivation of ACh results in cholinergic toxicity symptoms, with impairment of cognitive, respiratory, and muscle functions. Also, the interactions between neurotransmitters, such as the role of adenosine triphosphate (ATP) as an autonomic nerve co-transmitter, highlight the complexity of neurotransmission within the ANS (Cunha et al., 2000). The understanding of the acetylcholine pathways and mechanisms is essential for both the appreciation of normal autonomic processes and the development of therapeutic strategies for autonomic dysregulation-related disorders (Brust et al., 2014) (Figure 4.9).

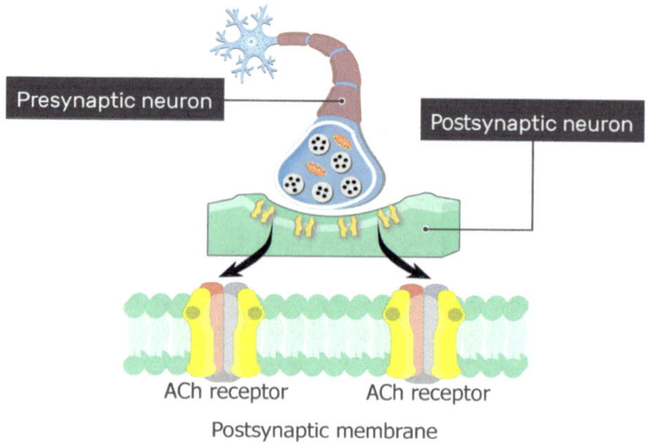

Figure 4.9. Acetylcholine (Ach) receptors.

Source: https://www.getbodysmart.com/wp-content/uploads/2017/09/Acetylcholine-Receptors-Labeled-1024x767.png.

4.3.2. Norepinephrine

Norepinephrine, the autonomic nervous system's central neurotransmitter, is also crucial in mediating the body's response to stress and homeostasis. As a significant component of the sympathetic nervous system, norepinephrine is responsible for facilitating the "fight or flight" response, characterized by increased heart rate, blood pressure, and energy expenditure. This life-threatening response allows individuals to respond rapidly to threatening situations. In the case of other conditions, such as postural orthostatic tachycardia syndrome (POTS), elevated norepinephrine levels underscore the complex interaction between autonomic control and neurotransmission. POTS patients, for instance, exhibit marked elevations in plasma norepinephrine with upright posture, indicative of increased sympathetic activity that underlies the symptomatology expressed in such patients, including fatigue and tachycardia (Raj et al., 2006). Understanding norepinephrine's complex roles in the autonomic nervous system is essential to the revelation of its significance in health and disease. Apart from its role in the acute stress response, norepinephrine is significant in the regulation of metabolic mechanisms, particularly in obesity and overfeeding. Research indicates that excessive calorie intake affects autonomic function, typified by modulation of both sympathetic and parasympathetic outflow. Increases in baseline plasma norepinephrine have been described in animal models subjected to hyperphagia, with suggestions that this is an adaptive response to preserve energy substrate homeostasis (Prins et al., 1996). This increased sympathetic tone is essential to the augmentation of lipolysis and energy mobilization during times of overindulgence in caloric intake. This adaptive response can be dampened and lead to decreased release of norepinephrine during exercise in overfeeding states.

Therefore, maintaining precise control over norepinephrine levels is vital to keep metabolism and prevent the ill consequences that typically result from obesity. Furthermore, dysregulation of norepinephrine transmission in the autonomic nervous system has a profound influence on cardiovascular well-being. The sympathetic nervous system, through the release of norepinephrine, not only controls heart rate but also vascular tone and blood pressure. Sustained elevation of norepinephrine levels, common among patients with conditions such as hypertension, can lead to excessive vasoconstriction and increased workload on the heart. This underscores the therapeutic importance of norepinephrine as a target for the management of cardiovascular disease and autonomic dysfunction. Furthermore, restoration of a normal ratio of norepinephrine can abrogate the functional abnormalities of many autonomic disorders, including POTS. Overall, understanding norepinephrine's multi-faceted impact on the autonomic nervous system is key to the resolution of the complex interplay between neurotransmission, metabolism, and cardiovascular health (Figure 4.10).

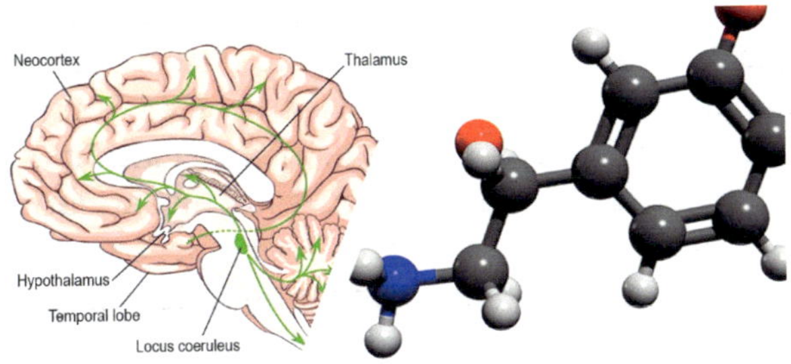

Figure 4.10. Norepinephrine function.

Source: https://draxe.com/wp-content/uploads/2019/07/norepinephrine-header.jpg.

4.3.3. Other Neuropeptides and Hormones

The ANS is primarily responsible for regulating various physiological processes, and its influence does not end with classical neurotransmitters but extends to a variety of neuropeptides and hormones. Notably, these molecules, such as neuropeptide Y (NPY) and vasoactive intestinal peptide (VIP), play critical roles in functions such as stress response, circulatory regulation, and gastrointestinal processes. NPY, produced primarily in sympathetic nervous system neurons, is a potent modulator of anxiety and stress by ensuring energy conservation under stress. Similarly, VIP is involved in gastrointestinal motility and vascular tone modulation, reflecting its role as a key coordinator between the nervous and gastrointestinal systems. Collectively, these neuropeptides illustrate the interconnected networks through which the ANS affects not only autonomic processes but also emotion and cognition, indicating the system's far-reaching implications. Research into other hormones, such as oxytocin and cortisol, continues to illustrate complex interactions within the ANS. Oxytocin, also referred to as the bonding hormone, illustrates the neuroendocrine connections of the ANS, influencing social behavior and emotional response. Conversely, cortisol, a key stress hormone, underscores the impact of the ANS on metabolic processes and cardiovascular health. Excess production of cortisol, typically secondary to chronic sympathetic activation, leads to allostatic load, which is linked to numerous diseases, including hypertension and metabolic syndrome. This intricate relationship emphasizes the need for further investigation into the impact of the regulatory processes of these hormones and their autonomic function, as their release and formation usually react to the same environmental stimuli that target the ANS. The interaction between neuropeptides, hormones, and the ANS is needed to comprehend the manyfold responses of the human body. Current evidence suggests an active nature in efficacy and deployment of such neurochemical signals, highlighting their ability to modulate the plasticity of neurons in response to environmental alterations and chronic stress. For instance, the neuroendocrine system is connected by positive and negative feedback loops, including channels between them, where disequilibrium leads to disease. This balance is worth knowing because it can create new pathways for the treatment of diseases like metabolic illness and anxiety disorders that are rooted in dysregulation of these systems. There has also been proposed a neurovisceral integration model, hypothesizing that autonomic circuits not only convey signals but actively modify states of neurochemicals and, therefore, affect gene expression and health outcomes (Martins et al., 2016; Domínguez Vías et al., 2021).

Test Your Knowledge

1. Which neurotransmitter is released by preganglionic neurons in both sympathetic and parasympathetic divisions?
2. What is the primary neurotransmitter released by postganglionic sympathetic neurons?

4.4. Autonomic Nervous System and Health

Learning Outcome

1. Identify the disorders related to autonomic dysfunction
2. Define the impact of stress on the autonomic system
3. Describe the role in chronic illnesses

ANS is needed to maintain homeostasis, upon which overall well-being relies. ANS is divided into sympathetic and parasympathetic branches, both of which have a contrasting effect on body function. The sympathetic branch triggers the "fight or flight" mechanism during stress, preparing the body to respond at once by increasing heart rate and redirecting blood flow to crucial muscles. The parasympathetic branch, on the other hand, initiates a "rest and digest" state with the possibility of relaxing and recovering processes. With the loss of balance between these systems, particularly chronic stress, adverse effects on health can ensue. Dysregulation from the loss of balance can lead to conditions such as hypertension, anxiety, and metabolic disease, thereby showing the ANS's important role in health maintenance and disease susceptibility. Habitual stress has proved to be a significant determinant of the activity of the ANS. Altered autonomic regulation can manifest in a broad spectrum of physical and mental disorders, ranging from emotional disturbances to cardiovascular illnesses. In line with recent research, there exists a profound correlation between the emotional status of an individual and the functional capacity of the ANS. Especially where stress is a chronic aspect of life, the sympathetic system will become overstimulated, leading to fatigue in mental and physical well-being. For this reason, understanding how the brain controls stress reactions and their consequent effects on body functions is essential. The imbalance between healthcare approaches focused on either psychological or physiologic causes serves to underscore the necessity for a more integrated perception of health and wellness, calling attention to the centrality of the ANS as an integrating force in this complex dynamic (Estrine et al., 2006). New approaches to crossing the interface between emotional well-being and the ANS have emerged on the horizon, including methods such as those outlined by the Institute of HeartMath. Their work sheds light on the physiological advantages of pleasant emotional states and how they might affect autonomic function. One key feature of their findings is that of physiological coherence as a distinctive pattern of functioning during prolonged positive emotions, which triggers positive health responses. Techniques such as Freeze-Frame® and Heart Lock-In® have proven effective in stress reduction through the induction of a coherent state, which impacts the mental, emotional, and physiological state of an individual. By altering the stress response and facilitating positive emotional experience, these methods highlight the importance of adding emotional health to strategies aimed at enhancing the health of the autonomic nervous system (Childre et al., 2002) (Figure 4.11).

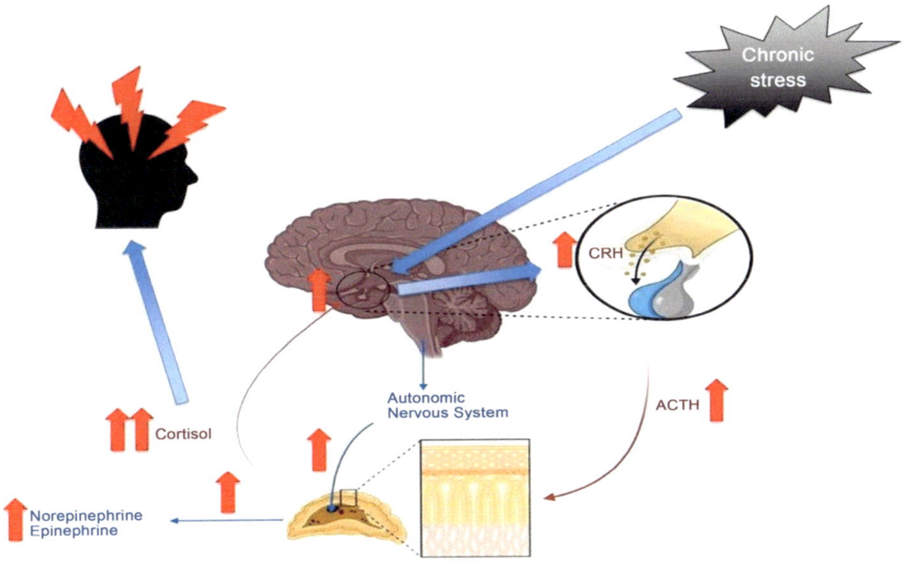

Figure 4.11. The role of the HPA axis and autonomic nervous system.

Source: https://www.mdpi.com/biomedicines/biomedicines-13-00463/article_deploy/html/images/biomedicines-13-00463-g002.png.

4.4.1. Disorders Related to Autonomic Dysfunction

Autonomic dysfunction disorders are a range of clinical manifestations that significantly influence quality of life. ANS regulates automatic physiological activities, such as heart rate, gastrointestinal peristalsis, and blood pressure. Dysregulation of the system may lead to a range of disorders, such as postural orthostatic tachycardia syndrome (POTS) and orthostatic hypotension. POTS is an inappropriately increased heart rate with standing, and most commonly, this leads to dizziness, fatigue, and palpitations. Orthostatic hypotension is a sudden drop in blood pressure on standing and may lead to falls and syncope. The widespread nature of these conditions is emphasized by findings showing that between 25% of children and nearly 70% of adults present with autonomic dysfunction symptoms, making it a significant public health problem that warrants recognition and further investigation into mechanisms and treatments (Simonenko et al., 2017). The relationship between central disorders and autonomic dysfunction, such as disorders that are characterized by hypersomnolence, also demonstrates the complexity of the ANS. Research has indicated that patients with type 1 narcolepsy and other sleep disorders frequently exhibit autonomic symptoms, ranging from abnormal cardiac functions to difficulties with thermoregulation. These symptoms not only interfere with everyday functioning but also lead to long-term health complications. The pathophysiological processes underlying such autonomic impairments remain largely unclear; however, even though studies have demonstrated that orexin/hypocretin neuronal deficits may be associated with such narcolepsy disturbances.

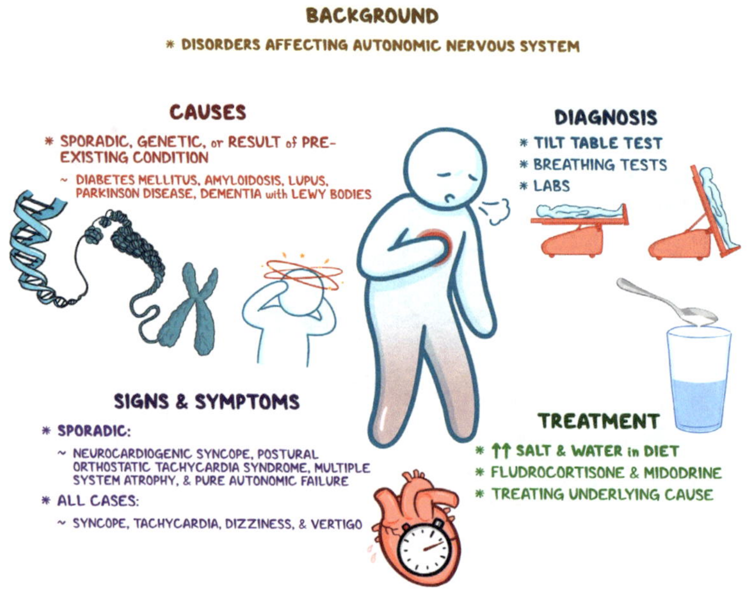

Figure 4.12. Disorders related to autonomic dysfunction.

Source: https://d16qt3wv6xm098.cloudfront.net/-r9bBRFoQ8qvuzJe-oa-sI-NRFe2vjU7/_.png.

Current treatments primarily focus on symptom alleviation with wake-promoting agents, but this raises issues of their impact on autonomic function and associated cardiovascular risks (Silvani et al., 2023). Detailed elucidation of such relationships is thus paramount in providing holistic patient care. Psychological processes also play a significant role in the formation of autonomic dysfunctions. Studies among groups such as medical students have shown associations between psychological traits and autonomic reactivity. Studies have shown that strongly extraverted students are likely to show non-stability of the higher nervous function, a condition associated with hyperergic autonomic reactions like sympathicotonia. This opens the door for the potential for psychological distress to exacerbate autonomic disorders, thereby potentially forming a self-perpetuating cycle of somatic symptomatology and psychological disturbance. The overlap between psychological health and autonomic dysfunction highlights the need to include psychological assessment as part of the diagnostic process. By doing so, clinicians become capable of understanding the intricate nature of autonomic disorders and creating interventions that touch both physiological and psychological aspects of patients' health (Simonenko et al., 2017) (Figure 4.12).

4.4.2. Impact of Stress on the Autonomic System

The ANS plays the central function in the body's physiological reaction to stress, directing the alterations necessary for survival. In response to a stressor, the sympathetic branch of the ANS is activated, providing the signal for fight or flight. This includes increased heart rate, raised blood pressure, and the discharge of stress hormones cortisol and adrenaline. These responses, no less critical in acute situations, become deleterious when stress is persistent. Chronic activation of the sympathetic system over a prolonged period can have adverse health effects, including cardiovascular disease, obesity, and anxiety disorders. The impact of stress on the ANS reveals a complex interplay between psychological and physiological events, reminding us of the significance of viewing health as an overall phenomenon, encompassing the mental as well as the physical experience (Estrine et al., 2006). Chronic stress powerfully alters the balance between the sympathetic and parasympathetic branches of the ANS, resulting in an autonomic dysfunction state. Under normal operating conditions, the parasympathetic nervous system, or rest and digest system, acts against sympathetic arousal. Chronic stress, however, will inhibit parasympathetic activity, producing a lack of recovery from stress and generating chronic physiological tension. This dysregulation is responsible for most disease, including gastrointestinal disease and immune system suppression. Also, the autonomic imbalance linked with stress highlights the importance of emotional health in maintaining physiological welfare. The body's capacity for physiological coherence, which is crucial for optimal functioning and emotional regulation, will deteriorate as chronic stress persists (Childre et al., 2002). Understanding the impact of stress on the autonomic system translates to creative interventions that can reverse its harmful effects. Techniques that promote relaxation and emotional regulation, such as the HeartMath techniques, have gained more popularity during recent decades.

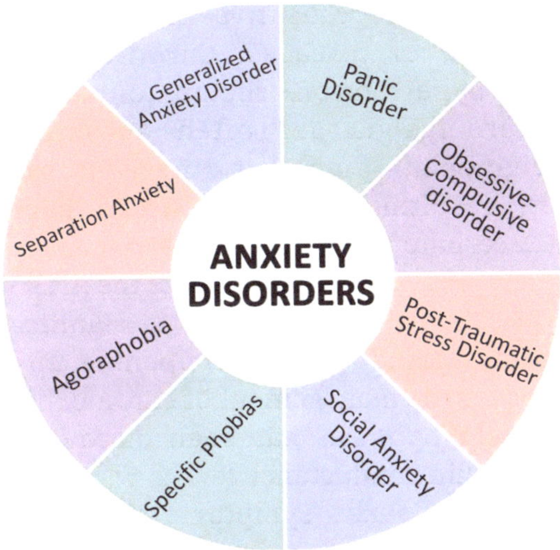

Figure 4.13. Understanding the different types of anxiety disorders and their symptoms.

Source: https://video.curegrid.co/dj/media/post_banners/Screenshot_2024-11-19_at_10.34.40AM.png.

Research has shown that the methods can enhance physiological coherence, which is characterized by synchrony in numerous body systems, leading to improved emotional and physiological well-being. Through the stimulation of positive emotions, people can engage the parasympathetic division of the ANS, which assists in recovery and health. Finally, this understanding speaks to the primary significance of the autonomic nervous system not only in responding to stressors but also in facilitating healing and resilience to life's challenges. As the relationship between stress and the ANS becomes increasingly understood, it is likewise crucial that healthcare systems embrace a holistic model that heals both emotion and body (Estrine et al., 2006) (Figure 4.13).

4.4.3. Role in Chronic Illnesses

Understanding the role of the ANS in chronic disease necessitates a detailed review of its regulatory function, particularly in sympathetic and parasympathetic predominance. The ANS plays a pivotal role in maintaining homeostasis but can also be causative in developing a wide range of diseases. Chronic illnesses such as hypertension, rheumatoid arthritis, and fibromyalgia are often accompanied by heightened sympathetic nervous system activity, resulting in chronic stress reactions that exacerbate the disease. Research has found that therapies that act to modulate the ANS, such as hypnosis, have been found to significantly reduce sympathetic outflow, opening up new avenues for the management of chronic disease. Specifically, hypnosis has been discovered to diminish skin conductance levels, which means that it can alleviate symptoms of conditions the severity of which is greatly determined by the sympathetic nervous system and redirect the treatment approaches utilized for chronic diseases (Kekecs et al., 2015). Application of stress management skills within the treatment plan of chronic diseases emphasizes the significant connection between emotional regulation and physiological well-being. Chronic stress not only makes the sympathetic nervous system work more, but also interferes with parasympathetic functioning required for recovery and restoration. Training programs in emotional self-management, like those involving police officers, have phenomenal reductions in unhealthy physiological responses caused by chronic stress. Interventions that bring emotional equilibrium and mental acuity can lead to the enhancement of aspects of life that are major contributors towards inducing stress, e.g., interpersonal relationships and organizational processes (Tomasino et al., 1999). The above evidence indicates that such interventions should be incorporated into chronic illness management to enable greater well-being as well as perhaps neutralize the vicious cycles of stress and physical deterioration. The potential for including ANS-focused interventions in chronic disease management is further supported by the nervous system's capacity for adapting to therapeutic interventions. As much as patients with chronic diseases are often caught up in vicious cycles of stress-mediated exacerbation, interventions focused on the ANS can not only result in symptom control but also in overall improvement in quality of life in the patient. The decline in sympathetic activation associated with therapies such as hypnosis highlights the critical role of the ANS in the control of chronic illness, with the inference that successful modulation of its response will pay dividends in the long term. Furthermore, ensconcing an overall integrated treatment approach and considering interlinked physical, psychological, and environmental factors is key to building systematic treatment regimens for chronic illness. Interaction with the subtlety of the ANS allows practitioners and patients access to resilience and healing in chronic disease, maximizing therapy efficacy as well as patient outcome.

Test Your Knowledge

1. How can dysregulation of the autonomic nervous system contribute to conditions such as hypertension or heart failure?
2. What are the common symptoms and physiological effects of autonomic neuropathy, and which diseases are commonly associated with it?

4.5. Diagnostic Tools for Autonomic Nervous System Assessment

Learning Outcome

1. Describe the heart rate variability analysis
2. Define the blood pressure response tests
3. Discuss the autonomic reflex testing

The measurement of the ANS is not just important for the study of body functions but also for the diagnosis of diseases in which there is autonomic dysfunction. A variety of diagnostic methods has been created, each providing useful information about the functioning of sympathetic as well as parasympathetic branches of the ANS. Traditional techniques like heart rate variability (HRV) analysis focus on the interrelationship between respiratory rhythms and heart rate, which can inform us regarding autonomic regulation in the numerous states of health and disease. Latest advances have also optimized the methods further, for example, in the use of biofeedback technology to enhance awareness and voluntary regulation of autonomic function, showing potential therapeutic directions for disorders like anxiety and stress disorders.

Providing precise diagnostics is crucial to determine the underlying causes of autonomic dysregulation to facilitate timely intervention. Micro-movement analysis has proven to be a useful tool in the assessment of the ANS, particularly in conditions such as elevated physiological sensitivity, e.g., autism spectrum disorder (ASD). Evidence demonstrates that small, involuntary movements are indicators of autonomic function that yield an objective quantification of systemic response not accessible with more traditional measures. Notably, the novel approaches combine continuous biometric data with observational ratings, exemplified in studies utilizing data extracted from databases like the autism brain imaging data exchange (ABIDE I-II). Through the observation of involuntary head movements and their correlated physiological rhythms, scientists have found it possible to dissect subgroups in the autistic population that differ in severity levels and contribute to our knowledge of movement behavior interaction with autonomic regulation.

These observations highlight the need for new analytical tools to uncover the subtle characteristics of autonomic functioning in heterogeneous populations. The integration of emerging diagnostic technologies makes it possible to comprehend the ANS in several dimensions, allowing for more effective clinical enhancements through specially tailored interventions. Computerized cluster analysis of behavioral data, for instance, can refine the diagnostic process by differentiating among various phenotypes within conditions like autism, facilitating the identification of nuanced differences in symptom expression. The confluence of observed behaviors with the more subtle autonomic rhythms enforces the utility of complete assessments based on both subjective and objective markers.

As can be understood from studies employing statistical models to separate data by gender in ASD, the applications of autonomic assessment are not only in the diagnosis of individuals but in informing larger discussions of developmental trajectories and the physiological underpinnings of neurodiversity. In conclusion, the creation of these diagnostic tools is meant to highlight the need for ongoing research and development aimed at improving our understanding of the autonomic nervous system's involvement in human behavior and illness (Figure 4.14).

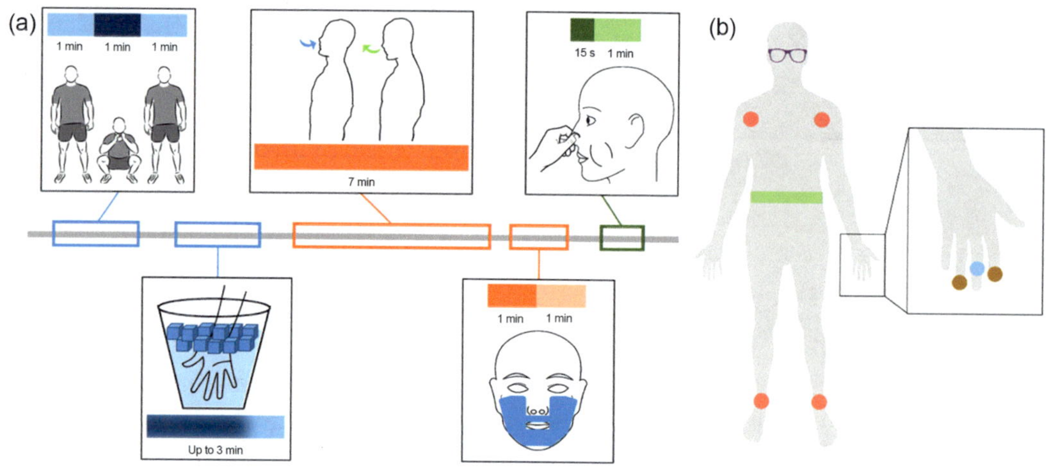

Figure 4.14. A method to quantify autonomic nervous system function in healthy.

Source: https://media.springernature.com/lw1200/springer-static/image/art%3A10.1186%2Fs42234-021-00075-7/MediaObjects/42234_2021_75_Fig1_HTML.png.

4.5.1. Heart Rate Variability Analysis

Heart rate variability (HRV) analysis is a critical component of the assessment of ANS activity and its sympathetic-parasympathetic balance. HRV refers to the body's capacity to recover from stressors, such as heart rate variability over time, and can potentially provide information about physiological and psychological health. By measuring HRV in both the time-domain and frequency-domain indices, researchers can gain insights into autonomic control and predict various health outcomes. Time-domain measures such as the standard deviation of NN intervals (SDNN) and root mean square of successive differences (RMSSD), for instance, inform about global autonomic tone. Conversely, frequency-domain measurements capture the distribution of power among oscillations of heart rate, which illuminates the interaction between parasympathetic and sympathetic limbs and thereby the dynamic nature of central nervous modulation of heart rate. Other investigations note the relationship of HRV to cognition, particularly in older individuals. A study with geriatric patients found a significant positive correlation between scores on tests of higher cognitive function, such as the mini-mental state examination (MMSE), and greater sympathetic activation reflected by various HRV indices, including SDNN and low frequency (LF) components. More significantly, in this study, increased sympathetic activation, rather than decreased vagal activity, was associated with better cognitive function in the elderly. These findings confirm that HRV is not only a cardiovascular health biomarker but also an essential measure for evaluating cognitive dynamics, hence providing a more integral picture of how autonomic function contributes to the total mental acuity with which individuals age, substantiating the significance of sympathetic influence in aging cognitive function (Dalise et al., 2020). Aside from cognitive applications, HRV analysis is also essential for understanding autonomic maturation in vulnerable populations, such as preterm infants. Evidence suggests HRV can be measurable quantitatively at birth and possibly indicate preterm infant ANS maturation. One longitudinal study reported considerable improvement in HRV measurements during hospital stay, suggesting improvement in parasympathetic and sympathetic activity. These results indicate that monitoring HRV could be a non-invasive way to assess autonomic maturation and predict long-term neurological status in preterm infants, as variations in the values of HRV describe their clinical course. This conforms to the overall view of ANS adaptation, suggesting that cardiac rhythm dynamics play a crucial role in evaluating developmental as well as maturation processes in various patient populations, thereby advancing predictive health strategies across multiple age groups (Martins et al., 2019).

4.5.2. Blood Pressure Response Tests

Blood pressure response tests are a valuable clinical tool for assessing the ANS's functional status. Tests that investigate the ability of the body to regulate blood pressure with an assortment of stimuli are indicative of sympathetic and parasympathetic system interaction. By employing methods such as stress testing for postural change or exercise, scientists can assess the ANS's proficiency at integrating cardiovascular responses. For instance, calibrated massage pressures were used and demonstrated significant results in rodent models, wherein varying pressure intensities brought measurable changes in systolic blood pressure. Specifically, pressures of 20 mm Hg and 40 mm Hg brought significant percentage reductions in blood pressure, which indicates the ANS's mediatory effect on cardiovascular control in the presence of external stressors that is similar to results attributed to autonomic control in human subjects. In addition to baseline and reflex blood pressure reactions, these measurements can diagnose illnesses like postural tachycardia syndrome (POTS). POTS is characterized by an inappropriate heart rate response to standing that is often accompanied by orthostatic intolerance and other disabling symptoms. Blood pressure response tests are helpful in the detection of the autonomic dysfunction present in patients with POTS, usually manifested by increased plasma norepinephrine and decreased blood volume. Coupled with clinical symptoms, blood pressure response assessments can provide a complete characterization of a patient's autonomic status and guide therapeutic interventions to normalize autonomic function and minimize symptoms. Thus, such tests are beneficial in clinical settings, facilitating the identification of autonomic dysregulation within various populations of patients. Furthermore, measurement of responses to blood pressure testing can provide underlying information regarding autonomic control mechanisms and their impact on health. As an example, the ratio of low-frequency to high-frequency activity, a crucial index of autonomic tone, was observed to rise considerably following specific massage pressures. This rise suggests greater sympathetic activity secondary to greater mechanical stimuli, indicating how the body may be manipulated in autonomic output to regulate cardiovascular requirements. Such findings not only enhance the pathophysiologic mechanisms of blood pressure regulation but also lay the ground for novel therapeutic strategies. Grasping the blood pressure response tests concerning the ANS essentially leads to a deeper appreciation of cardiovascular disease and health, with the importance of autonomic balance being key to maintaining homeostasis (Figure 4.15).

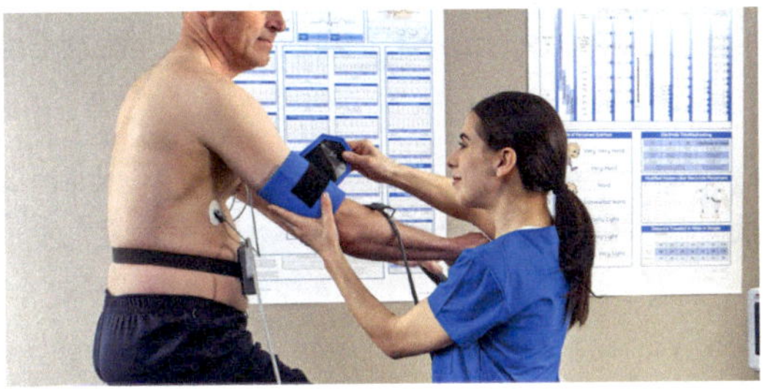

Figure 4.15. Blood pressure response during exercise stress testing.

Source: https://clinicalview.gehealthcare.com/sites/default/files/styles/hero_fallback/public/Man%20in%20a%20treadmill%20800x600.png?h=6416edf4&itok=YBdRzgNg.

4.5.3. Autonomic Reflex Testing

The subtlety of autonomic reflex testing is of key importance in evaluating ANS function. Examination comprises a battery of tests designed to assess sympathetic as well as parasympathetic responses to various stimuli. Cardiovascular measures like blood pressure and heart rate are recorded under controlled circumstances so that clinicians can be informed regarding autonomic regulation. These tests, like the Valsalva maneuver and the deep breathing tests, are standard components of autonomic testing, playing a significant role in patient diagnostics. Surprisingly, a single test cannot offer an integrated impression; thus, the application of more than one test is recommended to enhance diagnostic reliability and accuracy. As such, autonomic reflex testing emerges as a relevant diagnostic tool that sheds light on the neurophysiological status of patients, particularly when tailored to the individual situation and response (Siepmann et al., 2019). Among all the measures derived from autonomic reflex testing, sudomotor function emerges as a critical area to explore. Sudomotor reflex testing assesses the functional integrity of the sympathetic nervous system about sweat production, which may be compromised in a vast array of conditions like autonomic neuropathies and neurodegenerative disorders. Tests like the Sudoscan are not only indicative of the functioning of the sweat glands but are also markers of more generalized autonomic impairment at an earlier stage. This aspect of testing is particularly insightful, given the fact that impaired sweating can significantly impair a patient's quality of life. Therefore, sudomotor tests are a precious adjunct to cardiovascular assessments, providing a more holistic appreciation of autonomic health and the multi-dimensional ramifications of autonomic dysfunction (Siepmann et al., 2019). Improvements in autonomic reflex testing methods, driven by recent innovations, further attest to the ongoing refinement of diagnostic protocols for assessing autonomic nervous system function. Researchers are exploring tools like the Quantitative Direct and Indirect Axon Reflex Testing and the Sudoscan to minimize the technical challenges that have always accompanied such evaluations. Not only do these devices ensure greater diagnostic accuracy, but they also work to reduce interindividual variability, further facilitating patient evaluation. Early studies with conditions such as primary Sjögrens syndrome have demonstrated quantifiable correlations between symptoms of autonomic dysfunction and outcomes of cardiovascular reflex tests and implied diagnostic value for such tests in various clinical environments. As the body of work in this area grows, the role of advanced autonomic reflex testing in mapping and managing several pathologies may grow, ultimately leading to improvement in patient care and outcomes.

Test Your Knowledge

1. What is the purpose of the tilt table test, and how does it help diagnose autonomic dysfunction?
2. How are heart rate variability (HRV) measurements used to assess autonomic nervous system balance?

4.6. Treatment and Management of Autonomic Disorders

Learning Outcome

1. Describe the pharmacological interventions
2. Define the lifestyle modifications of the autonomic nervous system (ANS)
3. Understand the Alternative therapies of the autonomic nervous system (ANS)

The treatment and management of autonomic disorders are intricate and require an in-depth understanding of the complex functions of the autonomic nervous system. Various treatment modalities have been formulated for the management of these disorders, with each modality targeting specific dysfunctions along the autonomic pathways. Neuromodulation techniques, including vagus nerve stimulation (VNS) and sphenopalatine ganglion (SPG) stimulation, have been promising in treating conditions such as migraines, which predominantly involve autonomic dysfunction. These therapies work to modulate neural circuits, which may help alleviate symptoms of autonomic dysregulation. Current studies demonstrate that not only are these treatments effective treatment modalities but also for the most part well tolerated by the patient, representing a strategic shift in the treatment of autonomic disorders in clinical practice (Puledda et al., 2016). In addition to neuromodulation, pharmacologic interventions are also central to the management of autonomic disorders. Drugs targeting specific neurotransmitter systems can reduce symptoms and improve the quality of life of patients. For instance, beta-blockers are frequently used to manage the tachycardia of dysautonomia, and anticholinergic medications may be used to treat hypersecretion or gastrointestinal dysmotility. But these are only effective to the degree that they are grounded in an accurate understanding of the individual patient's autonomic profile and pathogenetic processes underlying their illness. Individualized care is essential, as it allows for medical professionals to craft treatment interventions that harmoniously blend pharmacological and non-pharmacological interventions. Finally, interaction between autonomic disease and psychological factors cannot be overlooked during treatment planning. The literature highlights how diseases such as anxiety can be a cause of autonomic dysfunction, particularly among atrial fibrillation patients, where anxiety has a significant role in the quality of life (Ceccacci et al., 2019). Therefore, anxiety control and psychotherapy are components of an autonomic disorder treatment program that deals with mental health. By identifying the interactive nature between autonomic nervous system functioning and psychological well-being, clinicians can design multimodal treatment protocols that maximize symptom management and improve patients' overall health status. This integrative strategy fosters an increased overall understanding of autonomic disorders and emphasizes the importance of interdisciplinary care in achieving optimal patient outcomes.

4.6.1. Pharmacological Interventions

Pharmacological therapy of the ANS is essential in treating hypertension and its cardiovascular complications. Antihypertensive drugs, particularly adrenergic beta-receptor blockers, have become an essential therapeutic choice due to their potential to dampen sympathetic nervous activity. Through blockade of catecholamine action of norepinephrine, these drugs decrease heart rate and blood pressure, thus lowering the cardiac workload. Literature indicates that modulation of the ANS using drugs effectively not only manages hypertension but also decreases the risk of atrial fibrillation and heart failure, leading to better overall cardiovascular health (Lisa et al., 2024). This approach thus emphasizes the application of

ANS targeting as a viable method of preventing end-organ damage among hypertensive patients. Aside from beta-blockers, other pharmacologic interventions have been placed in the spotlight owing to their potential to modify autonomic balance. For instance, those medications that amplify vagal tone, such as low-level vagal stimulation, are being explored for their therapeutic use in disease conditions marked by increased sympathetic predominance. Such treatments serve to enhance parasympathetic activity, thus allowing for a better autonomic output and cardiovascular variables. The outcomes of various studies suggest that such pharmacological interventions play a supportive role in enhancing outcomes for managing ANS dysregulation, a common condition observed in hypertensive patients (Lisa et al., 2024). As research advances, understanding how pharmacological interventions are connected to the ANS provides valuable information, paving the way for novel treatment options that can effectively target complex health problems. Besides, the integration of pharmacological treatment with non-pharmacological approaches highlights the multidirectional nature of ANS disorder treatment. As has been noted in recent studies, such interventions as sacroiliac joint manipulation have proven to be efficient in the restoration of autonomic balance, particularly in patients suffering from such ANS disorders as primary dysmenorrhea. The integration of such non-traditional treatments with traditional pharmacological therapy allows clinicians to reach results mostly related to autonomic dysfunction. The results show that such collaborative efforts pay off in the form of better pain management and general well-being, supporting the virtue of an integrated treatment approach to the conditions affected by the ANS. As more is learned about the autonomic nervous system, it is clearer than ever that new therapeutic strategies—combining pharmacological and non-pharmacological therapies—have immense potential for advancing patient care (Figure 4.16).

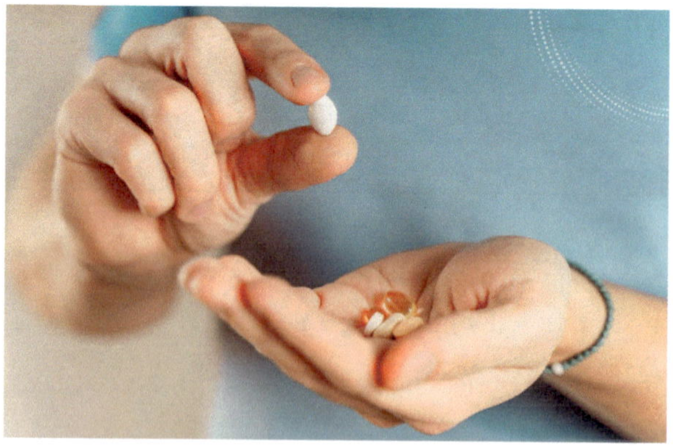

Figure 4.16. Treatment for autonomic dysfunction.

Source: https://lonestarneurology.net/wp-content/uploads/2023/06/1-Methods-of-Treatment-for-Autonomic-Dysfunction.webp.

4.6.2. Lifestyle Modifications

Lifestyle modifications are of vital significance in controlling the activity of the ANS and the general well-being of an individual. Of paramount importance among these modifications is habitual physical exercise, which has been demonstrated to have a beneficial influence on autonomic regulation. Exercise was revealed to bring about a revolution in autonomic function by its impact on promoting HRV, a significant marker of autonomous regulation. Particularly, research has indicated that with and after exercise, sympathetic activity can increase and parasympathetic activity can decrease, which implies dynamic interaction between these two systems when faced with physical stressors (Chiang et al., 2024). Through recurrent aerobic and resistance training, humans can adopt a lifestyle that is conducive to being resilient to stressors, resulting in improved cardiovascular health and intellectual clarity, which are integral parts of peak ANS upkeep. Aside from physical exercise, diet is another significant aspect of lifestyle change that aids in improving the ANS. Consumption of a well-balanced, nutrient-rich diet will mitigate the adverse effects of stress on autonomic function. Referencing omega-3 fatty acids, antioxidants, and fiber as examples, consuming these compounds will establish a healthy context for modulation of the ANS, as well as modulation of cardiovascular function. Type 2 diabetes patients, who are most susceptible to autonomic dysfunction, demonstrated better quality of life and treatment satisfaction when adhering to dietary management for metabolic control. Improvement not only empowers the patient but also reduces the somatic stress response to unhealthy food, indicating that diet can effectively modulate autonomic balance (Hecquet et al., 2024). An interdisciplinary strategy involving nutritional modifications can thus facilitate overall management of ANS-related illness. Psychological therapies, such as stress coping and mindfulness, have an equally crucial role in promoting a healthy autonomic nervous system. The impact of chronic stress on autonomic balance is a well-documented phenomenon as chronic stress can potentially lead to dysregulation of sympathetic and parasympathetic responses. The addition of behavioral strategies such as meditation, yoga, and biofeedback can reduce stress and promote relaxation and, therefore, augment parasympathetic activity. Not only do they encourage the state of relaxation, but also attention, emotional regulation, and physical healing, thereby strengthening a health-promoting lifestyle for ANS. In addition, interventions specifically constructed to reduce burdens on the autonomic system uncover sheer benefits for patients suffering from illnesses like type 2 diabetes, where empowerment and quality of health gains were defined within individuals actively engaging in such practices (Hecquet et al., 2024). Therefore, total ways of lifestyle alteration—spanning from exercise to diet to psychological well-being—are an intricate approach towards optimizing autonomic nervous system functioning.

4.6.3. Alternative Therapies

Other therapies have come to be of growing interest for their ability to affect the ANS, particularly in stress and enhancing well-being. Among these are reflexology, wherein pressure is applied to areas on the body, namely the hands and feet, that are thought to correspond to organs and systems of the body. It aligns with the belief that energy moves in predestined channels and obstruction leads to malfunction. By stimulating such areas of reflection, reflexology can normalize physiological processes and alleviate tension, thereby influencing the sympathetic and parasympathetic branches of the ANS. As a result, patients are relieved from pain and anxiety, thus emphasizing reflexology as an alternative to standard medicine in the treatment of conditions related to autonomic dysregulation. The therapeutic action of the practice is debated extensively in varied health settings, showing its relevance to modern holistic therapies of health (Quindlen et al., 2019). Breathing and meditation exercises have also come into the forefront in alternative treatment, particularly concerning their effects on the ANS. Recent studies have indicated that these exercises may reverse homeostatic alterations brought about by stress and anxiety. By emphasizing controlled breathing and awareness, such practices enable the process of moving from sympathetic dominance to parasympathetic arousal, increasing relaxation and emotional equilibrium. This approach is in contrast to traditional treatments that resolve neurotransmitter imbalance through pharmacological intervention. The hypothesis here is that drawing upon the body's natural capacity for self-regulation through control of the breath could prove more helpful in treating emotional disorders such as anxiety and depression. The interaction between respiration and emotional state also helps to highlight further the value of including such techniques in treatment programs for those who are seeking to optimize overall mental health and stress-resilience (Barnes et al., 2015) (Figure 4.17).

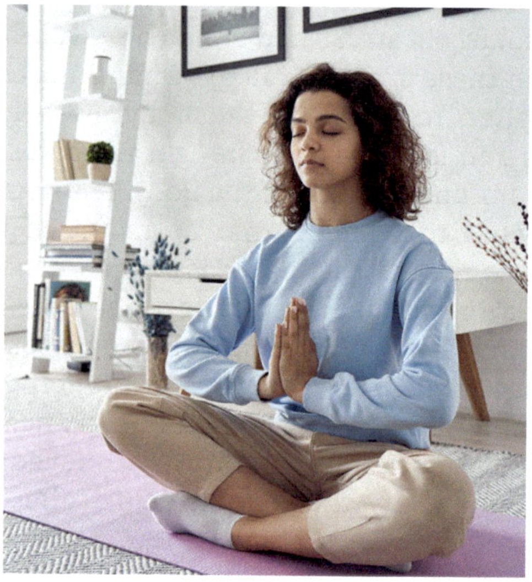

Figure 4.17. Woman practicing meditation as a stress management technique to promote mental well-being.

Source: https://www.santecenter.com/wp-content/uploads/2025/02/Top-6-Stress-Management-Techniques.jpeg.

As complementary therapies become more integrated into mainstream healthcare, their mechanisms must be known to practitioners and patients. Points of convergence among reflexology, meditation, and the ANS are critical to the body's response to psychological stressors. While the physiological processes behind the therapies are yet to be fully elucidated, evidence suggests their efficacy in enhancing wellbeing and reducing the incidence of stress-related disease. The combination of alternative therapies with a holistic approach can potentially empower people by allowing them to take charge of their health care. As there is growing interest in such non-surgical treatments, more studies must be conducted to elucidate the specific mechanisms by which they influence the ANS. This study not only identifies the capacity of alternative therapies to augment existing drugs but also deepens our understanding of the complex working relationships between mind and body within good health (Barnes et al., 2015; Quindlen et al., 2019).

Test Your Knowledge

1. What are the challenges in treating autonomic disorders that affect cardiovascular regulation, such as neurogenic hypertension?
2. How does patient education and multidisciplinary care contribute to the effective management of chronic autonomic disorders?

SUMMARY

In view of the intricate functions of the ANS, it is evident that its significance extends much beyond physiological control. The findings obtained from heterogeneous research highlight the need to understand the ANS in the context of different health illnesses, including psychiatric disease and cancer. For instance, abnormal functioning of the ANS, more precisely in schizophrenia, refers to an immediate necessity for particular therapeutic strategies. As illustrated, the difference between oral aripiprazole and long-acting injectable aripiprazole shows that formulation could have a significant effect on autonomic function, ultimately influencing treatment success and patient well-being. This finding emerges as critical in the quest for holistic management strategies targeting not only the symptomatology of mental disease but also the physiologic aberrations underneath (Hattori et al., 2023). Also included are the findings from the data about the ANSs involvement in cancer development and the efficacy of treatment. The enhanced activity of the β-2-adrenergic receptors in lung cancer and the possible benefits achieved with β-blocker therapy offer a further interesting dimension to this consideration. These revelations impact not only the pathology of lung cancer but also how we approach treatment options. The intersection of the ANS with pharmacological strategies indicates a new area of study that will provide improved patient care by possibly establishing integrative treatment pathways utilizing the internal regulatory mechanisms of the ANS to improve prognostic outcomes (Garramona et al., 2023). The autonomic nervous system takes center stage in the understanding of most health concerns, particularly in its intricate relationship with both mental and physical health challenges. With research continually de-mystifying the ANS, clinicians and researchers are presented with the possibility of refining treatment strategies that are more well-suited towards autonomic function. Correlations between ANS activity and therapeutic outcomes in illnesses such as schizophrenia and lung cancer illuminate the necessity for an interdisciplinary interface that interlinks neurology, psychiatry, and oncology. Future research is critical for bridging gaps in current knowledge and developing high-quality, prospective clinical trials that guide clinical interventions. Last but not least, a better understanding of the ANS could not only result in more efficient cures but even breakthroughs in managing complex health conditions (Hattori et al., 2023; Garramona et al., 2023).

To understand the ANS, it is essential to review several key points that highlight its elegance and significance in bodily functions. The ANS has the sympathetic and parasympathetic divisions, each of which has distinct roles in homeostasis and the regulation of several body processes. Sympathetic nervous system activation, for example, is responsible for the fight or flight response, which gets the body ready to react in a state of stress by distributing blood to the muscles and increasing heart rate. Alternatively, the parasympathetic nervous system triggers rest and digest functions, reducing the heart rate and facilitating healing processes. This delicate equilibrium maintained by the ANS is crucial in adapting to environmental demands, such that the body can respond efficiently to acute and chronic stressors. Besides that, research has established the relationship between the ANS and cardiac function with health implications. Autonomic control imbalances have been linked to many cardiovascular disorders, such as arrhythmias and heart failure. Unraveling the mechanisms through which autonomic stimulation regulates cardiac function is an elusive task due to the complex nature of neural interactions within different regions of the heart. Neurocardiac modeling has evolved in recent years to the extent that scientists now can predict the impact of sympathetic and parasympathetic stimulation on the heart. This progress could create new possibilities for therapeutic strategies. The modeling of this multiscale model incorporates several levels of biology, from cellular signal transduction to tissue responses, to a more complete explanation of how autonomic imbalance can set the stage for health complications and how interventions might reverse or block these complications (Clancy et al., 2023). In addition, clinical applications of methods of autonomic regulation have shown encouraging results in improving the quality of life and reducing impairments caused by stress. For instance, emotional self-regulation interventions have been evaluated in specific populations, such as police officers, and have been found effective in reducing physiological signs of stress and improving communication and interpersonal relations. These outcomes support the importance of stress management skills targeting the ANS as a means of facilitating emotional and physiological balance in stressful professions. By bridging the difference between theoretical research and actual practice, these techniques can contribute to enhanced mental clarity, functioning, and well-being, to illustrate the pivotal role of the autonomic nervous system in everyday life (Tomasino et al., 1999).

KEY TERMS FROM THIS CHAPTER

- Sympathetic Division
- Preganglionic Neurons
- Neuroeffector Junction
- Norepinephrine
- Fight-or-Flight Response
- Enteric Nervous System
- Heart rate
- Sexual arousal
- Parasympathetic Division
- Autonomic Ganglia
- Acetylcholine
- Dual Innervation
- Visceral Reflexes
- Autonomic Disorders
- Blood pressure
- Fibromyalgia

CRITICAL THINKING QUESTIONS

1. **Which division of the autonomic nervous system is responsible for the "rest and digest" response?**
   a. Sympathetic nervous system
   b. Parasympathetic nervous system
   c. Somatic nervous system
   d. Central nervous system
2. **What is the primary neurotransmitter released by postganglionic sympathetic neurons?**
   a. Acetylcholine
   b. Norepinephrine
   c. Dopamine
   d. Serotonin
3. **Which cranial nerve plays a major role in the parasympathetic nervous system?**
   a. Optic nerve (II)
   b. Vagus nerve (X)
   c. Trigeminal nerve (V)
   d. Facial nerve (VII)
4. **The "fight or flight" response is primarily mediated by which autonomic division?**
   a. Parasympathetic nervous system
   b. Enteric nervous system
   c. Sympathetic nervous system
   d. Somatic nervous system
5. **Which type of receptor does acetylcholine bind to in the parasympathetic nervous system's target organs?**
   a. Adrenergic receptors
   b. Nicotinic receptors
   c. Muscarinic receptors
   d. Dopaminergic receptors

Short Answer Questions

1. What are the two main divisions of the autonomic nervous system?
2. Which division of the ANS is responsible for "fight or flight" responses?
3. Name the neurotransmitter released by the parasympathetic nervous system at the target organ.
4. What is the primary function of the sympathetic nervous system?
5. Explain the physiological effects of sympathetic stimulation on various organs.
6. Discuss the role of the parasympathetic nervous system in regulating digestive processes.
7. Describe the pathway of autonomic nerve fibers from the CNS to target organs.
8. Compare the neurotransmitters and receptors involved in the sympathetic and parasympathetic nervous systems.

Answers to Critical Thinking Questions

1. (b); 2. (b); 3. (b); 4. (c); 5. (c)

REFERENCES

1. Robles, T. F., & Kane, H. S. (2013). The attachment System and Physiology in Adulthood: normative processes, individual differences, and implications for health. *Journal of Personality*, *82*(6), 515–527. https://doi.org/10.1111/jopy.12052
2. Alaerts, K., Brincker, M., Caballero, C., Caballero, C. C., Whyatt, C. P., Chai, C., et al. (2017). Stochastic signatures of involuntary head micro-movements can be used to classify females of ABIDE into different subtypes of neurodevelopmental disorders. https://core.ac.uk/download/287581413.pdf (accessed on 14th June 2025).
3. Alingh Prins, A., Scheurink, A., Steffens, A. B., et al. (1996). Overfeeding, autonomic regulation and metabolic consequences. https://core.ac.uk/download/pdf/12942087.pdf (accessed on 14th June 2025).
4. Ang, R., Opel, A., & Tinker, A. (2012). The role of inhibitory G proteins and regulators of G protein signaling in the *in vivo* control of heart rate and predisposition to cardiac arrhythmias. https://core.ac.uk/download/30697484.pdf (accessed on 14th June 2025).
5. Ashwini, D. L., & Raju, T. R. (2023). Autonomic nervous system and control of visual function. *Annals of Neurosciences, 30*, 151–153. https://www.semanticscholar.org/paper/55dff3850a9a22df614708e8e4debfec6da15998 (accessed on 14th June 2025).
6. Barnes, V. A., Crawford, M. W., & Jerath, R. (2014). Mind-body response and neurophysiological changes during stress and meditation: Central role of homeostasis. https://core.ac.uk/download/131210058.pdf (accessed on 14th June 2025).
7. Barnes, V. A., Crawford, M. W., Harden, K., et al. (2014). Widespread depolarization during expiration: A source of respiratory drive? https://core.ac.uk/download/131210052.pdf (accessed on 14th June 2025).
8. Barnes, V. A., Crawford, M. W., Harden, K., et al. (2015). Self-regulation of breathing as a primary treatment for anxiety. https://core.ac.uk/download/131210063.pdf (accessed on 14th June 2025).
9. Biesok, M., Lewoniuk, N., Macherski, M., et al. (2024). Analysis of the effects of regular yoga on the adaptive capacity of the nervous system. https://core.ac.uk/download/620863318.pdf (accessed on 14th June 2025).
10. Boundy, K., Cai, F. Z. J., Keen, H., et al. (2008). Mild autonomic dysfunction in primary Sjögren's syndrome: A controlled study. https://core.ac.uk/download/pdf/8114066.pdf (accessed on 14th June 2025).
11. Brincker, M., & Torres, E. (2017). Why study movement variability in autism? https://core.ac.uk/download/131210732.pdf (accessed on 14th June 2025).
12. Brust, P., Creeley, C., Feldman, R., Grandjean, P., Herken, H., Panzica, G., et al. (2014). Neurotoxicity. https://core.ac.uk/download/286729125.pdf (accessed on 14th June 2025).
13. Burnstock, G. (2009). Purinergic signaling: Past, present and future. https://core.ac.uk/download/1670991.pdf (accessed on 14th June 2025).
14. Ceccacci, A., Fedele, F., Lavalle, C., et al. (2019). Triggers for atrial fibrillation: The role of anxiety. https://core.ac.uk/download/188833222.pdf (accessed on 14th June 2025).

15. Chiang, J., Lin, Y. C., Hung, T. Y., Kao, H. H., & Kao, Y. H. (2024). The impact on autonomic nervous system activity during and following exercise in adults: A meta-regression study and trial sequential analysis. *Medicina, 60*. https://www.semanticscholar.org/paper/86e77d00199ec190289f8a8655267bab22b8ee89 (accessed on 14th June 2025).

16. Childre, D., & McCraty, R. (2002). The appreciative heart: The psychophysiology of positive emotions and optimal functioning. https://core.ac.uk/download/71342518.pdf (accessed on 14th June 2025).

17. Christensen, W. (2006). The evolutionary origins of volition. https://core.ac.uk/download/pdf/87234.pdf (accessed on 14th June 2025).

18. Clancy, C. E., Dawson, J. R. D., DeMarco, K. R., et al. (2023). A multiscale predictive digital twin for neurocardiac modulation. https://core.ac.uk/download/617744749.pdf (accessed on 14th June 2025).

19. Crawford, M. W., & Jerath, R. (2015). How does the body affect the mind? Role of cardiorespiratory coherence in the spectrum of emotions. https://core.ac.uk/download/131207333.pdf (accessed on 14th June 2025).

20. Cunha, R. A., & Ribeiro, J. A. (2000). ATP as a presynaptic modulator. https://core.ac.uk/download/12427071.pdf (accessed on 14th June 2025).

21. Curras-Collazo, M. C., Dobyns, A., Gutierrez, R., et al. (2017). A calibrated method of massage therapy decreases systolic blood pressure concomitant with changes in heart rate variability in male rats. https://core.ac.uk/download/286361424.pdf (accessed on 14th June 2025).

22. Dalise, A. M., Prestano, R., Fasano, R., Gambardella, A., Barbieri, M., & Rizzo, M. (2020). Autonomic nervous system and cognitive impairment in older patients: Evidence from long-term heart rate variability in real-life setting. *Frontiers in Aging Neuroscience, 12*. https://www.semanticscholar.org/paper/da600a28a975a351e556c42c74bda495378b6a68 (accessed on 14th June 2025).

23. Domínguez Vías, G., & Ramírez Sánchez, M. (2021). Brain asymmetry: Towards an asymmetrical neurovisceral integration. https://core.ac.uk/download/493007120.pdf (accessed on 14th June 2025).

24. Dorsher, P. (2008). Fibromyalgia: A unifying neuroendocrinology model for understanding its pathophysiology. https://core.ac.uk/download/pdf/288173.pdf (accessed on 14th June 2025).

25. Estrine, J., & DeLisle, L. (2006). Stress: Putting the brain back into medicine. https://core.ac.uk/download/71356692.pdf (accessed on 14th June 2025).

26. Federici, A., Zenzola, A., Xu, A., Akay, M., Aldroubi, A., Simone, F., Gonnella, G., et al. (2005). Response of autonomic nervous system to body positions: Fourier and wavelet analysis. http://arxiv.org/abs/physics/0310125 (accessed on 14th June 2025).

27. Garramona, F. T., Cunha, T. F., Vieira, J. S., Borges, G., Santos, G., de Castro, G., Ugrinowitsch, C., et al. (2023). Increased sympathetic nervous system impairs prognosis in lung cancer patients: A scoping review of clinical studies. *Lung Cancer Management, 12*. https://www.semanticscholar.org/paper/6fd58821e13984eed945c1686baa5401f57a2d14 (accessed on 14th June 2025).

28. Gottlieb, L. A., Mahfoud, F., Stavrakis, S., Jespersen, T., & Linz, D. K. (2024). Autonomic nervous system: A therapeutic target for cardiac end-organ damage in hypertension.

Hypertension (Dallas, Tex.: 1979), *81*, 2027–2037. https://www.semanticscholar.org/paper/e3432544b8a63aba6727392752bda65506eecf39 (accessed on 14th June 2025).

29. Grewal, S., & Gupta, V. (2011). Effect of obesity on autonomic nervous system. *International Journal of Current Biomedical Science*. https://core.ac.uk/download/pdf/14686.pdf (accessed on 14th June 2025).
30. Hattori, S., Suda, A., Kishida, I., Miyauchi, M., Shiraishi, Y., Noguchi, N., Furuno, T., et al. (2023). Differences in autonomic nervous system activity between long-acting injectable aripiprazole and oral aripiprazole in schizophrenia. *BMC Psychiatry, 23*. https://www.semanticscholar.org/paper/924ad99ec1e2d138a5a801d40f423c38e5378c79 (accessed on 14th June 2025).
31. Hecquet, S., Ballegaard, S., Eldrup, E., Hansen, C. S., Hansen, T., Harboe, G., Rossing, P., et al. (2024). New diabetic treatment by alleviation of autonomic nervous system dysfunction measured as periosteal pressure sensitivity at sternum improves empowerment, treatment satisfaction, and self-reported health of people with type 2 diabetes: A randomized trial. *Diabetes, Metabolic Syndrome and Obesity, 17*, 2519–2531. https://www.semanticscholar.org/paper/ace6b0308edd6218e01876ba84958becbd63222b (accessed on 14th June 2025).
32. Inhula, N. (2018). Variability of the heart rhythm as an additional marker for determining vegetative functions in patients with chronic cerebral ischemia. https://core.ac.uk/download/322516329.pdf (accessed on 14th June 2025).
33. Kekecs, Z., Szekely, A., & Varga, K. (2015). Alterations in electrodermal activity and cardiac parasympathetic tone during hypnosis. https://core.ac.uk/download/77011630.pdf (accessed on 14th June 2025).
34. Lange, K. A. (2025). *Physiology of Man and Animals in the Tenth Five-Year Plan: Proceedings of the Thirteenth Congress of the I. P. Pavlov All-Union Physiological Society*. https://core.ac.uk/download/pdf/42860886.pdf (accessed on 14th June 2025).
35. Li, H., Wang, H., & Wang, X. (2025). Psychedelics and the autonomic nervous system: A perspective on their interplay and therapeutic potential. *ACS Pharmacology & Translational Science, 8*(3), 899–902. https://www.semanticscholar.org/paper/5ddc94440df6424b0cf05f8e4c706089c6d0d931 (accessed on 14th June 2025).
36. Lisukha, L. (2017). The use of intermittent norm baric hypoxia in children's neurology (review). https://core.ac.uk/download/301580754.pdf (accessed on 14th June 2025).
37. Martins, I. J. (2016). Anti-aging genes improve appetite regulation and reverse cell senescence and apoptosis in global populations. https://core.ac.uk/download/84887634.pdf (accessed on 14th June 2025).
38. Motofei, I. G., & Rowland, D. L. (2017). Psycho-physiologic emergentism; four minds in a body. https://core.ac.uk/download/144553869.pdf (accessed on 14th June 2025).
39. Park, S., Kim, H., Jung, J., & Lee, S. (2024). Effects of sacroiliac joint manipulation on autonomic nervous system and lower abdominal pain in women with primary dysmenorrhea: A randomized controlled trial. *Medicina, 60*. https://www.semanticscholar.org/paper/eda21b5e5c39f9468e3bcd03ca68320dcf8a975b (accessed on 14th June 2025).
40. Puledda, F., & Goadsby, P. J. (2016). Current approaches to neuromodulation in primary headaches: Focus on vagal nerve and sphenopalatine ganglion stimulation. https://core.ac.uk/download/189244318.pdf (accessed on 14th June 2025).

41. Quindlen, K. A. (2019). Reflexology. https://cupola.gettysburg.edu/cgi/viewcontent.cgi?article=1840&context=student_scholarship (accessed on 14th June 2025).

42. Raj, S. R. (2006). The postural tachycardia syndrome (POTS): Pathophysiology, diagnosis & management. https://core.ac.uk/download/pdf/86508.pdf (accessed on 14th June 2025).

43. Siepmann, T., & Ziemssen, T. (2019). The investigation of the cardiovascular and sudomotor autonomic nervous system—A review. https://core.ac.uk/download/201288195.pdf (accessed on 14th June 2025).

44. Silvani, A., Heidbreder, A., Lambert, I., Barateau, L., & Dauvilliers, Y. (2023). Autonomic dysfunction in hypersomnia. https://core.ac.uk/download/611892825.pdf (accessed on 14th June 2025).

45. Simonenko, G. (2017). Detection of autonomic dysfunctions in complex neuropsychological examination of NMU students. https://core.ac.uk/download/301580770.pdf (accessed on 14th June 2025).

46. Souza Filho, L. F. M. de, de Oliveira, J. C. D., Ribeiro, M. K. A., Moura, M. C., Fernandes, N. D., de Sousa, R. D., Pedrino, G., et al. (2019). Evaluation of the autonomic nervous system by analysis of heart rate variability in the preterm infants. *BMC Cardiovascular Disorders, 19*. https://www.semanticscholar.org/paper/daa59fffe74007a94702375e951c801542055101 (accessed on 14th June 2025).

47. Steinhart, E. (2001). Persons versus brains: Biological intelligence in human organisms. https://core.ac.uk/download/287611886.pdf (accessed on 14th June 2025).

48. Tomasino, D., Sundram, J., Atkinson, M., & McCraty, R. (1999). Impact of the HeartMath self-management skills program on physiological and psychological stress in police officers. https://core.ac.uk/download/71342457.pdf (accessed on 14th June 2025).

THE CARDIOVASCULAR SYSTEM

5

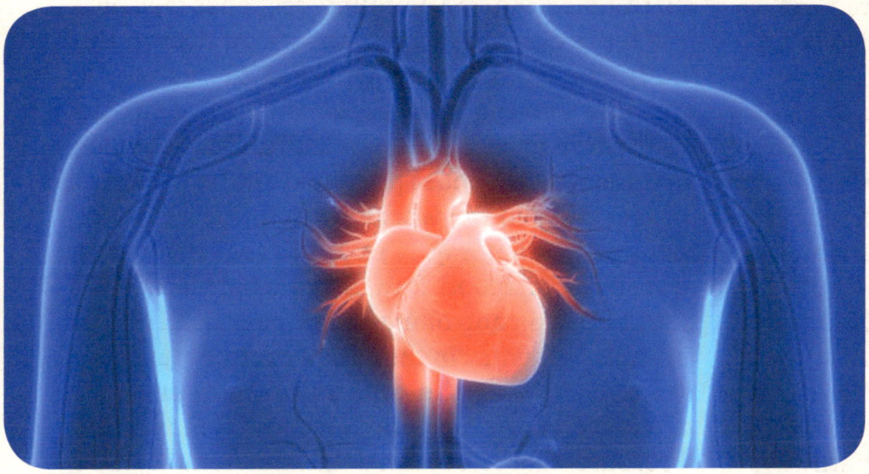

LEARNING OBJECTIVES

After studying this chapter, you will be able to:

1. Understand the cardiovascular anatomy
2. Identify the cardiovascular physiology
3. Describe the composition and role of blood
4. Highlight the common cardiovascular diseases
5. Define prevention and control of cardiovascular diseases
6. Discuss the development of cardiovascular research

Introduction

The cardiovascular system is the structural requirement for homeostasis in the human body and acts as an intermediary of transport for nutrients, gases, hormones, and waste products. It is primarily composed of the heart, blood vessels, and blood that all work together to distribute oxygenated blood to various tissues and organs. Knowledge of the cardiovascular system is vital, not just for understanding its importance, but also for dealing with the many challenges posed by cardiovascular diseases (CVDs). With the rising incidence of diseases such as hypertension, heart failure, and atherosclerosis, there is an urgent need for an in-depth study of the mechanisms of cardiovascular function. By examining physiological and pathologic processes, one can dissect the fine balance of this system and thus guide treatment choices and prevention. The latest progress in cardiovascular research emphasizes the pathophysiological function of noncoding RNAs (ncRNAs), i.e., microRNAs and long noncoding RNAs, in vascular disease and injury. These molecules have been established to be key regulators of vascular remodeling, particularly in conditions that are aggravated by inflammation and injury-induced vessel wall changes. Investigations have shown that miRNA manipulation can significantly reduce the weight of pathological vascular remodeling, hence promising therapeutic interventions. Additionally, the study of exosomal-derived ncRNAs emphasizes endothelial cell-vascular smooth muscle cell intercellular communication. With the revelation of the multifaceted roles played by ncRNAs in cardiovascular disease and health, researchers are opening up new ways to combat the increasing burden of CVDs in contemporary society (Baker et al., 2016). The family of natriuretic peptides (NPs) also appears as an essential factor in understanding cardiovascular physiology and pathology, together with ncRNAs. NPs play a key role in blood pressure regulation and maintaining heart and kidney function, and are part of our knowledge of different cardiovascular diseases like hypertension and heart failure. Significantly, molecular biology has enlightened the pathways along which NPs influence cardiovascular health and demonstrated that NPs possess therapeutic targetability for the treatment of CVDs. Through continuous research progress, the integration of NP-based therapies into clinical practice has the potential to offer new strategies for the treatment of cardiovascular disease. In the distant future, a very sophisticated understanding of NcRNAs as well as NPs will enhance the treatment of the complexities of cardiovascular disease, and this will be a landmark in optimizing patient outcomes and public health (Rubattu et al., 2019).

Definition of the Cardiovascular System

The cardiovascular or circulatory system is responsible for maintaining life by allowing the transport of waste products, oxygen, hormones, and nutrients around the body. The system, comprising blood vessels, heart, and blood, operates through a complex network that facilitates the effective distribution and exchange of necessary materials. The muscular heart acts as a pump to transport oxygenated blood through the arteries and receive deoxygenated blood through the veins. Double circulation not only maintains cellular metabolism but also maintains the body in homeostasis by controlling temperature and pH. Additionally, the circulatory system performs a vital function of transferring the immune response because the leukocytes present in the blood defend the body from pathogens. One has to realize its purpose and function, especially how it relates to the impact of cardiovascular diseases, which are some of the most prevalent primary causes of mortality in the world. Its definition extends beyond its anatomy to encompass the intricate dynamics of blood flow and the physiological mechanisms controlling it. The heart's electrical system presents rhythmic contractions, and the venous, arterial, and capillary system presents a closed loop in which blood's maximum pressure can be retained and nutrients can be provided. Co-operation of the two is essential to ensure health since the breakdown may result in catastrophic outcomes such as a heart attack or stroke. Comprehension of how this system functions means that diseases such as atherosclerosis directly affect the functioning of blood vessels and can significantly enhance cardiovascular disease threats. Systematic comprehension of these effects on health is thus necessary, particularly in establishing effective prevention and intervention strategies against cardiovascular disease. Cardiovascular medicine technological advances, such as decision aid systems and risk evaluation programs, are transforming the cardiovascular healthcare management practice. Recent work between clinicians and computer scientists has examined the efficacy of fuzzy rule-based systems utilizing advanced data analysis techniques in predicting cardiovascular risk. They not only enhance the accuracy of diagnosis but also assure using understandable guidelines capable of aiding clinicians a great deal in their decision-making process. As mentioned in recent studies, inclusion of such innovative methods in existing clinical practice will lead to improved results in cardiovascular care for patients. By providing more intimate understanding of the cardiovascular system, these discoveries form the foundation for individualized treatment modalities that can be shown to diminish risks and hazards of cardiovascular disease effectively and are therefore a fundamental component of modern clinical practice and research (Bohacik et al., 2013; Dimitrova et al., 2013) (Figure 5.1).

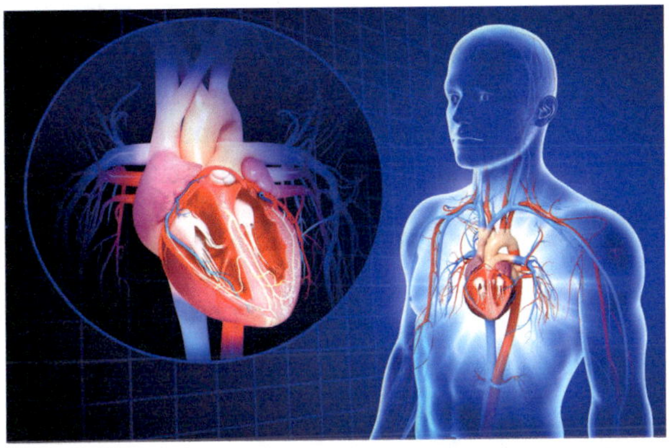

Figure 5.1. Cardiovascular system.

Source: https://www.thoughtco.com/thmb/rJ_oZzSWqIX4VfldjgU_xYSb49A=/1500x1003/filters:no_upscale():max_bytes(150000):strip_icc()/cardiovascular_system-57f6d56a3df78c690f77c7c7.jpg.

Importance of the Cardiovascular System in Human Health

The cardiovascular system plays a crucial role in maintaining homeostasis and human health through effective blood transport. The heart, blood vessels, and blood work together to provide tissues with necessary nutrients and oxygen and to remove products of metabolism. The efficiency of the transport system directly influences a great variety of functions of the body, including thermoregulation, pH balance, and immune function. As the core networking system of the body, the cardiovascular system is centrally involved in responses to physiological stressors and trauma. These interactions highlight the significance of an unbroken cardiovascular system to the general health status throughout life, particularly with the consideration of the reality that stress has been established to have effects on the cardiovascular system very much, a reflection of body systems' interdependence (Estrine et al., 2006). The second most significant characteristic of the cardiovascular system is its influence on the physiological welfare of other systems. Its operation must be understood within the framework of total human physiology, including cardiac function but also interaction with neuro-endocrine and immune mechanisms. The extended discussion of these systems, especially in Ayurvedic literature, describes the cardiovascular system as "Rasavaha Srotas," with attention given to its importance to body function (Patwardhan et al., 2008). Knowledge of how the cardiovascular system is interdependent with other physiological systems can be helpful in understanding its role in supporting life processes. For instance, the cardiovascular system supplies the delivery of growth and metabolism-regulating hormones, which indicates its essential interdependence with the endocrine system. The second implication of the cardiovascular system is in disease prevention. Poor cardiovascular function is linked to illnesses like hypertension, coronary heart disease, and stroke, and therefore requires preventive care as well as healthy living practices. The relationship between cardiovascular function and the stress response is also one that needs to be enhanced in terms of health performance. Enhanced cardiovascular function through exercise, good nutrition, and stress control can help avert the risk of cardiovascular disease. To this end, too, the cardiovascular system is a marker and facilitator of international health, once more necessitating ongoing research and public health programs for continued cardiovascular health, since the scope extends even beyond the heart to the realm of all-human health (Estrine et al., 2006).

5.1. Anatomy of the Cardiovascular System

Learning Outcome

1. Discuss the major components: heart, blood vessels, and blood
2. Understand the structure and function of the heart
3. Explain the types of blood vessels: arteries, veins, and capillaries

The anatomy of the cardiovascular system is a highly intricate integration of components working in unison in a bid to facilitate effective circulatory processes of the blood through the body. The heart, blood vessels, and blood form the core of the system. The heart is a muscular organ centrally located within the thoracic cavity and comprises four chambers: the right and left atria and ventricles. These chambers function cooperatively with one another so that deoxygenated blood may flow back from the body to the right atrium. Then the right ventricle forces it to the lungs to be oxygenated. At the same time, oxygenated blood flows into the left atrium and is ejected by the left ventricle into systemic circulation. This two-pump system shows that the systems work effectively and play a necessary role in physiological homeostasis. The vascular system continues to reveal the intricacy of the cardiovascular system. Arteries, veins, and capillaries all have different but associated functions; arteries carry oxygenated blood away from the heart, while veins carry deoxygenated blood to the heart. The most minute vessels, capillaries, provide the all-important exchange of waste products, nutrients, and gases at the tissue level. The vessel walls surprisingly vary in thickness and are thick and muscular in the arteries to be able to withstand high pressure upon ejection from the heart. Veins have thinner walls and backflow valves to ensure adequate return of blood under low pressure. Their singularity of structural features demonstrates how they uphold their specific functions, the final requirement to ensure the cardiovascular system is functioning in consonance and fulfilling its demands. Medical therapy and investigation must advance through a perception of the molecular and genetic processes that regulate the cardiovascular system. Only in the past has it been found that the function and integrity of numerous genes and proteins are crucial to maintaining cardiovascular health, as well as those disease processes which culminate in atherosclerosis and valvular disease. For example, gene expression for the integrity and assembly of the extracellular matrix is critical for the maintenance of cardiac structure and function.

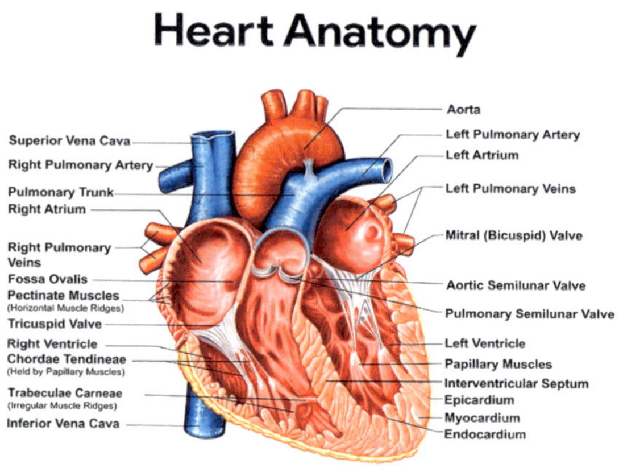

Figure 5.2. Anatomy cardiovascular system.

Source: https://nurseslabs.com/wp-content/uploads/2017/04/Heart-Anatomy-Cardiovascular-System-Anatomy-Charts.png.

Adversions like vascular calcification, however, preclude homoeostasis from taking place normally and hence influence the formation of cardiovascular disease. Using large animal models, e.g., sheep, researchers are investigating the transcriptome of cardiovascular tissue to determine the expression of genes related to development and disease. This novel approach not only contributes to the existing knowledge of cardiovascular anatomy but also lays a basis for the introduction of targeted therapies against cardiovascular disease, which appropriately answers the call of translational research to address the existing cardiovascular challenges (Bush et al., 2020; Abedin et al., 2016) (Figure 5.2).

5.1.1. Major Components: Heart, Blood Vessels, and Blood

The heart, an intricate organ, lies at the center of the cardiovascular system and is responsible for the continuous flow of blood throughout the body. The muscular pump, consisting primarily of cardiac muscle tissue, operates using a coordinated process of contraction and relaxation known as the cardiac cycle. Four chambers comprise the heart: the right atrium and left atrium, and the right ventricle and left ventricle.

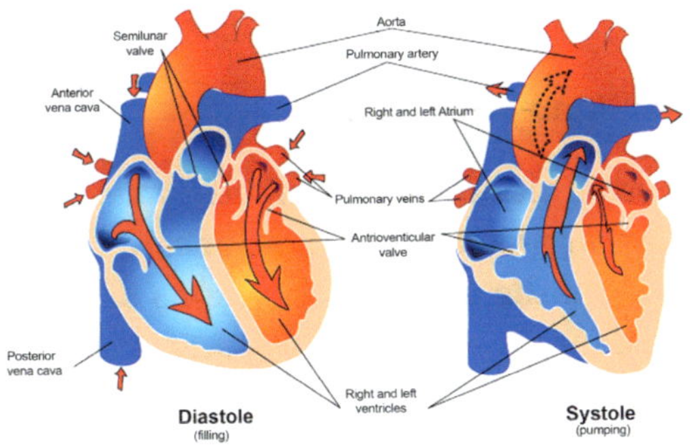

Figure 5.3. Ventricles.

Source: https://media.geeksforgeeks.org/wp-content/uploads/20220701103238/Diastolesystole.png.

The right side of the heart receives deoxygenated blood from the body through the superior and inferior vena cavae, which is circulated to the lungs to receive oxygen. The left side of the heart receives oxygenated blood from the lungs through the pulmonary veins and circulates it to the body through the aorta. Efficiency of the heart is necessary because a single fault can lead to severe cardiovascular diseases, which are a principal cause of death worldwide (Khan, 2024) (Figure 5.3).

In addition to the functioning of the heart, blood vessels form an extensive system that makes it possible for blood to be carried from the heart to organs. Three types of vessels exist: arteries, veins, and capillaries. Oxygenated blood is carried away from the heart by arteries via rigid, elastic walls with the capacity to handle high pressure. As the arteries branch into successively smaller arterioles and eventually capillaries, there is the exchange of wastes, gases, and nutrients. Capillaries are the small blood vessels that possess one-cell-thick walls through which effective diffusion can occur. Then, oxygen-poor blood returns through successively larger veins to the heart. This dynamic system relies on numerous mechanisms, including the contraction of muscles around it, the presence of valves in veins, and gravity forces to give a flow of blood against gravity (Tarnawski et al., 2022). Blood itself, being cells suspended in plasma, is a fundamental component of the cardiovascular system. It carries oxygen and carbon dioxide, nutrients, hormones, and waste products through a complex function. The blood has the following cellular components: red blood cells that carry oxygen, white blood cells that defend the body against infection, and platelets that help in clotting. The plasma component of the blood is water, and it contains vital proteins, salts, and nutrients. Alterations in blood composition also significantly impact cardiovascular wellbeing; for instance, high levels of low-density lipoprotein (LDL) cholesterol are responsible for atherosclerosis, a clogging and thickening of the arteries, which leads to heart attacks and strokes. So, understanding the properties and activities of blood is crucial for fighting cardiovascular illnesses as well as overall health (Khan, 2024).

5.1.2. Structure and Function of the Heart

The heart is the organ at the center of the cardiovascular system and functions as a powerful pump that pumps blood into the body. It is composed structurally of four chambers: the right and left atria, which receive blood, and the right and left ventricles, which eject blood to the lungs and the remainder of the body, respectively. This intricate structure facilitates effective oxygen-rich and oxygen-poor blood separation, maximizing efficiency in pulmonary and systemic circulation. The heart's muscular walls, such as the myocardium, rhythmically contract to supply equal blood flow, while the cardiac cycle effectively manages the time interval between heartbeats. Appreciating this organization not only highlights the heart's role as a pump but also underscores its reliance on intricate networks of electrical patterns and blood vessel connections to function optimally and maintain good cardiovascular health (Figure 5.4).

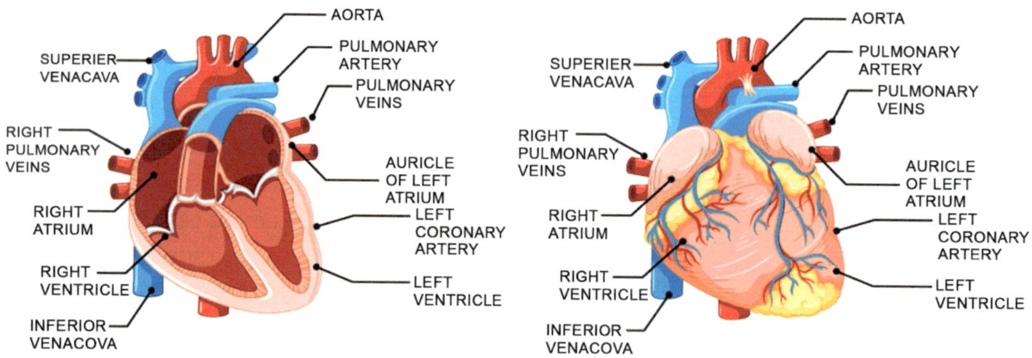

Figure 5.4. The labelled diagram of the human heart.

Source: https://www.geeksforgeeks.org/structure-and-functions-of-heart/.

The functional and structural design of the heart can be additionally explained by using fractal geometry and chaos theory, which recognize concealed biological patterns in charge of cardiac activity. Fractal concepts demonstrate how the His-Purkinje system and the branching systems of the blood vessels mirror natural patterns in other biological systems, thereby making the systems robust and adaptable. For instance, heart rate variability is not linear and exhibits chaotic behavior that emanates from complex interactions between the intrinsic nature of the heart and external stimuli. Perception of chaos in cardiac performance allows us to have a deeper understanding of irregularities in heart rhythm, highlighting the relevance of understanding these models toward a clearer perception of cardiovascular well-being and vulnerability in disease (Almog et al., 2025). The advancement in the knowledge of the cardiac structure and function has bearings on the development of new therapeutic options, particularly against the background of cardiovascular degeneration. The intrinsic poor repair capability of the cardiovascular system typically constrains standard pharmacological interventions. Scientists have therefore turned to bioengineering approaches to replicate heart tissues and functions in the lab. Techniques such as the fabrication of three-dimensional artificial heart muscle (AHM) models have emerged as highly prominent, showing a collective effort toward developing an environment where cardiac myocytes would survive and function optimally (Hogan et al., 2017). Employing scaffolds and mechanical conditioning, these models aim to more closely replicate heart muscle, paving the way for cardiovascular therapies that not only restore function but also provide long-term health for the afflicted.

5.1.3. Types of Blood Vessels: Arteries, Veins, and Capillaries

The human cardiovascular system includes three primary blood vessel types: arteries, veins, and capillaries, each of which has specific functions required to create homeostasis. Arteries are characterized by thick, muscular walls that enable them to withstand and control the high-pressure circulation of blood from the heart. These vessels transport oxygenated blood from the heart to various body tissues and are tasked with supplying organs with enough oxygen and nutrients. The structural make-up of arteries, for instance, possessing a dense elastin and smooth muscle layer, allows them to maintain the blood pressure as well as to support the pulsatile nature of blood flow. This structural solidity is of utmost importance, as any failure in the arteries can result in severe cardiovascular complications. In sharp contrast to the arteries, veins are the conduits for returning deoxygenated blood to the heart. Having a greater lumen and thinner walls, veins are equipped with one-way valves that prevent the retrograde flow of the blood, ensuring efficient circulation under lower pressure. Its reliance on skeletal muscle contractions and respiratory movements for easy venous return is particularly noteworthy; without these systems, blood flow through veins would be significantly diminished. Moreover, the fact that veins have lower pressure makes them more susceptible to afflictions such as varicose veins or deep vein thrombosis. It is worth noting the structural and functional distinctions between arteries and veins because they emphasize how the two vessels complement one another in the overall circulatory process. Capillaries, being the body's microvessels, are crucial sites for exchange between surrounding tissue and blood. They possess thin, permeable walls that facilitate adequate transportation of oxygen, carbon dioxide, nutrients, and waste products at a cellular level. Capillary beds are of different densities according to the metabolic needs of the tissues supplied; e.g., brain and muscle tissue have a dense capillary bed to supply their oxygen and nutritional requirements. Also, more recent findings have identified structures such as the endothelial cell protein C receptor (EPCR) with an irregular pattern in major arteries. They may be involved in hemostasis during embryonic and postnatal life (Crawley et al., 2002). These results cast an interesting light on vascular function and regulation in health and disease, demonstrating the intricate interplay typical of the cardiovascular system as a whole (Figure 5.5).

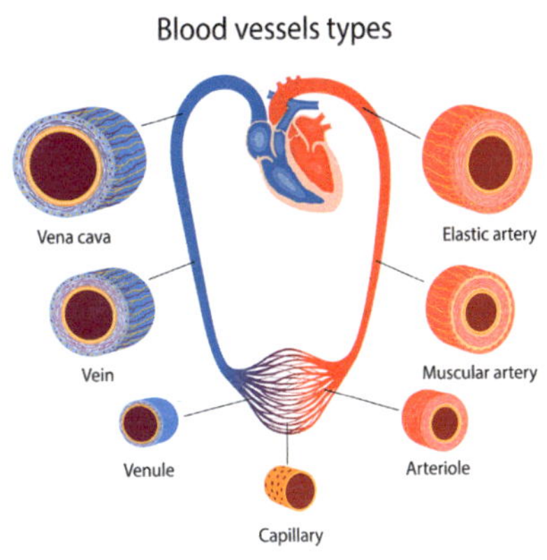

Figure 5.5. Blood vessel types.

Source: https://as1.ftcdn.net/v2/jpg/02/96/87/72/1000_F_296877237_HKkfA0spGpltpRVnxP8id8u08o7K5MjC.jpg.

Test Your Knowledge

1. Describe the basic structure and main function of the heart.
2. What are the differences between arteries, veins, and capillaries?

5.2. Physiology of the Cardiovascular System

Learning Outcome

1. Explain the blood circulation process
2. Describe the role of the heart in pumping blood
3. Define regulation of blood pressure and flow

Cardiovascular system plays a crucial role to maintain homeostasis by its intricate machinery of heart, blood vessels, and blood. The muscular organ, the heart, is at the center of this system that circulates blood to the body. The physiology of the heart involves intricate electrical and mechanical functions that facilitate efficient circulation. Cardiac autonomic innervation regulates heart rate and rhythm through sympathetic and parasympathetic channels, which are dynamically adjusted according to shifting physiological demands like exercise or stress. Information regarding this autonomic control is of extreme significance in the assessment of cardiac status, particularly in most cardiovascular illnesses, where imaging techniques like SPECT and PET to clarify the function of the sympathetic nervous system in the heart (Noordzij et al., 2021). This interaction of the mechanical and electrical systems of the heart is one instance of the elegant complexity that governs cardiovascular physiology. Outside the heart itself, the vascular components of the cardiovascular system have a significant role to play in modulating blood pressure and blood flow. Arteries, veins, and capillaries cooperate to perfuse tissues with oxygenated blood and to remove metabolic waste products. The resistance found in such vessels affects hemodynamics as a whole, and factors such as vessel diameter determine blood pressure and rate of flow. Mathematical modeling has provided explanations of such dynamics, which have allowed scientists to simulate cardiovascular response to varying conditions, including space flight (Leonard, 2025). The simulations help to explain interactions between divergent physiological systems and provide a basis from which to make predictions for cardiovascular responses to stressors. Such information has prognostic significance to diseases such as hypertension and in directing effective therapeutic interventions. Furthermore, the integration of cardiovascular physiology with other systems highlights its relevance in disease and health. The circulatory system profoundly interacts with the respiratory system to enable efficient gas exchange and oxygen delivery to tissues. The interaction between cardiovascular function and thermoregulation is also central in regulating body core temperature. The sophisticated feedback mechanisms offered in the cardiovascular system establish the necessity for a holistic understanding of human physiology. With research advances, particularly the use of technological innovation in data modeling and analysis, the systemic perspective of the cardiovascular system is revealed. This is not only advantageous on an academic basis but also on a clinical basis by rendering interventions appropriate to the sophisticated dynamics of the critical system (Leonard, 2025).

5.2.1. Blood Circulation Process

The circulation process of blood is a central aspect of the cardiovascular system, whose function is to transport essential materials, like oxygen, nutrients, hormones, and wastes, to and from the body. The heart is a muscular pump that propels blood through an intricate network of vessels, including arteries, veins, and capillaries. Arterial blood carries oxygen from the lungs to tissues, while venous blood carries deoxygenated blood and carbon dioxide to the heart. The concerted orchestration of these interactions not only sustains cellular metabolism but also aids in thermoregulation and immune responses. Understanding circulation mechanisms sheds light on its vital role in maintaining homeostasis and how disruptions to it could result in cataclysmic health consequences, such as hypertension and heart disease, and so keeping the cardiovascular system healthy is extremely important. To appreciate the mechanisms involved in the modulation of blood circulation, it is essential to think about how signaling pathways and some proteins, with their effects on vascular functions, are involved. For instance, PI3Kγ is a multifunctional protein that is essential in both the cardiovascular and immune systems, and it is central to regulating blood pressure alongside vascular tone. Current evidence highlights how PI3Kγ signaling integrates pathways fundamental to the maintenance of vascular homeostasis, particularly under the pathologic conditions of hypertension. The fact that this protein is bifunctional in immunity and vasculature regulation hints at a complex interplay between these two systems. With maturing research into the nuanced role of cellular signaling, it holds the potential to provide a window for therapies that could mitigate the effects of cardiovascular disease by exploiting the native physiological cross-talk contained within such pathways (Carnevale et al., 2016). Yet, managing the consequences of deleterious cardiovascular health is not only pharmacological but also requires lifestyle adjustments, particularly within the physical education system. Implementing specific training programs for individuals with cardiovascular diseases can significantly improve their health status. Research has proven that individualized fitness programs enhance the body's resistance to stressors, promote psychological tranquility and emotional balance, and refine physiological processes. For students suffering from cardiovascular diseases, engaging in appropriately designed physical activities enhances the level of motivation for adopting healthier lifestyles. It thereby improves their physical as well as mental condition. This identification with structured physical education and cardiovascular health also lends support to the crucial imperative for an integrated approach that nurtures body and mind alike, setting the stage for effective interventions in cardiac rehabilitation (Biletska et al., 2018) (Figure 5.6).

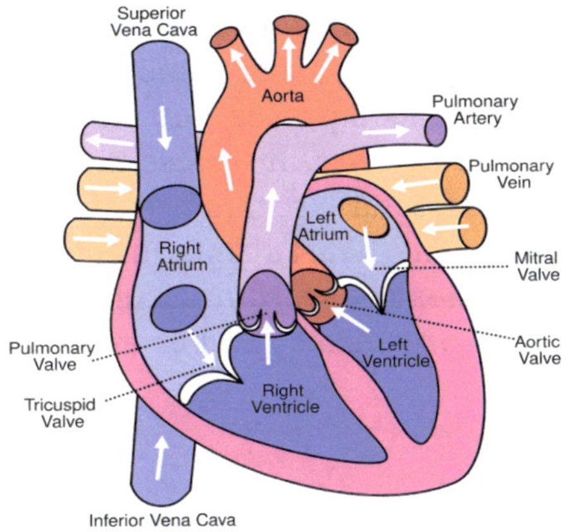

Figure 5.6. Blood circulation.

Source: https://i0.wp.com/gccexchange.com/blog/wp-content/uploads/2015/05/blood_circulation.gif.

5.2.2. Role of the Heart in Pumping Blood

The heart is the body's central pump, regulating the movement of blood around the body to supply life. It has four chambers: the left and right atria and the left and right ventricles, which allow this vital function to take place.

Blood from the body and lungs enters the heart via the atria. The deoxygenated blood from systemic circulation enters the right atrium, and oxygenated blood from pulmonary circulation enters the left atrium. The atrial walls pump and contract blood into the ventricles, preparing it for the next crucial phase of the cardiac cycle. This controlled filling and emptying, stimulated by the rhythmic contractions of the heart, ensures the delivery of oxygen and nutrients and the removal of waste products from tissues effectively, with the heart playing a critical role in the maintenance of homeostasis in the body. When in pumping mode, the heart generates pressure that pressures the blood into an extensive network of arteries and veins, demonstrating the dynamic interplay between vascular health and heart function. As the ventricle squeezes, blood is forced into the aorta, the largest artery, and then on into various tissues and back via the venous system. This pulse-like flow not only facilitates the transport of oxygen-rich blood but also helps venous return mechanisms, governed by muscle squeezes and valve systems, prevent backflow. However, cardiac dysfunction may lead to cardiac diseases such as atrial fibrillation (AF), which significantly negatively affects cardiac output and global hemodynamics. Investigation of AF has shown that impaired contractility of the heart and hemodynamics changes with AF point out the heart's crucial role in maintaining adequate circulation, thereby proving the connection between heart mechanics and systemic health (Camporeale et al., 2014). Also, the comprehension of cardiac function is embedded inextricably with its biological function in preserving life. John Searle's discourse on tasks in living organisms asserts the relevance of evaluating physiological roles in terms of goals of survival and health. For the heart, its primary function is to pump blood, thereby fulfilling the vital functions of nutrition, oxygen supply, and waste removal. In defining the performance of hearts, understanding of its functionality encompasses not only circulatory blood mechanics but also the larger picture of the organism's health. It necessitates a nuanced examination of dependency in cardiac function, whereby successful circulation of blood is needed to make tissues and organs viable within the body. Hence, the heart's pumping efficacy echoes a long history of biological processes, firmly linking the science of cardiovascular fitness to the ontological evaluation of physiological processes in biological organisms (Weber et al., 2017) (Figure 5.7).

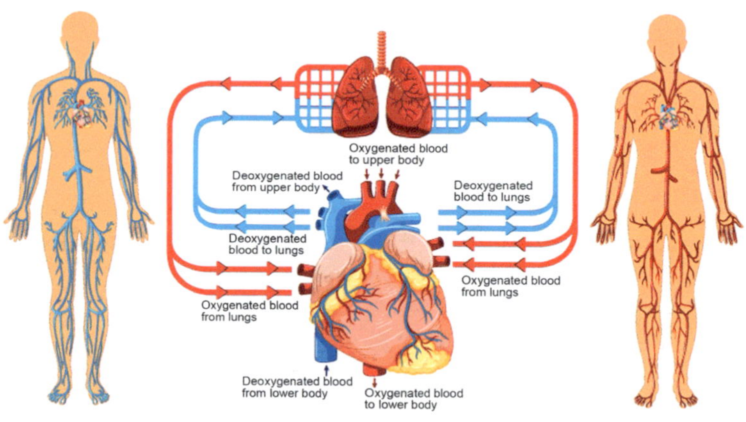

Figure 5.7. Heart pumping blood.

Source: https://external-content.duckduckgo.com/iu/?u=https%3A%2F%2Fcdn1.byjus.com%2Fwp-content%2Fuploads%2F2018%2F07%2Fheart-pump-of-the-circulatory-system.png&f=1&nofb=1&ipt=9644b0b679c1d9b752685a1307f7aadc759d23f8ee5ba8101016385039147fc7.

5.2.3. Regulation of Blood Pressure and Flow

The mechanism of blood flow and blood pressure regulation is a complex one, which is an integral part of the overall working of the cardiovascular system. Central to this regulation are mechanisms such as the renin-angiotensin-aldosterone system, the autonomic nervous system, and baroreceptor responses, which cumulatively keep the blood pressure at a sustainable range. New populations of sensory neurons, identified by TrkC and TH, play significant roles in regulating blood pressure and blood flow. Activation of TrkC+ TH+ neurons has been linked to increased blood pressure and heart rate variability, indicating their role in cardiovascular homeostasis. Of specific note, loss-of-function experiments demonstrate that ablation of the neurons can produce potentially fatal reductions in blood pressure and alterations in blood flow, pointing to their essential role in cardiovascular homeostasis (Morelli et al., 2020) (Figure 5.8).

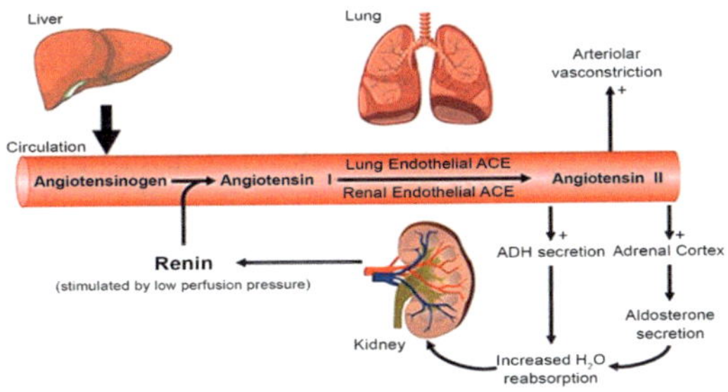

Figure 5.8. Renin–angiotensin–aldosterone system.

Source: https://www.cusabio.com/cardiovascular/Blood-Pressure-Regulation.html.

Also, the contribution of lifestyle determinants, such as dietary habits, cannot be exaggerated in the process of blood pressure maintenance. For example, prolonged intermittent fasting has gained popularity due to its likely benefits in cardiovascular health. It is proven to lead to reductions in arterial blood pressure; thus, there is an interaction between metabolic states and heart function. Experiments in acute fasting have revealed deep insights into the way the autonomic nervous system controls blood pressure and heart rate. Not only does fasting reduce overall blood pressure, but it also enhances vagal regulation of the heart, indicative of a change in autonomic tone that is conducive to cardiovascular health. These findings illuminate the intricate interaction between nutrition, autonomic function, and cardiovascular control, with avenues for further study in the regulation of blood pressure (Gonzalez et al., 2021). Furthermore, a general knowledge of blood pressure control necessitates an exploration of potential stressors and their effect on cardiovascular dynamics. Under mental stressors, patients are capable of having variability in neural and cardiovascular reactivity, which renders blood pressure regulation more difficult. While fasting reduced ambulatory blood pressure, it also added challenges in orthostatic tolerance, as can be seen using lower body negative pressure administrations. These responses highlight the critical role of the sympathetic nervous system in modulating vascular resistance and cardiac function in states of changing metabolism. The intricate process of sympathetic and parasympathetic balancing is highlighted in the dynamic cardiovascular regulation process, which demands more targeted interventions against lifestyle and physiological stressors to regulate blood pressure and overall cardiovascular management (Gonzalez et al., 2021).

Test Your Knowledge

1. What role does the heart play in pumping blood throughout the body?
2. How is blood pressure and flow regulated in the cardiovascular system?

5.3. Blood Composition and Function

Learning Outcome

1. Identify the components of blood: red blood cells, white blood cells, plasma, and platelets
2. Describe the functions of blood in the body
3. Understand the importance of maintaining a healthy blood composition

Its intricate composition of blood is fundamental to its diverse roles in the cardiovascular system. Blood consists of several components, including red blood cells, white blood cells, plasma, and platelets. Red blood cells or erythrocytes play an essential role in delivering oxygen from the lungs to tissues all over the body while facilitating the expulsion of carbon dioxide. This gaseous exchange is primarily influenced by erythrocyte morphology and hemoglobin content. Abnormalities in one or both can severely hamper oxygen delivery, which can lead to various cardiovascular complications. Understanding the precise composition of blood is crucial not only in diagnosing and curing disease but also in providing counsel on exercise and physical function within competitive environments, such as field hockey, where body loads can necessitate specific compensations in blood function and content (Van der Merwe et al., 2018). Other than red blood cells, plasma constitutes most of the blood and serves as the carrier of nutrients, hormones, antibodies, and waste materials. Water, electrolytes, proteins, and nutrients comprise the bulk of plasma, each playing an essential role in maintaining homeostasis. The proteins that are present in plasma, such as albumin, globulins, and fibrinogen, each serve individual purposes: albumin provides osmotic pressure, globulins play a part in the immune response, and fibrinogen plays a role in clotting. Plasma's fluid dynamic structure allows for the capability to adapt to various physiological needs, crucial to overall cardiovascular function. Above all else, alterations in the plasma can reflect underlying pathological states, highlighting the importance of blood examinations in cardiovascular status assessment (Gromova et al., 2016). Not only does the functionality of blood rely on its cellular and plasma components, but also on the interaction between erythrocytes and cardiovascular status. Current studies have highlighted that CVD patients exhibit marked changes in the structure of erythrocyte membranes and microviscosity, compromising the oxygen transport capacity.

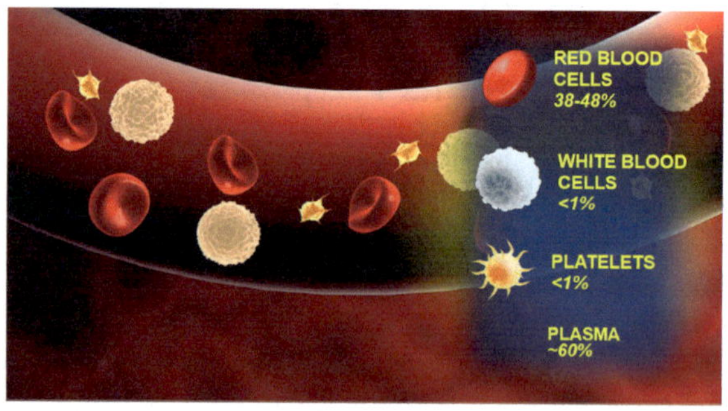

Figure 5.9. Blood components vessel.

Source: https://interactivebiology.com/wp-content/uploads/2022/01/Blood-components-vessel-1024x574.png.

These alterations complicate the process of transporting oxygen to tissues, particularly during stress or increased metabolic demand. Classic therapeutic approaches, such as antiaggregant and statin administration, may not fully restore functional properties of erythrocytes, suggesting the need for comprehensive treatment modalities considering both CVD and erythrocyte function (Gromova et al., 2016). It is because of this that blood composition knowledge is not only significant for pathology diagnosis but also for elaboration of combined treatment tactics in cardiovascular medicine (Figure 5.9).

5.3.1. Components of Blood: Red Blood Cells, White Blood Cells, Plasma, and Platelets

The human circulatory system contains numerous essential parts, each serving a unique function in the cardiovascular system as a whole. Red blood cells, or erythrocytes, are essential for carrying oxygen from the lungs to the body tissues, as well as carrying carbon dioxide back to the lungs for exhalation. Biconcave hemoglobin-stuffed cells are critical for maintaining cellular respiration, which contributes to generating energy in many physiological processes. They last about 120 days and are efficiently recycled by the spleen and liver. Balance and health in RBCs are very critical as any alteration can lead to anemia or other oxygen transport deficiencies, which would be of great importance in terms of overall cardiovascular health, illustrating how blood components rely on each other within the cardiovascular system. In contrast to red blood cells, white blood cells (WBCs) are primarily involved in the body's immune system, guarding it against infection and foreign invasion. Their heterogeneity consists of lymphocytes, neutrophils, monocytes, eosinophils, and basophils, each playing a special role. Lymphocytes are responsible for adaptive immunity, while neutrophils are most often the first responders to infection. There is interplay among these cells that makes their immune response strong and dynamic and plays a role in maintaining homeostasis (Figure 5.10).

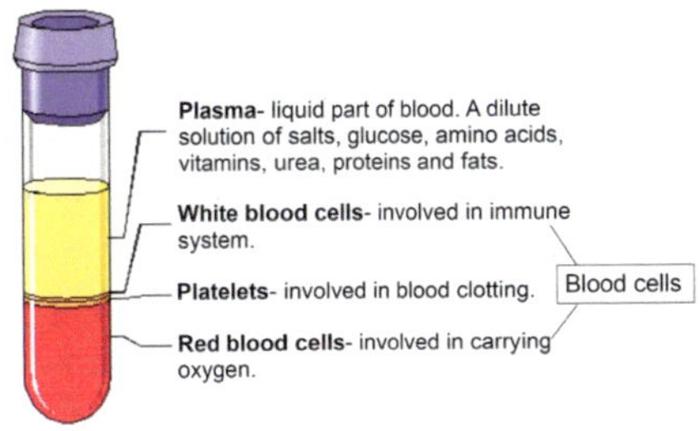

Figure 5.10. The four components in blood.

Source: https://www.westlab.com/media/amasty/blog/Components_of_Blood.png.

WBC well-being might be affected by several factors, such as environmental pollutants or exposure to micro- and nanoplastics (MNPs), which have been shown to initiate inflammation and compromise immune function through their interactions with these cells. Due attention should be given to the cardiovascular system's overall role in maintaining health and resisting disease (Rajendran et al., 2023). Plasma, the liquid component of blood, takes up about 55% of blood volume and is tasked with the transportation of most substances. Plasma has water, electrolytes, proteins, hormones, and waste products and serves as a medium for the transport of nutrients, excretion of waste, and heat dissipation. It also aids in controlling blood pressure and blood volume and carrying red and white cells and platelets through the circulatory system. Plasma proteins such as albumin, globulins, and fibrinogen have different roles, including blood coagulation and immune function. Moreover, recent studies highlight the antioxidant role of plasma constituents, e.g., platelet-rich plasma (PRP), suggesting a broader therapeutic use in the cardiovascular system. PRP has the potential to capture free radicals and may help reduce oxidative stress, making the plasma, besides functioning as a transport mechanism, also a potential therapeutic agent in the case of cardiovascular disease (Wienaldi et al., 2022).

5.3.2. Functions of Blood in the Body

Functions of blood are diverse and significant in the maintenance of homeostasis of the body as the medium of transportation of essential materials. Blood provides oxygen supply from the lungs to the tissues and organs, which is crucial for cell metabolism. A multi-component protein, hemoglobin, in red blood cells allows for the transportation of oxygen through binding with oxygen molecules. Besides, blood is also essential in transporting carbon dioxide, a byproduct of cellular respiration, to the lungs for exhalation. Nutrients absorbed from the gastrointestinal tract, such as glucose and amino acids, are also transported by the blood to offer energy and building blocks for cellular growth and repair. Blood is, thus, a multipurpose carrier whose functions are geared towards the preservation and regulation of body processes. Yet another crucial role played by blood is its support of the regulation of body heat and pH, which aid in homeostasis.

The circulatory system offloads metabolic heat and helps in the dissipation of excess heat using processes like vasodilation, wherein blood vessels dilate, leading to increased flow of blood to the skin. This thermoregulation is particularly significant in maintaining the ideal temperatures, therefore preventing heat illnesses, as revealed in recent research emphasizing the interplay between blood flow and thermoregulation (Fumimoto et al., 2024). Moreover, blood contains buffers such as bicarbonate ions, which serve to maintain pH levels within the tight range necessary for enzymatic and metabolic processes. As pH levels become disparate, this may induce severe physiological derangements, underlining the critical role of blood in maintaining overall body chemistry. Lastly, blood provides immune protection to shield the body from disease-causing pathogens and foreign invaders. White blood cells, or leukocytes, travel in the blood to seek out and destroy invading microorganisms, viruses, and other harmful agents. This function is vital to the immune process of the body, as it enables the immune system to effectively and speedily react to an invasion. In addition, blood elements such as antibodies are released from specialized white blood cells and circulated in the blood to neutralize specific antigens. The ability of the blood for both immune response and surveillance is augmented by its coagulation process, which prevents excessive bleeding from injury. Combined, these roles illustrate the reason why blood is , not only for the delivery of nutrients but also for the protection of body integrity and well-being during various physiological challenges (Kataoka et al., 2023).

5.3.3. Importance of Maintaining Healthy Blood Composition

Maintaining a healthy composition of the blood is of utmost importance for the efficient working of the cardiovascular system, as it directly governs systemic circulation and overall metabolic function. The blood is made up of various components like red blood cells, white blood cells, plasma, and platelets, which all have some significant functions in the body. Red blood cells, for instance, are responsible for the transport of oxygen, while white blood cells protect against infections. Disequilibrium among such constituents can lead to life-threatening illnesses such as hypertension and cardiovascular diseases. Some of these anthropometric dimensions, such as the neck circumference and fat-free mass index, are closely related to arterial stiffness, a precursor to cardiovascular complications. These results illustrate the intricate interplay between blood composition and cardiovascular well-being, and the need for regular checks on nutritional as well as physiological variables to prevent disease (Ib Aáñez et al., 2019) (Figure 5.11).

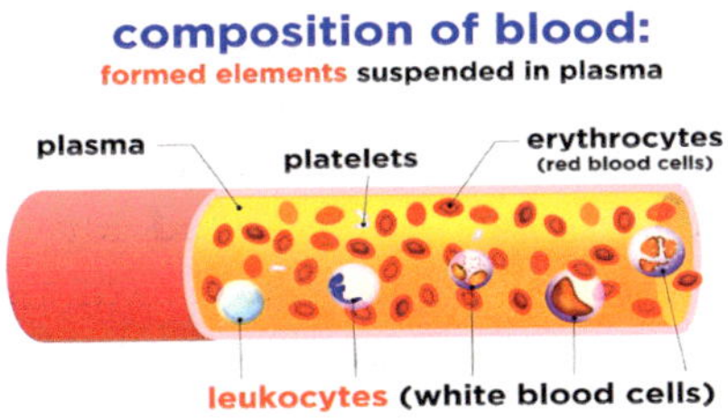

Figure 5.11. The composition of blood.

Source: https://external-content.duckduckgo.com/iu/?u=https%3A%2F%2Fi.ytimg.com%2Fvi%2Fyj7bfZKlIp8%2Fmaxresdefault.jpg&f=1&nofb=1&ipt=19b8c0497ac21af3882ac644a4567141e37bc95f704f683f1db6b226f5993b59.

Aside from its cellular composition, blood's biochemical composition is another significant determinant of cardiovascular health. Blood cholesterol levels, glucose, and inflammatory mediators are critically important in the diagnosis and management of metabolic diseases that have implications for the cardiovascular system. For example, metabolically unhealthy obesity patients are likely to have heightened risks of hypertension and cardiovascular disease. Experiments have demonstrated that lifestyle changes like supervised exercise and dietary modifications can significantly improve such biochemical markers. Surprisingly, transitioning from a metabolically unhealthy to a metabolically healthy profile decreases risk factors for high total cholesterol, hyperglycemia, and elevated blood pressure, hence enhancing cardiovascular well-being. However, without continued intervention, such positive effects may decrease over time, emphasizing the role of sustained health monitoring to maintain a healthy blood composition and, consequently, cardiovascular well-being (Aguirre-Betolaza et al., 2020). Healthy blood composition is not important merely for individual health but also mirrors public health issues. For high-risk populations for cardiovascular disease due to genetic, lifestyle, or socio-economic factors, preventive intervention in creating healthy blood profiles promises long-term reward. Consciousness of the interplay between blood composition and cardiovascular performance can inform public policy, health education, and prevention on the community level. Furthermore, as medical facilities have been trying to cope with the rising incidences of cardiovascular disease, emphasizing blood health as an intervention for prevention could enhance healthcare spending on chronic disease treatment. By raising awareness and launching programs that encourage healthy blood makeup, populations can enhance cardiovascular well-being overall, ultimately leading to reduced morbidity and quality of life (Ib Aáñez et al., 2019).

Test Your Knowledge

1. What are the main components of blood, and what is the primary function of each component?
2. Why is it important to maintain a healthy blood composition, and what can happen if the composition is imbalance?

5.4. Common Cardiovascular Diseases

Learning Outcome

1. Understand the overview of heart disease and its types
2. Describe the risk factors associated with cardiovascular diseases
3. Define symptoms and diagnosis of cardiovascular conditions

The sophistication of cardiovascular disease makes it a growing health problem globally. Atherosclerosis, or the deposit of plaque in artery walls, leads to compromised blood flow and an increased risk of heart attacks and strokes. The chronic condition plagues not just the elderly but also young individuals due to, among other factors, lifestyle issues such as inadequate diets and sedentary lifestyles. Besides, the inflammatory mechanisms underlying atherosclerosis have systemic aspects, linking cardiovascular disease to other diseases, such as psoriasis. It has been suggested that the sub-inflammatory state common to atherosclerosis and psoriasis could set patients at increased cardiovascular risk regardless of traditional risk factors, underlining the multifaceted nature of such conditions (Balduzzi et al., 2016). Hypertension is another prevalent cardiovascular disease that is characterized by elevated blood pressure, or what is commonly referred to as the silent killer because it is symptomless. Chronic hypertension can have damaging effects on most organs, including the heart and kidneys, typically resulting in heart failure or kidney dysfunction. The interdependence of cardiovascular and renal health becomes more evident, especially in the context of cardiorenal syndrome, where there is systemic dysfunction interfering with the other. Of note, patients with chronic kidney disease are at increased risk for mortality due to cardiovascular complications and therefore reaffirm the importance of blood pressure monitoring within a multifaceted health regimen (Bernthaler et al., 2011). The standard mechanisms and molecular pathways of the two conditions underscore the need for a unified approach to prevention and treatment. Heart failure, a syndrome resulting from the heart's inability to pump blood effectively, is a serious end point in the continuum of cardiovascular disease. Various etiologic factors, including ischemic heart disease, hypertension, and valve disease cause it. The presentation of heart failure is variable and can vary from breathlessness and fatigue to edema. Its management is equally varied and involves lifestyle modifications, drug therapy, and surgery. The prognosis for heart failure patients is, however, concerning with the observation that many have associated heart and renal disease, thus verifying the interrelatedness of cardiovascular disease. Understanding heart failure in the context of systemic cardiovascular health is vital because it involves understanding the various factors influencing patient outcomes in this complex disease process.

5.4.1. Overview of Heart Disease and Its Types

Heart disease is a collection of conditions that affect the heart's functioning, structure, and well-being. These complexities include coronary artery disease (CAD), heart rhythm disorders (arrhythmias), and diseases of the heart valves, among others. CAD, the most common one, is brought about by plaque buildup within the coronary arteries, narrowing down the blood supply to the cardiac muscle and ultimately leading to heart attacks. Arrhythmias, on the other hand, are abnormal heart rhythms that cause a variety of symptoms and can even be life-threatening. Heart valve disease consists of faulty valves that disrupt the normal circulation of blood, leading to stenosis or regurgitation, further complicating the functioning of the heart as a pump. Each of these conditions is treated with specific diagnostic and therapeutic measures, an indication of the multifaceted character of cardiovascular disorders in contemporary medicine. With the widespread occurrence and diversity of heart diseases, their pathophysiology is essential to know to develop efficient treatments. Groundbreaking research within the area has brought to the forefront advanced therapy medicinal products (ATMPs), with cell-based therapies using mesenchymal stem cells (MSCs) and induced pluripotent stem cells (iPSCs), holding great promise for myocardial regeneration. This method tries to restore function and regenerate damaged heart tissue, particularly in patients with long-term disease such as refractory angina and heart failure. Application of technologies, such as the three-dimensional NOGA-XP cardiac mapping system, further enhances the precision of therapy by allowing electromechanical analysis of myocardial viability. These advancements emphasize the integration of regenerative medicine strategies in the management of heart conditions, embracing a future for cardiovascular well-being (Caluori et al., 2023). Additionally, biomarker identification in cardiometabolic disease (CMD) is illuminating new possibilities for enhanced diagnosis and treatment of cardiac disease. CMD's multimodality necessitates a multi-omics approach that integrates genetics, epigenetics, and other biological factors, allowing for a more comprehensive understanding of disease processes. Scientists encourage the application of various types of omics to identify biomarkers that are capable of unequivocally defining the status of heart disease, enhancing predictions of outcomes as well as responses to therapy. Further, the significance of gender differences in heart disease also lends support to targeted methods of clinical practice, such that treatment is designed based on patient-specific profiles. Grasping that biological and sociocultural processes both influence heart disease expression gives a holistic perspective that can improve patient care in the long run (Argano et al., 2019) (Figure 5.12).

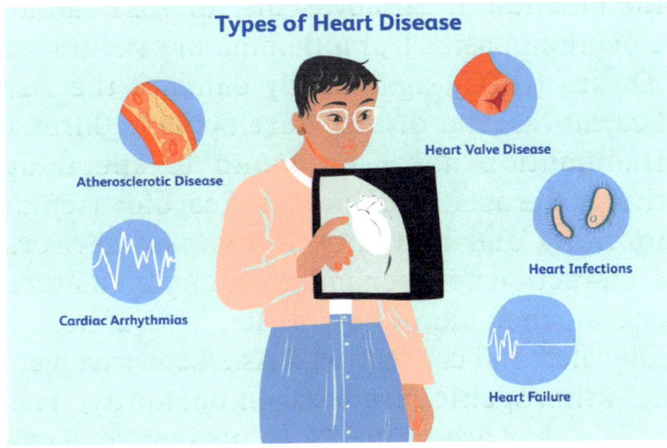

Figure 5.12. Heart disease and its types.

Source: https://www.verywellhealth.com/thmb/MT8bVVf0uHljl_9juoNxjZBISeg=/1500x0/filters:no_upscale():max_bytes(150000):strip_icc()/overview-of-heart-disease-4160961_final-152f46073f2242999b771e409973825b.png.

5.4.2. Risk Factors Associated with Cardiovascular Diseases

Understanding determinants of risk of cardiovascular diseases (CVD) is crucial for effective prevention and treatment policies. Among the most critical of them are metabolic derangements, which have become leading health problems worldwide. Obesity and insulin resistance are notable specifically as prime movers in the causation of CVD and significantly raise the burden of risk in them. These disorders induce a cascade of physiological changes that compromise cardiovascular well-being, ultimately leading to atherosclerotic complications. Additionally, mounting evidence indicates the interplay between deranged immune responses and traditional cardiovascular risk factors and foresees an integrated explanation of the pathogenesis of CVDs. This growing body of literature emphasizes the importance of addressing metabolic health to decrease cardiovascular complication incidence, representing a qualitative shift from purely physiological intervention to a more holistic understanding of health risk. The role of chronic inflammation in cardiovascular disease cannot be overemphasized, as inflammatory rheumatic diseases (IRDs) significantly enhance the risk of cardiovascular disease development. Chronic inflammation has been found to speed up atherosclerosis and increase cardiovascular morbidity and mortality. A complex network of interaction between inflammatory mediators, such as chemokines, cytokines, and adhesion molecules, and conventional risk factors triggers the atherogenic process. Importantly, risk models that are available at present may not entirely account for the unique profiles of IRD patients and thus lead to an underestimation of their cardiovascular risks. Consequently, a deep understanding of the interactions is essential for healthcare providers to create personalized plans of prevention and promote early cardiovascular disease diagnosis. Understanding selected risk factors peculiar to IRDs opens the way to more effective management and intervention activities. In-depth examination of cardiovascular risk demands the study of neural and immune system synergistic functions. Recent findings illustrate how the nervous system regulates immune function and influences metabolic and cardiovascular health. The central nervous system interacts with peripheral pathways to connect neural reflexes and immune response, thereby dictating initiation and progression of disease processes such as hypertension and obesity. Neuromodulatory activity brings into focus the role of the spleen as a primary location for pathophysiological communication among cardiovascular and immune systems. Elucidation of these mechanisms is essential for both clinicians and researchers because it can guide the development of novel therapeutic interventions that target metabolic as well as cardiovascular dysfunctions. Integration of knowledge from various fields of biology gives a more robust framework in handling the multilateral nature of risk factors of cardiovascular diseases, ensuring better health outcomes (Figure 5.13).

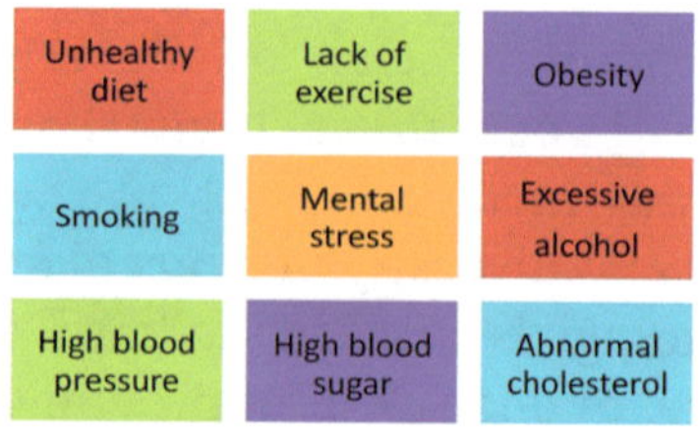

Figure 5.13. Cardiovascular risk factors.

Source: https://external-content.duckduckgo.com/iu/?u=http%3A%2F%2Fwww.cardiacwellnessinstitute.com%2Fheart-disease-treatment-prevention%2Fwp-content%2Fuploads%2F2019%2F12%2FSlide1.jpg&f=1&nofb=1&ipt=f551de504edc3721b229f9aa67fe9c8b4dcb3ac4c5b8be7e9b5cacf0a100806a.

5.4.3. Symptoms and Diagnosis of Cardiovascular Conditions

Symptom identification related to cardiovascular diseases is crucial in early diagnosis and management. Symptoms can be chest pain, dyspnea, palpitations, and fatigue. Symptoms vary significantly among patients, and the clinical presentation is complex. Patients, for instance, may present with atypical symptoms resembling conditions that are not cardiovascular, and it becomes difficult to distinguish. This lack of clarity in the diagnosis of cardiovascular emergencies ultimately reflects on bad outcomes, including increased morbidity and mortality. Clinicians should therefore embrace a comprehensive approach to evaluation, such as patient history and physical examinations in order to guide appropriate intervention and management of potential cardiovascular disease, according to literature studies (Anjum et al., 2018). An interaction of clinical examination and advanced diagnostic modalities governs correct diagnosis of cardiovascular ailments. Electrocardiogram, echocardiogram, and blood tests are standard techniques employed to identify underlying cardiac diseases. Research reveals the enormous burden of cardiovascular disease among elderly patients and identifies hypertension as a dominant condition (Kisenge et al., 2011) (Figure 5.14).

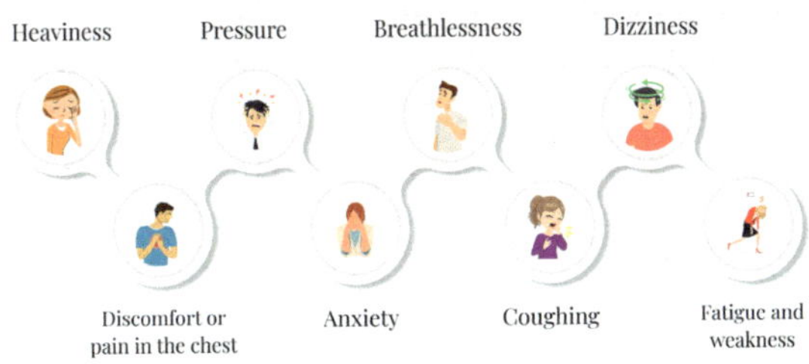

Figure 5.14. Symptoms of cardiovascular diseases.

Source: https://www.swasthyaclinics.com/images/heart%20disease%20symptoms_1657782394.webp.

Clinical presentations most frequently encountered are peripheral edema, chest pain, and shortness of breath, emphasizing the importance of meticulous screening among elderly groups. Also, the use of technology in diagnosis allows for adequate assessment and has dramatically changed the way healthcare providers treat cardiovascular conditions. As diagnostic methodologies continue to evolve, their application must also be set by clinical guidelines so as to identify the range of cardiovascular disorders effectively. In order to reduce the cardiovascular risks in at-risk populations like the elderly, a proactive symptom and diagnosis management is essential. Regular screening of hypertension and other cardiovascular risk factors is advised, particularly in elderly patients with non-specific symptoms. The evidence suggests that thorough investigations at hospital admission could be an efficient method for early detection of cardiovascular diseases, potentially reducing hospital admissions and improving patient outcomes. Second, patient education on early symptoms can allow patients to access medical treatment early. By creating awareness and implementing early diagnosis protocols, healthcare systems can more effectively counteract the rising prevalence of cardiovascular diseases, leading to better patient care (Kisenge et al., 2011).

Test Your Knowledge

1. What are the different types of heart disease, and how do they affect the cardiovascular system?
2. What are the common risk factors that increase the likelihood of developing cardiovascular diseases?

5.5. Prevention and Management of Cardiovascular Diseases

Learning Outcome

1. Identify the lifestyle changes for heart health
2. Define medical interventions and treatments
3. Understand the importance of regular health screenings

Cardiovascular diseases (CVDs) are a significant public health problem, impacting hundreds of millions of people globally and needing proper prevention and control. Prevention lies in the promotion of heart-healthy living through balanced dieting, regular physical activity, and abstinence from tobacco. Educational interventions on diet can also significantly reduce risk indicators of CVD; for instance, consumption of fruits, vegetables, and omega-3 fatty acids can lower cholesterol levels and enhance cardiac health as a whole. Physical activity programs at the community level—such as walking clubs or aerobic exercise classes—can also promote more active lifestyles among populations that traditionally exhibit sedentary habits. Because

CVD risk factors such as hypertension and obesity are typically preventable, public health programs that serve to educate and mobilize communities are necessary. Interventions that combine traditional dietary practices with modern nutritional guidance can enhance compliance with these prevention guidelines while being mindful of cultural sensitivities. Cardiovascular disease management is often a multi-factorial process that includes medical treatment, lifestyle modification, and psychosocial assistance. Pharmacologic interventions such as antihypertensives, statins, and anticoagulants can manage blood pressure, cholesterol levels, and prevent thromboembolic events. However, the efficacy of these drugs is greatly enhanced through nonpharmacologic interventions such as dietary modifications and exercise augmentation. Frequent patient education plays an important role here, encouraging the patient to become a partner in the therapeutic program. Health care providers must consider culture-sensitive variables that influence patients' perception of health and treatment adherence, particularly in the case of diverse populations. For example, women and men in Saudi Arabia have differences in cardiovascular health, risk factors, and access to healthcare, which need to be addressed through targeted interventions to be able to effectively counter such discrepancies (Clark et al., 2012). Finally, routine screening and early detection of risk factors for cardiovascular disease cannot be overstressed in the prevention and control of CVD. Early detection of hypertension, high cholesterol, and diabetes—conditions that typically precede more severe cardiovascular events—is facilitated by regular checkups. Screening programs, particularly in high-risk groups or among specific populations, are also essential in the prevention of morbidity and mortality due to heart disease. Technological advancements in telemedicine and mobile health applications have also emerged as practical tools for promoting regular surveillance and facilitating easy access to healthcare professionals. These technologies are particularly able to benefit the population with limited access to traditional health care, enabling timely interventions. Further, the integration of community participation in the surveillance of health supports an active strategy against CVD, causing empowered people who are actively engaged in their cardiovascular journey to good health (Kitsiou et al., 2013) (Figure 5.15).

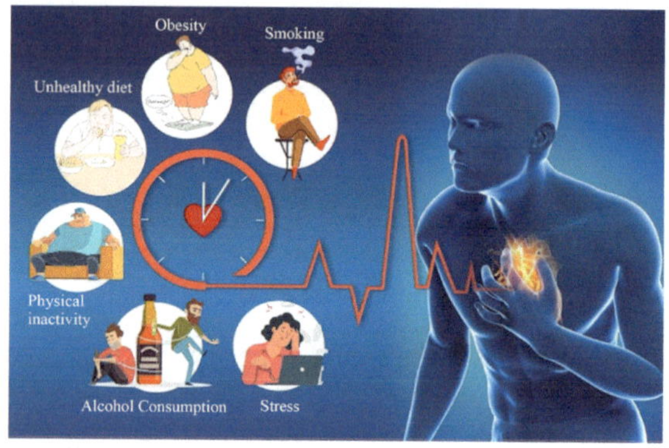

Figure 5.15. Prevent cardiovascular diseases.

Source: https://blog.thyrocare.com/wp-content/uploads/2021/11/prevent-cardiovascular-diseases.jpg.

5.5.1. Lifestyle Changes for Heart Health

In the management of heart health, the importance of lifestyle changes cannot be overemphasized. Regular exercise is an elementary component in maintaining cardiovascular well-being. Evidence indicates that the inclusion of exercise in everyday life can lead to dramatic improvements in the efficiency of the heart as well as general well-being. Physical exercise in the form of walking, swimming, or cycling not only contributes to physical well-being but also serves to reduce stress, which is the primary reason for cardiovascular disease. In addition, the communities promoting active lifestyles also have lower heart condition rates among their inhabitants, testifying to the common benefit of prevention strategies. The different programs, for example, the TEXTMe program in Detroit, aim at implementing such changes through outreach and education in the community to instill healthier habits in the residents with cardiovascular disease (Horton et al., 2021). All these changes pave the way for long-term changes that eventually result in improved cardiovascular health. Diet also plays a significant part in cardiovascular well-being, necessitating a comprehensive overhaul of one's diet. Research shows that diets rich in fruits, vegetables, whole grains, lean protein foods, and healthy fats significantly minimize the risk of cardiovascular disease. Conversely, overindulgence of processed food, sugar, and saturated fats can increase blood pressure and cholesterol levels, resulting in severe heart-related complications. Health education designed to make individuals aware of healthy eating habits has been effective, particularly among groups of people at risk of heart disease. For example, assessment of dietary behavior by different community programs allows health providers to offer targeted nutritional counseling that caters to the patient's health status and behavior. Besides, the integration of nutrition counseling with healthcare is successful in promoting healthy eating behavior and enhancing patients' cardiovascular disease metrics knowledge, as per a study on the long-term effectiveness of lifestyle modifications (Chen et al., 2020). Further, quitting smoking is vital for health improvement and the reduction in the occurrence of cardiovascular disease. Smoking is a well-documented risk factor for the occurrence of heart attacks, strokes, and other serious illnesses. Access to quit programs can thereby decrease these risks significantly. Extensive interventions with counseling, pharmacologic support, and community reinforcement can encourage smokers to quit smoking, leading to improved cardiovascular outcomes. The positive effects of quitting smoking are observed, with former smokers likely to show heart function improvement and a reduction in the risk of future cardiovascular events. Collaborations between clinicians and community organizations are crucial for implementing such interventions and fostering supportive lifestyles. This interrelated strategy not only elevates individual health levels but also contributes to the overall well-being of the population at large, making considerable strides in combating cardiovascular diseases (Horton et al., 2021) (Figure 5.16).

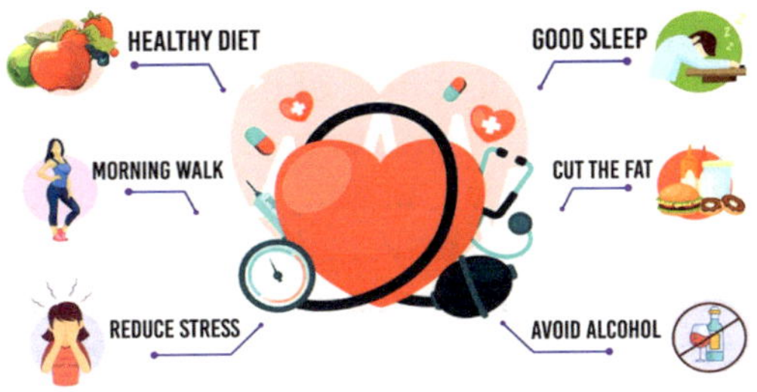

Figure 5.16. Lifestyle Changes Recommended by Cardiologists for a Healthy Heart.

Source: https://www.drashwanimehta.com/assets/image/blog/tips-from-cardiologist-for-healthy-heart.webp.

5.5.2. Medical Interventions and Treatments

The effective management of cardiovascular diseases largely relies on different forms of medical treatments and interventions directed at mitigating risks and complications. Pharmacological interventions constitute one standard method, which also involves the use of antihypertensive medication, statins, and antiplatelet drugs. These medications assist in managing blood pressure, lowering cholesterol levels, and preventing blood clotting, thereby resulting in a lower probability of acute cardiovascular events. According to recent studies, the implementation of these interventions has been successful, and an estimated 450 fewer deaths from cardiovascular disease were reported among targeted groups in 2009 compared to previous years. This highlights the significance of affordable drug treatment in the prevention of cardiovascular disease and indicates the role of timely intervention in altering patterns of disease. In addition to drug therapy, surgery plays a significant role in the treatment of various cardiovascular diseases as well. Treatment with CABG and PCI is employed to restore the blood supply in patients with a blocked artery. Such surgical treatment not only renders symptoms of diseases like coronary heart disease moot, but also significantly increases the quality of life as well as the life expectancy of patients. Evidence points to secondary prevention following acute myocardial infarction, usually involving surgery, as having significantly reduced death rates. Combine surgical methods with ongoing medical management to form a comprehensive treatment plan that yields optimal patient outcomes when faced with mounting cardiovascular risks. Lifestyle interventions are a highly integral component of comprehensive cardiovascular treatment plans as well. Interventions on diet, physical activity, and smoking cessation are the primary approaches to addressing the underlying risk factors leading to cardiovascular diseases. In various epidemiological surveys, including those in Tunisia, higher risk factor levels of obesity and inactivity have been identified to contribute to the cases of coronary heart disease significantly. So, appropriate interventions that promote healthy habits can have a substantial impact on the diminishment of such risk factors and consequently lead to better cardiovascular health outcomes. While drugs and surgery have an indispensable role, behavior change has a synergistic effect too, which cannot be undermined, as it offers a pathway for reducing the burden of cardiovascular diseases in the population worldwide.

5.5.3. Importance of Regular Health Screenings

Regular health checks are essential for the early detection of cardiovascular diseases, which are still the largest global killers. Employing screening, risk factors like hypertension, high levels of cholesterol, and diabetes are revealed—diseases that predominantly cause cardiovascular disease. Detection of these risks early allows practitioners to recommend lifestyle changes or interventions before the onset of advanced health issues. This health maintenance through preventive measures not only enhances the quality of one's life but also reduces healthcare costs in general by preventing the need for more serious medical interventions. As the incidence of cardiovascular illnesses rises, these tests cannot be overstressed because they contribute to the maintenance of long-term cardiovascular health. In addition, regular screening offers the potential for tailoring health advice and interventions based on someone's risks and lifestyle. For example, a comprehensive assessment during a health screening will likely convince individuals to adopt improved dietary habits and increased physical activity. These personalized recommendations are especially significant, as indicators such as family history and socio-economic status may significantly alter one's cardiovascular risk profile (Figure 5.17).

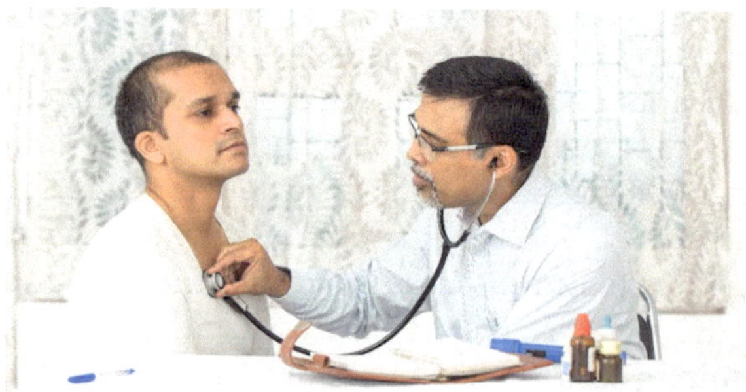

Figure 5.17. Doctor using a stethoscope to examine a patient's heartbeat during a clinical check-up.

Source: https://akm-img-a-in.tosshub.com/indiatoday/images/story/202505/mature-doctor-examining-a-young-patient-at-his-clinic-the-doctor-is-checking-his-heartbeat-with-a-s-20534684-16x9_0.jpg?VersionId=d0k66ogduNpHtNvNCELpbJMHckJMUG5S&size=690:388.

Such targeted health interventions not only give patients power but also instill a sense of increased responsibility for their health. Public health programs designed to generate awareness of the benefits of regular screening might engage communities more actively in cardiovascular health, ultimately working toward an education-based population. In specific communities, knowledge of the greater stakes at play in health screening may also make them more successful. For instance, variations in access to health facilities are likely to introduce unequal opportunities for screening, thereby leading to variations in health outcomes among populations. This situation mimics the evidence on the health impacts of natural disasters, whereby poor people have limited access to necessary services as reported in various studies (N/A, 2006). Similarly, when such screening programs are implemented fairly and equitably, they can help decrease these inequalities and provide appropriate cardiovascular assessments to all communities, particularly vulnerable populations. This agreement between healthcare providers and community organizations in advocating for such screenings becomes essential to bridge health equity gaps and ultimately improve community health outcomes for cardiovascular disease.

Test Your Knowledge

1. What lifestyle changes can help improve heart health and reduce the risk of cardiovascular disease?
2. What are some common medical interventions and treatments used for managing heart conditions?

5.6. Advances in Cardiovascular Research

Learning Outcome

1. Analyze recent innovations in treatment and technology related to cardiovascular health
2. Evaluate current research trends in the field of cardiovascular health
3. Discuss future directions and potential developments in cardiovascular studies

The field of cardiovascular research has seen tremendous advancements over the past few years, particularly in the domain of genetic understanding. Due to the advances in genotyping methods, researchers can now investigate deeper into the genetic underpinnings of cardiovascular diseases. Great emphasis has been placed on identifying candidate genes through the use of animal models, and converting them to human diseases remains a significant challenge. As suggested in recent literature, the direction towards genome-wide association studies of large size is growing stronger, with particular emphasis on high-quality standards for both genotyping and phenotyping processes. This not only raises the validity of the results of research but also provides an entry point for novel treatment modalities targeted against individual pathways involved in cardiovascular health. The focus on wider disease pathways instead of concentrating on single genetic variants is an integrative approach that may revolutionize our understanding of cardiovascular conditions (Abu-Amero et al., 2008). Advances in technologies have also pushed cardiovascular research to unexplored frontiers, especially about medical implants. The development of smart stent devices is an example of how engineering progress has a profound impact on clinical outcomes. The devices are now fitted with improved electrical characteristics that facilitate better disease diagnosis and treatment of conditions like atherosclerosis and central line access failure. The recent literature on this area presents a broad spectrum of innovations that not only address the condition of cardiovascular diseases but also enhance patient comfort and safety. The development of the implants explains the importance of multidisciplinary collaborations that bring together engineering, biology, and clinical expertise. With the development of these technologies further, they have significant implications for cardiovascular interventions. They can potentially reduce the incidence of heart attacks and strokes, which are still leading causes of death in today's society (Bussooa et al., 2018). Also, the intersection of technology and cardiovascular research has initiated an age of innovation that can transform the treatment strategy of cardiovascular diseases. Advances in the technology of designing, powering, and communicating in cardiovascular medical implants are enhancing their effectiveness and functionality. Some examples are devices that offer vascular access, which are crucial in the treatment of arterial diseases that are major precipitants of cardiovascular events. There are some drawbacks, however, particularly about manufacturing and compatibility of such devices within the human body. With the challenges overcome by research, the future for cardiovascular technology is bright and suggests that personalized design and high-performance engineering solutions will lead to improved outcomes. The intersection of such intelligent technologies has the potential to transform cardiovascular care and ultimately find its way to a healthier and improved quality of life for patients with these chronic diseases (Bussooa et al., 2018).

5.6.1. Innovations in Treatment and Technology

Recent advancements in cardiovascular treatment and technology have substantially improved patient outcomes and optimized healthcare delivery efficiency. Telemedicine and remote monitoring equipment are among the new technologies facilitating real-time data on patients' cardiovascular conditions for timely intervention. The technologies not only improve patient compliance with treatment programs but also empower individuals to participate in health management actively. Furthermore, the introduction of machine learning and artificial intelligence into diagnosis has revolutionized the identification and prediction of cardiovascular events.

The capacity of AI programs to process large data sets of health information enables clinicians to design focused treatment plans, hence enhancing the accuracy of interventions. Thus, the convergence of technology and cardiovascular therapy heralds an era of preventative cardiology, leading the field toward improved outcomes for diverse populations. In parallel with advancements in technology, pharmacological innovation has uncovered additional therapies for patients with cardiovascular disease. The introduction of new classes of drugs, such as PCSK9 inhibitors and SGLT2 inhibitors, has transformed the management of cholesterol and heart failure, respectively. Such therapies are part of a broader movement in clinical pharmacology whereby ongoing advancements in drug discoveries are impelled by intensive research and the need for medicines made to individuals' specifications. Most importantly, the role of platforms like Clinical Pharmacology & Therapeutics is characterized by continuous efforts at condensing and disseminating advanced knowledge informing clinical practice and regulatory guidelines. With the overcoming of traditional barriers to drug compliance through optimized dosing regimens and evidence-supported measures, such innovations align with the mission of enhancing therapeutic outcomes while reducing associated healthcare costs (Terzic et al., 2017) (Figure 5.18).

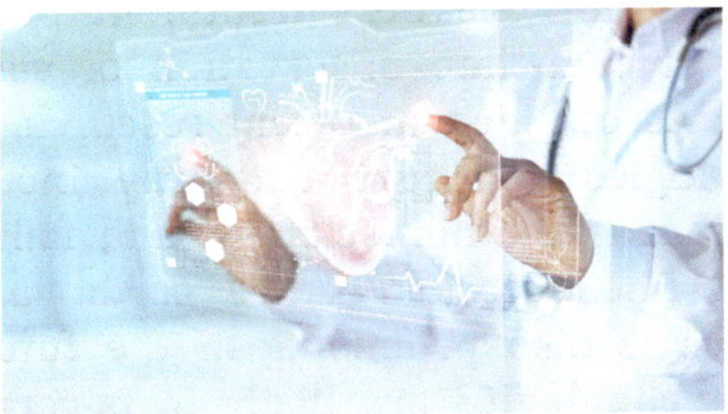

Figure 5.18. Doctor interacting with advanced cardiological technology displaying a digital heart and vital signs.

Source: https://revere-health.hqdemo.app/wp-content/uploads/2022/02/Cardiological_Technology_Advancements-scaled.jpeg.

Furthermore, the establishment of biotechnology has opened doors for groundbreaking treatments such as gene therapy and regenerative medicine that hold enormous promises for cardiovascular patients. Gene editing technologies such as CRISPR have unearthed new horizons in exploring genetic susceptibilities to heart disease to facilitate targeted interventions at the molecular level. Regenerative therapies, including stem cell therapy, aim to repair or replace injured cardiac tissue and regain function in patients with heart failure or myocardial infarction. Not only are they promising for regeneration and repair, but they are also a new model for curative as opposed to symptomatic-only therapy. As pharmaceutical and medical device companies aim to create shared value out of these innovations, they too have the potential to address unmet health needs among diverse populations and thereby create global health advancement (Peterson et al., 2012). It is a collaborative setup that fosters an environment in which innovative technology not only benefits clinical practice but also promotes fair access to healthcare across the world.

5.6.2. Current Research Trends in Cardiovascular Health

The evolving landscape of cardiovascular health research has expanded in size, particularly in research on risk factors contributing to cardiovascular disease (CVD). Current research indicates that established risk factors such as high blood pressure, high serum cholesterol levels, and smoking are the primary contributors to CVD-related deaths globally. High blood pressure is especially a leading cause of more CVD-related deaths than any other individual risk factor, citing the importance of targeted interventions. Current worldwide comparative risk assessment indicates that about 9.7 million CVD deaths annually are caused by a combination of known risk factors and conditions like excess body mass index and physical inactivity. However, irreplaceable uncertainty remains in these estimates because of insufficient population data on risk factor exposure and potential biases in observational studies. Closing these gaps is essential to developing efficient prevention strategies against CVD and policy alternatives to modify alterable preventable risk factors (Elliott et al., 2016). Contemporary analysis of trends in cardiovascular health also underscores the role of demographic factors in CVD risk profiles. New studies, including research on the cardiovascular disease risk profiles of Mexican-Americans by generation, reveal broad differences in terms of cultural, socioeconomic, and lifestyle differences. Outcomes indicate that second-generation Mexican-Americans experience higher rates of hypertension and lower smoking prevalence compared to their first-generation counterparts. Notably, the Framingham Risk Score, a widely utilized multicardiovascular risk index, did not indicate a generational difference, suggesting that interactions between genes and environment play an essential role in cardiovascular health. These studies underscore the need for sensitive analyses aware of demographic change and age cohort differences in risk factors to guide better public health interventions among at-risk groups (Escarce et al., 2011). Concurrent with demographic considerations, new approaches for the investigation of cardiovascular health are being created. Developments in data gathering and analytic methods are leading to more accurate tests of risk factor effects and interactions. For example, the use of big data approaches is enhancing epidemiologic studies through the capacity to analyze large data sets that represent diverse populations and risk exposures. Not only does this enhance the strength of findings, but it also allows for real-time monitoring of CVD trends and outcomes. Furthermore, the interactions across disciplines between fields such as genetics, nutrition, and behavioral science are leading to an inclusive understanding of cardiovascular health and unlocking potential interventions. Maintaining emphasis on such contemporary approaches and interdisciplinarity remains vital for further reinforcing the body of knowledge and addressing the global issue of cardiovascular disease (Elliott et al., 2016) (Figure 5.19).

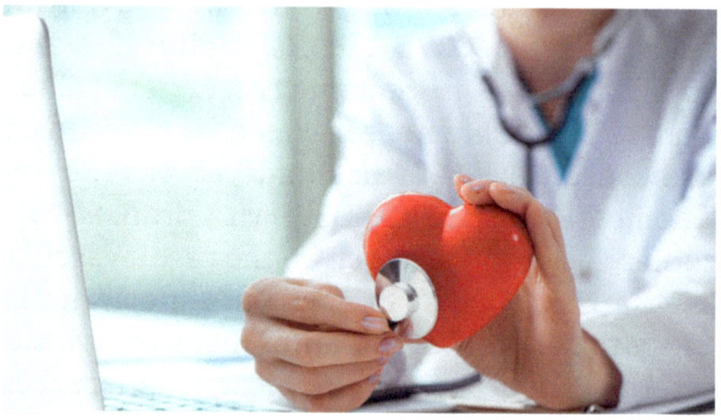

Figure 5.19. Cardiovascular-health-trends.

Source: https://lifesciences.enago.com/blogs/wp-content/uploads/2023/10/cardiovascular-health-trends.png.

5.6.3. Future Directions for Cardiovascular Studies

The evolution of cardiovascular science is increasingly driven by technological breakthroughs, particularly in medical implants. These innovative devices, such as intelligent stents, have the potential to revolutionize the diagnosis and treatment of a wide variety of cardiovascular diseases. These implants not only enhance the electrical characteristics necessary for the best treatment but also allow for real-time observation of vascular health. As outlined in recent research, these technologies can cure currently incurable conditions like atherosclerosis and failure of central line access. Further, cardiovascular research is also promising in the future as these technologies are likely to become the routine management of arterial disease, a significant cause of heart attacks and strokes. Hence, the integration of cutting-edge medical technology is probably going to be central to the promotion of patient outcomes in cardiovascular services (Bussooa et al., 2018). Coupled with technological advancements, interdisciplinary studies are likely to become increasingly common in cardiovascular research in the future. Multidisciplinary collaboration across disciplines such as physics and biology has been shown to result in better educational methods that can have a direct influence on health sciences. For instance, the inclusion of physics in biology curricula has allowed for enhanced understanding of intricate physiological phenomena, resulting in more holistic insights into cardiovascular health in students and future professionals. This pedagogical reform strikes sympathetic chords in education reforms around the world, such as those implemented under the Bologna Plan. Through the incorporation of their diverse areas of study and perspectives into cardiovascular research, discoveries and findings are greatly enhanced, calling for greater interdisciplinary investigation of heart disease and its system-wide effects (Cussó et al., 2019). Furthermore, future cardiovascular research emphasizes the call for personalized medicine and genetic research. Genomic and bioinformatics advances are providing opportunities for individualized therapies that consider the patient's profile, thereby changing therapy regimens. Understanding the genetic influences on cardiovascular conditions renders interventions and prevention more precise and complete, and therefore reduces the incidence and severity of cardiovascular disease. Ongoing research into the genetics of heart disease will assist in the identification of high-risk populations and, hopefully, mitigate cardiovascular disease health disparities. Last but not least, the coming together of personalized medicine and cardiovascular research is a paradigm shift of events that can lead to much-improved patient outcomes for heart disease patients (Bussooa et al., 2018).

Test Your Knowledge

1. What are some recent innovations in treatment and technology that have improved cardiovascular care?
2. What future directions are anticipated in cardiovascular studies to further enhance prevention and treatment?

SUMMARY

An integrative understanding of the cardiovascular system reveals not only its complexity but also the interrelatedness of various physiological components. At the forefront of this is vitamin D's role in cardiovascular disease, where recent findings indicate that vitamin D deficiency bears a high correlation with the prevalence of hypertension in vulnerable populations. For instance, a study found that among women with existing cardiovascular disease, those with diagnosed vitamin D deficiency had a significantly greater incidence of hypertension compared to their counterparts with normal levels of vitamin. Such a correlation stresses the need for health professionals to incorporate vitamin D status in cardiovascular risk evaluation and management strategies, further highlighting the pivotal role of micronutrients in maintaining cardiovascular well-being (Filipiak et al., 2016). Besides, the influence of therapeutic interventions on the cardiovascular system cannot be overlooked. Statins, initially prescribed to manage dyslipidemia, have manifested pleiotropic advantages over their mechanisms of lipid-lowering. The advantages can affect myocardial function, as evidenced by studies that reveal how statins influence caveolin expression and thus modulate cardiac contractility and adrenergic responsiveness. The outcomes of the research indicate that statin therapy is not just a prophylactic therapy of atherosclerosis but also an integrative treatment approach that can improve patient outcomes in cardiovascular disease, particularly in those with altered β-adrenoceptor signaling (Bist et al., 2014). This calls for further clinical research to understand the intricate roles of cardiovascular drugs fully. Ultimately, with our increasing comprehension of the cardiovascular system, we must take an integrated approach that unifies nutritional, pharmacological, and lifestyle factors with patient management. The coincidence of vitamin D deficiency and hypertension is an inherently modifiable risk factor, while the revolution in statin therapy emphasizes the use of drugs in treating cardiovascular disease. Subsequent studies will need to be large-scale to confirm such correlations and stimulate novel treatment strategies that take into account the complexity of cardiovascular disease. Through the collective understanding of several disciplines, we are more likely to advance patient care and enhance overall cardiovascular management.

The cardiovascular system, a highly complex network vital to human physiology, plays a crucial role in maintaining homeostasis and supporting every bodily function. Central to any discussion regarding this system is stress response, where the relationship between the brain and the cardiovascular system is emphasized. Physical or psychological stressors result in a cascade of physiological reactions that impact cardiovascular health. Understanding this connection is crucial as agents of health care often operate in isolated domains, either addressing neurological or cardiovascular issues without the proper synergy of both perspectives. A more holistic understanding is necessary to grasp the multifaceted implications of stress on cardiovascular function, thereby affirming the desirability of a holistic approach in enhancing disease prevention and control measures (Estrine et al., 2006). The contribution of environmental and genetic influences to cardiovascular health is another prominent theme in the discussion of the cardiovascular system. Research has increasingly accepted the role of disparities in genetic makeup, which are fostered by environmental variables, on the risk to cardiovascular disease. This has led to an understanding that has provided the foundation to explore epigenomics, which analyzes how external factors can modify gene expression without influencing the genetic code itself. Of special mention, advances in next-generation sequencing technology have made it possible to explore epigenomic landscapes increasingly deeply, uncovering the sophisticated interactions that shape cardiovascular health. This new perspective encourages a shift away from the most basic symptom alleviation towards an understanding of complex processes, potentially redesigning therapeutic interventions for the management of cardiovascular disease (McKinsey et al., 2018). Besides, the discourses call for an all-encompassing research agenda that combines the functions of genetics, environmental studies, and evolutionary biology in unraveling cardiovascular health intricacies. The focus on convergent principles marks the means through which diverse eukaryotic cells have standard genetic foundations with characteristic responses to environmental stimuli. Through the interfacing of these fields, scientists can develop an integrated appreciation of the impact of stress and overall health on cardiovascular outcomes throughout the lifespan. Integrative research like this is essential, not just for improving our understanding of the cardiovascular system, but also for developing novel methods to manage cardiovascular diseases in clinical care (Estrine et al., 2006; McKinsey et al., 2018).

KEY TERMS FROM THIS CHAPTER

- Heart
- Ventricles
- Septum
- Pulmonary Circulation
- Arteries
- Capillaries
- Cardiac Cycle
- Heart Rate
- Atria
- Valves
- Myocardium
- Systemic Circulation
- Veins
- Coronary Arteries
- Stroke Volume

CRITICAL THINKING QUESTIONS

1. **What is the primary function of the cardiovascular system?**
   a. Producing hormones
   b. Transporting oxygen, nutrients, and waste
   c. Controlling body temperature
   d. Breaking down food
2. **What is the largest artery in the human body?**
   a. Pulmonary artery
   b. Carotid artery
   c. Aorta
   d. Coronary artery
3. **Which chamber of the heart pumps oxygenated blood to the body?**
   a. Right atrium
   b. Right ventricle
   c. Left atrium
   d. Left ventricle
4. **What type of blood vessels carry blood back to the heart?**
   a. Arteries
   b. Capillaries
   c. Veins
   d. Arterioles
5. **What component of blood is responsible for clotting?**
   a. Red blood cells
   b. White blood cells
   c. Plasma
   d. Platelets

Short Answer Questions

1. What are the main functions of the cardiovascular system?
2. Describe the structure and function of the heart.
3. How does blood circulate through the heart, lungs, and body?
4. Explain the role of the sinoatrial (SA) node in regulating heartbeats.
5. How do lifestyle factors, such as diet and exercise, impact cardiovascular health?
6. What are common cardiovascular diseases, and how can they be prevented?
7. How does the autonomic nervous system regulate heart rate?

Answer to Critical Thinking Questions

1. (b); 2. (c); 3. (d); 4. (c); 5. (d)

REFERENCES

1. Tsang, H. G., Rashdan, N. A., Whitelaw, C. B. A., Corcoran, B. M., Summers, K. M., & MacRae, V. E. (2016). Large animal models of cardiovascular disease. *Cell Biochemistry and Function, 34*(3), 113–132. https://doi.org/10.1002/cbf.3173Abu-Amero, K., Aitman, T., Dominiczak, A. F., Benhamou, Y., Bhatnagar, A., Bowcock, A., Caulfield, M., et al. (2008). The genetics of cardiovascular disease. https://core.ac.uk/download/1395614.pdf (accessed on 14th June 2025).

2. Aguirre-Betolaza, A., Martínez, A., Arratibel-Imaz, I., Corres, P., et al. (2020). A metabolically healthy profile is a transient stage when exercise and diet are not supervised: Long-term effects in the EXERDIET-HTA study. https://core.ac.uk/download/322929946.pdf (accessed on 14th June 2025).

3. Alcaraz Ibáñez, M., García Artero, E., Hernández Martínez, A., et al. (2019). Influence of body composition on arterial stiffness in middle-aged adults: Healthy UAL cross-sectional study. https://core.ac.uk/download/286590321.pdf (accessed on 14th June 2025).

4. Almog, Y., Aon, M. A., Barabasi, A. L., Bhalla, U. S., Bigger, J. T., Boxenbaum, H., et al. (2025). Deterministic chaos and fractal complexity in the dynamics of cardiovascular behavior: Perspectives on a new frontier. https://core.ac.uk/download/pdf/8336146.pdf (accessed on 14th June 2025).

5. Anjum, S. (2018). Systematic approach to acute cardiovascular emergencies. https://core.ac.uk/download/322436228.pdf (accessed on 14th June 2025).

6. Argano, V., Balistreri, C. R., Giarratana, R. M., et al. (2019). On the road to accurate biomarkers for cardiometabolic diseases by integrating precision and gender medicine approaches. https://core.ac.uk/download/268910274.pdf (accessed on 14th June 2025).

7. Baker, A. H., Bradshaw, A. C., & Deng, L. (2016). Role of noncoding RNA in vascular remodeling. https://core.ac.uk/download/46558277.pdf (accessed on 14th June 2025).

8. Balduzzi, V., Bernardini, N., La Viola, G., et al. (2016). Cardiovascular risk evaluation through heart rate variability (HRV) analysis in patients with psoriasis before and after 12 weeks of etanercept therapy: A preliminary prospective study. https://core.ac.uk/download/481908477.pdf (accessed on 14th June 2025).

9. Bernthaler, A., Jandrasits, C., Mayer, B., et al. (2011). Integrative bioinformatics analysis of proteins associated with the cardiorenal syndrome. https://core.ac.uk/download/pdf/8500435.pdf (accessed on 14th June 2025).

10. Bist, A., Chesley, A., Reboulleau, A., Carozzi, A. J., Nussler, A. K., Norman, A. W., Aravamudan, B., et al. (2014). Caveolin contributes to the modulation of basal and β-adrenoceptor stimulated function of the adult rat ventricular myocyte by simvastatin: A novel pleiotropic effect. https://core.ac.uk/download/30270024.pdf (accessed on 14th June 2025).

11. Bohacik, J., & Davis, D. N. (2013). Fuzzy rule-based system applied to risk estimation of cardiovascular patients. https://core.ac.uk/download/151162747.pdf (accessed on 14th June 2025).

12. Briggs, A., Frank, B., Unal, B., Murray, C. J., Ford, E. S., Ben Romdhane, H., Ghozzi, H., et al. (2013). Analyzing recent coronary heart disease mortality trends in Tunisia between 1997 and 2009. https://core.ac.uk/download/17298046.pdf (accessed on 14th June 2025).

13. Bush, S., Clark, E., Corcoran, B., et al. (2020). Expression of calcification and extracellular matrix genes in the cardiovascular system of the healthy domestic sheep (*Ovis aries*). https://core.ac.uk/download/334415004.pdf (accessed on 14th June 2025).

14. Bussooa, A., Mercer, J. R., & Neale, S. (2018). Future of smart cardiovascular implants. https://core.ac.uk/download/161513601.pdf (accessed on 14th June 2025).

15. Caluori, G., Dobrolinska, M. M., Follin, B., et al. (2023). Induced pluripotent stem cells and allogeneic mesenchymal stem cell therapy in cardiovascular diseases. https://core.ac.uk/download/620186233.pdf (accessed on 14th June 2025).

16. Camporeale, C., Guala, A., Ridolfi, L., et al. (2014). Impact of atrial fibrillation on the cardiovascular system through a lumped-parameter approach. https://core.ac.uk/download/pdf/76524032.pdf (accessed on 14th June 2025).

17. Carnevale, D., Lembo, G., & Perrotta, M. (2016). The multifaceted roles of PI3Kγ in hypertension, vascular biology, and inflammation. https://core.ac.uk/download/98335835.pdf (accessed on 14th June 2025).

18. Carnevale, D., Lembo, G., Lori, A., et al. (2017). The spleen: A hub connecting nervous and immune systems in cardiovascular and metabolic diseases. https://core.ac.uk/download/98347401.pdf (accessed on 14th June 2025).

19. Chen, T., Li, W., Wang, Y., et al. (2020). Effect of lifestyle changes after percutaneous coronary intervention on revascularization. https://core.ac.uk/download/287724707.pdf (accessed on 14th June 2025).

20. Clark, R., Rawas, H., Windsor, C., et al. (2012). Cultural challenges to secondary prevention: Implications for Saudi women. https://core.ac.uk/download/10909715.pdf (accessed on 14th June 2025).

21. Crawley, J. T., Esmon, C. T., Ferrell, G., et al. (2002). Distribution of endothelial cell protein C/activated protein C receptor (EPCR) during mouse embryo development. https://core.ac.uk/download/77002979.pdf (accessed on 14th June 2025).

22. Cussó, F., Del Romero, A., Herrera-Melle, L., et al. (2019). Physics for non-physicists – Two bio-degrees reforms in Spanish universities: Health Biology and Biology. https://repositorio.uam.es/bitstream/10486/691103/1/physics_cusso_jop_2019.pdf (accessed on 14th June 2025).

23. Dimitrova, D. S., Haberman, S., & Kaishev, V. K. (2013). Dependent competing risks: Cause elimination and its impact on survival. https://core.ac.uk/download/42629183.pdf (accessed on 14th June 2025).

24. Elliott, P., Ezzati, M., Kontis, V., et al. (2016). Worldwide exposures to cardiovascular risk factors and associated health effects: Current knowledge and data gaps. https://core.ac.uk/download/77013626.pdf (accessed on 14th June 2025).

25. Escarce, J. J., Leng, M., & Morales, L. S. (2011). Risk of cardiovascular disease in first and second generation Mexican-Americans. https://core.ac.uk/download/323079775.pdf (accessed on 14th June 2025).

26. Estrine, J., & DeLisle, L. (2006). Stress: Putting the brain back into medicine. https://core.ac.uk/download/71356692.pdf (accessed on 14th June 2025).

27. Filipiak, K. J., Kotkowski, M., Krzowski, B., et al. (2016). Association between vitamin D levels and arterial hypertension in women at very high cardiovascular risk. https://core.ac.uk/download/268453381.pdf (accessed on 14th June 2025).

28. Fumimoto, K., Okada, S., Manno, M., Sakaue, Y., & Makikawa, M. (2024). Non-contact assessment of cardiovascular and thermoregulatory function during exercise after sleep deprivation. *2024 46th Annual International Conference of the IEEE Engineering in Medicine and Biology Society (EMBC)*. https://www.semanticscholar.org/paper/480f2055cee9f4daa2907f10a2611ab15aa63079 (accessed on 14th June 2025).

29. Gonzalez, J. (2021). Short-term fasting and autonomic control. https://core.ac.uk/download/482030008.pdf (accessed on 14th June 2025).

30. Gromova, N. V., Imarova, O. G., Martynova, M. I., et al. (2016). Role of membrane lipids in the regulation of erythrocytic oxygen-transport function in cardiovascular diseases. https://core.ac.uk/download/228177833.pdf (accessed on 14th June 2025).

31. Haralanova, P., Kisheva, A., & Momcheva, I. (2023). Subclinical atherosclerosis and cardiovascular risk in inflammatory rheumatic diseases. https://core.ac.uk/download/599136500.pdf (accessed on 14th June 2025).

32. Hogan, M. K. (2017). A heart artificial: Building the foundation for the development and maintenance of *in vitro* tissue mimetic cardiovascular models. https://core.ac.uk/download/235095042.pdf (accessed on 14th June 2025).

33. Irwin, M. R. (2014). Sleep and inflammation in resilient aging. https://core.ac.uk/download/323076827.pdf (accessed on 14th June 2025).

34. Kataoka, Y., Fukuda, Y., Peterson, J., Yokota, S., Uemura, K., Saku, K., Alexander, J., et al. (2023). Analytical representation of four-dimensional hemodynamics for drug therapy simulation in acute heart failure treatment. *2023 45th Annual International Conference of the IEEE Engineering & Biology Society (EMBC)*. https://www.semanticscholar.org/paper/67426070abc69f0a8bde62e12918dc8f150222e9 (accessed on 14th June 2025).

35. Khan, F. (2024). Role of dietary fiber & cardiovascular diseases. *The Journal of Cardiovascular Diseases*. https://www.semanticscholar.org/paper/d5b1cd18cdb3eb3f84ee5739037bd243e8d394df (accessed on 14th June 2025).

36. Kisenge, P. R. (2011). Pattern of cardiovascular diseases among elderly patients admitted in medical wards at Muhimbili National Hospital Dar es Salaam, Tanzania. https://core.ac.uk/download/pdf/16666639.pdf (accessed on 14th June 2025).

37. Leonard, J. I. (2025). An integrated analysis of the physiological effects of space flight: Executive summary. https://core.ac.uk/download/pdf/42844718.pdf (accessed on 14th June 2025).

38. McKinsey, T. A., Morimoto, T., Poller, W., Turner, B. M., & Wang, Y. (2018). Epigenomes in cardiovascular disease. https://core.ac.uk/download/323078188.pdf (accessed on 14th June 2025).

39. Morelli, C. (2020). Identification of a new population of TrkC+ sensory neurons that regulates blood pressure. https://core.ac.uk/download/359888429.pdf (accessed on 14th June 2025).

40. Noordzij, W., Slart, R. H. J. A., & Stegger, L. (2021). Hybrid imaging of the autonomic cardiac nervous system. https://core.ac.uk/download/589896310.pdf (accessed on 14th June 2025).

41. Patel, T. (2002). Quantitative assessment of reflex blood pressure regulation using a dynamic model of the cardiovascular system. https://core.ac.uk/download/232275536.pdf (accessed on 14th June 2025).

42. Patwardhan, K. (2008). Concepts of human physiology in Ayurveda. https://core.ac.uk/download/pdf/87482.pdf (accessed on 14th June 2025).
43. Peterson, K., Rehrig, M., Stamp, M., & Kim, S. (2012). Competing by saving lives: How pharmaceutical and medical device companies create shared value in global health. https://core.ac.uk/download/71359569.pdf (accessed on 14th June 2025).
44. Rajendran, D., & Chandrasekaran, N. (2023). Journey of micronanoplastics with blood components. *RSC Advances, 13*, 31435–31459. https://www.semanticscholar.org/paper/a1ab942766bcfb33b172570d0dae887c44b8aed1 (accessed on 14th June 2025).
45. Rubattu, S., & Volpe, M. (2019). Natriuretic peptides in the cardiovascular system: Multifaceted roles in physiology, pathology and therapeutics. https://core.ac.uk/download/231746948.pdf (accessed on 14th June 2025).
46. Saunders, P. (2018). Getting ahead of the curve: Screening and early detection of scoliosis in adolescents to prevent progression of spinal deformity. https://core.ac.uk/download/215153739.pdf (accessed on 14th June 2025).
47. Terzic, A., & Waldman, S. A. (2017). *Clinical Pharmacology & Therapeutics*: Past, present, and future. https://core.ac.uk/download/83049656.pdf (accessed on 14th June 2025).
48. Van der Merwe, F. H. (2018). GPS analysis of a team competing at a national under-18 field hockey tournament. https://core.ac.uk/download/187724717.pdf (accessed on 14th June 2025).
49. Weber, M. (2017). How objective are biological functions? https://core.ac.uk/download/131213862.pdf (accessed on 14th June 2025).
50. Wienaldi, I. N. E. L., & Sihombing, B. (2022). Antioxidant activity of platelet-rich plasma Wistar rats with DPPH and ABTS test. *International Journal of Health and Pharmaceutical (IJHP)*. https://www.semanticscholar.org/paper/0c0255d7ea0a16e6b2e069ca698f372ab79e9601 (accessed on 14th June 2025).

BLOOD VESSELS AND CIRCULATION

6

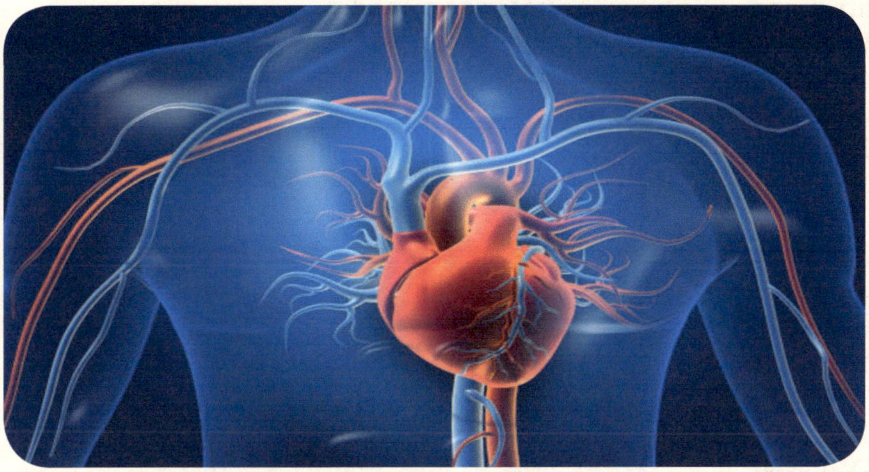

LEARNING OBJECTIVES

After studying this chapter, you will be able to:

1. Identify and differentiate the types of blood vessels and their function
2. Describe the structural characteristics of various blood vessels
3. Describe the circuits of systemic and pulmonary blood circulation
4. Explain the mechanisms of cardiovascular control
5. Recognize prevalent vascular diseases and their clinical relevance
6. Discuss recent advances and developments in vascular medicine

Introduction

The circulatory system is critical to sustaining life since it ensures the continuity of blood within the body. Blood vessels such as arteries, veins, and capillaries form a complex network that allows the exchange of oxygen, nutrients, and waste materials among organs and tissues. The dynamics of blood flow and the physiological characteristics of vessels can significantly affect the overall condition. Moreover, factors including blood pressure, vessel elastic properties, and systemic resistance have crucial roles to play when it comes to circulatory efficacy. Worth mentioning is that hypertension, which is a condition of blood pressure above 140/90 mmHg, is a widespread condition that impacts a considerable number of people globally, especially adults between 30-79 years old, with 1.28 billion people having been reported to have this disease by the World Health Organization (Alivian et al., 2024). Understanding the pathophysiology of blood flow and how various interventions impact it is essential for the management of hypertension. Other treatments, for example, like foot soak therapy using warm ginger water, have been researched for their beneficial effect on blood flow. Such interventions are particularly vital in elderly individuals, where age-related physiological changes—like decreased vessel compliance and heart failure—can exacerbate hypertension. Case study research indicates promising results, with mean decreases in blood pressure in older adults following such therapies. This illustrates how non-invasive treatments can be of great benefit to blood pressure control and vascular health (Alivian et al., 2024). This is also in addition to the investigation into blood flow for the impact of lifestyle components, such as smoking, on hemodynamics. The most recent research focused on female smokers has evidenced widespread alteration in cerebral blood flow and vascular tone, suggesting potential hypoxia within the brain. This concurs with the appreciation of environmental etiology impairing vascular integrity, leading to reduced levels of blood flow and increased arterial resistance. By analyzing such profound physiological changes, researchers are better able to comprehend the complexity of blood vessel function and circulation and, therefore, inform prevention and rehabilitation efforts among affected populations. Ultimately, this data, based on such studies, highlights the importance of vascular integrity in overall health and aging.

Definition of Blood Vessels

The building blocks of the circulatory system are blood vessels, which are vessels in which blood circulates through the body. Blood vessels are essentially classified into three types: arteries, veins, and capillaries, each playing a specific role in circulation. Arteries are responsible for carrying oxygenated blood from the heart to tissues, demonstrating thick, muscular walls to withstand high pressure. Meanwhile, veins carry deoxygenated blood back to the heart and possess thinner walls with the additional framework of valves to prevent backflow. The tightest and smallest vessels of blood are capillaries, which permit exchange among nutrients, gases, and waste between blood and tissues. This complex network of blood vessels is essential to the process of homeostasis and supports the metabolic demands of each organ system of the body. The structural and physiological features of the blood vessels are essential to their role in the circulatory system. The endothelium, a layer of endothelial cells lining the interior surfaces, plays a vital role in the modulation of vascular tone and blood flow (Figure 6.1).

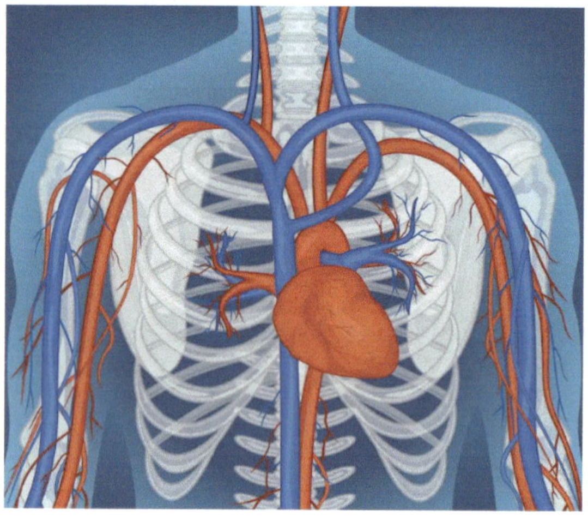

Figure 6.1. Human cardiovascular system showing the heart, arteries, and veins in the upper torso.

Source: https://www.metropolisindia.com/upgrade/blog/upload/2023/08/xray-human-body-with-internal-organs_1308-110356-1.webp.

Moreover, endothelial dysfunction will also predispose the subject to a variety of cardiovascular ailments. For instance, the association between desquamated endothelial cells (DECs) in ischemic stroke highlights the importance of vascular functionality and integrity for body health preservation. Research on the association between DECs and markers of endothelial dysfunction suggests a significant association between the vascular system and various pathophysiological conditions. The insight into these mechanisms not only points to the delicate balance that is maintained by blood vessels but also betrays the repercussions when this system collapses (Kosheleva et al., 2017). On a larger scale, the definitions and functions of blood vessels extend to their implications in disease conditions. Myocardial infarction (MI) is an example of how blood vessels can make a significant impact on health. MI, through the occlusion of blood to the heart muscle, causes cell death and subsequent complications. The dynamic process of ischemia involves complex mechanisms, where irreversible damage develops over time from reversible damage. Understanding the pathobiology of MI reveals basic information about the vascular response to injury and therapeutic interventions (Bello et al., 2015). Lastly, the multifunctionality of blood vessels is finally explained, not only for their vital functions in circulation but also for their prominence in cardiovascular health and disease regulation.

6.1. Types of Blood Vessels

Learning Outcome

1. Discuss the arteries and their functions
2. Define the veins and their role in circulation
3. Understand the capillaries and nutrient exchange

The human circulatory system contains three large categories of blood vessels: arteries, veins, and capillaries, all of which play a critical role in maintaining homeostasis. Arteries are elastic and muscular vessels that transport oxygen-rich blood from the heart to the tissues. Arterial walls contain muscle, which makes them thick and enables them to withstand the high blood pressure pumped by the heart. Beyond this, arteries can dilate and constrict in a way that allows them to regulate the flow of blood. This is necessary in the regulation of various physiological needs so that oxygenated blood can be delivered to organs with efficiency. If arteries did not work in this manner, tissue oxygenation would be compromised, with detrimental effects on overall health. Veins, however, carry out the vital function of bringing deoxygenated blood back to the heart. Compared to arteries, veins are less muscular and thinner due to containing much lower pressure. The addition of one-way valves ensures one-way blood flow and the prevention of backflow in gravity. This body readjustment is significant in the extremities, where blood needs to be actively pumped against gravity. Additionally, veins carry more blood volume and act as a circulatory reservoir of blood. This storage capacity of blood becomes important in states of augmented demand, i.e., exercise, when circulation can be diverted from reserve to the contracting muscle for efficient circulation. Capillaries are the most abundant and smallest of the blood vessels and serve as the vital link between tissues and the circulatory system. Capillaries possess one layer of endothelial cells, which facilitates the smooth diffusion of waste products, gases, and nutrients. This enables the exchange of gases, nutrients, and waste products, which is fundamental in the maintenance of cellular metabolism and organ function. The structural elements of capillaries make their surface area greater than their volume, thus making them very effective in gas and nutrient exchange. Besides, the latest research has demonstrated that hemodynamic forces such as blood flow-generated shear stress have a significant role in capillary remodeling and function, e.g., in yolk sac growth in mice. The information records the intricate relationship between vascular adaptation and blood flow dynamics to maintain tissue homeostasis, recording the intricacy of the circulatory system in health and disease (Chen et al., 2007) (Figure 6.2).

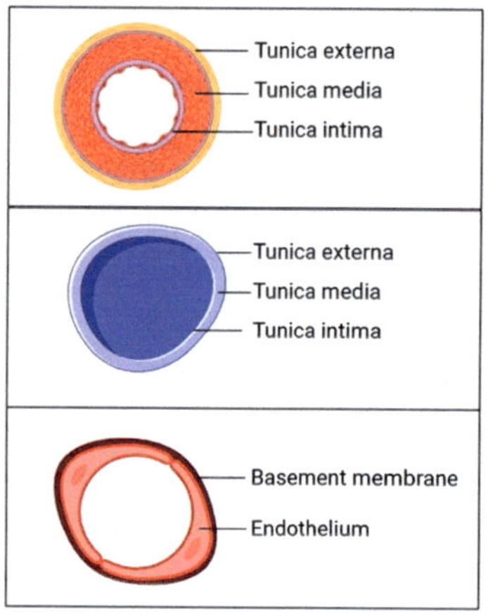

Figure 6.2. Types of blood vessels.

Source: https://blogger.googleusercon tent.com/img/b/R29vZ2xl/AVvXsEj01y2E1jh6V7TL2rD8NILzq94nLYTgvzGPKLH192IOlt8Up1_D5KtD9l 6ZjRj8jNoEsvQhBSA6fuPh bYEBsIzVhc5lkELHbXpRvzWLKhbrVr4ue RLD1Z3Aicy fPSC8eCRbjPhxctLZIU7Yj cDxllbJGcAV2f CWP1J9ge4 PfX7TKxB tyjPcuZnl oluXN8c/w1200-h630-p-k-no-nu/ What% 20are %20the%20 Main%20Types %20of%20Blood% 20Vessels.webp.

6.1.1. Arteries and Their Functions

Arteries form the core part of the circulatory system as the primary vessels for carrying oxygenated blood to distribute essential nutrients from the heart to various tissues within the body. Arteries possess thick, elastic walls with many layers, including the tunica intima, tunica media, and tunica externa. This unique structure not only helps them withstand the powerful pressure of blood flow created by heart contraction but also enables them to adapt to variations in blood volume. The elastic nature of the arterial wall facilitates a process known as the arterial rebound, which helps maintain constant blood flow despite the heart being in diastole, i.e., resting. Lastly, the structural specialization of arteries accounts for their effectiveness in transmitting blood and regulating circulation to various physiological demands. Beyond their physical characteristics, arteries are involved in several regulatory mechanisms that enhance blood flow according to the needs of the body. For instance, vasodilation and vasoconstriction alter the size of arteries directly, thereby impacting the pressure and rate of blood flow. These include the production of nitric oxide and sexual hormones such as testosterone, whose effects on arterial function have been demonstrated (Figure 6.3).

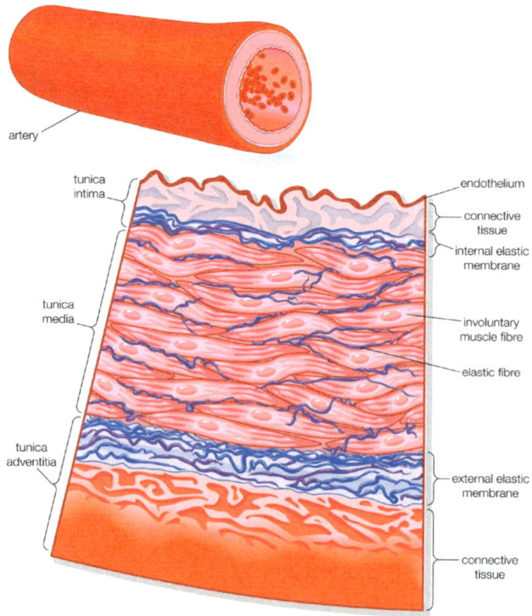

Figure 6.3. Transverse section of an artery.

Source: https://www.britannica.com/science/artery.

Testosterone has been found to induce relaxation in coronary arteries to allow for variation in the supply of blood to the myocardium. Specifically, studies indicate that the side branches and the left anterior descending artery exhibit heterogeneous responses to testosterone, which suggests a multilevel interaction between hormone levels and vascular responsiveness existing in vivo. These regulatory functions play a key role in sustaining homeostasis and ensuring adequate tissue perfusion. Besides, functional implications of arterial health extend beyond mere blood transport; they play crucial roles in general cardiovascular health. Atherosclerosis, or the status of plaque accumulation in the arterial wall, may impair arterial function and lead to dire consequences such as heart attack and stroke. Arterial interactions, as research spurred by hormonal activity, imply potential avenues for therapeutic inventions that can mitigate these risks. For example, information regarding how different segments of arteries respond to testosterone at an individual level may paint a picture of customized plans for the treatment of cardiovascular disease. Therefore, the intricate role of arteries in circulation, as well as their physiology in response to stimuli, is essential for understanding cardiovascular well-being and disease treatment, and underscores the importance of ongoing research.

6.1.2. Veins and Their Role in Circulation

Veins are critical to the circulatory system, with their primary role being the return of oxygen-depleted blood to the heart. Unlike arteries, which deliver oxygenated blood from the heart, veins typically have thinner walls and greater luminal diameters to accommodate the transmission of varying amounts of blood. They have valves to prevent backflow of the blood, particularly in the extremities, where gravity is a significant problem. The efficiency of venous return is also increased by contractions of skeletal muscle and respiratory movement, enabling the movement of blood in these vessels. This relationship between the physiological function and anatomical organization emphasizes the importance of veins in providing effective circulation and helping to ensure adequate return of blood to the heart for oxygenation. In detail, venous anatomy is relatively diverse throughout the body, adapting to specific functional requirements. For instance, the systemic veins drain blood from the body, and the pulmonary veins drain oxygenated blood from the lungs to the heart. One of the most important examples of a venous drainage abnormality is total anomalous pulmonary vein drainage (TAPVD) or congenital malformation in which the pulmonary veins fail to drain to the left atrium but drain into a systemic vein. This circumstance can lead to serious complications, highlighting the crucial role of optimal venous structure in maintaining cardiovascular health. Venous connectivity and integrity are not only critical for normal physiological function but also to effective therapy of vascular disease, one with surgical implications as discussed in some clinical observations of congenital cardiac defects (Adamczyk et al., 2018) (Figure 6.4).

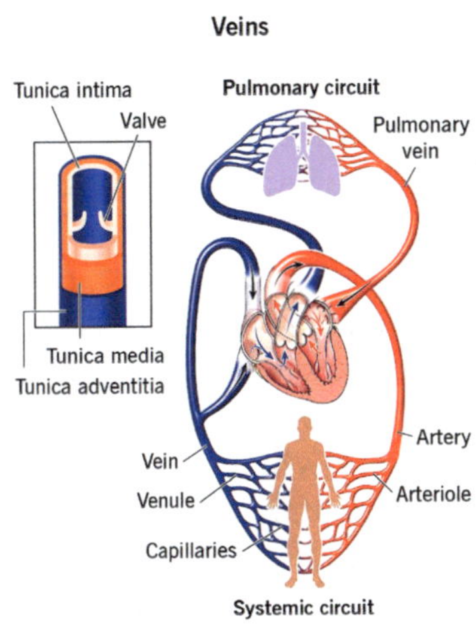

Figure 6.4. Your veins are part of a complex network of blood vessels that carry blood throughout your body.

Source: https://my.clevelandclinic.org/-/scassets/images/org/health/articles/23360-veins.

Furthermore, venous study has historical significance and directly relates to vascular physiology and anatomical development. Early attempts to conceptualize the circulatory process based on Galen's work marked a duality of blood circulation that was later disputed with the developments in anatomical dissection.

The discovery of the lymph system, together with extensive study on veins, has significantly reorganized contemporary knowledge, emphasizing the fact that the blood does not solely produce in the liver, but instead flows through a highly developed system that is tasked with the transport of nutrients and waste (Tonetti et al., 2017). Such scientific milestones not only enhance the vein's importance in circulation but also demonstrate the dynamic process of scientific discovery, whereby discoveries are continuously reverberating back into and further shaping existing frameworks of knowledge in cardiovascular physiology.

6.1.3. Capillaries and Nutrient Exchange

The intricate network of capillaries forms the critical frontier between the circulatory system and the tissues that surround it, facilitating the essential exchange of vital nutrients. Capillary walls are composed of single layers of endothelial cells, which are permeable to facilitate the effective exchange of oxygen, carbon dioxide, nutrients, and waste products. The fact that this structure is thin decreases the distance over which the diffusion occurs, and thus the rate at which the substances are exchanged is higher.

The size of capillaries is vast, several orders of magnitude greater than that of large vessels, which again enhances the possibility of functional ability in the transfer of nutrients. When blood is perfused through capillaries, hydraulic pressure generated by the heart pushes plasma into adjacent interstitial fluid, a phenomenon that is the foundation of transcapillary exchange. Such an exchange is essential in sustaining tissue homeostasis and supplying cells with adequate nutrition for metabolic processes. In addition, nutrient exchange is primarily regulated by dynamic interactions among capillary walls and red blood cells. As emphasized in recent studies, the endothelial glycocalyx—a gel-like coating on endothelial cells—is a key player in regulating these interactions. It remodels blood flow patterns and dictates the transport of solutes and fluid across the capillary membrane. Specifically, since red blood cell and capillary lumen sizes are similar to each other, the dynamics of the exchange become highly complex. Understanding these interactions better promises innovations in tissue engineering and regenerative medicine, as the formation of vascular networks under physiological conditions is instrumental for engineered tissue functionality and survival (de Boer et al., 2008) (Figure 6.5).

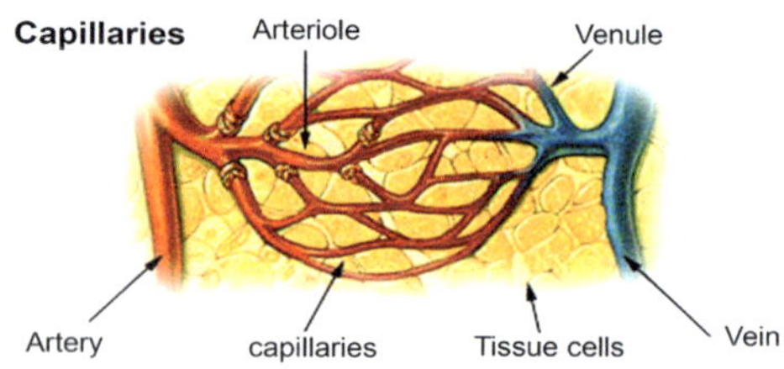

Figure 6.5. Capillary.

Source: https://simple.wikipedia.org/wiki/Capillary#/media/File:Illu_capillary_en.jpg.

This complexity must be approached both in research and clinical application, particularly with therapies that enhance the delivery of nutrients to impaired tissues. Secondarily, fluid and solute exchange processes through capillaries are regulated by several anatomical properties, including the counter-current structures present in certain microvessels. This body shape not only facilitates the delivery of nutrients but also plays a central role in mechanisms such as the renal concentrating mechanism, which is crucial in water homeostasis. Studies have shown that particle transport across capillary walls is enabled by transcapillary pressures, where hydrostatic and osmotic gradient forces dictate the exchange rate and direction (Lu et al., 2010). Understanding of such physiological mechanisms is essential as they are the basis for the overall efficacy of circulatory mechanisms and the well-being of tissue. As scientists continue to decipher the physiology of capillary dynamics, insights gained will undoubtedly guide the creation of better medical protocols and technologies aimed at facilitating the supply of nutrients and oxygen into vital organs.

Test Your Knowledge

1. What are the primary functions of arteries in the circulatory system, and how are they structurally adapted to perform these functions?
2. How do veins contribute to blood circulation, and what features help them return blood to the heart?

6.2. Structure of Blood Vessels

Learning Outcome

1. Discuss the layers of blood vessel walls
2. Understand the differences between arteries and veins
3. Describe the role of smooth muscle in blood vessels

The structure of blood vessels is of utmost significance to their function in the circulatory system. Blood vessels are primarily categorized as arteries, veins, and capillaries with varying structural features that enable them to perform their respective tasks in circulation. Arteries transport oxygenated blood from the heart and possess thick, muscular walls that can withstand high pressure. Their elasticity allows them to expand and contract with each heartbeat, providing a smooth blood flow. Veins return deoxygenated blood to the heart; thus, their walls are less thick and are equipped with valves to prevent backflow. This structural characteristic is required to help venous return, especially against the force of gravity. The microstructure of these vessels, for instance, the endothelium layer, is significantly responsible for the functionality, thereby emphasizing the significance of structural integrity to guarantee circulatory proficiency. Capillaries are another pivotal element in the structure of blood vessels and are functional units that are in charge of exchange operations between blood and tissues. These small vessels, sometimes only one cell in thickness, possess a unique structure that maximizes their surface area and minimizes the diffusion distance for the waste and nutrients. The thinness of the endothelium facilitates quick exchange, with oxygen, carbon dioxide, and metabolic waste being transported efficiently. Furthermore, the capillaries differ in types—continuous, fenestrated, and sinusoidal—and each type possesses a particular function in different tissues such as the brain, kidneys, and liver. With mathematical modeling used to address such dynamics, researchers can visualize how hemodynamics in the vascular network are affected by structural changes. Here, structure-function interaction recognizes the central role of capillary structure in systemic circulation (Audi et al., 2006). Emerging new approaches introducing biological mechanisms into computational algorithms reveal the intricate relationship between vessel structure and blood flow dynamics. For instance, hybrid models of cellular and blood flow behavior draw inspiration from nature in modeling the way that vessels respond to circulatory demands and pressures. These models mimic the behaviors of swarming organisms, which are akin to circulating blood cells. The dynamics of such interactions can be applied in offering insights into hemodynamic change in pathological circumstances, ultimately resulting in therapeutic interventions. In addition, advancements in computational power may allow for investigating the various environmental factors that influence the shape of blood vessels. This is critically important to vascular adaptation considerations to stresses like hypoxia and its role in conditions of disease like pulmonary hypertension (Aber et al., 2012).

6.2.1. Layers of Blood Vessel Walls

The structure of the vessel is complicated, composed of three distinct layers: the tunica intima, tunica media, and tunica externa, each functioning with different tasks to maintain vascular health and function. The tunica intima, the innermost layer, is composed of one layer of endothelial cells that line the lumen, forming a smooth surface for blood flow and functioning as a border to facilitate interaction between flowing blood and surrounding tissues. This layer not only ensures hemodynamic stability but also prevents bacterial and fibrinogen thrombosis.

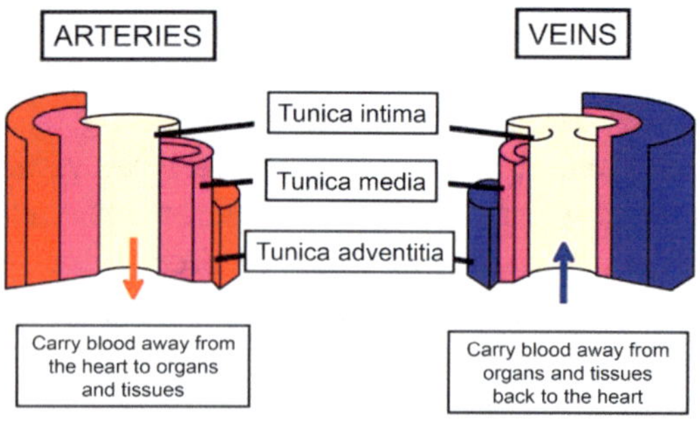

Figure 6.6. Schematic representation of the three layers of the blood vessel wall in an artery and a vein.

Source: https://www.researchgate.net/figure/Schematic-representation-of-the-three-layers-of-the-blood-vessel-wall-in-an-artery-and-a_fig2_6597677.

The endothelial cells are part of the signaling pathways that regulate blood vessel tone and overall cardiovascular health, such that any failure of this layer would result in severe pathological conditions such as atherosclerosis. Beyond the tunica intima, the tunica media consists primarily of smooth muscle cells and elastic fibers and plays a role in controlling blood pressure and flow. The muscular layer enables the vessels to constrict and dilate when the physiological demands of the body vary (Figure 6.6).

The make-up of the tunica media between different blood vessels varies; for instance, muscular arteries possess a thicker tunica media compared to elastic arteries, as per their respective functions within the cardiovascular system. The presence of elastic fibers in the media is particularly significant in the case of large arteries, as this allows them to withstand and absorb the pressure waves generated by the heart's beat. This function is of extreme importance in maintaining the ceaseless flow of blood in the circulatory system.

The outermost layer, or the tunica externa or adventitia, is made primarily of connective tissue, which imparts structural strength and integrity to the blood vessel. This layer contains collagen and elastin fibers that contribute to the tensile strength of the vessel and allow it to withstand outer pressure. The vasa vasorum, the small blood vessels that supply oxygen and nutrition to the major vessel, particularly when diffusion from the lumen is insufficient, are also located within the tunica externa. The role of the tunica externa and the blood vessel function as a whole cannot be overstated, since it will dictate the stability and health of the vascular system. Abnormalities in any of them can lead to dangerous pathological states, which corresponds to the need to become acquainted with their structure and function in the blood circuit (Wilde et al., 2016; 4th Micro and Conference NF (MNF2014), 2014).

6.2.2. Differences Between Arteries and Veins

The human body's circulatory system is composed of many vessels with essential functions in maintaining homeostasis. Of these vessels, arteries and veins play roles in other functions driven by their unique structural characteristics. Arteries have the function of distributing oxygenated blood from the heart to various tissues in the body, except pulmonary arteries, which deliver deoxygenated blood to the lungs. Walls of arteries are thicker and more elastic than those of veins to sustain the high-pressure blood flow resulting from cardiac contraction. This physical characteristic not only serves to maintain blood pressure constant but also aids in controlling blood flow during physiological regulation, facilitating the fundamental roles performed by arteries within systemic circulation and overall cardiovascular health. Conversely, veins are responsible for the return of oxygen-depleted blood to the heart at much lower pressure than arterial flow. Veins possess thinner walls and wider luminal diameters to accommodate the lower pressure of returning blood. Several veins valves that can ensure that the blood does not backflow, providing unidirectional blood flow towards the heart. These valves are critical in the extremities, where blood must move against gravity. The differences in the structure of arteries and veins also reflect their respective functions in the circulatory system, showing an individualized adaptation to blood carriage to suit the contrasting demands of oxygen supply and nutrient transfer in the body. The relationship of arteries and veins is also seen in some vascular circuits, such as pulmonary circulation. For instance, a recent study designed a computational model that can effectively replicate both arterial and venous pressure and flow in this system and prove how various vessels coordinate to provide good blood circulation (Burton et al., 2014) (Figure 6.7).

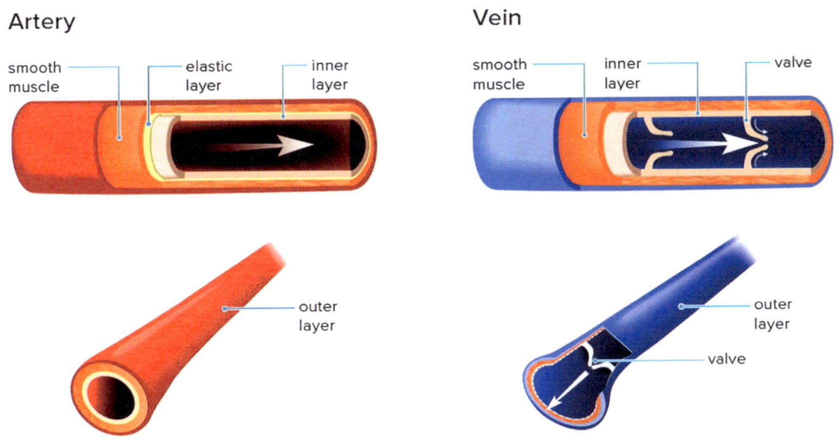

Figure 6.7. The difference between an artery and a vein.

Source: https://post.medicalnewstoday.com/wp-content/uploads/sites/3/2020/04/Artboard-3.jpg.

Furthermore, advances in imaging technology in imaging systems, including swept-source optical coherence tomography, have enabled researchers to image choroidal and retinal vascular beds, which provide information regarding microscopic structural disparity and functional implications of arteries and veins (Fraser et al., 2012). It is crucial to understand these disparities not only to comprehend normal physiological function but to diagnose and treat circulatory diseases, further attributing the importance of arteries and veins in disease and health.

6.2.3. Role of Smooth Muscle in Blood Vessels

Smooth muscle plays a crucial role in the functioning of blood vessels, enabling the control of vascular tone and blood distribution throughout the body. Smooth muscle exists in arterial and venous walls and is capable of contraction and relaxation when stimulated. This function is required for blood pressure maintenance and ensuring tissues receive enough oxygen and nutrients. The shortening of smooth muscle fibers constricts the blood vessels, a phenomenon referred to as vasoconstriction, and is induced by certain stimuli like sympathetic nervous stimulation or specific hormones. In contrast, relaxation of such smooth muscles, referred to as vasodilation, enables more blood flow and is regulated by endothelial agents and other vasoactive substances.

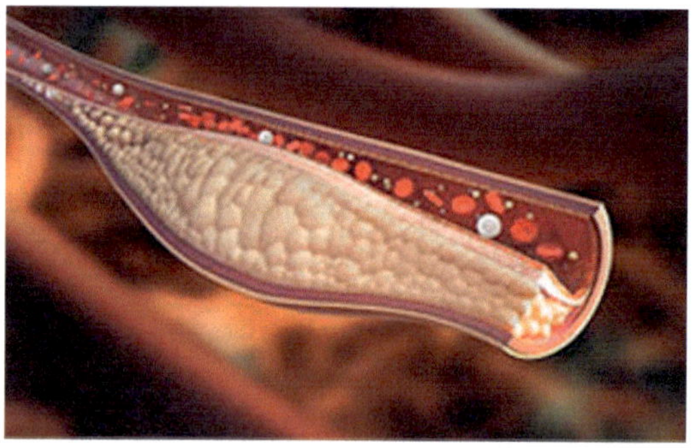

Figure 6.8. Vascular smooth muscle cells.

Source: https://www.lifelinecelltech.com/wp-content/uploads/2017/09/calcified-vein-V2.jpg.

The active balance of relaxation and contraction is what ensures cardiovascular system homeostasis, thereby demonstrating the prominence of smooth muscle in blood vessel function. As well as its simple mechanical roles, blood vessel smooth muscle contributes to an enormous number of physiological processes that affect cardiovascular health. For instance, smooth muscle not only responds but is implicated in the pathophysiology of vascular disease. Vascular smooth muscle dysfunction, which is often linked to inflammation and oxidative stress, may cause disorders such as hypertension and atherosclerosis (Figure 6.8).

Of interest, perivascular adipose tissue (PVAT) around the vessels plays a significant role in regulating smooth muscle function. If PVAT is impaired, it secretes inflammatory mediators with a deleterious impact on smooth muscle, thereby exacerbating vascular pathologies. This interaction emphasizes the role of smooth muscle as not just a structural component, but as an active contributor to vascular disease and homeostasis, and underscores the importance of cardiovascular research (Guzik et al., 2017). The study of the effect of sex hormones such as testosterone on smooth muscle reaction in blood vessels further illustrates its nuance. For example, it has been shown in research that testosterone induces vasorelaxation in coronary arteries, a phenomenon seen not only under in-vitro conditions but also under physiological conditions. Significantly, the size of this effect varies across different segments of the coronary vascular tree, with side arteries presenting distinct responses compared to major arteries like the LAD. The differential expression of androgen receptors in these vessels suggests that smooth muscle responsiveness may be under hormonal modulation, impacting global vascular reactivity. These findings underscore the multiscale character of smooth muscle and indicate the complexity of signaling pathways regulating its function and the potential implications in cardiovascular disease understanding and management (Madanu et al., 2012).

Test Your Knowledge

1. What are the three main layers of blood vessel walls, and what are the functions of each layer?
2. What are the key structural and functional differences between arteries and veins?

6.3. Blood Circulation Pathways

Learning Outcome

1. Explain the systemic circulation and pulmonary circulation
2. Define coronary circulation and heart health

The complexity of the pathway of blood circulation is at the heart of understanding the intricate network that sustains human life. All the vessels in the blood are arteries, veins, and capillaries, each serving a unique function within the circulatory system. Arteries carry oxygenated blood from the heart to the smaller arterioles and eventually to capillaries, where exchange at a cellular level of gases, nutrients, and waste occurs. Conversely, veins transport deoxygenated blood back to the heart through the use of valves in order to prevent backflow and facilitate adequate return flow against gravity. This circularity in blood movement highlights the dynamic interaction among various vessel types, which facilitates the effective delivery of nutrients and waste removal essential for maintaining homeostasis. The interaction between blood flow and body health cannot be overstressed, particularly regarding obesity and its cardiovascular consequences. Local adipose tissue deposits, which are usually found near arterioles, have been found to have a significant role in the regulation of the vessels. For instance, in obese individuals, insulin signaling pathways are dysregulated, leading to reduced production of nitric oxide, which is supposed to be vasodilatory. Instead, an overproduction of adipocytokines such as tumor necrosis factor-α can be a cause of unopposed arteriole vasoconstriction and hence prevent maximal blood flow (Eringa et al., 2005) (Figure 6.9).

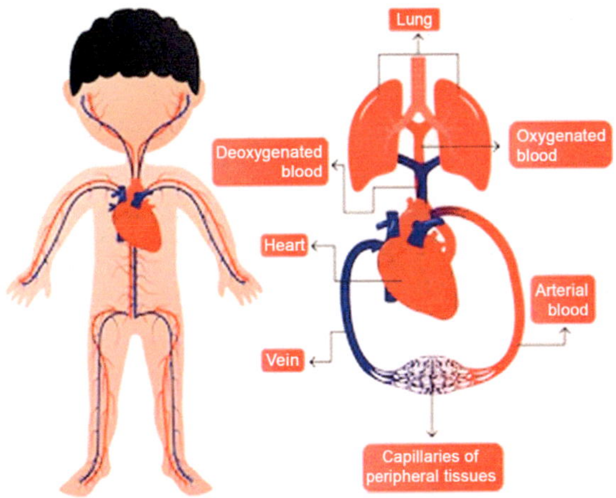

Figure 6.9. Circulatory pathways system.

Source: https://www.geeksforgeeks.org/circulatory-pathways-class-11-notes/.

This is a demonstration of how metabolic disease can complicate blood flow and highlight the significant interaction between fat tissue and vascular health. Additionally, the return of blood flow after injury demonstrates the adaptive functionality of vascular pathways. With healing processes, such as tendon trauma, there is a significant need for revascularization to supply reparative material from the blood supply. The first response is an expansion of endothelial cells leading to neovascularization, which is critical for the restoration of blood supply and tissue repair (Fenwick et al., 2002). The regeneration process not only underscores the need for adequate blood supply during healing but also illustrates the intricate remodeling of the blood vessel in response to demand. Such identification contributes to our understanding of vascular health and how it applies to broader clinical situations, so the necessity for more research on patterns of blood circulation is highlighted.

6.3.1. Systemic Circulation Explained

Central to the circulatory system is systemic circulation, a complex process where oxygen-rich blood is dispersed to the body. The route of circulation begins as oxygenated blood departs the left ventricle of the heart and is pushed into the ascending aorta. From this central artery, the blood circulates through a network of arteries that branch down to smaller arterioles and capillaries, where exchange of nutrients and gases occurs at the cellular level. The systemic circulation plays a significant role in homeostasis because it acts to supply all body tissues with the necessary oxygen and nutrients and to assist in the removal of metabolic waste, such as carbon dioxide. This intricate process is vital to organ and systemic function, testifying to the importance of healthy circulation to overall health. Along the course of its passage through the systemic circulation, blood makes contact with a variety of vessels having distinct structural and functional properties. The muscular, thick walls of arteries prepare them to meet increased pressures as they carry blood from the heart outward in all directions. In contrast, veins have thinner walls and larger lumina for the return of deoxygenated blood to the heart under reduced pressure. The conversion of arteries to veins is done through a broad network of capillaries, where the actual exchange of gases, nutrients, and wastes between tissues and blood takes place. Also, the fact that veins are lined with valves prevents backflow, which enhances unidirectional blood flow and maximizes efficiency in the whole circulatory process. As such, systemic circulation is not only the best example of the complexity of vascular architecture but also represents the essential roles of these vessels in general circulatory health (Figure 6.10).

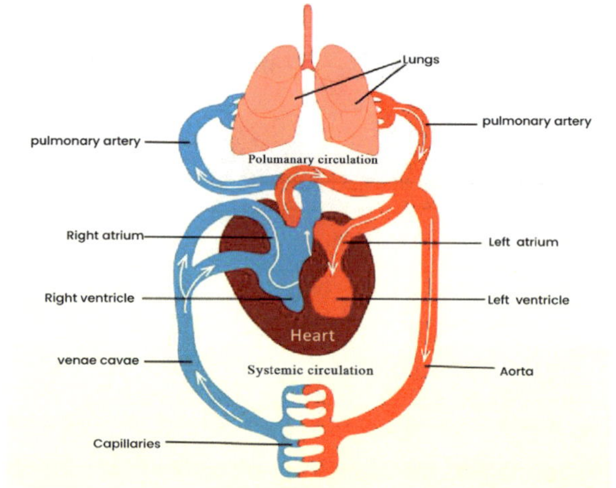

Figure 6.10. Systemic circulation of the heart.

Source: https://sunfox.in/wp-content/uploads/2024/05/16.2-understanding-Systemic-Circulation-of-the-Heart.webp.

Secondly, systemic circulation is also intensely associated with a variety of physiological responses, particularly during stress or heightened activity. For instance, during conditions of exercise, the body induces neural as well as hormonal control that enhances blood delivery to muscles at the cost of less vital functions. This active regulation is necessary to maximize oxygen supply where it is most required, thereby increasing performance and duration. Nonetheless, alterations in systemic circulation may result in serious health issues, such as hypertension or atherosclerosis, that are commonly associated with lifestyle and genetic predispositions. Evidence also exists that conditions of blood vessels can have systemic effects, as exemplified by the interactions between inflammatory reactions and the circulatory system (Goetz et al., 1999; Asimaki et al., 2006). This highlights the need for ongoing research and public health interventions targeted towards the promotion of vascular health and the prevention of circulatory disorders.

6.3.2. Pulmonary Circulation Overview

Pulmonary circulation is a segment of the entire cardiovascular system that has the chief role to perform gas exchange in the lungs. Pulmonary circulation begins with the transportation of deoxygenated blood from the right ventricle of the heart through pulmonary arteries to the lungs. The blood continues through a small series of vessels, ultimately to the alveoli, where carbon dioxide is expelled and oxygen is taken in. The process has to be highly efficient since any minute impediment can lead to severe health issues like pulmonary hypertension or chronic obstructive pulmonary disease (COPD).

It is crucial to understand the dynamics of blood pressure and flow in this singular circuit since it is central to physiological adaptation to effect efficient gas exchange and overall respiratory function, demonstrating how interdependent the harmony between blood vessels and systemic circulation is. Extensive research on pulmonary circulation has revealed the complex interplay of venous and arterial pressure and blood flow. New mathematical models have been developed to examine the interactions, which better understand this circulatory pathway than previous research. With the use of patient-specific information gained from advanced imaging techniques like magnetic resonance imaging (MRI), researchers can simulate and predict the behavior of the flow of blood in pulmonary arteries and veins accurately.

These models incorporate several variables, including material properties and vessel geometry, which play a central role in identifying how vessel stiffening and vascular rarefaction affect flow dynamics. Thus, these discoveries can find utility in helping to diagnose and treat various cardiovascular and respiratory diseases effectively, pointing to the importance of pulmonary circulation in the general study of human physiology (Burton et al., 2014) (Figure 6.11).

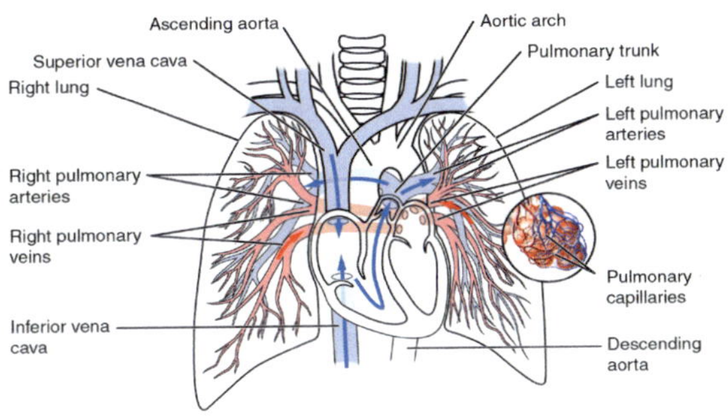

Figure 6.11. Pulmonary circulation in the heart.

Source: https://en.wikipedia.org/wiki/Pulmonary_circulation#/media/File:2119_Pulmonary_Circuit.jpg.

Furthermore, mathematical modeling is not restricted to adult pulmonary circulation and can have application to circulatory dynamics of some groups, including the fetus. Doppler ultrasound techniques are applied routinely to quantify fetal cardiovascular status, although velocity-based indices that correspond to precise physiological states remain difficult to associate. By using mathematical models that simulate velocity wave propagation through the fetal circulatory system, clinicians can study how growth patterns and vessel resistance influence hemodynamic profiles. This process facilitates improved clinical judgment regarding fetal health and highlights the continued need for new techniques to explore vascular dynamics. Lastly, such advances in both pulmonary and overall circulatory modeling reiterate the indispensable nature of continuous research toward enhancing healthcare delivery based on blood vessel function and circulatory health (Bovendeerd et al., 2024).

6.3.3. Coronary Circulation and Heart Health

Coronary circulation is the key feature of maintaining overall cardiac health as it provides oxygen-rich blood to the myocardium, enabling the cardiac muscle to function effectively. Coronary arteries form a part of this vascular network, which branches off from the aorta and encircles the heart, whereas coronary veins return deoxygenated blood to the right atrium. Normal coronary perfusion is required to prevent ischemic heart conditions, where the diminished blood flow leads to myocardial infarction or angina. Hypertension and elevated cholesterol have an adverse effect on coronary perfusion, predisposing conditions such as endothelial dysfunction. Since elevated blood pressure has been linked with various cardiovascular disorders, including heart failure and ischemic heart disease, information about the regulatory mechanisms of coronary circulation enhances the promise for effective preventative and therapeutic interventions of heart disease (Cameron et al., 2016). The relationship between endothelial function and coronary circulation highlights the importance of preserving vascular health to guarantee cardiac performance. Endothelial cells line the coronary arteries and are responsible for regulating blood flow, maintaining vascular tone, and reacting to shear stress. When there is endothelial dysfunction, as would typically be caused by complications like hypertension, the heart struggles to respond normally to physiological need, hence affecting coronary vasodilation. Interventions such as antihypertensive medication have been effective in improving endothelial function, which is crucial for maximum coronary circulation. More significantly, though, are the calcium channel blockers and the angiotensin converting enzyme inhibitors, which have proven beneficial in this sense, as these increase the availability of nitric oxide and thus improve endothelial response (Cameron et al., 2016) (Figure 6.12).

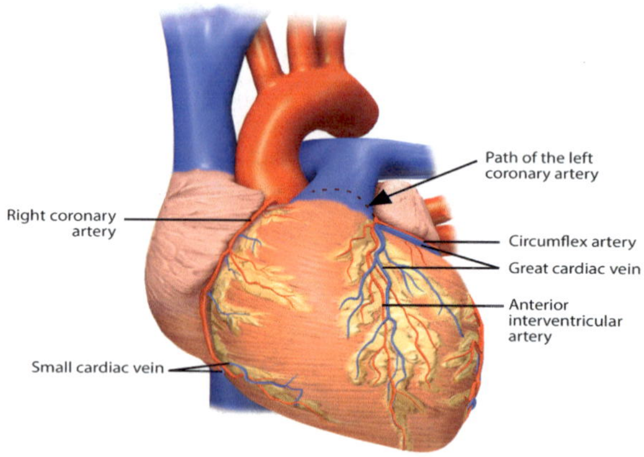

Figure 6.12. Coronary circulation.

Source: https://med.libretexts.org/@api/deki/files/51771/Coronary_Vessels_Anterior_View.png?revision=1&size=bestfit&width=530&height=447.

Thus, there is a need to address endothelial health through pharmacologic and lifestyle measures to prevent heart-related disease. New research has tested new therapies that aim to correct endothelial dysfunction in patients with coronary atherosclerosis. For instance, l-arginine supplementation has been found to enhance coronary vasodilation, particularly under conditions of stress such as cardiac exercise. By its role as substrate for the production of nitric oxide, l-arginine can increase coronary flow by facilitating blood flow and reducing epicardial and microvascular segment constriction. These findings suggest that l-arginine may be of therapeutic value, especially to patients who experience ischemic events initiated through endothelial dysfunction. In summary, the understanding and optimization of coronary perfusion through pharmacologic and lifestyle treatments can be an important determinant of heart health, neutralizing risks associated with coronary artery disease and promoting cardiovascular resilience.

Test Your Knowledge

1. What is systemic circulation, and how does it function to supply oxygenated blood to the body?
2. How does pulmonary circulation work, and what is its role in the exchange of gases in the lungs?

6.4. Regulation of Blood Flow

Learning Outcome

1. Describe the role of the autonomic nervous system
2. Explain the hormonal influences on blood vessel diameter
3. Identify the impact of physical activity on circulation

Perfusion of blood is a sophisticated process where several physiological mechanisms are involved in keeping tissues well-perfused. Central to the process is the regulation of vessels, which constrict or dilate to local and systemic stimuli. Regulation is primarily done by the smooth muscle of vessel walls, which responds to stimuli such as ischemia, metabolic demand, and neural regulation. Moreover, end blood distribution is also controlled finely by the mechanism of autoregulation, which enables tissues to adjust their blood supply according to their metabolic need. For instance, in exercise, muscle tissue releases metabolites that cause vasodilatation and lead to increased blood flow to support enhanced oxygen demand, thereby emphasizing the dynamic nature of vascular control. An essential aspect of control of blood flow is found in Murray's law, the assumption that can be made for an ideal geometric pattern of blood vessels to minimize power loss in the circulatory system. Murray's law ideally shows that the flow rate is a function of the cube of the vessel radius, highlighting the significance of vessel size in the maintenance of diverse physiological functions.

While initially observed in macrocirculation, subsequent studies have shown that the laws of principle hold for microcirculation too, with modifications for shear-dependent viscosity, as described by Alarcón et al. This development of knowledge underlines the importance of both blood rheology and vessel morphology in delineating wall shear stress and hence the overall efficiency of blood flow. The findings serve to bridge traditional hemodynamic principles with current knowledge of fluid dynamics in vascular networks to enhance our comprehension of blood flow (Figure 6.13).

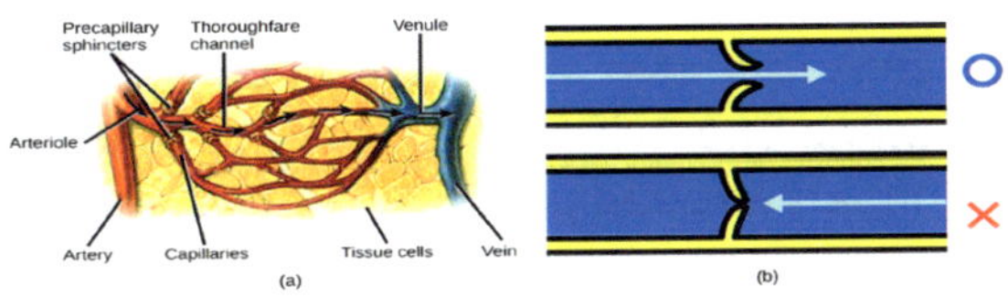

Figure 6.13. (a) Precapillary sphincters are rings of smooth muscle that regulate the flow of blood through capillaries; they help control the location of blood flow to where it is needed; and (b) Valves in the veins prevent blood from moving backward.

Source: https://courses.lumenlearning.com/suny-wmopen-biology2/chapter/blood-flow-and-blood-pressure-regulation/.

One can not disregard the role of external factors in maintaining blood flow, especially in professions with high demands like air aviation. Data show that the intensified physical and psychological load on pilots raises the danger of cardiovascular pathologies and their causal potential consequences on performance and safety. Statistics reveal that there is a troubling trend: an increasing number of flight accidents caused by such medical conditions, combined with a growing percentage of pilots discovered to be unqualified for duty due to silent cardiac illnesses. These trends warrant increased active tracking and intervention to avoid cardiovascular risk among flight crews. By fine-tuning the regulation of blood flow and the management of developing pathologies, the aviation industry can optimize its employees' health and performance, providing safer flight conditions. The intersection of body demands, cardiovascular health, and regulatory management is a critical area of ongoing research and applied practice in maintaining adequate blood circulation in stressful field operations.

6.4.1. Role of the Autonomic Nervous System (ANS)

The ANS plays a central part in regulating the vascular activity of the blood vessels and, consequently, the intricacies of human circulation. The ANS is principally composed of the sympathetic and parasympathetic branches, each of which exerts various impacts on vascular dynamics. While the sympathetic nervous system promotes vasoconstriction and thus higher blood pressure and reduced peripheral blood flow, the parasympathetic system inclines towards vasodilation and reduced heart rate. These combined actions guarantee that the body adequately responds to varying physiological requirements, balancing the demand for oxygenated blood in oxygen-hungry situations against saving energy when at rest. This dynamic relationship highlights the central role of the ANS in the control of hemodynamic stability and homeostasis during diverse activities. Additionally, its relationship with specific clinical conditions highlights the relevance of this system to vascular health. Conditions such as postural tachycardia syndrome (POTS), for instance, highlight how autonomic dysregulation leads to obvious cardiovascular manifestations such as tachycardia and intolerance to exercise (Raj et al., 2006) (Figure 6.14).

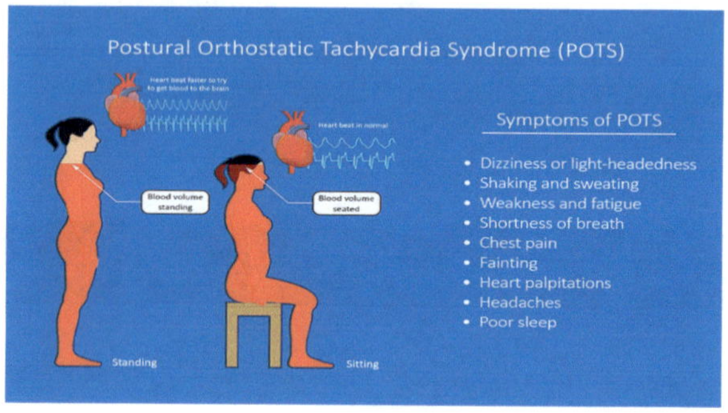

Figure 6.14. Postural tachycardia syndrome (POTS).

Source: https://www.yorkrehabclinic.ca/media/mediahub/generic-media/POTS-Postural-Orthostatic-Tachycardia-Syndrome.png.

In patients with POTS, the inappropriate activation of the sympathetic nervous system is manifested as elevated heart rates and disturbed blood volume distribution, resulting in symptoms of dizziness and fatigue. Treatment of this imbalance with tailored therapies can demonstrate how crucial the ANS is in managing circulation and ultimately patient outcomes. The description of these conditions is utilized to emphasize the ANS's central role in regular physiology and pathology of blood vessels and circulation in general. Contributing to the ANS's function's complexity in circulation is differential sympathetic nerve activity (SNA) across various vascular beds during stress responses. Research using methods like photoplethysmography indicates that SNA plays a significant role in peripheral and central blood vessel responses to stimulation, such as cold exposure (Ainslie et al., 2019). For instance, research indicates augmented response in peripheral vessels during freezing conditions, indicating a focus on the regulation of blood flow according to environmental requirements. These findings bring to light the sophisticated mechanisms engaged to conserve heat and protect core organs while regulating peripheral circulation. Such a detailed understanding of the autonomic nervous system's control function is imperative in the design of effective interventions to improve circulatory-related disorders in a clinical environment.

6.4.2. Hormonal Influences on Blood Vessel Diameter

The tone of blood vessels is strongly regulated by many hormones, which also regulate vascular tone and blood delivery. Estrogen and progesterone are two significant hormones, particularly in physiological states such as pregnancy, when the uteroplacental blood requirement rapidly increases. Experiments confirm that vasodilation and blood vessel growth are tightly controlled adaptations during pregnancy, with blood flow increased more than tenfold to support the expanding small fetus. Imbalance of the hormones can lead to complications, such as intrauterine growth restriction and precclampsia, reflecting the susceptibility of the blood vessel function and diameter to fluctuating body hormones (Glessner-Fischer et al., 2018). The effect of these hormones, combined with other variables such as wall shear stress, illustrates the multifactorial aspect of vascular adaptation for good circulation at this stage of life. Besides estrogen and progesterone, other biochemical mediators of blood vessel size are worth mentioning. The balance between vasodilators and vasoconstrictors, such as nitric oxide and endothelin, respectively, is under the control of hormonal activity. For instance, rises in estrogen are associated with increased production of nitric oxide, causing vasodilation and relaxation of vascular smooth muscle. Conversely, vasoconstrictive mechanisms can be increased by elevated cortisol or certain peptide hormones during stress responses, resulting in adverse effects on blood pressure and overall circulation. These hormonal actions emphasize the necessity for homeostatic mechanisms to maintain vascular function and integrity, and they illustrate how the control by hormones is an intrinsic component of vascular biology and the dynamics of blood flow (Cardon et al., 2025). The complexity of the power of blood vessel diameter by hormones is extended to other physiological states, beyond pregnancy, to both health and disease conditions.

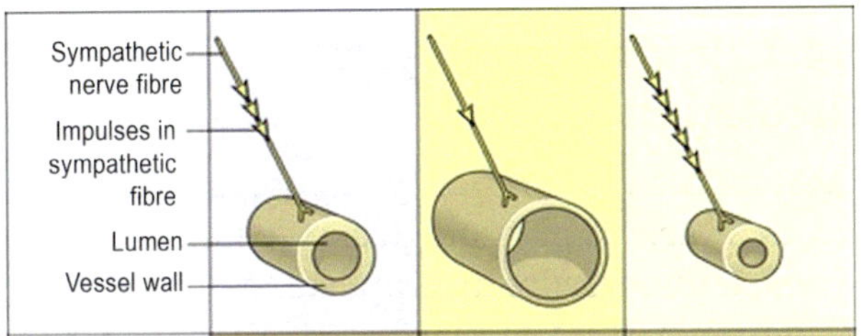

	Baseline (resting)	Vasodilation	Vasoconstriction
Sympathetic stimulation	Moderate	Decreased	Increased
Smooth muscle	Moderate tone	Relaxed	Contracted
Thickness of vessel wall	Moderate	Thinner	Thicker
Diameter of lumen	Moderate	Increased	Decreased
Peripheral resistance in arterioles	Moderate	Decreased	Increased

Figure 6.15. The relationship between sympathetic stimulation and blood vessel diameter.

Source: https://basicmedicalkey.com/the-cardiovascular-system-2/.

For instance, the effect of hormonal contraceptives on vascular function remains under active investigation, as changes in hormone levels have the potential to alter endothelial function and vessel reactivity. Given that hormones play such a fundamental role in vascular remodeling and responsiveness, insight into their mechanisms holds the potential to guide the treatment of diseases such as hypertension and atherosclerosis, in which the diameter of blood vessels is compromised. Studies of the signaling pathways activated by such hormones can provide insights into potential therapeutic targets. Therefore, an interdisciplinary effort to elucidate hormonal actions on the circulatory system must be done to guide both preventive and therapeutic interventions for vascular disease (Glessner-Fischer et al., 2018) (Figure 6.15).

6.4.3. Impact of Physical Activity on Circulation

Physical activity primarily supports circulation through various physiological mechanisms, most of which underscore the importance of achieving maximum cardiovascular health. During aerobic exercise, such as running or pedaling a bicycle, the body's increased heart rate results in augmented blood flow, providing oxygen and nutrients to contracting muscles. Augmented perfusion not only sustains the performance of exercise but also plays a crucial role in sustaining vascular health. Over time, habitual exercise results in adaptations such as greater endothelial function, reduced arterial stiffness, and increased vascular remodeling, which are all vital in ensuring the presence of a healthy blood pressure profile. As quoted by Cameron et al. (2016), lifestyle factors such as exercise are significant in the prevention of undesirable vascular changes that are associated with hypertension and in reducing cardiovascular risk. In addition, physical exercise helps to sustain blood pressure by virtue of its effect on the vascular bed and general cardiovascular function. Regular exercise has been shown to lower systemic blood pressure by increasing peripheral vascular resistance and decreasing the workload on the heart. This is particularly relevant in the management of hypertension, a condition characterized by vascular insufficiency and increased arterial stiffness. The addition of aerobic and strength exercise to one's routine not only aids in weight management but also leads to pronounced structural and functional alterations within the blood vessels. As noted in (Cameron et al., 2016), antihypertensive therapy with a vascular focus represents the central approach to reducing cardiovascular risk, and physical exercise will likely augment these drug-based interventions to achieve maximum health benefit. Apart from its direct effect on blood flow, exercise is also a preventive action against the prevalent cardiovascular diseases. Through increased endothelial function, frequent exercise causes adaptive responses of the vascular system, resulting in improved circulation and decreased risk of atherosclerosis, among others. State-of-the-art investigations using mathematical modeling have made exercise a central component to reveal the interaction between cardiovascular stressors and vascular form, particularly in diseases like pulmonary hypertension. The interactive relationship between physical exercise and cardiovascular wellness underscores the importance of medical professionals advocating for exercise as a foundational element of cardiovascular care. This approach offers a non-invasive means of enhancing circulation while mitigating the risk of hypertension and its associated complications, as evidenced by recent studies.

Test Your Knowledge

1. How does the autonomic nervous system regulate heart rate and blood vessel function in the circulatory system?
2. What hormonal factors influence blood vessel diameter, and how do they affect blood pressure and flow?

6.5. Common Disorders of Blood Vessels

Learning Outcome

1. Define atherosclerosis and its effects
2. Define varicose veins and their causes
3. Discuss hypertension and its implications

Among the various blood vessel abnormalities, one of the most prevalent ones is atherosclerosis, which has significant implications for cardiovascular health. It's the defining feature of plaque accumulation in arterial walls that results in blood vessel narrowing and limits blood circulation, hence leading to many complications in the form of heart attacks and strokes. Risk factors for atherosclerosis include hyperlipidemia, hypertension, smoking, and diabetes, all of which worsen endothelial injury and promote inflammatory responses in the vascular bed. As disease progression occurs, arterial stiffness increases, contributing to elevated systolic blood pressure and further impairing perfusion. The systemic manifestations of atherosclerosis can be dramatic and necessitate the use of multifaceted treatments, including lifestyle changes and medications aimed at suppressing lipid profiles and inflammation. Another significant disorder is peripheral artery disease (PAD) that accompanies atherosclerotic changes in the peripheral arteries, particularly those supplying the limbs. The impaired blood supply in the context of PAD manifests as claudication symptoms, pain, or cramping of the legs while one is exercising. During the progression of the disease, the patients may develop critical limb ischemia, wherein the blood supply is so minimized that it jeopardizes tissue viability and can lead to gangrene or amputation. PAD may be diagnosed with a non-invasive assessment of blood supply and could necessitate further intervention in the form of angioplasty or bypass surgery. The harmful effects of PAD extend beyond the temporary physical symptoms, increasing cardiovascular morbidity and mortality risk, and necessitating early diagnosis and treatment interventions. Cerebral SVD is another critical disorder of blood vessel pathology, primarily affecting the small perforating arteries in the brain. This illness is directly associated with hypertension and is a vital component of the development of stroke and cognitive impairment through the causation of diffuse brain injury over time. Animal model studies, such as the spontaneously hypertensive stroke-prone rat, have elucidated the mechanisms of pathophysiologic events in SVD, revealing gene expression defects in relation to endothelial function and vascular reactivity. The interplay between inflammation and endothelial dysfunction underscores the virulence of SVD, which provokes both the vascular and neurological pathway disturbances. With the growing understanding of SVD, comprehensive management practices accounting for both vascular health and cognition become increasingly vital in thwarting the adverse effects of this disorder on world health and quality of life (Bailey et al., 2014; Berry et al., 2019).

6.5.1. Atherosclerosis and Its Effects

Atherosclerosis is a long-term disease characterized by the buildup of plaques in the walls of arteries, leading to a variety of cardiovascular morbidities. Pathogenesis of atherosclerosis involves the complex interaction between genetic, lifestyle, and molecular factors impinging on endothelial injury and secondary inflammation. Insulin resistance, a manifestation of metabolic illness, has been identified as a significant etiology of endothelial dysfunction, with tertiary promotion of atherosclerotic processes. Additional evidence suggests that insulin has a direct impact on the cardiovascular system, specifically controlling endothelial generation of nitric oxide and endothelin-1 in an active state. However, the consequences to cardiovascular health are less clear. As the diabetes epidemic grows, the negative impact of impaired vascular insulin action on atherosclerosis becomes increasingly evident, suggesting that particular treatments would be capable of decreasing vascular complications (Salt et al., 2013). One of the most significant effects of atherosclerosis is its contribution to hypertension, which has been described as the most prevalent preventable risk factor for cardiovascular morbidity and mortality.

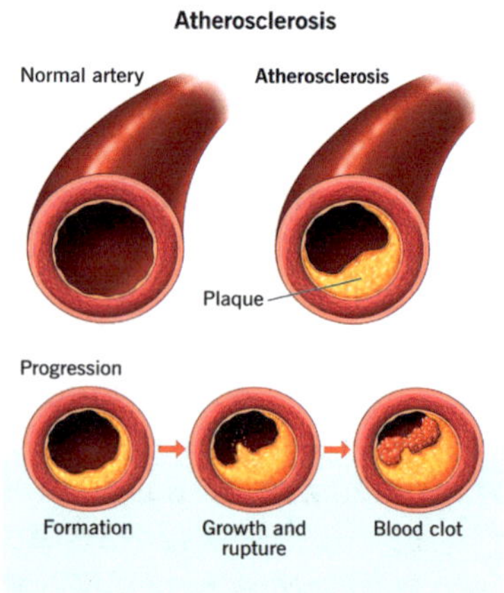

Figure 6.16. Atherosclerosis involves gradual plaque buildup inside your artery.

Source: https://my.clevelandclinic.org/health/diseases/16753-atherosclerosis-arterial-disease.

The vascular process associated with atherosclerosis includes endothelial dysfunction, arterial remodeling, and increased stiffness, adding to elevated blood pressure and subsequent target organ damage. Atherosclerotic lesions deteriorate blood flow, creating a state of turbulence that aggravates vascular inflammation and is involved in the pathogenesis of hypertension. In addition, these vascular disorders significantly elevate the risk of major cardiovascular events such as stroke, heart failure, and ischemic heart disease. Recent evidence shows that pharmacologic intervention of these vascular changes improves cardiovascular outcomes, underlining the importance of treating atherosclerosis in the management of hypertension (Cameron et al., 2016) (Figure 6.16).

Due to its multifactorial nature, the effect of atherosclerosis extends beyond isolated vascular dysfunction and exerts a critical influence on health and quality of life in general. Dietary, physical inactivity, and smoking factors augment the progression of atherosclerosis and typically result in harmful events necessitating holistic clinical management. Lifestyle modification is an essential determinant in reducing the effect of atherosclerosis since interventions for management that encourage heart-healthy lifestyles can significantly influence vascular health. Furthermore, integration of lifestyle elements into treatments will be crucial to optimize patients' outcomes and reduce cardiovascular risk. Clinicians are being called on more and more to create comprehensive treatment paradigms that include pharmacologic and lifestyle interventions to effectively counteract the effects of atherosclerosis and enhance circulation and long-term cardiovascular well-being.

6.5.2. Varicose Veins and Their Causes

The vascular system is tasked with the regulation of blood flow, and varicose veins directly affect this function. Varicose veins refer to enlarged, curved veins, typically with a blue or deep purple color, that generally appear in the legs. The primary cause of varicose veins is the inability of the valves within the veins to function correctly. These valves generally act against the backward flow of blood towards the heart. When such valves become faulty or degenerated due to the effects of prolonged standing, obesity, and heredity, blood begins to accumulate within the veins, leading to their dilatation and development of varicosities. Knowledge of the pathophysiology of varicose veins is essential for developing effective treatment strategies and managing the potential complications of this condition, which include pain, ulcers, and thrombophlebitis. Apart from mechanical failure of the venous valves, there are certain intrinsic factors that could be responsible for the occurrence of varicose veins. Age is a significant factor, as vein wall elasticity deteriorates with time, making the veins more susceptible to failure. Hormonal changes, particularly in women due to pregnancy or menopause, also have an impact on vein health by relaxing the smooth muscle of the vein wall. Some occupations that consist of long-standing or sitting have a similar effect, increasing pressure on the venous system. Even recent studies have gone as far as suggesting the existence of genetic predisposition, the suggestion being that heredity may play an essential role in one's susceptibility to developing varicosities.

These multivariate determinants attest to the complexity of varicosity pathogenesis and are a call for further studies into effective prevention and management measures. The clinical implications of varicose veins extend beyond aesthetics, as they may lead to serious health complications if left unaddressed. For instance, chronic venous insufficiency secondary to varicosities may cause extreme discomfort, swelling, and ulceration of the skin. Clinicians should be most concerned with venous anatomy and pathophysiologic understanding of varicosities, especially about diagnostic approaches such as venography. Venography is extremely valuable in determining the competence of the deep venous structures versus varicose changes in the superficial venous system. The findings can guide therapy, e.g., operative techniques to remove incompetent veins, which will minimize the risk of ulcers and other complications. Further investigation into the etiology of varicose veins, backed by widespread venographic studies, aims to enhance clinical results and patient quality of life in the treatment of venous disease (Curr et al., 1945; Dow et al., 1949) (Figure 6.17).

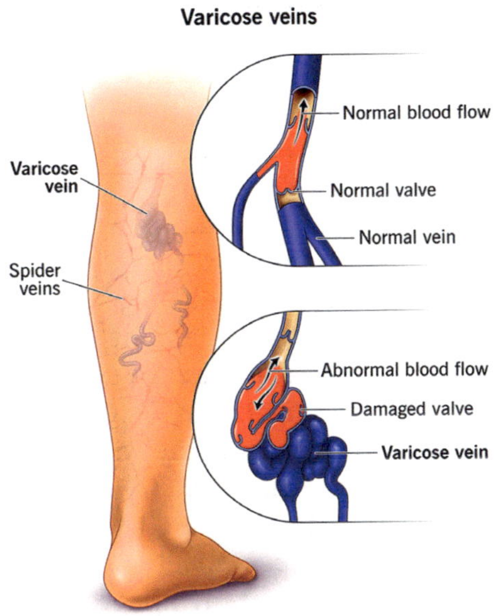

Figure 6.17. Varicose veins look blue or purple below the skin.

Source: https://my.clevelandclinic.org/-/scassets/images/org/health/articles/4722-varicose-veins-illustration.

6.5.3. Hypertension and Its Implications

Hypertension, or high blood pressure, has severe health implications beyond its fundamental physiological effects. Hypertension is the most prevalent preventable risk factor for cardiovascular disease and mortality across the world. The impact of hypertension is catastrophic and results in target organ damage such as cerebrovascular accidents, heart failure, ischemic heart disease, and renal failure. While many conditions could cause hypertension, effects on the vascular system are most dangerous. Vascular damage due to hypertension is manifested as endothelial dysfunction, arterial remodeling, and increased stiffness, which together enhance cardiovascular risk. Therefore, the control of hypertension requires an appropriate comprehension of its vascular factors and the need to satisfy the demand for adequate clinical interventions and lifestyle modifications to reverse these hazards of high levels of blood pressure (Cameron et al., 2016). The association with age-related vascular modifications further makes the clinical picture more complex. With increasing age, structural and mechanical alterations in arteries are akin to those occurring in patients with hypertension, including endothelial dysfunction and enhancement of arterial stiffness. The same could be present in young subjects with hypertension, suggesting that the disease accelerates the normal aging process of the vasculature. In addition, the interaction between biological aging and hypertension enhances the character of the vascular injury present in affected subjects. Both conditions have molecular mechanisms of pathways, such as oxidative stress and inflammation, that are responsible for causing and worsening vascular pathologies. Therefore, deciphering and recognizing compounded aging and hypertension effects is essential in developing targeted therapeutic interventions that ensure vascular health in a growing population of geriatric patients (Harvey et al., 2015). Controlling hypertension is successful through an integrative approach with both pharmacotherapy and lifestyle management. The current antihypertensive medications, including angiotensin II receptor blockers and angiotensin-converting enzyme inhibitors, not only lower blood pressure but also possess a positive effect on vascular function, lowering the risk of cardiovascular events. At the same time, lifestyle modifications—dietary modification, exercise, and stress control—are also just as crucial in preventing adverse vascular changes associated with hypertension. Data indicate that individuals who practice an integrated method of managing blood pressure can attain more beneficial health outcomes. It is, therefore, the responsibility of clinicians and scientists to give prominence to both pharmacologic and non-pharmacologic approaches in the management of hypertension such that a holistic effort towards improving vascular health and ·ducing the complications associated with this widespread problem (Cameron et al., 2016) (Figure 6.18).

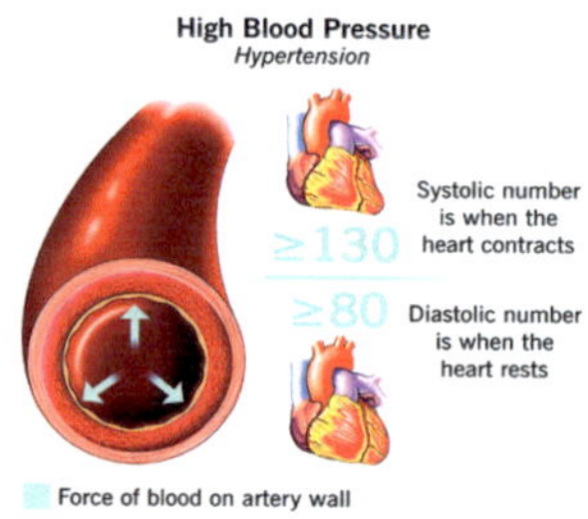

Figure 6.18. High blood pressure.

Source: https://my.clevelandclinic.org/-/scassets/images/org/health/articles/4314-high-blood-pressure-illustration.

Test Your Knowledge

1. What is atherosclerosis, and how does it affect blood flow and overall cardiovascular health?
2. What causes varicose veins, and how do they impact the function of the circulatory system?

6.6. Advances in Vascular Medicine

Learning Outcome

1. Understand the innovations in diagnostic techniques
2. Discuss the treatments for vascular diseases
3. Explain the future research directions in circulation

Recent progress in vascular medicine has significantly enhanced our understanding of blood vessel biology and pathophysiology, and consequently, more specific therapeutic strategies. The study of vascular endothelial function has demonstrated the crucial role of endothelial cells in regulating blood flow and vascular homeostasis. Endothelial dysfunction contributes to most cardiovascular diseases, including hypertension and atherosclerosis. As mechanisms of endothelial dysfunction become better understood by scientists, targeted therapies await in the form of those that will increase nitric oxide bioavailability or restrict inflammation. These strategies have not only potential for the treatment of established disease but, importantly, for the prevention of disease progression in the general vascular population. Lastly, an enhanced knowledge of the physiological and disease mechanisms within blood vessels provides the possibility of new therapies to improve circulatory function and outcomes for patients. As a parallel to the appreciation of endothelial function, research is increasingly focusing on the role of vascular reactive oxygen and nitrogen species (RONS) in the pathogenesis of vascular disease. Although firm experimental evidence abounds, highlighting their role in hypertension and related diseases, clinical utilization of these findings has lagged. It has increasingly become evident that redox stress and aberrant redox signaling may play a role in the development of serious vascular complications. Therefore, a thorough review of these biochemical pathways is indicated. This review emphasizes the need for clinical studies that define the contribution of oxidative stress to disease in human tissues, particularly in small-vessel diseases, which are often overlooked. By bridging the bench-to-bedside divide, the promise of mechanism-based treatments could revolutionize the treatment of cardiovascular disease and ultimately advance patient care and outcomes (Liang et al., 2017). Moreover, technological advances in imaging and biomarker detection over the last few decades have revolutionized the diagnosis and observation of vascular diseases. Developments such as non-surgical imaging modalities allow assessment of vascular status and blood flow patterns without surgery. Moreover, the discovery of new biomarkers facilitates earlier diagnosis, risk stratification, and targeted interventions based on individual patient profiles. This precision medicine approach not only enhances our knowledge of vascular health but also allows for more tailored therapy programs. Furthermore, as researchers continue to examine the genetic basis of vascular disease, the potential for gene-based remedies emerges, and hope is placed in the prospect of future disease management that has bedeviled us for millennia. These developments represent a landmark turning point in vascular medicine, toward a day when individualized approaches dramatically minimize morbidity and mortality from vascular disease (Figure 6.19).

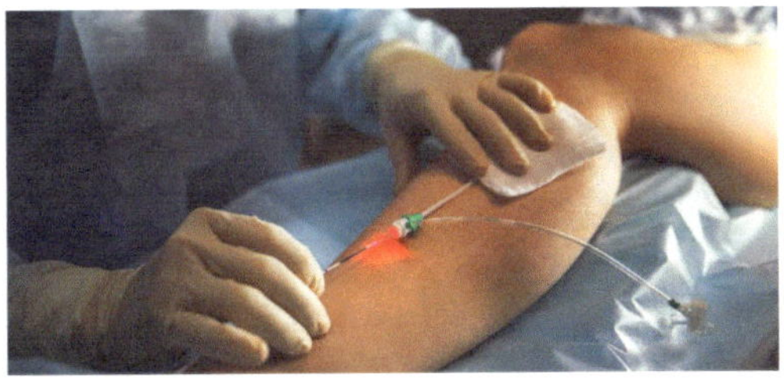

Figure 6.19. Advanced vascular surgery.

Source: https://preethihospitals.com/wp-content/uploads/2025/05/Vascular-Surgery-Big-Image-1024x504.png.

6.6.1. Innovations in Diagnostic Techniques

Diagnostic technology advancements have significantly enhanced the control and knowledge of cardiovascular health, particularly in the areas of blood vessels and circulation. Technologies have evolved in instrumentalities such as electrodes for improved skin compatibility to enable more comfortable use over extended periods of monitoring. The advancements have facilitated more precise gathering of data about the status of the heart, necessary in the early diagnosis and control of hypertension and arteriosclerosis. Moreover, procedures such as contourography provide instant electrocardiogram (EKG) images, thereby allowing for immediate clinical interpretation. Such integration of advanced diagnostic modalities not only enhances patient care but also facilitates a more integrated approach to cardiovascular diagnostics, picking up potential issues before they develop into full-blown health crises (Schafer, 2025) (Figure 6.20).

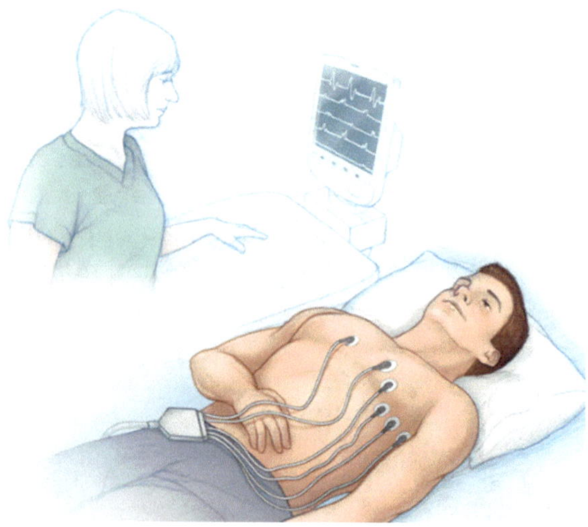

Figure 6.20. Electrocardiogram (ECG or EKG).

Source: https://www.mayoclinic.org/-/media/kcms/gbs/patient-consumer/images/2016/10/11/18/07/mcdc7_electrocardiogram-8col.jpg.

Still another breathtaking development in diagnostic techniques is the application of optical coherence tomography (OCT), particularly in the study of retinal vasculature. Studies demonstrate how OCT can accurately measure retinal nerve fiber layer (RNFL) thickness and vessel density, providing essential data regarding ocular health, which has a direct association with vascular disease. For instance, analysis by cpVD and wiVD has been constructive in differentiating normal eyes from open-angle glaucoma (OAG) eyes. Noted diagnostic performance in which the area under the receiver operating characteristic curves (AUROC) showed eminent power to distinguish accounts for the potential of OCT in identifying early disease.

This evolution reflects the way in which diagnostic innovations outperform traditional techniques, ultimately culminating in a comprehensive image of vascular health, which is crucial in managing systemic circulatory illnesses (Belghith et al., 2016). Further, the role of automated, noninvasive devices in blood pressure monitoring constitutes a principal revolution in cardiovascular diagnosis. The devices facilitate uninterrupted and trustworthy tracking, allowing real-time analysis with fewer intrusions and greater patient comfort. This technology is most valuable for an ongoing illness that requires them to be monitored consistently. By eliminating human error and enhancing the precision of readings, these technologies create a preventive system in circulatory management. Rechargeable pacemakers for the heart are also an area where technology has made significant innovations through its aid in patient mobility and reduction of device-related surgery. Together, these technologies are a paradigm shift in diagnostic procedures, refining overall knowledge of blood vessels and circulation and enhancing patient health with targeted care approaches (Schafer, 2025).

6.6.2. Treatments for Vascular Diseases

Therapeutic management of vascular disease involves various strategies to restore the blood supply and improve overall vascular health. Salvage is typically in the form of pharmacologic therapy addressing etiologic factors behind vascular compromise. Antithrombotic medications such as aspirin and anticoagulants are crucial to avoid thrombus formation within the arteries, thereby ensuring improved circulation. In more complicated cases, surgical interventions such as angioplasty and bypass surgery are required to facilitate blood flow through damaged blood vessels. These interventions not only relieve symptoms but also minimize the risk of complications secondary to chronic vascular disease. As further advances continue in research, newer treatments such as gene therapy and regenerative medicine have the potential to further enhance outcomes by repairing or replacing damaged vascular tissue. In a recent experiment with a pig model of avascular osteonecrosis, ligatures were utilized to induce a reduction in the blood supply in the femoral head, illustrating the value of targeted therapy (Kim et al., 2010). This research demonstrated that some arterial structures close to the femoral neck were significant regarding blood supply, and that therapies that focused on increasing blood flow through these structures in the local vasculature networks could potentially be beneficial for patients with concomitant vascular disease. Augmentation of blood flow through these arteries can enhance recovery from necrotic conditions, and is an exciting field to explore for future therapeutic intervention. The study emphasizes the importance of addressing localized deficiencies in blood flow since reperfusion can facilitate healing and prevent worsening of vascular disease associated with osteonecrosis. Also, utilizing probiotics in dietary treatment has been known as a new adjunct therapy for vascular health, particularly in specific groups like poultry. Strikingly, a pilot study indicated that the incorporation of probiotic PoultryStar® resulted in a significant reduction of lameness incidence, which means higher overall health and mobility in stress-exposed broiler chickens (Stark et al., 2013). Even though this finding is avian in nature, it offers an opportunity to explore how nutritional interventions may add to vascular and circulatory well-being in human populations as well. The intersection point of nutrition and vascular therapies underscores the importance of comprehensive interventions that involve not only direct therapeutic approaches but also diet and lifestyle modifications aimed at optimizing vascular function, ultimately resulting in better circulatory efficiency and outcome for the patient.

6.6.3. Future Research Directions in Circulation

With continued research on blood vessels and circulation, an important focus is on new therapeutic technologies that aim to enhance vascular health. The field has seen significant advancements, particularly in the development of drug-eluting stents and bioresorbable stents, which have revolutionized coronary artery disease treatment. Complications, however, cling to such treatments as risks, both acute and chronic. Future research must explore alternative materials and methods that minimize these risks while maximizing the efficacy of existing technologies. Exploration of novel macromolecular coatings and their potential for promoting healthy vascular repair after interventions such as balloon angioplasty will be significant. Maximizing both the mechanical and biological responses in the circulatory system can significantly improve patient outcomes and quality of life for cardiovascular disease patients (Panitch et al., 2014). In addition to treatment advancement, understanding the mechanisms of hypertension is essential for future guidance on circulation research. The vascular system also plays a significant role in hypertension, both as a cause and an effect. Scientific research must delve deeper into the vascular phenotype of hypertension, including endothelial dysfunction, arterial remodeling, and enhanced arterial stiffness. This information is crucial for the development of new antihypertensive drugs that will treat these vascular changes rather than simply reducing blood pressure. Incorporating lifestyle changes, which are helpful in the management of hypertension, into treatment plans will be equally crucial. This direction of research underscores the need for an overarching strategy for cardiovascular wellness, with the importance of dealing with vascular dysfunction placed alongside pharmacological interventions (Cameron et al., 2016). Finally, there should be a multidisciplinary approach with consideration of the overlap of vascular biology, pharmacology, and patient lifestyle to confront the complexities of circulation and blood vessel health. Future research would be improved by multimodal cooperative research among distinct branches of science investigating the influences of disparate factors, including genetics, dietary intake, and physical activity, on vascular remodeling and cardiovascular well-being. For instance, understanding the process of inflammation in the vascular system can open up new therapeutic targets to enhance vascular function. Additionally, studies on how cutting-edge technologies, such as wearable sensors for tracking real-time blood pressure or artificial intelligence for predicting cardiovascular events, can change patient treatment. This holistic approach, which integrates diverse research interventions and patient-centered interventions, will undoubtedly play a key role in preventing and managing cardiovascular diseases and hence improving health outcomes at a broader level.

Test Your Knowledge

1. What are some recent innovations in diagnostic techniques used to detect vascular diseases?
2. What are the standard treatment options available for managing vascular diseases?

SUMMARY

With the discovery of circulation and blood vessels comes the realization that the intricate workings of circulating blood are a key element in maintaining overall cardiovascular wellness. The interplay of factors such as vessel morphology, blood viscosity, and disease state can play a significant role in determining the efficiency of blood transportation throughout the body. For example, CAD conditions point out how an incremental buildup of plaque can cause a decrease in blood supply, which has severe physiological consequences. Outward remodeling, as evidenced by experiments with coronary epicardial adipose tissue removal, points out the compensatory mechanisms of the body against such blockages. These adaptive responses are crucial in dictating how blood vessels can maintain their integrity against pathological challenge, hence their importance in the broader context of circulation and overall well-being. Further investigation of the rheological properties of blood reveals greater complexity in the circulatory system. The non-Newtonian behavior of blood, for instance, viscoelasticity, yield stress, and deformation-rate dependence, challenges traditional models of fluid dynamics in vascular biology. These characteristics directly influence the blood-vessel wall interaction and thus how perfusion rates are modified, as well as the chances of thrombus formation. It is essential to comprehend all these mechanisms, particularly in relation to thinking about therapeutic options for treating cardiovascular disease. As has been implied in many studies, including CAD analysis, these rheological properties may have the potential to influence disease course and surgical availability and therefore indicate the potential for further research to optimize treatment protocols. Lastly, knowledge advancement in this area is essential to the development of effective interventions to improve circulatory health. Blood vessel and circulatory pathophysiology is a dynamic field that requires an integrative approach to understand its complexity. The data in CAD research, including outcomes of surgical procedures, can reveal the potential for both local and systemic influences on vascular function. While the compensatory mechanisms that minimize immediate effects of atherosclerosis in cases, in instances, may bring relief only temporarily, failure of significant change with therapies raises fundamental questions about the effectiveness of current approaches. Over and above this, increased understanding of blood's non-Newtonian character should serve to make models of blood flow dynamics more accurate, thereby better outlining the circulatory system's reaction to pathology. As we continue to explore these blended components, we are brought closer to innovative solutions capable of addressing the challenges of cardiovascular diseases, supporting the importance of continued research in this critical area of healthcare.

The intricate network of blood vessels plays a highly significant role in ensuring efficient circulation within the body. Blood vessels are divided into arteries, veins, and capillaries with distinct structural and functional attributes. Arterial system vessels, being capable of transporting high-pressure blood flow, have strong elastic walls to supply oxygen-rich blood from the heart to peripheral tissues. Veins, conversely, possess thin walls and valves that prevent backflow to facilitate the return of deoxygenated blood to the heart. Capillaries, the smallest vessels, are highly permeable, with nutrient and gas exchange occurring at a cellular level. Understanding the similarities and differences between these vessels of different types gives insight into the complexities of the circulatory system. It highlights the importance of vascular function on overall physiological performance. Current studies have shed light on the function of the extracellular matrix (ECM) in vascular homeostasis and how it plays a key role in keeping blood vessels intact. Specifically, research has revealed that the lysyl oxidase enzyme responsible for cross-linking collagen has been identified in all cells within the blood vessels and plays a crucial role in maintaining vessel structure. In vivo experiments using β-aminopropionitrile (BAPN) showed that lysyl oxidase inhibition results in prompt regression of vascular networks, continuing to alter the ultrastructure of collagen fibers of vessel basement membranes. Regression is not a passive process but instead occurs through controlled mechanisms like apoptosis and cell extrusion, which preserve vessel integrity but allow necessary cellular remodeling. These findings bring to light control mechanisms between ECM changes and homeostatic reactions within the vascular compartment, hence contributing to vascular dynamics and reactivity. In microcirculation, vessel-to-vessel interactions are of profound importance in the distribution of blood flow as well as pressure regulation. Microvessels like arterioles, capillaries, and venules make up intricate networks that supply tissue with oxygen and nutrients. Mathematical modeling of these networks shows how the resistances of individual vessels and their geometry affect global hemodynamics. By using a computational model, researchers have been able to simulate the flow of blood under various conditions and measure significant responses to interstitial pressure change. The model includes the structural differences between arterioles and venules to address vessel deformation and potential collapse issues. Collectively, they highlight the significance of systemic and local determinants in the explanation of microcirculatory dynamics, paving the way to advanced paradigms to treat vascular diseases and optimize therapeutic intervention in the clinic (Causin et al., 2016; Boyer et al., 2017).

KEY TERMS FROM THIS CHAPTER

- Aorta
- Capillary Beds
- Pulmonary Arteries
- Coronary Circulation
- Circulatory system
- Capillaries
- Endothelial cells
- Blood Flow
- Arterioles
- Venules
- Pulmonary Veins
- Systemic Circulation
- Hypertension
- Endothelium
- Desquamated endothelial cells (DECs)
- Vascular Resistance

CRITICAL THINKING QUESTIONS

1. **Which blood vessels carry blood away from the heart?**
   a. Veins
   b. Arteries
   c. Capillaries
   d. Venules
2. **What type of blood vessel is responsible for the exchange of gases, nutrients, and waste between blood and tissues?**
   a. Arteries
   b. Veins
   c. Capillaries
   d. Arterioles
3. **Which blood vessels have valves to prevent backflow of blood?**
   a. Arteries
   b. Capillaries
   c. Veins
   d. Arterioles
4. **The largest artery in the human body is the:**
   a. Pulmonary artery
   b. Aorta
   c. Carotid artery
   d. Coronary artery
5. **Which of the following is the correct order of blood flow through the circulatory system?**
   a. Veins → Heart → Capillaries → Arteries
   b. Heart → Arteries → Capillaries → Veins → Heart
   c. Arteries → Heart → Veins → Capillaries
   d. Capillaries → Arteries → Veins → Heart

Short Answer Questions

1. What are the three main types of blood vessels in the circulatory system?
2. How do the structures of arteries, veins, and capillaries differ?
3. What are the two major blood circulation pathways in the human body?
4. How is blood flow regulated within blood vessels?
5. Name two common disorders that affect blood vessels.
6. What are the symptoms of peripheral artery disease (PAD)?
7. Mention one recent advancement in the field of vascular medicine.

Answer to Critical Thinking Questions

1. (b); 2. (c); 3. (c); 4. (b); 5. (b)

REFERENCES

1. Al-Rifaie, M. M., Aber, A., & Bishop, J. M. (2012). Cooperation of nature and physiologically inspired mechanisms in visualisation. In *IGI Global eBooks* (pp. 31–58). https://doi.org/10.4018/978-1-4666-0942-6.ch003
2. Adamczyk, P., Czekajska-Chehab, E., Drop, A., et al. (2018). Total anomalous pulmonary vein drainage in a 60-year-old woman diagnosed in an ECG-gated multidetector computed tomography: A case report and review of literature. https://core.ac.uk/download/160736705.pdf (accessed on 14th June 2025).
3. Ainslie, D., Anderson, M., Appelhans, M., Billman, G., Budidha, K., et al. (2019). Photoplethysmography for quantitative assessment of sympathetic nerve activity (SNA) during cold stress. https://core.ac.uk/download/169434493.pdf (accessed on 14th June 2025).
4. Alivian, G. N., Iskandar, A., Salis, K. F., et al. (2024). The effect of complementary foot soak therapy using red ginger boiled water to lower blood pressure in the elderly: Case study. https://core.ac.uk/download/617687415.pdf (accessed on 14th June 2025).
5. Aponchuk, L., & Shevchuk, T. (2017). The analysis of indices of cerebral blood circulation in women-smokers. https://core.ac.uk/download/301580911.pdf (accessed on 14th June 2025).
6. Asimaki, A., Ebrahim, H. Y., Elliott, P. M., et al. (2006). Clinical expression of plakophilin-2 mutations in familial arrhythmogenic right ventricular cardiomyopathy. https://core.ac.uk/download/1676798.pdf (accessed on 14th June 2025).
7. Audi, S. H., Clough, A. V., Krenz, G. S., et al. (2006). Lung circulation modeling: Status and prospect. https://core.ac.uk/download/213071954.pdf (accessed on 14th June 2025).
8. Bailey, E. L., Crawford, W., Dominiczak, A. F., et al. (2014). Differential gene expression in multiple neurological, inflammatory and connective tissue pathways in a spontaneous model of human small vessel stroke. https://core.ac.uk/download/19182593.pdf (accessed on 14th June 2025).
9. Belghith, A., Diniz-Filho, A., Fatehee, N., et al. (2016). Optical coherence tomography angiography vessel density in healthy, glaucoma suspect, and glaucoma eyes. https://core.ac.uk/download/323064405.pdf (accessed on 14th June 2025).
10. Bello, S., Fineschi, V., Neri, M., et al. (2015). The meaning of different forms of structural myocardial injury, immune response and timing of infarct necrosis and cardiac repair. https://core.ac.uk/download/54248087.pdf (accessed on 14th June 2025).
11. Berry, C., Ford, T. J., Hainsworth, A. H., et al. (2019). Small vessel disease in the heart and brain: Current knowledge, unmet therapeutic need and future directions. https://core.ac.uk/download/186332724.pdf (accessed on 14th June 2025).
12. Bovendeerd, P. H. M., Huberts, W., van de Vosse, F. N., et al. (2024). A multiscale mathematical model for the fetal blood circulation of the second half of pregnancy. https://core.ac.uk/download/636392170.pdf (accessed on 14th June 2025).
13. Boyer, S. W., Braden, B. P., Calhoun, C., et al. (2017). *In vivo* manipulation of the extracellular matrix induces vascular regression in a basal chordate. https://core.ac.uk/download/323063488.pdf (accessed on 14th June 2025).

14. Burton, A. C., Peacock, A. J., Peacock, A. J., Pries, A. R., Levy, B. I., Steele, B. N., Figueroa, C. A., et al. (2014). Numerical simulation of blood flow and pressure drop in the pulmonary arterial and venous circulation. https://core.ac.uk/download/19502793.pdf (accessed on 14th June 2025).
15. Cameron, A. C., Lang, N. N., & Touyz, R. M. (2016). Drug treatment of hypertension: Focus on vascular health. https://core.ac.uk/download/46559725.pdf (accessed on 14th June 2025).
16. Cannon, R. O., Dakak, N., Diodati, J. G., et al. (1997). Effect of L-arginine on human coronary endothelium-dependent and physiologic vasodilation. https://core.ac.uk/download/pdf/82535140.pdf (accessed on 14th June 2025).
17. Cardon, S. Z., Ehrenberg, M. H., & Iberall, A. S. (2025). General dynamics of the physical-chemical systems in mammals. https://core.ac.uk/download/pdf/85249008.pdf (accessed on 14th June 2025).
18. Causin, P., & Malgaroli, F. (2016). Mathematical modeling of local perfusion in large distensible microvascular networks. https://core.ac.uk/download/187977482.pdf (accessed on 14th June 2025).
19. Chen, J., Dickinson, M. E., Fraser, S. E., et al. (2007). Vascular remodeling of the mouse yolk sac requires hemodynamic force. https://core.ac.uk/download/4879546.pdf (accessed on 14th June 2025).
20. Coderre, K. (2017). Assessment of coronary artery outward remodeling in consequence of excision of epicardial adipose tissue in Ossabaw swine. https://core.ac.uk/download/212824266.pdf (accessed on 14th June 2025).
21. Conrad, J., & Gillen, A. L. (2019). Life is in the blood. https://core.ac.uk/download/225132022.pdf (accessed on 14th June 2025).
22. Curr, J. F. (1945). Congenital arterio-venous fistulae and other vascular anomalies. https://core.ac.uk/download/429722122.pdf (accessed on 14th June 2025).
23. de Boer, J., Liu, J., Rivron, N. C., et al. (2008). Engineering vascularized tissues *in vitro*. https://core.ac.uk/download/pdf/11472201.pdf (accessed on 14th June 2025).
24. De Wilde, D., Gijsen, F. J. H., McCann, G., et al. (2016). Contrast-enhanced micro-CT imaging in murine carotid arteries: A new protocol for computing wall shear stress. https://core.ac.uk/download/91389700.pdf (accessed on 14th June 2025).
25. Dow, J. D. (1949). An investigation into the value of venography with special reference to varices in the lower limb. https://core.ac.uk/download/287590228.pdf (accessed on 14th June 2025).
26. Eringa, E., Stehouwer, C. D. A., & Yudkin, J. S. (2005). Hypothesis: 'Vasocrine' signaling from perivascular fat–a mechanism linking insulin resistance and vascular disease. https://core.ac.uk/download/1668998.pdf (accessed on 14th June 2025).
27. Fenwick, S. A., Hazleman, B. L., & Riley, G. P. (2002). The vasculature and its role in the damaged and healing tendon. https://core.ac.uk/download/2756790.pdf (accessed on 14th June 2025).
28. Fraser, S. E., Motaghiannezam, R., & Schwartz, D. M. (2012). *In vivo* human choroidal vascular pattern visualization using high-speed swept-source optical coherence tomography at 1060 nm. https://core.ac.uk/download/4895349.pdf (accessed on 14th June 2025).

29. Glessner-Fischer, A. D. (2018). The role of sex hormones in inducing maternal uterine remodeling and vasodilation during pregnancy. https://core.ac.uk/download/215153958.pdf (accessed on 14th June 2025).

30. Goetz, A. E., Groh, J., Kiefmann, R., et al. (1999). Leukocyte sequestration in pulmonary micro vessels and lung injury following systemic complement activation in rabbits. https://core.ac.uk/download/16432557.pdf (accessed on 14th June 2025).

31. Guzik, T. J., & Nosalski, R. (2017). Perivascular adipose tissue inflammation in vascular disease. https://core.ac.uk/download/77600990.pdf (accessed on 14th June 2025).

32. Harvey, A., Montezano, A. C., & Touyz, R. M. (2015). Vascular biology of ageing—implications in hypertension. https://core.ac.uk/download/42363485.pdf (accessed on 14th June 2025).

33. Hobbs, A. J., Moyes, A. J., Ahluwalia, A., Rebstock, A. S., Brown, C. F., Sánchez Ferrer, C. F., et al. (2014). Endothelial C-type natriuretic peptide maintains vascular homeostasis. https://core.ac.uk/download/30696975.pdf (accessed on 14th June 2025).

34. Kim, H., Liang, Y., Yokota, H., et al. (2010). Evaluation of a pig femoral head osteonecrosis model. https://core.ac.uk/download/323269724.pdf (accessed on 14th June 2025).

35. Kosheleva, A. (2017). The structural features of vascular endothelium in acute cerebral ischemia. https://core.ac.uk/download/322516288.pdf (accessed on 14th June 2025).

36. Liang, M., Montezano, A. C., Rios, F., et al. (2017). Redox stress defines the small artery vasculopathy of hypertension: How do we bridge the bench-to-bedside gap? https://core.ac.uk/download/84148299.pdf (accessed on 14th June 2025).

37. Lu, Y., & Wang, W. (2010). Multiscale modelling of fluid and solute transport in soft tissues and micro vessels. https://core.ac.uk/download/46170774.pdf (accessed on 14th June 2025).

38. Madanu, S. (2012). The acute responses of different-sized coronary arteries to testosterone. https://core.ac.uk/download/10683771.pdf (accessed on 14th June 2025).

39. Mauroy, B., & Moreau, B. (2015). Murray's law revisited: Quemada's fluid model and fractal trees. https://core.ac.uk/download/47087169.pdf (accessed on 14th June 2025).

40. Panitch, A., & Scott, R. A. (2014). Macromolecular approaches to prevent thrombosis and intimal hyperplasia following percutaneous coronary intervention. https://core.ac.uk/download/323070882.pdf (accessed on 14th June 2025).

41. Raj, S. R. (2006). The postural tachycardia syndrome (POTS): Pathophysiology, diagnosis & management. https://core.ac.uk/download/pdf/86508.pdf (accessed on 14th June 2025).

42. Salt, I. P. (2013). Examining the role of insulin in the regulation of cardiovascular health. https://core.ac.uk/download/9652225.pdf (accessed on 14th June 2025).

43. Schafer, G. (2025). A case study of technology transfer: Cardiology. https://core.ac.uk/download/pdf/42897756.pdf (accessed on 14th June 2025).

44. Sochi, T. (2014). Non-Newtonian rheology in blood circulation. http://arxiv.org/abs/1306.2067 (accessed on 14th June 2025).

45. Stark, J. M. (2013). Efficacy of probiotics for reducing the incidence of lameness in broilers grown on wire flooring. https://core.ac.uk/download/72842771.pdf (accessed on 14th June 2025).

THE LYMPHATIC SYSTEM AND IMMUNITY

7

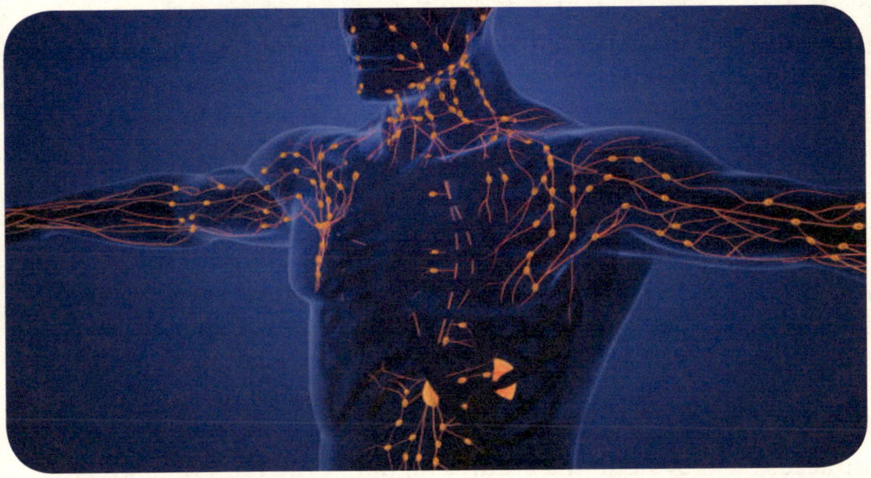

LEARNING OBJECTIVES

After studying this chapter, you will be able to:

1. Explain the anatomy and key structures of the lymphatic system
2. Explain the key roles of the lymphatic system in maintaining the body healthy
3. Provide an overview of the immune system
4. Explain the role of lymphocytes in immunity.
5. Explain how the immune system responds to pathogens
6. Explain key diseases of the lymphatic system and how they impact health

Introduction

The lymphatic system is the core component of the immune defense of the human body, acting as a conduit for the transport of lymph, an immune cell-bearing fluid, throughout the body. A sophisticated network of vessels, nodes, and organs, the lymphatic system plays two roles: not only to drain interstitial fluid but also to sense and react to infection. This system operates largely through many of the immune processes to facilitate the body's ability to recognize and destroy foreign invaders. The intricate architecture of lymph nodes serves as a platform for activation and maturation of lymphocytes, highlighting the importance of the lymphatic system to immune homeostasis and resistance to disease in humans and other animals. Recent studies have revealed the lymphatic system's reaction to environmental changes, particularly those generated by seasonal cycles that potentially affect immune function. For example, environmental change is succeeded by fluctuations in glucocorticoid levels that can impair immune reactions.

This is something to be learned about; it could reveal how organisms predict and prepare for immunological threats introduced by changing seasons. As suggested by research, short-day season during winter and autumn is also the season of low immune function, indicating that the lymphatic system can expect seasonal modulation from factors such as melatonin and hormonal regulation (Demas et al., 1995). This information supports the need for overall knowledge concerning the effects of seasonal influences on the health and resistance of the lymphatic system. Imaging advances have significantly enhanced our understanding of lymphatic function and its immunological role. The presence of non-invasive imaging techniques allows for the real-time observation of lymphocyte dynamics in lymph nodes, yielding information of great benefit to the study of immune activation mechanisms. By enabling longitudinal studies without invasive procedures, scientists can observe the trafficking and interactions of immune cells in a way that could not be done before (Andrea et al., 2012). These advances not only provide greater access to the lymphatic system's functional operations but also create doors for future therapeutic interventions that can modulate immune responses. As we delve into the complexity of the lymphatic system, it is clear that an integrated understanding of its structure and function is essential to deciphering the code of immunity and disease control.

Definition of the Lymphatic System

The lymphatic system, one of the circulatory and immune systems, serves various vital roles crucial to body homeostasis. It is comprised of a network of lymphatic vessels, nodes, and lymph organs like the spleen and thymus. The lymph, which is a watery fluid flowing through this system, contains lymphocytes and other immune cells that play a significant role in innate and adaptive immunity. The lymphatic system facilitates the transport of these immune cells to tissues so that an immediate response to pathogens is possible, and the removal of interstitial fluid, proteins, and waste products from tissues. Thus, it is essential to comprehend the intricacy of the system to understand its function in metabolic processes and protective immunity mechanisms. One of the key functions of the lymphatic system is the filtering and screening of lymphatic fluid by lymph nodes, which are crucial locations for immune activity. Lymph nodes trap pathogenic invaders to facilitate the stimulation of lymphocytes that play a vital role in coordinating immune responses. Dendritic cells, the key antigen-presenting cells, also travel via lymphatic vessels into lymph nodes, where they activate T-cells and B-cells and hence produce a robust immune response. This demonstrates the role of the lymphatic system not only in the travel of immune cells but also in allowing them to communicate with one another. More recent studies have characterized the migrating intestinal lymph DC subsets as having varying functional characteristics, indicating heterogeneity in function for the system; the studies highlight the immunological complexity of lymphatic function (Allan et al., 2010). The lymphatic system is also a central mechanism for the maintenance of fluid balance and tissue health. By removing excess water from interstitial spaces and pumping it back into the bloodstream, the lymphatic system prevents edema and ensures overall tissue hydration. Any disruption of this system may cause crippling pathological states like lymphedema and chronic inflammation. Specifically, an imbalanced immune response within the lymphatic system can lead to chronic conditions such as dry eye disease (DED), where the balance between innate and adaptive immunity is lost, and this leads to inflammation of the ocular surface (Lin et al., 2020). It is, therefore, paramount that the function and integrity of the lymphatic system are preserved for not just immune protection but to achieve homeostasis and avoid pathological conditions in the whole body.

Importance of Immunity in Human Health

Immunity plays a pivotal role in upholding human health by serving as the body's first line of defense against diseases and pathogens. A healthy immune system requires the ability to detect and destroy infectious agents, such as bacteria, viruses, and fungi, that cause damage to human health. The lymphatic system, an essential component of the immune system, assists in the movement of immune cells and the removal of toxins from the body. It has lymphocytes, such as T cells and B cells, which are in charge of adaptive immunity, yielding specific responses for individual pathogens. In a normal immune system, it protects from infection, decreases infection susceptibility, and provides general homeostasis. A malfunctioning immune response, however, leads to increased susceptibility to infection, autoimmune illnesses, and chronic disease, showing the significant effect of immunity on human health. Lymphatic involvement is also key in the formation of tertiary lymphoid organs (TLOs), which form secondary to chronic inflammation or infection. These ectopic tissues facilitate local immune responses by clustering antigen-presenting cells and lymphocytes within peripheral tissues. TLOs enhance the activity of immune cells to engage with antigens, causing a swift and localized immune response, which is essential for control of infection and the initiation of healing of tissues. A deeper understanding of how such lymphoid tissues process antigens might illuminate novel therapeutic strategies in conditions of compromised immunity, such as chronic inflammatory diseases and cancer. Experiments on TLOs demonstrate the immune system's plasticity, underlining the importance of local immunological processes for maintaining systemic health and protecting against pathogenic threats, as discussed in recent reviews on the subject (Bedaj et al., 2016). Furthermore, the richness of the immune system is not only innate and adaptive but also involves a rich diversity of cell types, such as mast cells, which might play a significant role in disease as well as in health. Mast cells, traditionally recognized for their contribution to allergic disease, also play a role in multifaceted functions in tissue homeostasis and tumorigenesis. These cells often possess typical subpopulations that have protective or pro-inflammatory actions, depending on the extrinsic environment in the human body. Their positioning at strategic locations within various tissues, for example, the myocardium and in atheromatous plaques, suggests their role in normal as well as pathological processes. Recognition of the two-sided functions of mast cells in immunity could unlock new therapeutic approaches aimed at leveraging their beneficial roles without decreasing favorable effects and minimizing adverse consequences (de Paulis et al., 2019). This two-sided view of immune function is crucial for furthering our understanding of immunity's critical role in human health.

7.1. Anatomy of the Lymphatic System

Learning Outcome

1. Describe the major components: lymph nodes, vessels, and organs
2. Describe the role of the spleen and thymus
3. Explain the interaction with the circulatory system

The anatomy of the lymphatic system is very complex, consisting of a vast network of lymphatic vessels, lymph nodes, and accessory organs. The lymphatic vessels, running parallel to the circulatory system, serve to transport lymph—a fluid filled with lymphocytes and waste substances—throughout the body. They start as blind-ending capillaries within interstitial spaces, which facilitate the uptake of interstitial fluid and solutes. As lymph travels through vessels of increasingly larger diameter, it passes through lymph nodes in which immune cells filter out pathogens and foreign substances. Such filtering is crucial, as lymph nodes are one of the most critical sites of adaptive immune responses, facilitating lymphocytes' encounter with antigens. Hence, the anatomical organization of the lymphatic system is essentially connected to its function of immune surveillance and maintenance of body fluid equilibrium. At the center of lymphatic anatomy are the lymph nodes, which are found at sites of convergence of lymphatic vessels. Typically, there is a cluster of lymph nodes in the cervical, axillary, and inguinal groups to filter lymph systematically as it returns to the bloodstream. Each lymph node holds an external cortex and an internal medulla, which are packed with distinct subpopulations of immune cells, including B and T lymphocytes, macrophages, and dendritic cells. This organization enhances the lymph nodes' efficiency in reacting with immunity; when pathogens are present, a cascade of cellular activation occurs, as seen with the onset of cytokine release. This local immune response establishes the primary role of lymph nodes in preventing systemic infection spread and reinforces their position as functional sites of innate and adaptive immunity (Germain et al., 2012). The spleen and thymus are also other notable components of the lymphatic system, whose roles considerably contribute to the body's immune function. The spleen, for instance, filters blood and not lymph, disposing of aged red blood cells and serving as a reservoir of immune cells. Its white pulp is highly packed with lymphocytes. It interacts with blood-borne antigens and thus serves as a crucial site for the activation of immune responses to systemic infections. The thymus, on the other hand, is primarily involved in T cell maturation for adaptive immunity. The communication between these organs is critical, e.g., that the thymus will stimulate healthy T cell maturation, which will then flow to lymph nodes and the spleen so that there is an effective and organized immune response (Barril et al., 2014). This anatomy organization is a reflection of the sophistication and plasticity of the lymphatic system in immune homeostasis (Figure 7.1).

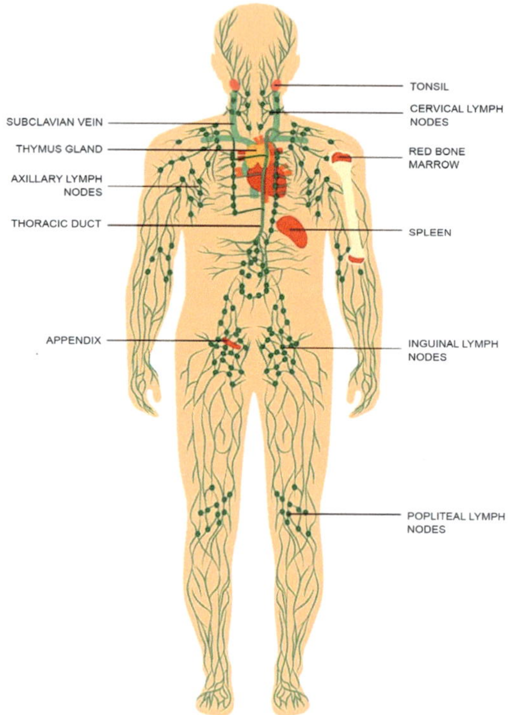

Figure 7.1. Anatomy of the lymphatic system.

Source: https://nurseslabs.com/wp-content/uploads/2017/08/Lymphatic-System-Lymphatic-System-Anatomy-and-Physiology.jpg.

7.1.1. Major Components: Lymph Nodes, Vessels, and Organs

The lymphatic system is critical to the maintenance of immune function, and lymph nodes are critical components of the system. Lymph nodes are strategically positioned throughout the body to catch pathogens and foreign material. They have high densities of lymphocytes, B and T cells, which are a distinctive feature of adaptive immunity. When they come into contact with antigens, these lymphocytes can proliferate and differentiate rapidly and thus induce an immune response.

Structural organization within the lymph nodes permits coordination of cell-to-cell interactions and is vital in activating the immune cells. Further, the structure of lymph nodes facilitates proper antigen processing to enable the immune system to act rapidly against infections. Thus, the operation of lymph nodes is not just vital for filtering lymphatic fluid but for initiating robust immune responses to different pathogens (Figure 7.2).

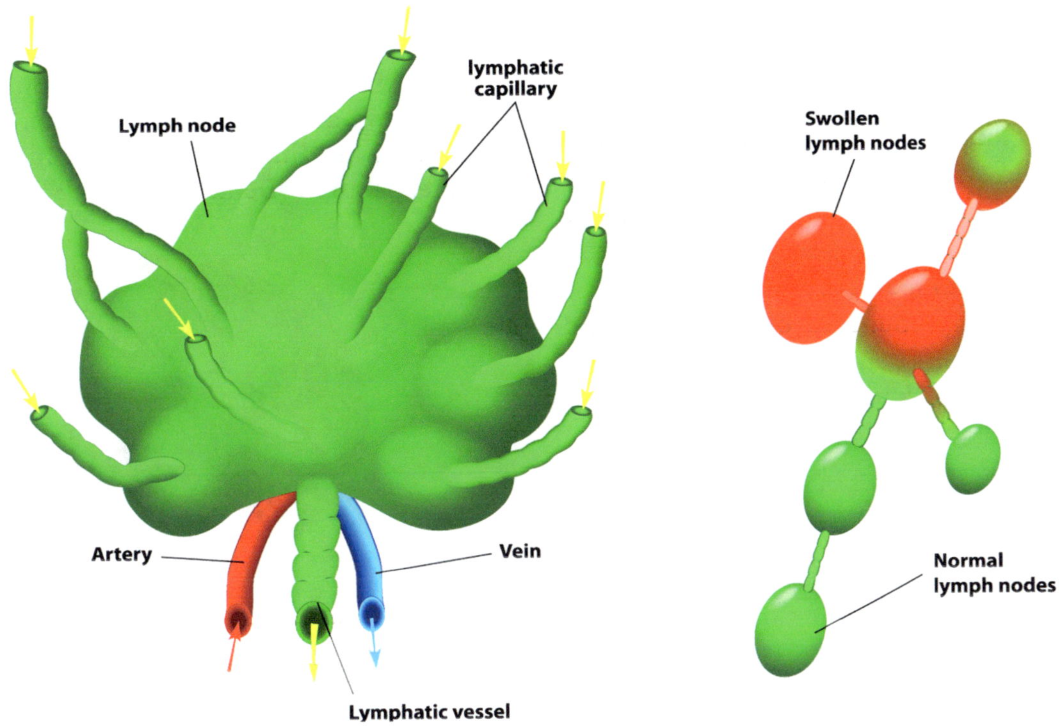

Figure 7.2. Lymph Nodes.

Source: https://nurseslabs.com/lymphatic-system-anatomy-physiology/.

Underlying the entire anatomy of the lymphatic system, lymphatic vessels play a similarly important function, forming an extensive network for the transport of lymph and immune cells throughout the body. Vessels are for one-way travel towards lymph nodes and ultimately to the bloodstream, serving as conduits for the return of interstitial fluid and mobilization of immune cells. Flow through the tubes relies on a combination of intrinsic contractions along with extrinsic properties, including contraction of the skeletal muscles. The lymphatic vessels also serve to present antigens to lymph nodes in a step that facilitates efficient immune surveillance. Pathology of the lymphatic vessels leads to edema and compromised immune capability, further substantiating their function in both fluid balance and immune capability. Therefore, it is necessary to understand the dynamic role of lymphatic vessels to understand how the lymphatic system is involved in immune health and responding to insult. In addition to lymph nodes and vessels, tertiary lymphoid organs (TLOs) are significant components of the lymphatic system, particularly in peripheral tissues. TLOs arise as a response to inflammation and provide localized niches for immune cell activation and expansion, often arising in the context of antigens. Their organization is similar to that of the healthy lymph nodes in allowing effective antigen presentation and organization of immune responses. The existence of antigen-presenting cells in the TLOs is essential in maintaining appropriate immune activity, demonstrating their role as central immune-modulating compartments. Considerably more, though, remains to be uncovered about mechanisms that govern antigen handling within these ectopic structures. As it evolves further, understanding of TLO development and function may unveil new therapeutic avenues for the treatment of immune-associated disease and further our comprehension of tissue-specific immune regulation (Bedaj et al., 2016) (Figure 7.3).

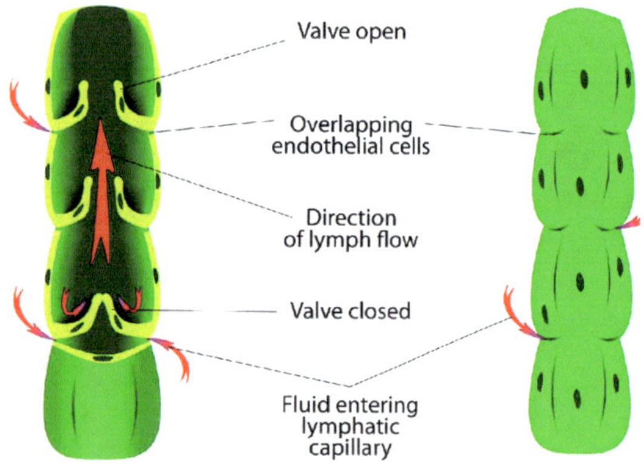

Figure 7.3. Lymphatic vessels.

Source: https://nurseslabs.com/lymphatic-system-anatomy-physiology/.

7.1.2. The Role of the Spleen and Thymus

The spleen and thymus are both components of the lymphatic system, but have widely differing but complementary roles to enhance and assist immunity. The spleen, the largest of the lymphatic organs, is primarily a filter for blood. It screens the blood to see if there are pathogens or other foreign matter present, draining out old or damaged red blood cells and reusing the iron from them. It is within the white pulp of the spleen that immune responses are initiated, since it contains a dense population of lymphocytes, which are in charge of identifying and responding to infecting pathogens. This organizational structure enables the spleen not only to observe the circulation of blood-borne pathogens but also to enable immune memory formation, leading to a better response upon later exposures (Demas et al., 1995).

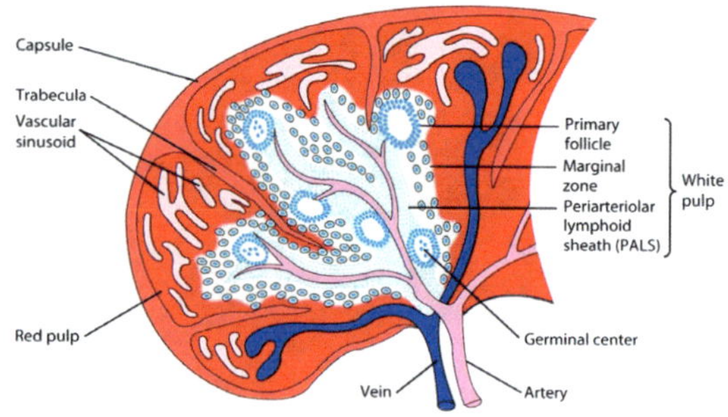

Figure 7.4. Spleen.

Source: https://nurseslabs.com/lymphatic-system-anatomy-physiology/.

The thymus, however, is responsible for the development of T-lymphocytes, key to the adaptive immune response. Found in the upper part of the chest, the thymus is most functional and largest in children and adolescents and declines in function and size into adulthood. T-cells are positively and negatively selected during their maturation to ensure that only cells that can view foreign antigens and not self-antigens are allowed to be released into the blood. So rigorous selection becomes essential to prevent autoimmune reactions, wherein the immune system will attack the body's own tissues based on incorrect identification. The thymus, therefore, plays an important training site for T-cells, ultimately resulting in immune tolerance and the body's ability to fight back against pathogens without inflicting self-damage (Demas et al., 1995) (Figure 7.4).

Together, the spleen and thymus are indicative of the dual nature of the lymphatic system's role in immunity. Their functions not only show the complexity of immune processes but also express the importance of their harmony in defense processes in the body. While the thymus educates T-lymphocytes and the spleen facilitates recognition and reaction towards pathogens, they reinforce the organism's capacity to address both internal and external challenges collectively. Understanding how these organs enhance immune competence is crucial in comprehending multifarious immunological illnesses and diseases, demonstrating the significance of thorough knowledge regarding lymphatic system structure and function (Gallucci et al., 1995) (Figure 7.5).

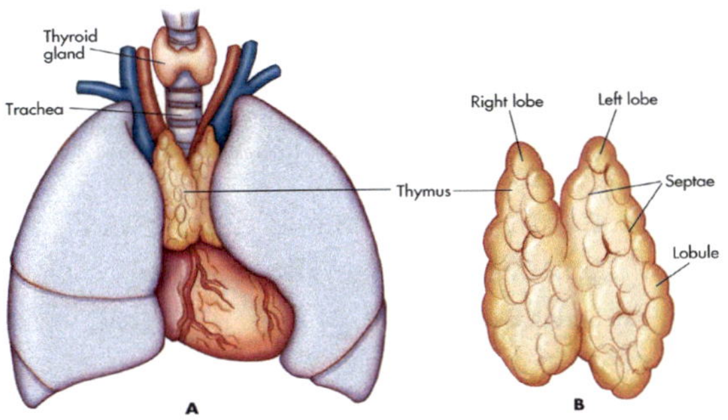

Figure 7.5. Thymus gland.

Source: https://nurseslabs.com/lymphatic-system-anatomy-physiology/.

7.1.3. Interaction with the Circulatory System

The lymphatic system plays a starring role in the interaction with the circulatory system as an essential component of the immune system. It appears as a drainage system that reclaims excess interstitial fluid and directs it back into the bloodstream, and in so doing, ensures fluid balance in the body. This is essential for efficient circulation and homeostasis of the tissues. As the lymphatic fluid traverses the lymphatic vessels, it conveys various immune cells, such as lymphocytes and antigen-presenting cells, to the immune surveillance of the potential pathogens. The coordination of these two systems is most evident during infection times, as the lymphatic system acts as a route for immune responses, from local immune response to systemic circulation, thus allowing coordinated protection against the invading pathogens. The role of the lymphatic system extends beyond fluid transport; it is also a principal player in the systemic immune response. In lymph nodes, the lymph and circulatory systems interact closely, removing antigens and pathogens from the lymph fluid and presenting them to immune cells. This enables activation of the adaptive immune responses, which are required for long-term protection. The lymph nodes are enriched with diverse immune cell populations, including natural killer cells and T cells, which are strategically positioned to respond to these signals rapidly. Recent studies have highlighted how cytokines, particularly IL-18, induced by pathogens trigger quick activation of innate lymphocytes, representative of dynamic interaction between lymphatic and circulatory systems as they coordinate to increase effective immune responses to infection (Germain et al., 2012). Temporal factors also impinge on the interaction between lymphatic and circulatory systems, particularly seasonal changes influencing immune function. Research indicates that photoperiod alterations can cue the body to alter its immune response, impacting the size and function of lymphatic tissue. For instance, during autumn and winter seasons, environmental stressors induce decreased immune activity that can compromise an organism's ability to fight infection. The role of melatonin as a mediator of this transition between seasons provides one interesting link, suggesting that anticipation and reaction to environmental cues is essential for immune proficiency. Studying these interactions and variation points to the significance of looking at both systems holistically because change in their functioning can have a very significant impact on global health and the ability to ward off disease (Demas et al., 1995).

Test Your Knowledge

1. What are the major components of the lymphatic system, and what roles do lymph nodes, vessels, and organs play?
2. What are the specific functions of the spleen and thymus in the lymphatic and immune systems?

7.2. Functions of the Lymphatic System

Learning Outcome

1. Discuss the fluid balance and tissue drainage
2. Define absorption of dietary fats
3. Explain the immune response facilitation

The lymph system has several very crucial functions required to the maintenance of immune homeostasis and overall body health. Primarily, it is responsible for the carriage of lymph, which is a circulating fluid within and through the lymph vessels, transporting not only excess fluid from the tissues but also proteins and waste products. By the recovery and return of the fluid to the circulation, the lymph system prevents edema and sustains a healthy fluid economy in the body. Moreover, the lymphatic vessels also serve as pathways for immune cells, predominantly lymphocytes, to enable their migration to and from lymphoid organs, wherein the immune response is triggered. Such circulatory action of lymphatic circulation is essential for effective immune surveillance and response to infection. The functions of the lymphatic system are thus crucial to both homeostasis and regulation of the body defense mechanisms against infections and disease. Apart from the regulation of fluids and transport of lymphocytes, the lymphatic system also plays a significant role in the filtration and removal of pathogens. Lymph, within lymph nodes, which are natural filters, is exposed to various immune cells such as macrophages and dendritic cells. These cells are essential in identifying and capturing foreign substances, like bacteria and viruses. The interaction of lymphocytes with antigen-presenting cells plays a crucial role in initiating adaptive immune responses that enable the body to build a specific defense against pathogens. Interestingly, tertiary lymphoid organs (TLOs) also contribute towards such a filtering process, which occurs after antigens in tissues peripheral to the lymphoid organs. These ectopic tissues enable localized immunity generation, which emphasizes the adaptive role of the lymphatic system in various pathological processes (Bedaj et al., 2016). The role of the lymph system in immune function is broader than the filtration of pathogens; it also affects the maturation and development of diverse immune cells. Lymphatic vessels and organs facilitate the trafficking of T and B lymphocytes, central to the adaptive immune response. Moreover, the formation of such cells is also based on interactions within the lymph environment as well as stromal cell signals around them. Such complex interactions not only ensure effective immune response but also create immunological memory, allowing for quicker responses to familiar pathogens. Furthermore, it is proposed that mast cells, which interact with lymphatic tissue, may be capable of performing several functions in host protection and healing of tissue, highlighting the sophistication of the lymphatic system (de Paulis et al., 2019). Understanding these processes can help shed light on the development of novel immunotherapies and targeted treatments for numerous ailments, further suggesting the role of lymphatic systems in disease and health.

7.2.1. Fluid Balance and Tissue Drainage

Fluid balance and adequate tissue drainage are key functions of the lymphatic system and are in direct association with its immunological function. The lymphatic vessels act to drain interstitial fluid, proteins, and waste products from the tissues and thus prevent edema as well as create a stable environment for cellular processes. In fluid buildup due to injury or inflammation, lymphatic drainage plays a crucial role in helping the body return to homeostasis. This is an active process rather than one in which the lymphatic system sits back, and the immune response is controlled. Lymphatic transport can carry antigens and immune cells throughout the body. Understanding fluid balance dynamics within the lymphatic system illuminates its essential function both in the inflammatory process as well as tissue integrity, and highlights the importance of the system for overall health.

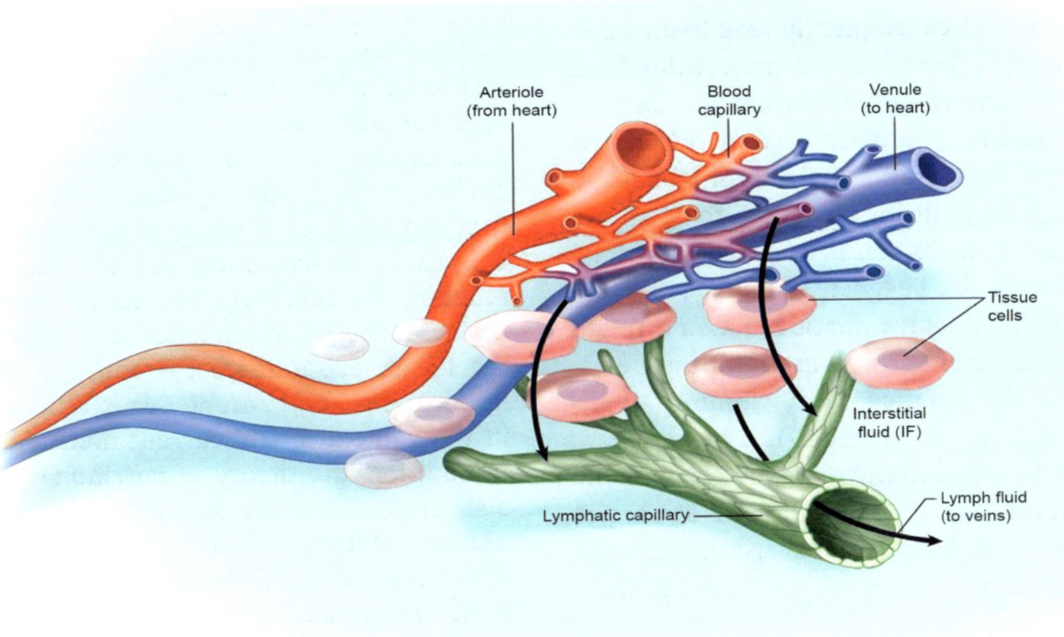

Figure 7.6. Role of the lymphatic system in fluid balance.

Source: https://basicmedicalkey.com/lymphatic-system/.

The relationship between fluid balance and lymphatic function encompasses more than drainage mechanisms, such as the system's role in immune modulation. It is discovered that the lymph vessels play a critical role in modulating immune cell trafficking to calibrate immune responses appropriately to clear infections without causing excess tissue damage. As discussed in recent studies, such a regulatory function is especially relevant in chronic inflammation, where dysregulation can lead to autoimmunity or increased susceptibility to infection. In this manner, then, the lymphatic system acts as a crucial checkpoint, modulating the interface between peripheral tolerance and activation of immunity. The intricate relationship between immune regulation and fluid regulation justifies the lymphatic system's double role as a mechanism for drainage of fluid as well as for the immune response, described in its connection with inflammation and tumor immunity (Lund et al., 2018) (Figure 7.6).

Further, the implications of lymphatic dysfunction are massive, particularly with regard to ailments such as obesity and cardiovascular disease when fluid balance is critical. Damage to the lymphatic vasculature can lead to poor fluid homeostasis and, consequently, lead to diseases such as lymphedema, where interstitial fluid overload results in severe pathology. Current research on the lymphatic system reveals its role in lipid uptake and cholesterol transport, implicating its multifunctionality to facilitate physiological homeostasis in tissues. At the same time, evidence also suggests immune cells' role in the modulation of lymphatic function through mechanisms such as lymphangiogenesis, merging fluid balance with immune well-being (Anisimov et al., 2019). Consequently, an insight into lymphatic dynamics is valuable for the development of therapeutic strategies to recover fluid balance and sustain immune system function in many disease conditions.

7.2.2. Absorption of Dietary Fats

The emulsification of dietary lipids is a complex physiological process of central importance to general nutrition and immunocompetence. Following ingestion, lipids are emulsified within the gut by the activity of bile salts and digestive enzymes. This results in the formation of micelles, which enhance the solubility of fatty acids and monoglycerides so that they can be absorbed into intestinal epithelial cells. Once inside the enterocytes, fatty acids are re-esterified back into triglycerides and packaged in the form of chylomicrons. The chylomicrons are then released into lymphatic circulation, a critical juncture at which dietary lipids intersect with the immune system. In addition to being carried through the lymphatic system, nutrients actually influence immune cell function, illustrating the intricate interaction between metabolism and immunological health. The role of saturated fatty acids (SFAs) in immunological function exemplifies the importance of dietary fats beyond energy supply. Recent studies have elucidated how SFAs like palmitic acid modulate innate immunity, which may affect monocytes and macrophages. Such modulation occurs when SFAs are being transported within the lymphatics, which means the lymphatic system plays a key role in immune memory and inflammatory responses within the body. Specifically, palmitic acid has also been shown to induce a hyper-inflammatory state upon secondary microbial challenge in model systems, which implies that ingestion of these types of dietary lipids can exert far-reaching impacts on immune function. Cumulatively, the above observations underscore the importance of understanding the fat absorption process and the associated implications for immune regulation, especially in the context of the current dietary situation. In addition, the theory of nutritional immunity also emphasizes the interaction of dietary fat uptake and immune function regulation. At times of infection or inflammation, the body tends to limit the availability of nutrients to pathogens, resulting in a competitive situation where the host is required to modulate nutrient uptake in support of immune function while restricting access to invaders. Of note is that although the micronutrient absorptions may be inhibited in inflammatory states, mechanisms for dietary fat absorption are maintained, emphasizing the lymphatic system's importance. Clinical trials of the lymphatic system's function in fat absorption, particularly with ketogenic or antioxidant diets, are promising avenues of research into the reversal of inflammation and better health outcomes. As the interaction of diet, immunity, and the lymphatic system continues to evolve, further research will be needed to bridge these gaps for improved public health.

7.2.3. Immune Response Facilitation

The facilitation of the immune system plays an essential role in defining the extent to which the body can resist pathogens and disease. At its heart are specialized molecules and cells that travel the lymphatic system, an access route for immune cells to communicate and respond to threats. Dendritic cells, for example, recognize and present antigens to T cells and hence trigger a successful adaptive immune response. This is made possible by a network of lymphatic vessels transporting the immune cells along with antigens to lymph nodes, where a local immune response is elicited. These processes underscore the importance of proper lymphatic system function in immune control and suggest how such dysfunction can compromise overall immunity, with heightened risk of infection and disease. The molecules involved in signaling to enable immune function, such as cytokines and chemokines, are also key to bringing together the various components of the immune system. They are released upon the recognition of pathogens and influence the function of different immune cells to promote proliferation, differentiation, and T cell polarization. For instance, the inflammatory cytokine interleukin-6 enables the transition from innate to adaptive immunity, allowing a more targeted and efficient response. Besides that, recently it has been suggested that microRNAs, namely miR-132 and miR-212, contribute to immune functions by regulating the immune response at the genetic level. In contrast, their deficiency has been demonstrated not to lead to apparent immune dysfunction, as in murine models (Ucar et al., 2013) (Figure 7.7).

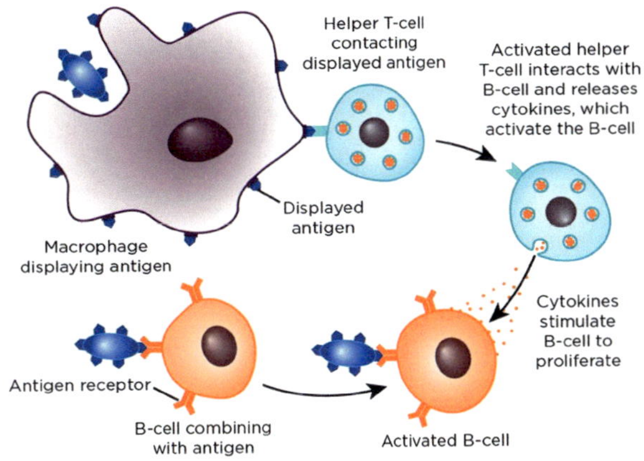

Figure 7.7. Immune reactions inside a lymph node.

Source: https://cdn.ps.emap.com/wp-content/uploads/sites/3/2020/11/Fig2-Immune-reaction-inside-a-lymph-node-1024x799.jpg.

Hence, a realistic perception of these molecules aids in the development of new immunotherapeutic strategies. Besides, the bioconjugates have emerged as game-changing entities in the field of immunotherapy by providing targeted immunity. These engineered complexes combine antigens and adjuvants to enhance the immunogenicity of vaccines, providing a strategic strategy for directing immune responses against specific pathogens. The ability of bioconjugates to mimic the structural properties of native pathogens while simultaneously communicating with important immune cells emphasizes their potential use in vaccine design. For example, recent evidence has unveiled that these molecular immunomodulators can significantly enhance vaccine potency by stimulating T and B cell activation and therefore long-term immunity (Irvine et al., 2015). With the development of new fields, investigating the structure-function relationships of such materials can potentially not only deliver safer vaccines but also contribute to overall strategies against infectious disease combat and enhanced immune surveillance.

Test Your Knowledge

1. How does the lymphatic system contribute to fluid balance and the drainage of excess tissue fluid?
2. What role does the lymphatic system play in the absorption of dietary fats?

7.3. The Immune System Overview

Learning Outcome

1. Define components of the immune system
2. Explain the types of immunity: innate and adaptive
3. Understand the role of white blood cells in immunity

The immune system is the body's first defense against germs and other foreign invaders, with an absolutely critical role in maintaining overall wellness and homeostasis. It is an advanced system consisting of various components, including white blood cells, lymph nodes, and antibodies, that work together to identify and destroy harmful agents. Notably, the immune response is commonly classified into innate and adaptive immunity. While innate immunity provides a rapid but nonspecific defense through barriers and phagocytic cells, adaptive immunity offers a more specific defense that improves with repeated exposure to the same pathogen. Understanding these distinct yet integral systems is key to knowing the immune system's function, especially in terms of developing new ways of disease treatments for diseases such as cancer and autoimmune diseases, as seen about biotherapy in today's studies (Gallucci et al., 1995). The lymphatic system, which is involved in immunity, permits the transportation of lymph, a fluid full of immune cells, throughout the entire body. Lymph nodes are sentinel stations where lymphocytes, particularly T cells and B cells, can meet pathogens and initiate immune reactions. To this end, the lymphatic system plays a central role in infection monitoring and immune regulation. In addition, it transports lipid absorbed from the diet in the intestine via specialized lymphatic vessels, the lacteals. However, the dialogue between the immune response and the lymphatic system is not merely for defense mechanisms. In the pre-Fall world, the immune response might have been operating with a second intention of promoting body growth and microbial balance upkeep, suggesting that the function would have been multifaceted beyond simply defense (Conrad et al., 2014).

A close examination of the immune system illustrates its potential for complexity and specialization, which is necessary to grasp immune health. The system utilizes an array of immune cells, such as macrophages, neutrophils, and natural killer cells, to identify and destroy pathogens efficiently. Further, the higher-order mechanisms of memory response facilitate quicker and more efficient responses to antigens seen before, and this shows the beauty of evolutionary design in immunology. However, mistakes in this system can prove fatal, leading to autoimmune diseases or cancer when the body's own immune reactions become directed against itself or are unable to recognize cancer cells. With pioneering work being done in immunotherapy as well as biotherapy, understanding of the fundamental functioning of the immune system's interaction with the lymphatic system, as well as various pathogens, is needed for the sake of breaking new ground for therapy (Gallucci et al., 1995).

7.3.1. Definition and Components of the Immune System

The immune system is the body's defense system, orchestrating a concerted response to infections by microorganisms like bacteria, viruses, and parasites. It is usually classified into two types: the innate immune system and the adaptive immune system. The innate immune system provides the first line of defense and includes physical barriers like skin and mucous membranes, and cellular components like macrophages and neutrophils. These cells respond quickly and non-specifically to threat. The adaptive immune system, by contrast, is characterized by specificity in antigen recognition and by memory development, allowing for a more effective and specific response following repeated exposure. The dual organization of these systems underscores the importance of both immediate and persistent immune responses in securing health and battling infection. Understanding these parts is crucial to creating effective immunotherapies and vaccines. The lymphatic system is the core of the operation of the immune system, facilitating the transport and maturation of immune cells. The lymph nodes, dispersed throughout the body, are critical organs where lymphocytes, i.e., T-cells and B-cells, become activated and proliferate upon antigen exposure. This facilitates the adaptive immune response since it enables the body to specifically react to the pathogens effectively. Furthermore, the lymphatic system contributes to the elimination of toxins and pathogens from the extracellular space, thus highlighting its contribution to homeostasis. A functional lymphatic system not only enhances immune surveillance but also allows for the interaction between various immune components, such that immune coordination against infection is achieved. The coordination between the lymphatic system and immune response imposes an imperative for ongoing progress in immunology and lymphatics (Figure 7.8).

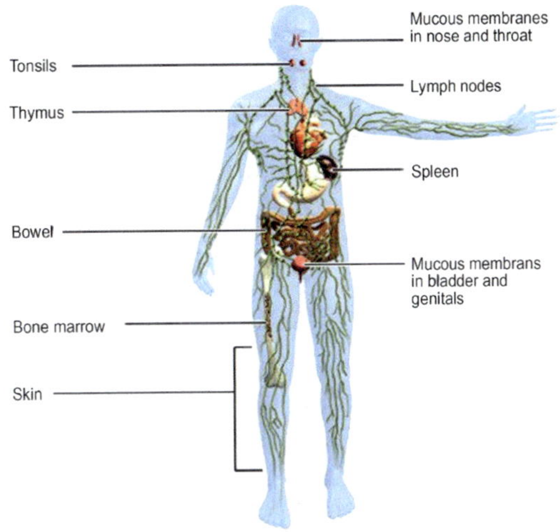

Figure 7.8. Parts of the immune system.

Source: https://www.healio.com/hematology-oncology/learn-immuno-oncology/the-immune-system/components-of-the-immune-system.

Other external parameters and microbial interaction dynamics in human body also condition efficiency of the immune system. The gut microbiota, for example, plays a pivotal role in immune shaping, with its structure affecting the innate and adaptive immune functions. Evidence indicates that the manipulation of such microbial communities can have long-term impacts on immunity and suggests approaches such as microbial resource management (MRM) towards improved health.

Additionally, advances in vaccine technologies for particular pathogens, particularly helminths, depict the importance of information regarding immune mechanisms. Ongoing patent landscape analysis reports growing interest in the development of vaccines to enhance protective immunity against such parasites and projects the potential future of immunological science and treatment possibilities essential for the combat of global health challenges, as outlined by the latest research (Alma et al., 2011; Burke et al., 2013).

7.3.2. Types of Immunity: Innate and Adaptive

There are two broad types of immunity in the immune system: innate and adaptive. Innate immunity is the initial defense of the body against infection, providing immediate yet nonspecific protection. It is composed of physical barriers, such as the skin and mucous membranes, and cellular components, like phagocytes and natural killer cells, that can respond quickly to invaders. It is the system that can recognize general features of pathogens to trigger rapid immune reactions without exposure. The innate immune response is highly conserved between species and plays a crucial role in activating the adaptive immune response, which is specialized but slow to react. In this manner of interaction, the innate immune system creates an environment supportive of the specific and directed action of adaptive immunity, even as it emphasizes the critical coordination between the two branches of the immune system (Figure 7.9).

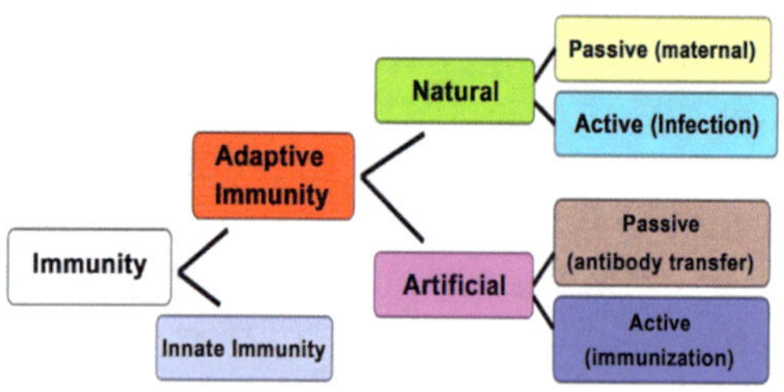

Figure 7.9. Types of immunity.

Source: https://external-content.duckduckgo.com/iu/?u=https%3A%2F%2Fwww.onlinebiologynotes.com%2Fwp-content%2Fuploads%2F2018%2F02%2FImmunity-and-its-types.gif&f=1&nofb=1&ipt=333bd79d2d2f1c4174656bcc28cb0022d84fe909df403874747b52f1966ce183.

Adaptive immunity is specific and has memory, which is achieved by exposure to unique pathogens. Adaptive immunity is primarily mediated by lymphocytes like T cells and B cells, which get activated and differentiated upon exposure to their respective antigens. T cells are responsible for cell-mediated immunity, infecting and killing infected host cells or stimulating other immune cells. In contrast, B cells are responsible for humoral immunity through the production of antibodies that neutralize the pathogens in the blood system. Not only does the adaptive immune response provide specific protection against pathogens, but it also forms long-term immunological memory, enabling rapid and more intense responses to subsequent challenge with the same antigen. This process highlights the advantage of adaptive immunity from an evolutionary perspective, as it enhances immunity to subsequent infection. The interchange between innate and adaptive immunity is a dynamic, highly complex process essential for health protection. The innate response, in several ways, has the potential to modulate the activation and efficiency of the adaptive response. For example, occupational antigen-presenting cells, including dendritic cells, bridge the two systems by capturing and processing antigens and presenting them to T cells to initiate the adaptive response. Second, signaling pathways for leukocyte migration, including those that involve G-protein-coupled receptors, have essential roles in directing immune cells toward sites of infection or inflammation (Boneschansker et al., 2019). The examination of these interactions is essential in immunology research, particularly regarding the development of therapeutics that harness these responses effectively, like biotherapies that modulate immune function and also cure disease (Gallucci et al., 1995). The data on the cooperation between innate and adaptive immunity reveal the redundancy and delicate balance of the human immune system.

7.3.3. The Role of White Blood Cells in Immunity

The intricate interaction between white blood cells, or leukocytes, and the immune system reflects the biological nature of immunity in the lymphatic system. White blood cells are essential in defending the body against pathogens, finding, and responding to foreign invaders such as bacteria, viruses, and parasites. White blood cells are classified into several different types, such as lymphocytes, neutrophils, monocytes, and macrophages, each differing in their functions during immune responses. Lymphocytes, of which T cells and B cells are a part, are essential for adaptive immunity, as they can create a specific response to a particular pathogen. Activation of these immune cells is a complex process that includes signaling pathways crucial to the initiation of appropriate types of physiological response to combat breaches in the body's integrity, as attested by breakthroughs in biotherapy to utilize such immune responses against cancer and autoimmune diseases (Gallucci et al., 1995) (Figure 7.10).

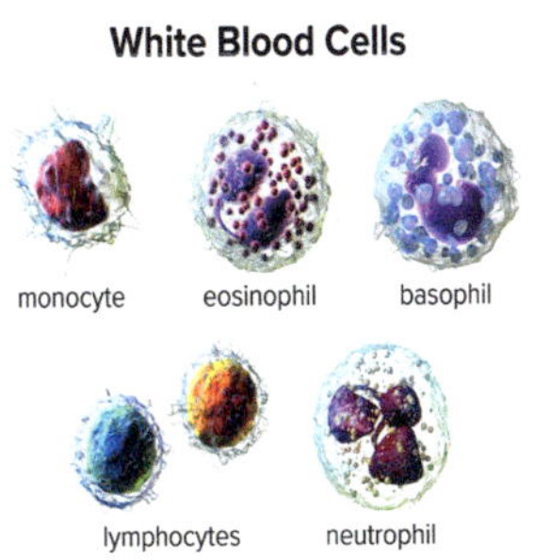

Figure 7.10. Types of white blood cells.

Source: https://www.medicalnewstoday.com/articles/327446#types-and-function.

Communication among white blood cells is of most tremendous significance in ensuring correct immune function. Several mechanisms of signaling, entailing the action of cytokines and chemokines, trigger the activation and recruitment of leukocytes at the site of inflammation or infection. For instance, chemokines direct specialized subsets of leukocytes to tissues that are inflamed and thus enable a rapid and coordinated immune response. Recent research highlights the role of G-protein-coupled receptors (GPCRs) in controlling the dynamics of leukocyte migration, which is essential for tissue navigation in immune responses. Directed migration, regulated by several signaling pathways, not only fine-tunes the immune response but also enables the leukocytes to arrive at their targeted location efficiently. Explanation of these signaling networks is significant in the planning of therapeutic strategies that can enhance or modulate immune responses, and thereby improve the effect of treatment of many diseases (Boneschansker et al., 2019). Beyond their direct role in capturing and killing pathogens, white blood cells play a role in overall immune surveillance and homeostasis in the body. Macrophages, for instance, phagocytose not only pathogens but also aid in the clearance of debris and initiate repair of the tissue following infection. White blood cell surveillance at all times maintains an expectant immune state, warding off infections before establishing a foothold. Furthermore, leukocyte interactions with other immune and non-immune cells of the lymphoid system form the foundation for systemic immunity coordination. With our expanding knowledge about leukocyte behavior, especially their signaling and navigation in tissues, it promises the construction of new therapies that take advantage of these inherent processes to enhance immunity to infectious disease and maximize responses to cancer therapy (Gallucci et al., 1995).

Test Your Knowledge

1. What are the main components of the immune system, and how do they work together to protect the body?
2. What is the difference between innate immunity and adaptive immunity?

7.4. The Role of Lymphocytes

Learning Outcome

1. Discuss the types of lymphocytes: B cells and T cells
2. Define mechanisms of action in the immune response
3. Explain the memory cells and long-term immunity

Lymphocytes are a category of white blood cells that are critical to the body's immune response. Lymphocytes are generally categorized into three groups: B cells, T cells, and natural killer (NK) cells. B cells produce antibodies, proteins that attach to and destroy pathogens, which then cannot cause disease. T cells, on the other hand, are responsible for directly killing infected cells and organizing other immune processes. This intricate interaction between forms of lymphocytes enables the immune system to be efficiently responsive to a vast array of pathogens. Recent findings show that the organization and mass of lymphoid tissues exhibit seasonal oscillations, reflecting the physiological responses of the body to environmental stress, and emphasize the predominance of lymphocytes for imparting intense immune protection throughout the year (Demas et al., 1995). The development and differentiation of lymphocytes within the lymphoid system are closely linked to their function. To be able to carry out their particular tasks, lymphocytes must go through specialized maturation processes, beginning with pluripotent hematopoietic stem cells in the bone marrow. For instance, while B cells mature in the bone marrow, T cells migrate to the thymus. This differentiation is necessary because it enables the lymphocytes to be equipped with the specific receptors for the recognition of specific antigens. Aside from that, their ability to generate memory cells allows the immune system to react faster and more efficiently during subsequent exposures to previously seen pathogens. This means that lymphocytes not only contribute to active defense in the present, but are also a form of immunological memory, something that underlies current vaccine strategies and advances in immunotherapy (Gallucci et al., 1995). Moreover, lymphocytes are deeply affected by a large number of physiological and environmental factors, whose effects may enhance or impede their role. Photoperiod changes, especially seasonal ones, regulate lymphocyte function, illustrating the close relationship between immune response and environment. During times of lower photoperiod, such as in winter, research indicates immune performance is compromised, leaving organisms more vulnerable to infection (Demas et al., 1995). Furthermore, biotherapies involving lymphocyte modulation are promising to unlock new avenues in treating cancer and autoimmune disease. Through the utilization of lymphocyte functions, researchers hope to create a therapy that not only strengthens immune function but also manipulates cellular mechanisms at a molecular level, adding further emphasis on the central role of lymphocytes in sustaining health and resisting disease (Gallucci et al., 1995).

7.4.1. Types of Lymphocytes: B Cells and T Cells

It is necessary to understand the forms of lymphocytes to value the immune response delivered by the lymphatic system. Leading the immune response are B cells and T cells, two types of lymphocytes that originate from bone marrow hematopoietic stem cells. B cells are primarily concerned with the production of antibodies, proteins that identify and bind specifically to antigens such as bacteria and viruses. When they encounter their corresponding antigens, B cells proliferate and develop into plasma cells that secrete such antibodies to identify foreign invaders for destruction. This process is central to humoral immunity, highlighting B cells' function to provide long-lasting protection in the form of memory cells capable of responding quickly to infections in the future. Their function in the adaptive immune response showcases how B cells coordinate defense, with significant implications for vaccine design and therapeutic strategies in immunology. T cells, however, have diverse functions in cellular immunity, differentiating into various subtypes, including helper T cells (CD4+ T cells) and cytotoxic T cells (CD8+ T cells). Helper T cells strengthen the immune response by producing cytokines that stimulate B cells and other immune cells, creating a significantly coordinated attack on pathogen invaders. CD8+ T cells, on the other hand, kill infected or malignant cells directly and play an essential role in clearing threats that have escaped the humoral immune response. In their separate functions, T cells are not only central to infection control but also implicated in tumor immunosurveillance. The dynamic interaction between T and B cells illustrates the complex nature and effectiveness of adaptive immune function, and how these lymphocytes cooperate to bring about homeostasis as well as adaptive immunity against constantly and dynamically shifting pathogens (Figure 7.11).

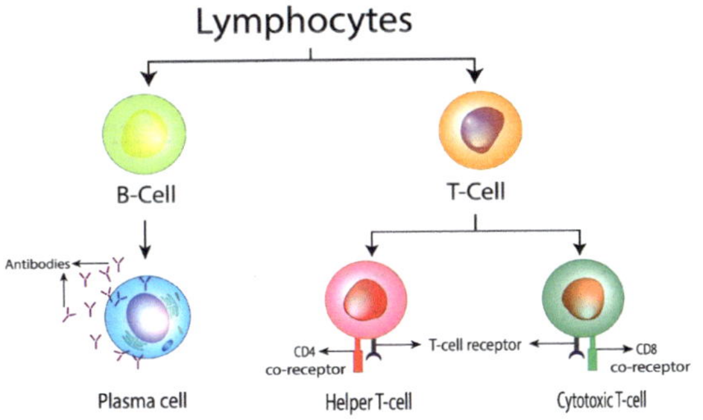

Figure 7.11. Types of lymphocytes.

Source: https://www.narayanahealth.org/blog/lymphocytes-function-definition-levels-ranges.

Recent progress in immunology has illustrated the sophisticated behaviors of T cells and B cells in the context of the lymphatic system. Recent advances in imaging technologies, as seen in experiments with non-invasive in vivo imaging techniques, have made it possible for scientists to track the activity of lymphocytes within lymph nodes and achieve a better understanding of their dynamics during immune response. This technique, which permits longitudinal observation without resorting to invasive methods, has unlocked how cells migrate, proliferate, and carry out their function in real time. This understanding at the cellular level not only enhances the scientific community's awareness of immune system function but also holds important implications for the design of targeted immunotherapies. Such advances represent a turning point in the manipulation of lymphocyte responses to therapeutic advantage, particularly in the fields of autoimmune disease and cancer treatment, highlighting the importance of examining lymphocyte subsets in relation to the general immune system (de Paulis et al., 2019; Andrea et al., 2012).

7.4.2. Mechanisms of Action in Immune Response

The immune response is a complex interplay of signaling molecules and cells that work together to recognize and eliminate pathogens. This intricate system is rooted mainly in the lymphatic system, which provides the pathway for the immune cells to travel to sites of infection. Lymphocytes—B cells and T cells—are key to this process, their individual but complementary functions working to activate the response. B cells secrete antibodies that neutralize the foreign antigens, whereas T cells directly kill infected cells or assist other immune cells to carry out their functions. Activation and proliferation of these lymphocytes are carefully regulated by several cytokines and chemokines, molecules that orchestrate the immune response. Hence, the mechanisms of action in this system are not merely reactive but are actually reflective of an evolved ability to enhance survival through state-dependent modulation of immune function (Demas et al., 1995). Further study of immune mechanisms illustrates the effect of environmental and physiological states on the efficiency of the immune system. Literature indicates that season changes have the potential to significantly influence immune function, with specific conditions, such as decreased daylight, having been linked to impaired immune response efficacy. This is mediated by melatonin, which is involved in circadian rhythm and regulation of immune function. For example, while laboratory experiments typically show improved immune function on shorter days. Field experiments are more complicated, and it appears that immune response can be compromised in the field as winter approaches. Acknowledging such seasonal fluctuations not only accounts for the adaptive nature of immune responses but also emphasizes the necessity of organisms to be capable of forecasting and preparing repeated immune challenges throughout their life cycles (Demas et al., 1995) (Figure 7.12).

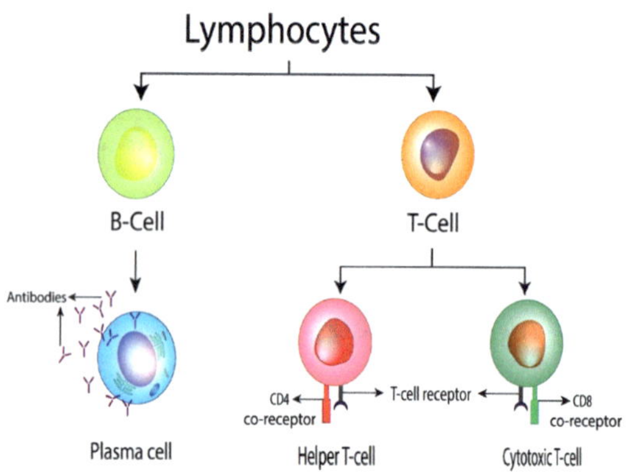

Figure 7.12. Immune response.

Source: http://www.immuneresponse.org/wp-content/uploads/2016/08/bigstock-127354466.jpg.

In addition, improvements in biotherapy have assisted in uncovering mechanisms by which therapy drugs can affect immune reactions to combat disease, e.g., cancer and autoimmune disease. Modern biotherapeutics, made by gene engineering, are agents that trigger the immune system or change gene expression, enhancing the body's inherent capacity to combat disease. This evolution from nonspecific immunostimulants to particular biological modifiers is a significant advance in the field of understanding immune phenomena. By identifying the molecular mechanisms concerned with oncogenesis and immunity, researchers open new avenues to therapy and disease control. This book further validates the central interaction between the lymphatic system and the immune system. It highlights the relevance of comprehending both cellular processes in question, as well as greater implications for health and disease.

7.4.3. Memory Cells and Long-Term Immunity

Memory cells play an essential role in long-term immunity and serve as the foundation of immunological memory established on first exposure to pathogens. Upon initial contact with an antigen, the naive B and T cell is activated by the immune system and mature into effector cells responsible for organizing a response to an immune stimulus. Upon removal of the pathogen, activated cells persist as memory cells. In comparison to effector cells, memory cells have a long life span. They are strategically positioned in the lymphatic system such that on repeated exposure to the same antigen, they can generate a rapid and effective response. This state places greater emphasis on the function of memory cells in vaccination procedures, as this enables the body to react faster and better to the infectious disease, thereby reducing morbidity. The mechanisms by which memory cells confer long-term immunity are complex and multifactorial. Memory T cells have been generally divided into central memory T cells and effector memory T cells with distinct immune recall functions. Central memory T cells reside in lymphoid tissues and expand on re-exposure to an antigen, while effector memory

T cells reside in the periphery and provide for immediate defense. Similarly, memory B cells contribute to long-term immunity by rapid differentiation into plasma cells capable of producing antibodies upon re-exposure to the antigen. Affinity maturation, being a component of the germinal center response, increases the effectiveness of memory B cells, leading to a more specific antibody response. This dynamic interplay among heterogeneous immune cells, like the involvement of antigen-presenting cells discussed in recent research on tertiary lymphoid organs, indicates the complexity of immunological memory, an area of significant interest in immunology (Bedaj et al., 2016) (Figure 7.13).

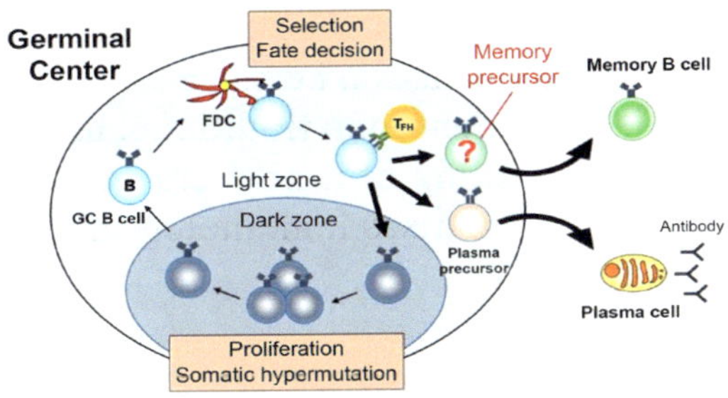

Figure 7.13. The making of memory B cells and long-term immune responses.

Source: https://resou.osaka-u.ac.jp/en/research/2020/20201012_1.

The therapeutic applications of memory cells, particularly in modern biotherapy, have bright prospects for enhancing immune responses against conditions such as cancer and autoimmune disease. The developments in genetic engineering enable the production of targeted therapy aimed at unleashing the innate power of the immune system, specifically through utilizing memory cells and their rapid response function. Current research is exploring biological agents that not only stimulate the immune system but also modify gene expression to enhance immune memory. Understanding the intricacies of memory cell dynamics is essential to designing proper interventions able to leverage these processes, ultimately translating to better patient outcomes in immunological therapy. With expanding overlap between oncology and immunology, further investigation of the interaction between immune cells, oncogenes, and the controlling mechanisms of long-term immunity will be crucial in optimizing therapy models in immunotherapy (Gallucci et al., 1995).

Test Your Knowledge

1. What are the primary differences between B cells and T cells in terms of their roles in the immune response?
2. How do B cells and T cells function to identify and eliminate pathogens during an immune response?

7.5. Pathogens and the Immune Response

Learning Outcome

1. Explain the types of pathogens: bacteria, viruses, fungi, and parasites
2. Define how the lymphatic system identifies pathogens
3. Describe the process of inflammation and its significance

The communication between the immune response and the pathogens is a fundamental mode of operation of the lymphatic system's efficiency and performance. While the pathogens invade the host, they might utilize the lymphatic system to travel across the body. The network of lymph acts as a route for interstitial fluid and antigens to be transported to lymph nodes, which are primary sites in which an immune response is initiated. Lymph nodes are more than mere passive points of filtering but are instead active participants in immune surveillance. This is illustrated by the location of various lymphoid cells, including natural killer cells and γδ T cells, near sentinel macrophages in the lymphatic sinuses. This positioning facilitates rapid communication and response to pathogens, emphasizing the significance of spatial structure in the lymphatic system for combat against infection (Germain et al., 2012). The intricate cellular interaction occurring in lymph nodes is paramount to ensuring the immune response against pathogens functions properly. Upon detection of an infection, a heterogeneous population of lymphocytes mobilizes in response to stimulants such as IL-18 released by the phagocytic macrophages, identifying pathogens. The process is crucial for resistance to antimicrobial development, as quick release of cytokines such as IFNγ from these natural lymphocytes enhances the activation of macrophages and their killing activity against pathogens. However, when such communication is interrupted, it may evolve into systemic spread of pathogens, impairing the immune response. Such a finding highlights the importance of local intercellular communication in lymph nodes and further illustrates their role as dynamic immune centers for defensive action against infectious agents (Germain et al., 2012). Immunotherapy innovations illustrate how immune system research and pathogen interaction can lead to therapeutic advances. Modern biotherapy involves the application of biological agents that modulate immunity, promising therapeutic management of multiple diseases, including cancer and autoimmune diseases. The therapies themselves are generally a product of engineered biological products that enhance or regulate immune function. Detailed knowledge of mechanisms of immune response, including knowledge of pathology of disease, is essential to develop effective therapy. Such biotherapeutic means can be more effective and targeted in treatment than traditional methods, marking the opening of a new era in medical science that harmonizes immunological insight with utility.

7.5.1. Types of Pathogens: Bacteria, Viruses, Fungi, and Parasites

In pathology, there is a significant differentiation between bacteria, viruses, fungi, and parasites, all requiring the lymphatic system to mount different immune reactions. Bacteria are single-cell organisms with the ability to replicate independently, often eliciting a vigorous immune response accompanied by inflammation. For instance, bacteria such as Streptococcus or *Escherichia coli* are capable of inducing acute immune responses by stimulating lymphocytes and the release of cytokines that provide a maximally effective response. Another immunological strategy is caused by viruses that infect host cells in order to replicate. The role of lymphatic systems is primarily to contribute to the formation of antibodies and activate T-cells when responding to viral infections, demonstrating the requirement for adaptive immune mechanisms (Besedovsky et al., 2019) (Figure 7.14).

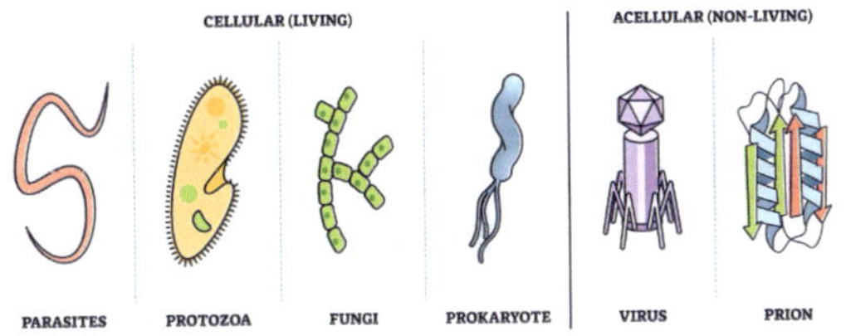

Figure 7.14. Types of pathogens.

Source: https://as1.ftcdn.net/jpg/04/56/01/02/1000_F_456010270_HmpUAnaEs2UOcuHbfFlZTp4xxlLM96f0.jpg.

The nature of the pathogenic invasion determines the body's defense mechanisms, which are indicative of the complexity of host-pathogen interactions. Fungi are yet another category of pathogens that vary from innocuous organisms to pathogenic organisms, primarily exploiting immunocompromised hosts. They possess specialized structural elements, like chitin, which are recognized by the immune system as foreign and cause the activation of numerous immune cells. Specifically, macrophages and dendritic cells play primary roles in fungal infection detection and resistance, and then antigen presentation to T-cells. The lymphatic system plays a crucial role in coordinating immune responses to fungi by ensuring immunocompetence of antigen-presenting cells (APCs) and their interaction with immune cells. As the spleen cleanses blood and contributes towards the adaptive immune response, its role becomes of paramount significance in controlling systemic mycotic infections (Steven et al., 2019). Hence, the understanding of the complex nature of fungal pathogens needs to be developed in order to elicit effective immunological responses. Parasites, including protozoa and helminths, provide immunity with unique challenges and represent a significant research area within the field of immunology. The lymphatic system is a central battlefield, with immune outcomes decided by parasites' ability to avoid being detected and often manipulate host immunity pathways. As illustrations, certain parasites can trigger regulatory T-cells that suppress effective immunity, showing a sophisticated degree of evasion. The parasitic infection typically invokes an immune response, both cell-mediated and humoral (antibody-mediated) in nature, which requires concerted effort by more than one lymphoid organ. Parasitic infections can also lead to chronic disease, resulting in sustained inflammation, which affects the health and immunity of the hosts (Besedovsky et al., 2019). The understanding of the mixed strategies employed by various pathogens allows more exhaustive research into the lymphatic system's contribution to immunity.

7.5.2. How the Lymphatic System Identifies Pathogens

The lymphatic system plays a critical role in pathogen detection and immune response activation within the body. The lymph vessel network and lymph nodes provide a route for lymph fluid, which transports immune cells such as lymphocytes and macrophages throughout the body. When invading pathogens approach, they are likely intercepted by resident immune cells such as macrophages within tissues. These cells recognize pathogen-associated molecular patterns (PAMPs) and respond by phagocytosis of the pathogens, a process critical for pathogen recognition. In addition, upon recognition, the macrophages and dendritic cells migrate to lymph nodes and present antigens to T cells, which subsequently trigger adaptive immune responses. This pathway emphasizes the lymphatic system's unifying role in not only detecting pathogens but also organizing a sophisticated response integrating both innate and adaptive immunity. Within the lymphatic system, heterogeneous populations of immune cells have specific contributions to the detection and processing of pathogens (Figure 7.15).

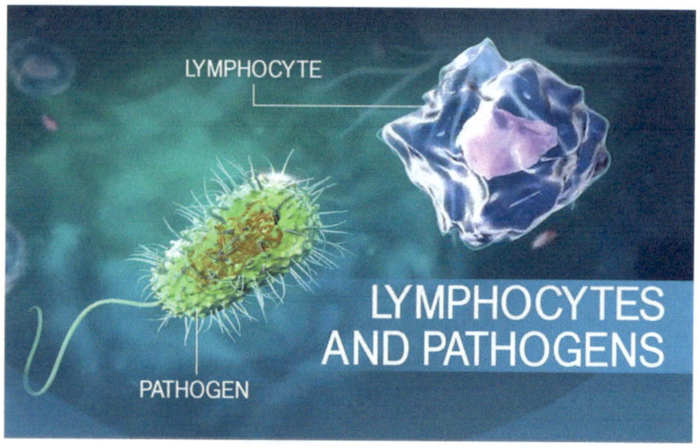

Figure 7.15. Illustration of a lymphocyte interacting with a pathogen as part of the immune response.

Source: https://www.visiblebody.com/hubfs/Learn_Articles/Lymphatic_System/1B-Lymphocyte-and-Pathogen.jpg.

For instance, dendritic cells (DCs) are significant antigen-presenting cells that degrade subtle details of the pathogens to which they are exposed. Present in various compartments of the lymphatic system, such cells internalize antigens and present them to draining lymph nodes, where they stimulate naïve T cells. Some recent observations have indicated that migrating intestinal DC subsets in the lymphatic system possess different functional properties, suggesting specialization for these immune cells. This specialization enables a more nuanced immune response because individual subsets of DCs can promote unique paths toward tolerance or full immune activation. This functional plasticity is valuable, particularly in heavily pathogen-exposed locations, where the capacity to quickly and efficiently detect pathogens is critical to allow homeostasis to be preserved and infection not to be initiated (Allan et al., 2010). These interactions are complemented by the existence of various pattern recognition receptors (PRRs) on immune cells that facilitate recognition of pathogens at the molecular level. These receptors facilitate lymphatic tissues—particularly lymph nodes and mucosal sites like the intestines—to very quickly respond to pathogens through the use of innate immune responses. For example, resident immune cells in the middle ear, like monocytes and macrophages, exhibit rapid expression of innate immune genes in response to pathogens, establishing themselves as frontline defenders in immediate immunity. This swift response is a departure from the delayed adaptive immunity responses, which accentuates the lymphatic system's double function in pathogen recognition. These productive mechanisms establish the capability for the body to be able to effectively respond adequately to entering pathogens and set the stage for an extended adaptive response (Draf et al., 2020).

7.5.3. The Process of Inflammation and Its Significance

Inflammatory process is an important defense mechanism in the body that enables the immune system to respond to harmful stimuli such as pathogens, injured cells, or irritants. When tissues are injured or infected, a multicellular phenomenon known as the inflammatory response occurs, which entails the release of signaling molecules for augmented blood supply to the area where injury has taken place. This allows for the invasion of immune cells, particularly leukocytes, into the infected or damaged tissue, where they can function to kill invaders or assist with healing tissue. Such initial responses underscore the importance of inflammation as not only an adaptive mechanism but as part of an essential process in healing, setting the stage for a possible resolution of the existing immune challenge. Resolution of inflammation is as essential as its initiation, emphasizing that inflammation must be strictly regulated to prevent chronic conditions. Chronic inflammation may result from repeated stimuli or breakdown in resolution mechanisms and leads to different diseases, including autoimmune diseases. For example, in the absence of proper resolution pathways, psoriasis has become a developing disease, as seen in

D6-deficient mice models where exaggerated inflammatory responses mimic human disease. To understand the intricacies of such regulatory mechanisms, involving the activities of such critical mediators as chemokines and cytokines, is crucial to therapeutic approaches against avoiding or fighting inflammation-associated disease. The research into these processes also more accurately outlines how dysregulation can contribute to severe conditions such as rheumatoid arthritis and inflammatory bowel disease, further establishing the role of inflammation in pathology. The relationship between inflammation and the lymphatic system is an essential component of immune reactions. The lymphatic circulation plays a significant role in transmitting immune cells from and to the inflamed areas, thus maintaining tissue fluid balance and facilitating the easy removal of inflammatory debris. It has been observed that tertiary lymphoid organ-like structures have been emerging in chronic inflammation, which provide niches for the activation of B and T cells in the central nervous system, like in multiple sclerosis (MS). These aggregates not only highlight the lymphatic system's involvement in sustaining inflammatory reactions but also pose essential questions as to what their implications are for disease evolution. By exploring interactions between the lymphatic system and inflammation pathways, researchers can gain insight into therapeutic targets in modulating immune function effectively and treating long-term inflammatory illnesses (Baldwin et al., 2013; Mitsdoerffer et al., 2016).

Test Your Knowledge

1. What are the main types of pathogens that can cause disease in the human body, and how do they differ from one another?
2. How does the lymphatic system detect and respond to the presence of harmful pathogens?

7.6. Disorders of the Lymphatic System

Learning Outcome

1. Explain the causes and effects of lymphedema.
2. Describe lymphoma and other cancers that impact the lymphatic system
3. Identify autoimmune diseases affecting the lymphatic system

The lymphatic system plays a vital role in immune homeostasis and fluid balance, but is susceptible to various disorders that can disrupt its functions. Of these, lymphedema deserves mention since it represents the abnormal accumulation of lymph fluid caused by poor lymphatic drainage. Lymphedema is a common occurrence after surgery and radiation therapy, particularly in cancer treatment, in which lymph nodes are removed or destroyed. The subsequent swelling poses not only a risk to the physical appearance of affected limbs but also elevates the risk of infection and chronic inflammation. Further, psychological harm has to be observed in that most patients face challenges in adjusting to both the physical and social effects of the condition, illustrating the multifaceted impacts of lymphatic diseases that go beyond mere physiological effects. Another critical disorder of the lymphatic system is lymphangitis, an outcome of lymphatic vessel inflammation, typically caused by bacterial infection. The presentation generally involves redness, swelling, and pain along the involved route, typically with fever and chills, which means systemic illness. This is an acute process that occurs due to the immune reaction of the body to combat the infection and is responsible for the symptoms of lymphangitis. If left unchecked, the infection may exacerbate and require more serious medical treatment. Furthermore, awareness of the underlying etiology and pathophysiology of lymphangitis is essential in order to manage it successfully since it is a sign of potential complications like cellulitis or sepsis. Thus, early diagnosis and treatment of lymphangitis is crucial to maintain the integrity of the lymphatic system and general health. Furthermore, tertiary lymphoid organ (TLO)-associated disorders represent a complex field of lymphatic disease that often develops as a response to chronic inflammation or infection. TLOs are ectopic secondary lymphoid tissues that are similar to lymph nodes and allow localized immunity through the organization of lymphocytes and antigen-presenting cells at the location of chronic insult. However, they can also be indicators of dysregulated immune responses to promote disorders such as autoimmune diseases or chronic infections. Recent research emphasizes the role of antigen presentation within such structures, providing insight into lymphatic and immune interaction. As researchers examine drivers of TLO development and function, this arena of investigation promises new treatment options, particularly regarding immunological disorders prevalent in more prosperous societies. The possible therapeutic applications of information about TLOs can bridge the divide between lymphatic disease and overall immunity problems in contemporary medicine (Araujo et al., 2016; Bedaj et al., 2016).

7.6.1. Lymphedema and Its Causes

Lymphedema, or tissue swelling resulting from compromised lymphatic drainage, is the result of a variety of underlying causes. Lymphatic circulation is responsible for fluid homeostasis, immunity, and the absorption of ingested lipids. The system may become dysfunctional due to primary lymphedema, in which lymph vessel development and/or function is abnormal as a result of mutations in genes. Secondary lymphedema is most often due to external factors such as trauma, surgery, or cancer treatment, and obesity and malignancy. For instance, lymph node removal surgery or radiation therapy can damage lymphatic vessels, resulting in interstitial fluid accumulation and, subsequently, lymphedema. Understanding the etiology of lymphedema is crucial to the successful prevention and treatment of the condition, especially in patients with a history of lymphatic disturbance or pathologies of this nature (Detmar et al., 2018) (Figure 7.16).

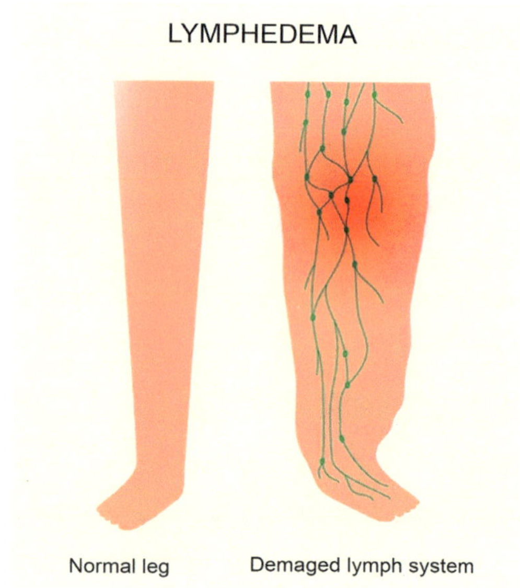

Figure 7.16. Normal leg versus leg with lymphedema caused by a damaged lymphatic system.

Source: https://external-content.duckduckgo.com/iu/?u=https%3A%2F%2Fimages.onlymyhealth.com%2Fimported%2Fimages%2F2023%2FAugust%2F17_Aug_2023%2FLymphedema.jpg&f=1&nofb=1&ipt=adad3dc4eaf40896b452d72d74eefda1a081789aefb8f14181b1cf6546242092.

The progressive nature of lymphedema can significantly decrease the quality of life in patients. The ongoing swelling leads to pain, restricted mobility, and increased susceptibility to infections, particularly cellulitis. As the condition advances, it not only causes physical impairment but also disturbs psychological well-being due to changes in appearance and function. Conservative management is primarily focused on symptom alleviation and places a special emphasis on compression therapy and physiotherapy. However, advances in surgery interventions, such as lymph node transfer and lymphaticovenous anastomosis, are promising interventions. These interventions aim to revive the lymph function and promote drainage of the fluids, bringing significant relief in symptom control and patient satisfaction (Rannikko et al., 2024). The progression of such treatments underscores the need for more research and advancements in the treatment of lymphedema. Additionally, the recent discovery of the lymphatic system's function in inflammation and immunity has opened the door for targeted therapies. Developments in the discovery of lymphatic endothelial cell-specific markers and growth factors have uncovered new avenues for new treatments that will increase lymphatic function and reduce lymphedema's impairing impact. Investigation of lymphatic growth factor use, including VEGF-C, has shown potential for initiating lymphatic regeneration and function, but with definitive results still to be investigated (Detmar et al., 2018). Such evolving information positions the health of the lymphatic system at the forefront of total lymphedema care, with specific significance acknowledged both therapeutically and in value for understanding lymphatic system-connectedness with immunity. The complex interaction between inflammatory mechanisms and lymphatic incompetence entails that treatment of lymphedema could potentially exert a positive effect on a patient's immune status, highlighting the importance of integrated management approaches for this multi-factorial disease (Figure 7.17).

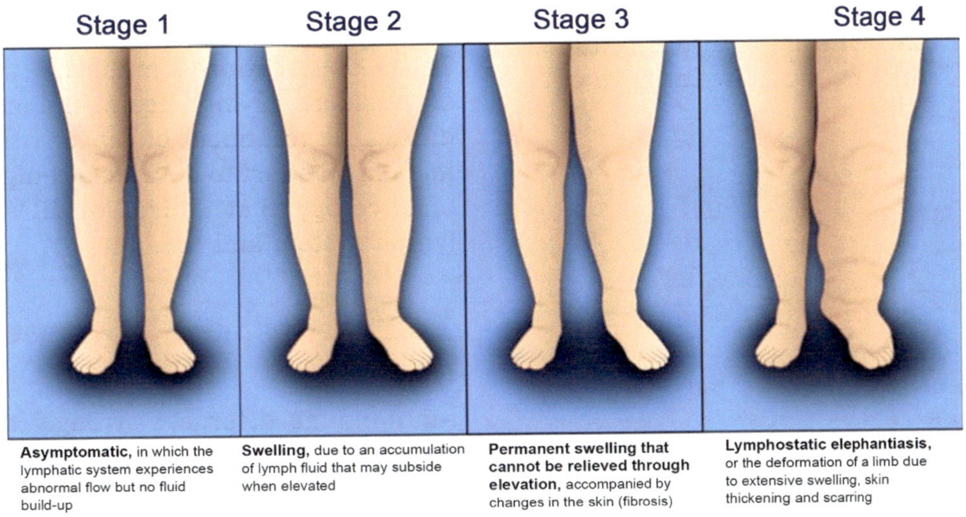

Figure 7.17. Stage of lymphedema.

Source: https://external-content.duckduckgo.com/iu/?u=https%3A%2F%2Fsurgery.wustl.edu%2Fwp-content%2Fuploads%2F2021%2F09%2F7_-four-Stages-of-Lymhpedema-768x594.jpg&f=1&nofb=1&ipt=c429dfae56ccc753e30e6f4d87ba1b3bd9a4d044efe96bcebbc57d2531591269.

7.6.2. Lymphoma and Other Cancers

The lymph system plays a crucial role in the body's immune response and is seriously involved in all forms of cancer, particularly lymphomas. Lymphoma, a cancer of lymph system origin, can significantly impair immune function since it impinges upon lymphocyte growth and development. Such a situation is mainly divided into Hodgkin lymphoma and non-Hodgkin lymphoma, which are so diverse in pathology and treatment response. Tumorigenicity of higher risk has been described by scientists after the disruption of lymphatic homeostasis, with the system proving to be crucial for the movement of immune cells that can identify and kill cancerous cells. The relations between the lymphatic microenvironment, such as with cytokines and growth factors, further complicate the role of the lymphatic system in cancerogenesis. CDKs like CDK5 have also been implicated by recent findings to modulate lymphocyte function and carcinogenesis. CDK5's new mechanism of activation, which is independent of the typical cyclin binding, allows it to be engaged in various signaling pathways with implications in cancer formation and immune evasion (Casimiro et al., 2017) (Figure 7.18).

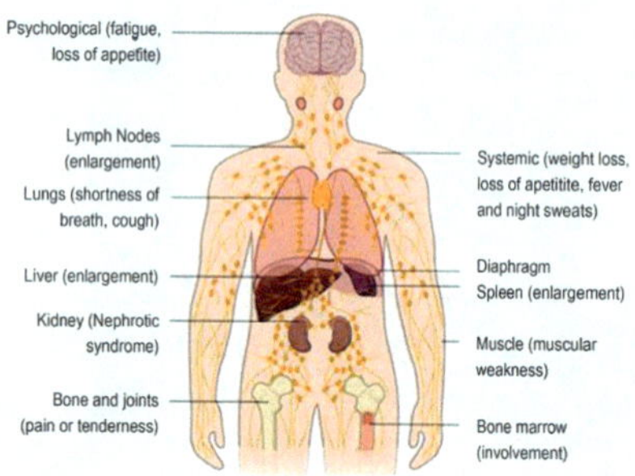

Figure 7.18. Symptoms of lymphoma.

Source: https://external-content.duckduckgo.com/iu/?u=https%3A%2F%2Ftse4.mm.bing.net%2Fth%2Fid%2FOIP.AwrtMSy309bjQ6GE9LalcAHaGU%3Fpid%3DApi&f=1&ipt=25346c52ac500105671547fb5e091d2cf8a4178890ae3286a199a183343f81e9.

Evidence indicates that abnormality in the activity of CDK can predispose one to develop lymphomas and perhaps other cancers. Control of CDK5 levels of activity by its binding to different proteins demonstrates the complexity of cellular signaling, particularly in malignancy. As a promising area of interest, understanding CDK's role in lymphatic as well as immune system dynamics could potentially provide insight into the therapeutic targets for treating lymphomas and other cancers. In addition, the association between viral infections, i.e., human immunodeficiency virus (HIV), and the onset of non-AIDS-defining cancers is an area that is critical to explore. Research proves that HIV patients are at greater risk of acquiring diseases such as glioblastoma multiforme, which is the cause of the impaired immune state that defines the disease process (Bui et al., 2016). The complex nature of cancer treatment in immunocompromised hosts indicates the importance of antiviral therapies like highly active antiretroviral therapy (HAART), which has been linked to improved survival rates among patients with HIV-associated malignancies. These observations emphasize the necessity of considering lymph health and immune status during the treatment of cancer risk and cancer itself in an effort to develop a complete practice of oncology that addresses all facets of the lymph system and immunity.

7.6.3. Autoimmune Diseases Affecting the Lymphatic System

Autoimmune disorders strongly influence the lymphatic system, leading to a large number of immune disorders. The lymphatic system can become dysfunctional in certain autoimmune disorders, such as systemic lupus erythematosus (SLE) and rheumatoid arthritis. This further promotes the inflammation process. Dysfunction is caused by the failure of the lymphatic vessels to properly transport immune cells and drain interstitial fluid, which is critical in keeping systemic homeostasis. Consequently, IHI and pro-inflammatory cytokines inflow into the target tissues, leading to an additive cycle of tissue damage and inflammation. Moreover, the disrupted lymphatic flow can interfere with immune surveillance, whereby the body is not able to effectively clear the pathogens and become susceptible to secondary infections and a variety of malignancies. It has been proven in studies that the lymphatic vasculature plays a critical role in inducing and developing autoimmune diseases. For instance, tertiary lymphoid organs (TLOs) that arise in the presence of chronic inflammation are implicated in autoimmune disease etiopathogenesis. TLOs are ectopic lymphoid tissues where immune cells can accumulate, proliferate, and engage with antigens and thereby perpetuate inflammatory processes. Understanding antigen presentation pathways within such organs underscores their role in disease aetiology. Explaining how antigen-presenting cells function in TLOs may provide pathways for targeted therapeutic interventions to manage the immune dysregulation of autoimmune diseases, emphasizing the lymphatic system's contribution to general immunity and inflammation regulation (Bedaj et al., 2016). The connection between autoimmune disease and the lymphatic system is further applied to the therapeutic potential that lymphatic functions may exert in controlling disease. New evidence accentuates the utilization of the immunoregulatory role of helminth parasites, suggesting their ability to dampen inflammation and evoke immune tolerance. Evidence from research indicates that helminths sustain the regulatory arm of the immune system, which may potentially balance the hyperreactivity associated with autoimmune reactions. This strategy is initiating an open dialogue about the use of helminth products as novel therapeutic agents for inflammatory and autoimmune disorders prevalent in resource-abundant communities. By elucidating the complex relationship between lymphatic function, immune regulation, and autoimmune pathology, not only is there the potential to manage such diseases more effectively, but to improve our comprehension of mechanisms of immune response at a systemic level (Araujo et al., 2016).

Test Your Knowledge

1. What is lymphoma, and how does it differ from other types of cancer affecting the lymphatic system?
2. How do autoimmune diseases impact the lymphatic system, and what are some examples of such conditions?

SUMMARY

The given discussion of the lymphatic system mapping and its closely engaged relation with immunity demonstrates that this network takes a pivotal position in sustaining the body's defensive mechanisms. The lymph system is not just a conduit for lymph and immune cells but also an extremely significant site for immune surveillance and reaction. Understanding of fluid dynamics and cellular interactions within the system provides insight into how lymphocytes, and specifically T and B cells, are activated and trafficked to the point of infection or inflammation. Additionally, progress in imaging methods, such as the novel method of transplanting lymph nodes for repeated noninvasive in vivo imaging, has dramatically expanded our understanding of lymphatic function and lymphocyte behavior over time (Andrea et al., 2012). This study signifies the dynamic nature of lymphatic architecture and circulation-regulated immune responses, showing complexity in systems. The significance of leukocyte dynamics within the lymphatic system cannot be overstated, as they are the ones to blame for both innate and adaptive immune responses. Spatiotemporal regulation of leukocyte migration will allow for the accurate immune interactions with pathogens, and hence, an elevated understanding of how these cells move through lymphatic tissues is needed. Leukocyte motility mechanisms, controlled by biochemical signals and physical lymph node structure, uncover the harmony of biological and biophysical mechanisms in initiating immune responses and immune response regulation. Homeostatic lymphocyte trafficking is significant in present research, which contributes to successful immune responses during infection and returns to pre-inflammatory states (Germain et al., 2014). Thus, the lymphatic system seems to play a central role not just in the delivery of immune cells but also in orchestrating their function. Finally, integration of the development of both basic and translational research can lead to more therapeutic strategies targeting the lymphatic system in disease, particularly where immune competence is compromised. Advances in lymphatic targeting or promotion of lymphatic drainage may hold tremendous advantages for immunotherapy in diseases such as cancer and chronic inflammatory conditions. As our knowledge becomes more profound, the promise to engineer lymphatic routes and leukocyte actions brings new possibilities for intervention and healing. Future studies must reaffirm the significance of evaluating lymphatic function along with immune response to optimize treatment effects properly. Thus, the lymphatic system occupies a focal point in immunological research, an essential interface of health, disease, and therapeutics.

The lymphatic system plays an essential role in the immune response of the body by providing a system in which immune cells can be transported and activated. The intricate system consists of lymphatic vessels, nodes, and organs such as the spleen and thymus that are essential to homeostasis as well as the war against disease-causing organisms. Lymph vessels provide a means for the circulation of lymph, a fluid containing immune cells, proteins, and waste, throughout the body. Lymph nodes are major sites of filtering for tissue damage or infection, where the lymph is filtered for pathogenic antigens. Stimulation of lymphocytes, particularly T and B cells, occurs primarily in these nodes, which points to the lymphatic system's role as an immunocyte cell division and differentiation center. This combined system ultimately allows immune responses to be rapid and effective, highlighting the lymphatic system's simple role in immunity. Further, the lymphatic system's linkage to mast cells adds complexity to its role in immune protection. Mast cells, situated in tissues in a strategic location, respond to tissue injury and inflammation by secreting mediators that regulate immune responses. Recent studies have indicated that cells can exhibit diverse subsets, i.e., MC1 and MC2, which are more than likely to exert anti-tumor or pro-tumorigenic activities, demonstrating their multifaceted roles in health and disease, as described in the newest studies in immunology (de Paulis et al., 2019). This versatility is characteristic of the versatile nature of mast cells and attests to the dynamic interaction in the lymphatic system. Through their coordination of local immune responses and systemic inflammation, mast cells significantly augment the overall function of the lymphatic system in protecting the body against infection and malignancy. Furthermore, advances in biotherapy have made possible new therapies that leverage the power of the immune system, particularly for cancer and autoimmune disorders. As biotherapy has evolved over the years, it has moved from using nonspecific immune stimulators to more specific treatments, with a greater emphasis on regulating the immune response to make it stronger in fighting disease, as evidenced by modern medical journals (Gallucci et al., 1995). By accessing the knowledge accrued through knowing the lymphatic system and its components, researchers are better placed to develop treatments that result in maximized immune responses. This integration of biotherapy with the clinic illustrates the increasing paradigm of immunity and the lymphatic system's interaction, opening up new avenues for therapy. Awareness of these interactions not only deepens our knowledge of immunological mechanisms but also directs future therapeutic strategies aimed at harnessing the immune system's potential to combat disease.

KEY TERMS FROM THIS CHAPTER

- Lymph
- Lymph Nodes
- Spleen
- Bone Marrow
- B Cells
- Natural Killer Cells
- Antibodies
- Innate Immunity
- Lymphatic Vessels
- Thymus
- Tonsils
- Lymphocytes
- T Cells
- Antigens
- Immune Response
- Adaptive Immunity

CRITICAL THINKING QUESTIONS

1. **What is the primary function of the lymphatic system?**
   a. Transport oxygen to tissues
   b. Return excess tissue fluid to the bloodstream
   c. Produce red blood cells
   d. Carry nutrients from the digestive system
2. **Which organ is a primary lymphoid organ where T cells mature?**
   a. Spleen
   b. Thymus
   c. Lymph nodes
   d. Bone marrow
3. **What are lymph nodes primarily responsible for?**
   a. Filtering lymph and trapping pathogens
   b. Producing blood cells
   c. Transporting oxygen
   d. Storing fat
4. **Which type of immunity is acquired after exposure to a pathogen?**
   a. Innate immunity
   b. Passive immunity
   c. Active immunity
   d. Mechanical immunity
5. **Which cells are responsible for producing antibodies in the immune response?**
   a. T cells
   b. B cells
   c. Macrophages
   d. Neutrophils

Short Answer Questions

1. What are the key anatomical structures of the lymphatic system?
2. Describe two main functions of the lymphatic system.
3. How is the lymphatic system connected to the immune system?
4. What types of lymphocytes are involved in the immune response?
5. Explain the role of B cells and T cells in fighting pathogens.
6. What are pathogens, and how does the immune system detect them?
7. List two common disorders that affect the lymphatic system.
8. How does lymphatic system dysfunction contribute to the development of lymphedema?

Answer to Critical Thinking Questions

1. (b); 2. (b); 3. (a); 4. (c); 5. (b)

REFERENCES

1. Allan, J., Anjuere, F., Anjuere, F., Bedoui, S., Belz, G., Bimczok, D., Blazquez, A. B., et al. (2010). Subsets of migrating intestinal dendritic cells. https://core.ac.uk/download/81091.pdf (accessed on 14th JuneCrotti, E., Balloi, A., Hamdi, C., Sansonno, L., Marzorati, M., Gonella, E., Favia, G., Cherif, A., Bandi, C., Alma, A., & Daffonchio, D. (2011). Microbial symbionts: a resource for the management of insect-related problems. *Microbial Biotechnology*, *5*(3), 307–317. https://doi.org/10.1111/j.1751-7915.2011.00312.xAnisimov, A., Aspelund, A., Dashkevich, A., Dashkevich, A., Dashkevich, A., Louveau, A., Ratajska, A., et al. (2019). Cardiac lymphatics in health and disease. https://core.ac.uk/download/287761839.pdf (accessed on 14th June 2025).
2. Araujo, M. I., Asher, L., Babu, S., Bager, P., Benzel, E. C., Bourke, C. D., Broadhurst, M. J., et al. (2016). Parasitic helminth infections and the control of human allergic and autoimmune disorders. https://core.ac.uk/download/42371598.pdf (accessed on 14th June 2025).
3. Baldwin, H. M., Carballido, J. M., Graham, G. J., Jamieson, T., et al. (2013). Microarray analyses demonstrate the involvement of type I interferons in psoriasiform pathology development in D6-deficient mice. https://core.ac.uk/download/18492467.pdf (accessed on 14th June 2025).
4. Barril, C., Cardona, P. J., Díaz, J., López, M., et al. (2014). To achieve an earlier IFN-γ response is not sufficient to control *Mycobacterium tuberculosis* infection in mice. https://core.ac.uk/download/41777878.pdf (accessed on 14th June 2025).
5. Bedaj, M., Benson, R. A., Hughes, C. E., Maffia, P., et al. (2016). Antigen-presenting cells and antigen presentation in tertiary lymphoid organs. https://core.ac.uk/download/74229920.pdf (accessed on 14th June 2025).
6. Berni Canani, R., O'Mahony, L., Peroni, D., Roth-Walter, F., et al. (2023). Nutrition in chronic inflammatory conditions: Bypassing the mucosal block for micronutrients. https://core.ac.uk/download/597780063.pdf (accessed on 14th June 2025).
7. Besedovsky, L., Lange, T., & Haack, M. (2019). The sleep-immune crosstalk in health and disease. *Physiological Reviews, 99*, 1325–1380. https://doi.org/10.1152/physrev.00010.2018 (accessed on 14th June 2025).
8. Boneschansker, L., Brandt, S. L., Chan, E. C., Filippo, K., Freedman, N. J., Hjorto, G. M., Hons, M., et al. (2019). Concepts of GPCR-controlled navigation in the immune system.
9. Bui, T. T., Choy, W., Lagman, C., Lee, S., et al. (2016). Impact of human immunodeficiency virus in the pathogenesis and outcome of patients with glioblastoma multiforme. https://core.ac.uk/download/323076887.pdf (accessed on 14th June 2025).
10. Burke, R., Cavicchi, J. R., Kowalski, S. P., Michaud-King, C., et al. (2013). Patent landscape of helminth vaccines and related technologies. https://core.ac.uk/download/72052224.pdf (accessed on 14th June 2025).
11. Casimiro, M. C., Pestell, R. G., & Shupp, A. (2017). Biological functions of CDK5 and potential CDK5 targeted clinical treatments. https://core.ac.uk/download/83049850.pdf (accessed on 14th June 2025).
12. Conrad, J., & Gillen, A. L. (2014). Our impressive immune system: More than a defense. https://core.ac.uk/download/220159125.pdf (accessed on 14th June 2025).

13. de Paulis, A., Galli, S. J., Marone, G., Varricchi, G., et al. (2019). Future needs in mast cell biology. https://core.ac.uk/download/323062505.pdf (accessed on 14th June 2025).
14. Demas, G., Klein, S., Kriegsfeld, L., Nelson, R., et al. (1995). The influence of season, photoperiod, and pineal melatonin on immune function. https://core.ac.uk/download/323081880.pdf (accessed on 14th June 2025).
15. Detmar, M., & Jurisic, G. (2018). Lymphatic endothelium in health and disease. https://core.ac.uk/download/159154476.pdf (accessed on 14th June 2025).
16. Draf, C., Fisch, K. M., Kurabi, A., Nasamran, T., et al. (2020). Single-cell transcriptomes reveal a complex cellular landscape in the middle ear and differential capacities for acute response to infection. https://core.ac.uk/download/323308745.pdf (accessed on 14th June 2025).
17. Gallucci, B. B., & McCarthy, D. O. (1995). The immune system. https://core.ac.uk/download/213081395.pdf (accessed on 14th June 2025).
18. Germain, R., & Lämmermann, T. (2014). The multiple faces of leukocyte interstitial migration.
19. Germain, R., Kastenmüller, W., Lämmermann, T., et al. (2012). A spatially-organized multicellular innate immune response in lymph nodes limits systemic pathogen spread. https://core.ac.uk/download/294828981.pdf (accessed on 14th June 2025).
20. Irvine, D. J., & Liu, H. (2015). Guiding principles in the design of molecular bioconjugates for vaccine applications. https://core.ac.uk/download/83231429.pdf (accessed on 14th June 2025).
21. Lewis, S. M., Williams, A., & Eisenbarth, S. C. (2019). Structure and function of the immune system in the spleen. *Science Immunology, 4*. https://doi.org/10.1126/sciimmunol.aau6085 (accessed on 14th June 2025).
22. Lin, M. C., Neri, P., Perez, V. L., Periman, C., et al. (2020). The immunological basis of dry eye disease and current topical treatment options. https://core.ac.uk/download/323083122.pdf (accessed on 14th June 2025).
23. Lund, A., & Swartz, M. (2018). Role of lymphatic vessels in tumor immunity: Passive conduits or active participants? https://core.ac.uk/download/159154967.pdf (accessed on 14th June 2025).
24. Mitsdoerffer, M., & Peters, A. (2016). Tertiary lymphoid organs in central nervous system autoimmunity. https://core.ac.uk/download/210651370.pdf (accessed on 14th June 2025).
25. Napier, B. A., & Seufert, A. L. (2023). A new frontier for fat: Dietary palmitic acid induces innate immune memory. https://core.ac.uk/download/576491548.pdf (accessed on 14th June 2025).
26. Rannikko, E. (2024). Vascularized lymph node transfer and lymphatic growth factors in the treatment of lymphedema. https://core.ac.uk/download/619888802.pdf (accessed on 14th June 2025).
27. Ucar, A., Ucar, A., Wingate, A. D., Macdonald, A., Nudelman, A. S., Frenguelli, B. G., Frenguelli, B. G., et al. (2013). miR-132/212 knockout mice reveal roles for these miRNAs in regulating cortical synaptic transmission and plasticity. https://core.ac.uk/download/16663002.pdf (accessed on 14th June 2025).

INTRODUCTION TO RESPIRATORY SYSTEM

8

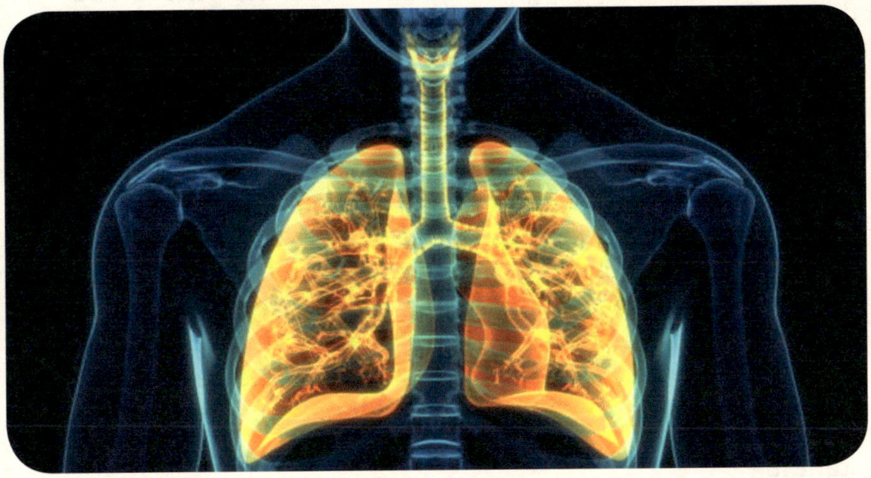

LEARNING OBJECTIVES

After studying this chapter, you will be able to:

1. Discuss the function of the respiratory system
2. Explain the structural anatomy of the respiratory system
3. Explain the primary organs of the respiratory system
4. Describe the types of respiration
5. Describe areas of the respiratory system

Introduction

The respiratory system is a critical component of human physiology, giving essential functions to sustain life. The intricate system of organs and structures is primarily responsible for gas exchange, whereby oxygen enters the bloodstream while carbon dioxide is released. Apart from its essential function in respiration, the system plays a part in other important functions like voice production, thermoregulation, and smell perception. The intricate interaction of different organs, such as the lungs, trachea, and diaphragm, emphasizes the need to know this system's anatomy and functions. Since the respiratory system closely interacts with the cardiovascular system, any impairment in these functions can severely affect general health and well-being. Therefore, an introductory understanding of the respiratory system's function and structural anatomy offers a basic knowledge required for understanding its different parts in more detail. There is a detailed explanation of the respiratory system that highlights several crucial anatomical features that allow for its diversified functions. The structural pattern can be differentiated into conducting areas and respiratory areas, both with varied functions in the process of breathing. The conducting area includes the nasal cavity, pharynx, larynx, trachea, bronchi, and bronchioles, all of which ensure the passage of air to and from the lungs. The respiratory zone, however, is comprised of the alveoli in which gas exchange is made. This makes evident the intricacy of the respiratory system: to know these zones is to know how airflow and gas exchange are regulated. Furthermore, the respiratory epithelium, including its cilia and mucous secretions, plays a critical function in filtering and humidifying inhaled air and thereby protecting against pathogens and allergens. This is echoed in the ongoing scientific investigation into disease and health of the respiratory system, a recognition of the significance of knowing the structural complexity of this system. The significance of the respiratory system is not just an indication of fundamental function; it is also at the center of the prevention and control of disease. For instance, understanding the interaction of respiratory and environmental factors can point to how exposure to pollutants or allergens affects lung function, leading to asthma or COPD. Furthermore, advances in medical research seek to clarify the underlying drivers of respiratory diseases to unlock new therapies and treatments. As mandated by extensive medical literature, including data on the physiological and pathologic aspects of respiratory well-being, there is a continued need for integrative approaches to respiratory education and public health. Detailed analysis of the respiratory system not only contributes to our knowledge of its structure and function but also informs respiratory health improvement activities and solutions to new health problems, ultimately contributing to better results for individuals and populations (Bekish et al., 2014; N/A, 2025).

Definition of the Respiratory System

The respiratory system can be technically defined as a complex system of organs and structures that allows the body to exchange gases with the external environment. In essence, it is the system that brings in oxygen into the bloodstream while at the same time expelling carbon dioxide, which is a byproduct of cellular metabolism. This intricate interaction occurs primarily in alveoli, tiny air sacs in the lungs, where oxygen is transferred into the blood and carbon dioxide is expelled. Further, the respiratory system comprises other structures such as the nasal cavity, trachea, bronchi, and lungs, each having an extremely crucial function to provide proper ventilation and gas exchange. Therefore, the respiratory system definition goes one step further than anatomy to include the morphology of physiological functions that enable its vital function, which makes it an essential system for the preservation of life. As a complex system, the respiratory anatomy contains conducting and respiratory zones, which have various but complementary functions. The conducting region, comprising the nasal passages, pharynx, larynx, trachea, and bronchi, has the primary function of warming, filtering, and humidifying air entering, thereby protecting the lung's sensitive structures. The respiratory region, made up of respiratory bronchioles, alveolar ducts, and alveoli, is where the critical gas exchange takes place. This division not only demonstrates the intricacy of the respiratory system structure but also highlights how each part has to work in harmony so that homeostasis may be achieved. In devising the definition of the respiratory system, one has to grasp that its function and structure show deep evolutionary adaptations that have allowed organisms to meet their metabolic demands in various environments successfully. Research into the respiratory system continues to reveal intricate relationships between its structure and function, claiming its fundamental role in human health. An understanding of how the components of the respiratory system act in harmony to influence sufficient exchange of gases and support metabolic processes is needed in order to understand its definition. Complexity is further brought out by medical language applied in explaining various aspects of the system, with some of these words employed in clinical practice previously being scientifically controversial. For instance, the requirement of correct nomenclature brings to the fore the significance of accuracy in communicating science, as the language has to distinctly represent the anatomy and function of the respiratory system (AlMehzaa et al., 2019). Therefore, ongoing debate in medical semantics demands an enhancement of the utilization of terms towards suggesting a more rational and pragmatic terminology in keeping with advances in respiratory science and clinical practice so that greater integration and comprehension are achieved across contiguous disciplines (N/A, 2025) (Figure 8.1).

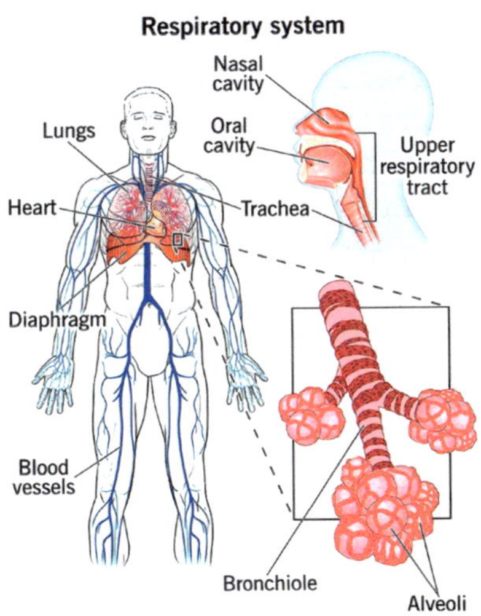

Figure 8.1. Respiratory system.

Source: https://my.clevelandclinic.org/-/scassets/images/org/health/articles/respiratory-system.

Importance of the Respiratory System in Human Physiology

The breathing system has a central role in the maintenance of homeostasis and the support of cellular operations through the exchange of gases. For aerobic metabolism, the overall energy generation process in human cells, oxygen is essential. Inhalation brings air containing oxygen into the lungs, where it permeates into the walls of the alveoli and into the blood. Exhalation removes carbon dioxide, a cellular respiration waste product. This function is not just crucial for the production of energy but also for the regulation of blood pH levels, hence offering a balance in the body's acid-base homeostasis. The understanding of the intricate mechanics involved in such functions supports the respiratory system's role in maintaining general health and well-being, as abnormal gas exchange leads to metabolic changes and numerous complications, emphasizing its irreplaceable nature in human physiology. Another vital role of the respiratory system is the protective function, which guards the body against pathogens and toxins. The system employs various anatomical structures and reflexes to filter, humidify, and warm the air before it gets into the lungs. Nasal hair and mucus trap particulates as well as microbes, and the lining cilia on the airways propel mucus towards the head so that it can be coughed up or swallowed. This mechanism for defense is essential in preventing respiratory infections and illnesses such as pneumonia and bronchitis. The respiratory system also assists the immune system through the provision of special immune cells in the lung tissues that react to inhaled pathogens in the respiratory system. The respiratory system, thus, is not only a mere passive channel of air; it's also an active participant in the defense of the body against disease, thereby once more demonstrating its importance in human physiology (Bekish et al., 2014; Bekish et al., 2017). Further, the respiratory system is closely entwined with other organ systems, demonstrating its multifaceted role in human physiology. Cardiovascular and respiratory systems work in collaboration during the process of gaseous exchange; oxygenated blood is delivered to organs and tissues, while deoxygenated blood is transported back to the lungs to be re-oxygenated. Such dependency signifies the role of the respiratory system in metabolic processes across the body. Furthermore, the ability to manage respiration rates based on physical activity or emotional state indicates the system's role in physiological adaptation. An increased need for oxygen during exercise invokes a rise in the rate and depth of respiration to accommodate metabolic needs. Interconnectedness of systems highlights the respiratory systems tremendous significance, not only for oxygen supply but also for physiological coordination and concord as a whole (Bekish et al., 2014; Bekish et al., 2017).

8.1. Functions of the Respiratory System

Learning Outcome

1. Define gas exchange: oxygen and carbon dioxide
2. Analyze the regulation of blood pH
3. Define protection against pathogens and irritants

The respiratory system carries out several very significant functions that are critical to homeostasis maintenance in the human body. The foremost is gas exchange, where oxygen (O_2) is absorbed into the body, and carbon dioxide (CO_2) is expelled from the body. All of these take place primarily in the alveoli, where oxygen is absorbed into the bloodstream and carbon dioxide is exhaled. Additionally, the respiratory system plays a crucial role in maintaining blood pH through the bicarbonate buffer system that adjusts levels of CO_2 in the blood. Such adjustment is critical since it allows for acid-base balance, which affects overall cellular metabolism and function. Lastly, gas exchange and pH regulation functions define the best role of the respiratory system in sustaining physiological balance and maintaining cellular processes in the body. In addition to gas exchange, the respiratory system also serves to provide various ancillary functions that enhance overall well-being and interaction with the environment, such as olfaction, or the sense of smell, which is reliant on specific receptors in the nasal passage. This sense is helpful for the perception of environmental stimuli and influences behaviors such as appetite and social behavior. Furthermore, the respiratory system aids in thermoregulation through warming or cooling air entering the lungs to match body temperature. This process is essential in preventing harm to sensitive pulmonary tissues. Furthermore, the mucociliary escalator, a mechanism employing mucus and cilia, aids in trapping and expelling foreign particles and pathogens, thus contributing to immune protection and lung health. Hence, these additional functions illustrate the multifaceted importance of respiratory systems beyond basic gas exchange. The immune function of the respiratory system is vital, as it is a crucial frontline defense against pathogens. The bronchus-associated lymphoid tissue (BALT) is the predominant component of such immune defense, as it helps coordinate defense against inhaled pathogens, particularly in birds (Dalamani et al., 2006). In human beings, these protective measures are there in the sense that numerous macrophages and other immune cells are found within the respiratory tract, actively looking for and eliminating infections. Furthermore, the occurrence of secretory immunoglobulin A (IgA) on mucosal surfaces provides humoral defense against viruses and bacteria. This interaction between structural elements, such as BALT and mucosal immune elements, optimizes the respiratory system's response to infection, thus preserving general well-being. By human immune functions of this sort, we are more able to understand the human respiratory system's overall function in protecting the human body from disease (Bekish et al., 2017).

8.1.1. Gas Exchange: Oxygen and Carbon Dioxide

The gas exchange is at the core of the function of the respiratory system, where it is the diffusion of oxygen and carbon dioxide from the alveoli of the lungs to the blood. The oxygen, which is utilized in cellular respiration, diffuses from the alveoli to the capillaries by a concentration gradient; this is facilitated through the large surface area of the alveoli with thin walls to enable the distance of diffusion to be minimized. Conversely, carbon dioxide, a product of cellular metabolism, is passed from the bloodstream to the alveoli to be excreted during exhalation. The two-way exchange sustains cellular metabolism and the acid-base balance of the body, revealing the imperative for efficient gas exchange through the respiratory system. The efficiency of gas exchange is based on several factors, including partial pressures of gases and the diffusion surface area available. The gradients of partial pressures allow carbon dioxide and oxygen to move; a higher partial pressure of oxygen in the alveoli compared to the blood allows it to diffuse into the circulation. Likewise, the increased carbon dioxide level in the blood relative to that in the alveolar space makes it easier for it to be expelled from the body. Pneumonia or pulmonary edema can interfere with such gradients, causing inefficient gas exchange and resultant hypoxia, emphasizing the fragile equilibrium that the respiratory system needs to sustain to efficiently deliver oxygen and remove carbon dioxide during varying states of physiology. Various types of respiration contribute to the alteration in gas exchange, which not only involves external respiration—the exchange within the lungs—but internal respiration, i.e., utilization of oxygen and production of carbon dioxide at the cellular level. Moreover, organisms also have various areas of respiration based on their adaptations to multiple conditions. For example, aquatic mammals possess specialized mechanisms to maintain prolonged breath-holding durations and efficient gas exchange during dives. These diverse mechanisms raise our knowledge of the diverse physiology between species and express the sophisticated interaction between structural structure and functional capacity of the respiratory apparatus in the supply of gas exchange in varying conditions, as expounded in comprehensive studies of respiration mechanisms and their driving forces (N/A, 2025; Bekish et al., 2014) (Figure 8.2).

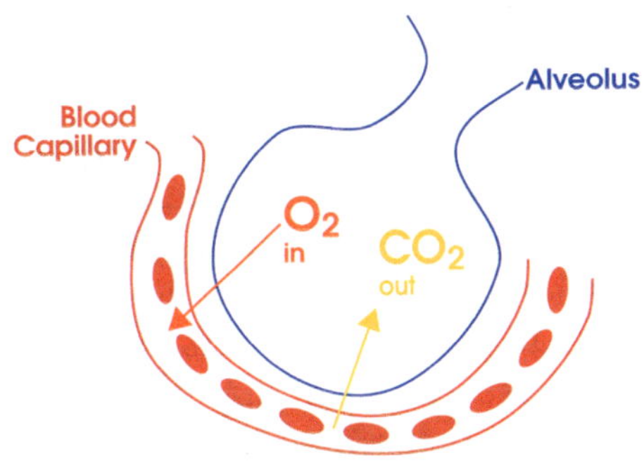

Figure 8.2. Gas exchange in humans. Oxygen and carbon dioxide switch places between a capillary (part of the bloodstream) and an alveolus (an air sac in the lungs).

Source: https://upload.wikimedia.org/wikipedia/commons/thumb/c/c4/Gas_exchange_in_the_aveolus_simple_%28en%29.svg/1024px-Gas_exchange_in_the_aveolus_simple_%28en%29.svg.png.

8.1.2. Regulation of Blood pH

One of the key roles that homeostasis plays within the human body is the regulation of blood pH, and it is regulated by the respiratory system. Blood pH is tightly regulated between 7.35 and 7.45, and these are levels crucial for providing enzymatic activity and metabolic function to function optimally. Regulation of carbon dioxide

(CO_2) concentration by the respiratory system is one of the key contributions to this level of control, as CO_2 is the cellular respiratory waste. When CO_2 levels increase, it combines with body water to form carbonic acid, which lowers blood pH and leads to acidosis. Conversely, the removal of CO_2 through respiration increases pH levels, towards alkalosis. Therefore, the ability of the respiratory system to adjust ventilation rates is a vital mechanism for controlling blood acidity and attaining homeostasis. The coupling of the respiratory system and the renal system again highlights the need for pH regulation of blood. While the respiratory system can make rapid changes in CO_2 concentration, the kidneys are responsible for maintaining long-term pH balance through the excretion or reabsorption of bicarbonate and hydrogen ions. This buffering system complements the respiratory changes and allows for ongoing pH homeostasis. When pulmonary function is impaired, as in the case of chronic obstructive pulmonary disease (COPD), the failure to vent CO_2 results in respiratory acidosis. These cases emphasize the need for an integrated understanding of how the two systems work together to regulate blood pH within the relatively narrow window necessary for physiological equilibrium. This synergy demonstrates the sophistication of human biology and the importance of multiple organ systems playing roles in establishing balance. Derangements in pH homeostasis may have severe consequences for health, illustrating the role of the respiratory system in achieving metabolic homeostasis. Acidosis and alkalosis have systemic effects on cellular functions and can affect all the way from conduction in nerves to muscle contraction. Symptomatology can present itself as respiratory distress, confusion, or changes in muscle function and must be treated by a physician immediately. It is an understanding of these mechanisms that informs healthcare practitioners regarding the development of treatment protocols in response to conditions of pH imbalance. Therefore, the operation of respiratory systems transcends mere gas exchange, and it is a crucial element with a critical function in blood pH fine-tuning required to sustain life and achieve optimal health. With the continued growth of education in physiology, texts such as lab manuals and updated bibliographies assist us in our comprehension of these intricate biological processes (Beebe et al., 2019; N/A, 2025) (Figure 8.3).

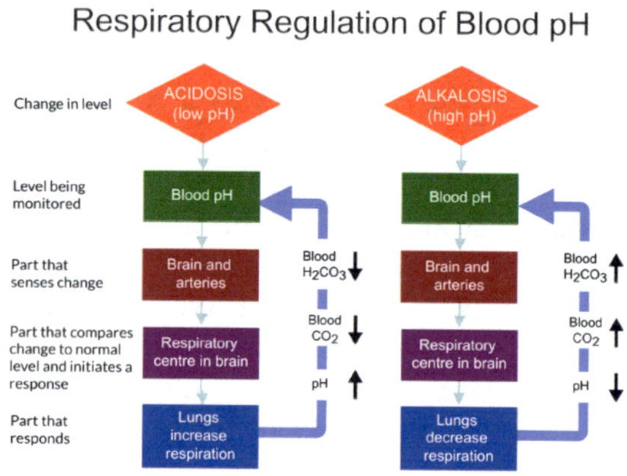

Figure 8.3. Respiratory regulation of blood pH.

Source: https://letstalkscience.ca/sites/default/files/styles/width_800px/public/2021-11/Respiratory-regulation-of-blood-pH.png?itok=Wp77tX9E.

8.1.3. Protection Against Pathogens and Irritants

The respiratory system is a key defense against environmental pathogens and irritants, utilizing several anatomical and physiological pathways to protect pulmonary health. The nasal passages are a significant site of air filtration, where mucous membranes capture particulate, dust, and microorganisms. Ciliated epithelial cells augment this protective function by sweeping captured particles toward the throat, allowing their clearance by swallowing or coughing. Besides, the presence of immune cells in respiratory tissues, such as macrophages and lymphocytes, provides an adaptive immune response, allowing rapid identification and inactivation of potential pathogens before infection. These initial lines of defense are vital in maintaining a healthy respiratory tract and reducing the likelihood of respiratory disease, thus highlighting the importance of the structural anatomy in defense against impending threats. In addition to mechanical filtration, the respiratory system also has biochemical mechanisms to protect against irritants and pathogens. In addition to trapping harmful particles, mucus contains antimicrobial compounds like lysozyme and defensins. These substances are used to neutralize bacteria and viruses that may find their way into the respiratory tract. Secondly, there cannot be an underestimation of the impact of oxidative stress on respiratory health since exposure to inhaled air contaminants aggravates conditions such as asthma or chronic obstructive pulmonary disease (COPD). It is proven that oxidative stress will result in severe lung damage, undermining the protective capacity of the respiratory system, necessitating the preservation of antioxidant levels to mitigate these consequences (Sabuncuo et al., 2022). Thus, a multi-modal strategy combining structural and biochemical defense is necessary to offer consistent protection against inhaled pathogens and irritants. Pathologic states such as cystic fibrosis (CF) illustrate the consequences of compromised protective mechanisms in the airways. In cystic fibrosis patients, mucus plugging creates an environment conducive to the growth of specific pathogens, particularly Pseudomonas aeruginosa, which causes severe lung tissue destruction. The interaction of host defenses, dysbiotic microbiota, and environmental factors renders the pattern of infection complex, leading to a chronic inflammatory vicious cycle and lung injury (Anjali et al., 2016). Such complexity calls for the limitation of single-modality therapy approaches, suggesting that multifactorial approaches are necessary for management and treatment. An understanding of the intricate interaction between pathogens and the protective barriers of the host ultimately informs the development of new therapies to enhance lung function and resistance to infection. Protection against irritants and pathogens thus serves to underscore the imperative of continued research and development in the field of respiratory health.

Test Your Knowledge

1. How does gas exchange occur in the lungs, and what roles do oxygen and carbon dioxide play in this process?
2. How does the respiratory system help regulate blood pH levels, and why is this critical for homeostasis?

8.2. Structural Anatomy of the Respiratory System

Learning Outcome

1. Define upper respiratory tract components
2. Discuss the lower respiratory tract components
3. Define supporting structures: thoracic cavity and diaphragm

The structural body of the respiratory system is a component of its entire function, enabling efficient gas exchange and homeostasis. The system is dispersed from the external nasal passages to the alveoli of the lungs, which are primarily the site for the exchange of carbon dioxide and oxygen. The upper respiratory system is composed of the nasal cavity, larynx, and pharynx, which filter, warm, and humidify air before it reaches the lungs. In contrast to this, the trachea, bronchi, and bronchioles make up the lower respiratory tract, extending down to the alveolar sacs. Each of these structures is delicately designed to optimize airflow as well as keep the respiratory surfaces in a moist state, enhancing effective gas exchange (Bekish et al., 2014). Furthermore, the respiratory system's architecture is highly specialized as it progresses from wider airways to very intricate alveolar structures. The trachea is supported by C-shaped cartilaginous rings that serve to prevent collapse without obstructing the airways. When the bronchi enter the lungs, they further branch out into smaller bronchioles, which end in the alveoli; these tiny air sacs significantly increase the surface area exposed to gas exchange. The alveolar walls are fragile, a single layer of epithelial cells, and covered with surfactant, a substance that reduces surface tension. This body structure enables oxygen to diffuse rapidly into the bloodstream and carbon dioxide to escape, highlighting how efficient the system is (Bekish et al., 2017). The intricate design of the respiratory system is not just functional but also symbolic of the evolutionary processes that have developed to meet metabolic demands. Each segment and structure is an evolutionary adaptation responding to environmental pressure, optimizing respiratory efficiency, and supporting varied physiological functions. For instance, the increased surface area provided by the alveoli facilitates the exchange of gases necessary for sustaining higher metabolic processes, particularly in active organisms. The structural support provided by connective tissue helps to keep the airways open during the cycle of respiration, thereby facilitating continuous airflow. In general, respiratory system structural anatomy is a complex interplay of form and function that is conducive to the essential respiration and gas exchange processes. As such, it is a seminal area of research in human physiology (Bekish et al., 2014).

8.2.1. Upper Respiratory Tract Components

The upper respiratory tract is critical to the first level of gas exchange, being integral to conditioning, filtering, and humidifying air. The main constituents of the upper respiratory tract are the nasal cavity, pharynx, and larynx, each making substantial contributions to the act of respiration. The nasal cavity, covered by mucosa and cilia, is the primary defense mechanism against airborne pathogens and particles. Not only does it warm and moisten inhaled air, but it also facilitates olfactory functions to allow survival-relevant odors to be sensed. The intricate anatomy of the nasal turbinates greatly increases the surface area for these processes so that efficiency in air processing is maximized before it enters into the lower respiratory system. Following the nasal cavity, the pharynx is shared by air and food passage, illustrating the complex interaction between the digestive and respiratory systems. The pharynx itself is separated into the nasopharynx, oropharynx, and laryngopharynx, each of which carries out specific functions in breathing. The nasopharynx, located posterior to the nasal cavity, is mainly responsible for air passage, and it houses the adenoids that assist with immunity. The oropharynx and laryngopharynx serve as conduits for food and air, allowing for the act of swallowing. It is this multiplicity of function that provides aspiration to be avoided and air to be directed accurately towards the larynx, where it is used in vocalization, eventually connecting respiratory activity and communication, a function that has become highly developed in humans as described in recent research on motor evolution (John, 2008). The larynx or voice box is an essential organ of the upper respiratory system that not only allows for phonation but also serves as a protective device for the lower respiratory system.

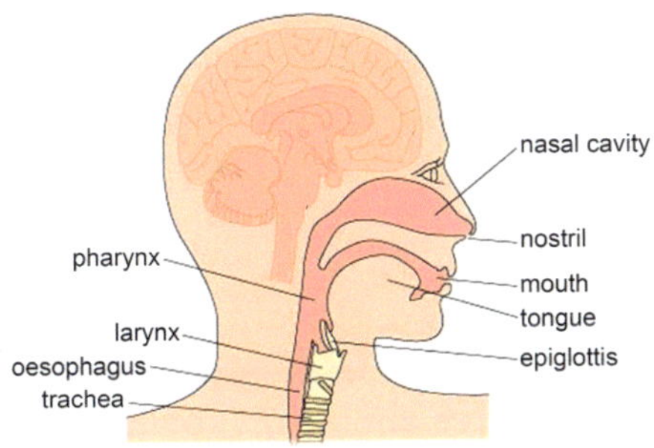

Figure 8.4. Structures of the upper respiratory tract.

Source: https://www.open.edu/openlearn/science-maths-technology/blood-and-the-respiratory-system/content-section-1.1.1.

The larynx is made up of several cartilaginous elements, of which the vocal cords are housed, and is actively involved in the generation of sound through the processes of vibration and modulation. Besides, as swallowing occurs, the epiglottis, which is part of laryngeal anatomy, moves to cover the trachea to prevent food from entering the airway, thereby demonstrating the synchronized aspect of respiratory and digestive interaction. The accurate coordination of the processes is central to the maintenance of airway patency and best communication, which requires emphasis on upper respiratory components in the overall context of respiratory system function (Beebe et al., 2019) (Figure 8.4).

8.2.2. Lower Respiratory Tract Components

The lower respiratory tract encompasses significant anatomical structures involved in gas exchange and the respiratory process as a whole. This respiratory component goes on from the trachea, branching into the main bronchi and again into the secondary and tertiary bronchi inside each lung. The complex network of bronchial structures facilitates air passage to all regions of the lungs with maximum surface area for oxygen and carbon dioxide exchange. Surrounding these airways are supporting structures essential to the patency of the airway, including cartilage and smooth muscle, which allow for alterations in airway diameter during the respiratory cycle. Understanding the structural anatomy of the lower respiratory tract is essential in the diagnosis and management of respiratory illness because disease of this region has the potential to have a significant impact on the efficiency of respiration, an essential role of the respiratory system. The terminal of the bronchial apparatus is the alveoli, which are the primary units for gas exchange. Alveoli are minute, balloon-like structures in clusters, with a vast surface area for the absorption of oxygen and the removal of carbon dioxide. The walls of the alveoli consist of complex single epithelial cells to ensure efficient gas diffusion. Of particular importance, the surfactant complex of lipoproteins, secreted by type II alveolar cells, reduces surface tension in the alveoli, preventing collapse of the latter on exhalation and enhancing lung compliance. The interactive structure of alveoli and the pulmonary capillaries is of utmost significance; any derangement can result in ineffective gas exchange, which causes a variety of lung diseases. As highlighted by recent studies, addressing the burden of lung diseases is imperative because of their rising prevalence and limited therapeutic interventions (Cryan et al., 2015). Moreover, knowledge of the pathophysiology of the lower respiratory tract is central in designing treatment strategies and promoting patient outcomes. Asthma and COPD are examples that illustrate the influence of structural changes and inflammation on lung function. In the past decade, interest has been expressed in whether tissue engineering has any future as a treatment option to repair damaged airway tissues and promote improved lung function. Therapies and techniques that involve biomaterials and stem cell treatments are aimed at not just restoring the structural function but also enhancing the functional capacity of the lower respiratory tract (Cryan et al., 2015). With the tremendous health burden entailed by lower respiratory conditions, it becomes more and more essential to develop an in-depth knowledge of underlying anatomy as well as mechanisms so that therapeutic strategies can be designed to impact respiratory health outcomes (Figure 8.5) significantly.

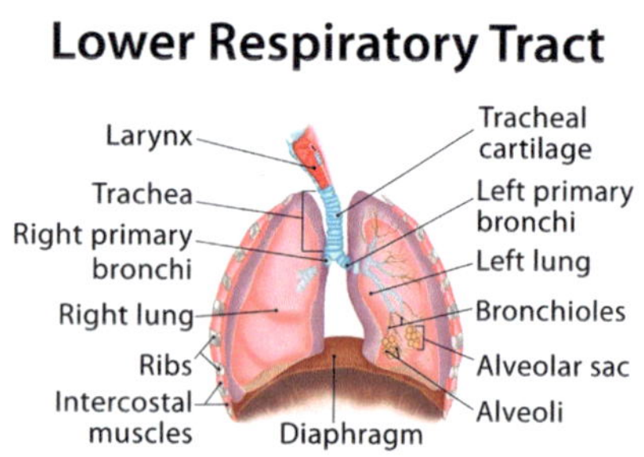

Figure 8.5. Lower respiratory tract.

Source: https://i0.wp.com/student-nurse-life.com/wp-content/uploads/2021/02/Lower-Respiratory-Tract.jpg?resize=750%2C536.

8.2.3. Supporting Structures: Thoracic Cavity and Diaphragm

The thoracic cavity is also a significant supportive framework of the respiratory system, with vital organs such as the heart and lungs. The thoracic cavity is housed within the rib cage, which offers protection and allows for mechanical movement as part of the process of breathing. Made up of 12 pairs of ribs, vertebrae, and the sternum, the rib cage protects the organs of the thorax but is also an active participant in the expansion and contraction of the thoracic cavity when respiring. The lungs, which reside in the neck of the cavity, are covered by a double-membrane pleura, which carries negative pressure to prevent collapse of the lungs. In addition, the shape and spatial structure of the thoracic cavity facilitate the process of gas exchange. The mechanics of respiration are heavily dependent on the structural organization, which promotes changes in volume and pressures within the thoracic cavity, thereby creating a passage for air to be inhaled and expelled from the lungs. The diaphragm, a dome-shaped muscle separating the thoracic cavity from the abdominal cavity, is central to the mechanics of respiration. Its function forms part of the process of breathing as it contracts and becomes flattened when the body is filling up with air, hence creating a vacuum that draws in air into the lungs. It not only increases the thoracic cavity volume but also ventilates the lungs for maximum gas exchange. As it exhales, the diaphragm relaxes, and the lungs deflate to expel air. Studies emphasize the necessity of proper positioning of the diaphragm to achieve maximum respiratory efficiency, particularly in clinical settings. For instance, patient positioning will necessarily influence pulmonary aeration and effective bronchial secretions elimination, thus locating the function of the diaphragm outside of breathing and suggesting its relevance in patient care within the context of the intensive care unit (ICU) environment, as revealed through evidence on optimal patient postures towards increased respiratory competency (Grigoriadis et al., 2009). The functional relationship between the thoracic cavity and diaphragm is also explained by realizing the diffusion process that occurs in the alveoli. The efficiency of gas exchange relies heavily on the structural stability and functional dynamics of these support structures. Changes in red blood cell distribution can have a substantial impact on lung-diffusing capacity, according to a mathematical model of gas diffusion in alveolar areas. This highlights the significance of both anatomical and physiological factors for respiratory health (Kulish et al., 2006). Such an intricate interdependence between thoracic supporting structures and diaphragmatic action underscores their mutual role in the effectiveness and efficiency of the respiratory system. As such, any injury to these structures could lead to compromised respiration, highlighting their importance in health and in clinical recovery cases (Figure 8.6).

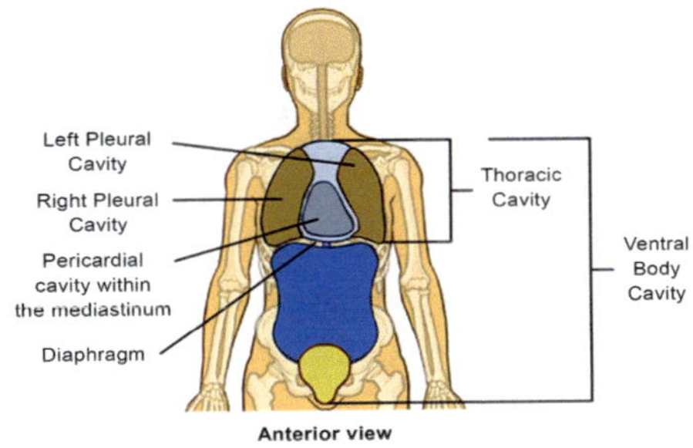

Figure 8.6. The thoracic cavity is the superior cavity in the ventral body cavity.

Source: https://images.my.labster.com/v2/BPS/52977293-f6f5-4177-b41d-6467b5129fb7/BPS_ThoracicCavity.en.x512.png.

Test Your Knowledge

1. What are the main components of the upper respiratory tract, and what functions do they serve in respiration?
2. Which structures make up the lower respiratory tract, and how do they contribute to gas exchange?

8.3. Major Organs of the Respiratory System

Learning Outcome

1. Define nose and nasal cavity
2. Discuss the lungs and alveoli
3. Explain the trachea and bronchi

The respiratory system is comprised of a series of vital organs functioning together to facilitate gas exchange, a critical process for the sustenance of life. The key organs are the lungs, trachea, bronchi, and diaphragm, each responsible for a specific function. The lungs, which are the primary organs of respiration, oxygenate blood and eliminate carbon dioxide. The trachea serves as an air passage, branching into bronchi to supply the lungs directly. Bronchi and bronchioles consist of a series of airways that progressively narrow to create an effective exchange of gases. The funnel-shaped physical structure ensures that air is effectively filtered, warmed, and humidified before reaching sensitive alveoli where the critical gas exchange occurs. In addition to their original respiratory functions, these organs also have immune defenses against airborne pathogens that are required. The bronchus-associated lymphoid tissue (BALT) of the bird lung is a prime example of how respiratory organs can be both respiratory and immunological in function. As stated, the anatomy of BALT is well-established and matures with age, displaying an adaptive immune response that is more potent as the organism becomes older. The presence of lymphocytes and tissue macrophages in lung interstitial tissues also highlights the principal role of immune cells in the health of the respiratory system and infection-fighting ability. Having this dual role implies that there must be a comprehensive understanding of respiratory anatomy as well as physiology because disruption of either may pose critical problems concerning health, such as excessive vulnerability to respiratory infections (Dalamani et al., 2006). Additionally, understanding the respiratory zones is crucial in the identification of how such organs operate as part of greater systems of physiology. The respiratory system functions most effectively when divided into conducting and respiratory zones. The conducting zone, which comprises organs such as the trachea and bronchi, is mainly responsible for conducting air. In contrast, the respiratory zone has the alveoli, where exchange of gases takes place. It highlights the respiratory system's complexity, which must function not just in moving air but also in gas exchange effectively. There are several anatomical features, including the vast surface area of alveoli and the thinness of the alveolar membrane, that are specifically designed for the process. As knowledge of respiratory organs expands, it is increasingly evident how much they are intertwined with overall health, facilitating not just respiration but also critical functions in immune protection and homeostasis (Bekish et al., 2014).

8.3.1. Nose and Nasal Cavity

The nasal cavity and nose are key structures of the respiratory system, used to aid in proper breathing and initial processing of air before it enters the lungs. The nasal cavity has a complex anatomy with a system of turbinates, which are bony structures that provide an increased surface area for air filtering, humidification, and temperature adjustment. When the air passes through the nasal passages, it is humidified and warmed up to the level necessary for entry into the lungs. This process is critical to the maintenance of the integrity of the respiratory tract as well as the optimization of gas exchange. Furthermore, mucus membranes in the nasal cavity trap pathogens and particulate material, contributing to the body's immune defense system. Accordingly, nasal structure health is essential for respiratory effectiveness as a whole and against environmental poisons.

Apart from their function of respiration, the nose and nasal cavity play significant roles in the sense of smell, or olfaction, an integral part of human experience and conduct. Olfactory epithelium, located in the upper part of the nasal cavity, contains specialized smell receptors that detect airborne chemical particles and are accountable not only for the sense of smell but also for modifying taste and the pleasure of eating. It is vital for survival as it allows dangerous substances, such as spoiled food or poisonous substances, to be detected. Also, the coupling of the olfactory signal with emotional response emphasizes the function of the nasal cavity in relation to neurological processes. The possibility of intranasal drug delivery for the management of some conditions further reiterates the function of the nasal cavity in neuroscience since it offers access to the central nervous system without the barriers encountered with systemic delivery pathways (Keller et al., 2021; Erd et al., 2018). The evolution of research on intranasal drug delivery has also pointed the finger at the nose and nasal cavity as pathways for drug delivery directly to the central nervous system (CNS). This is a series of advantages, including bypassing the blood-brain barrier, maximizing drug bioavailability, and minimizing the frequency of systemic side effects with reduced doses compared to oral delivery. Since most of the neurological disorders are challenging to treat due to the poor penetration of drugs, employing the nasal route is a new technique that exploits the anatomical and physiological properties of the nasal tract (Keller et al., 2021). Research highlights the importance of understanding the nasal barrier structure and function, and optimizing the formulation for better drug absorption, which can be a breakthrough for therapeutic intervention in neurodegenerative and psychiatric disease patients (Erd et al., 2018). More information about the incredibly intricate relationship between respiratory management and neurological health is being unveiled from such research (Figure 8.7).

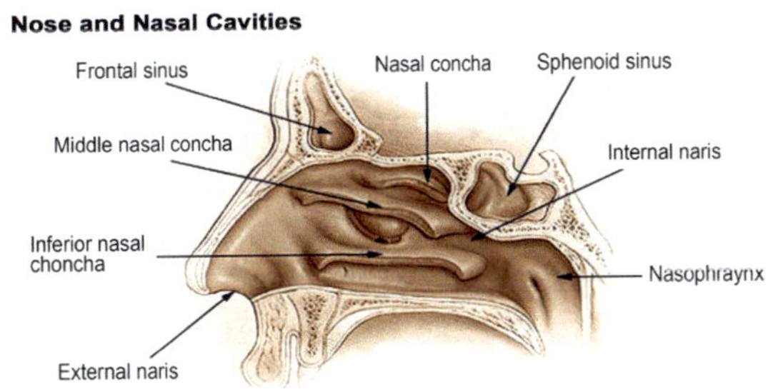

Figure 8.7. Nose and nasal cavity.

Source: https://training.seer.cancer.gov/images/anatomy/respiratory/nose_nasal_cavities.jpg.

8.3.2. Lungs and Alveoli

The lungs are the primary organs of respiration, tasked with gas exchange and homeostasis in the body. Comprising a very complex structure of tissue and alveoli, the lungs efficiently facilitate oxygenation into the blood while evacuating carbon dioxide out of the body. This level of complexity enables a vast surface area, which maximizes diffusion efficiency in the mechanism of respiration. Alveoli, the small air bladders that cover the lungs, play an essential role in this gaseous exchange process, providing a medium between the air and blood. The organization is functionally adapted to have alveoli that consist of a thin layer of epithelium through which gases can be passed rapidly , facilitating the efficient oxygenation of blood. Understanding the anatomical and functional connection between the alveoli and the lungs is essential to comprehending the mechanics of respiratory physiology in general. A vast network of capillaries surrounds alveoli, further highlighting their role in gas exchange. Surfactant, a covering that reduces surface tension and prevents collapse during exhalation, covers each alveolus. This surfactant is essential to maintaining alveolar stability and patency for proper gas exchange. The immune system also plays a vital role in protecting the alveoli from infection and toxic debris. Bronchus-associated lymphoid tissue (BALT) is responsible for the adaptive immune response within these areas, responding to various exposures to the environment, as described in recent literature. Such proof further emphasizes the importance of alveolar health in the prevention of respiratory disease, given that malfunction in this equipment can lead to catastrophic complications and chronic disorders like chronic obstructive pulmonary disease or asthma, which bear seriously on public health (Ak et al., 2021) (Figure 8.8).

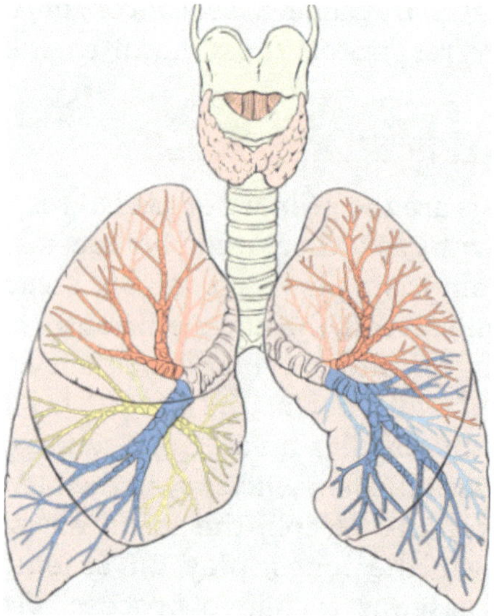

Figure 8.8. Lungs diagram with internal details.

Source: https://upload.wikimedia.org/wikipedia/commons/thumb/a/a1/Lungs_diagram_detailed.svg/800px-Lungs_diagram_detailed.svg.png.

Research into the engineering of lung tissue has been an exciting field of therapy for respiratory disease. Chronic respiratory diseases have become increasingly prevalent, and there is a need for innovative modes of treatment to improve patient outcomes. These include engineered constructs that replicate the structural and functional characteristics of lung tissue. These advances not only aim to enhance recovery from airway injury but also attempt alternatives to traditional modes of therapy and organ transplantation. Relevant engineering of alveolar and other structures is the foundation for functional integration in the respiratory system. Ongoing investigation into biomaterials and the cellular signaling processes that promote healing has immense potential for regenerative medicine, as it avails time-dependent solutions for effective intervention in managing respiratory diseases (Cryan et al., 2015). Such trailblazing techniques promise paradigm-breaking treatments that irreversibly alter the way lung-related health issues are addressed (Figure 8.9).

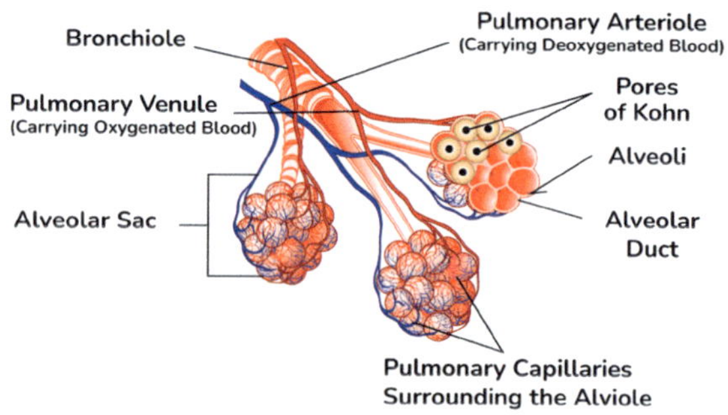

Figure 8.9. Diagram of alveoli.

Source: https://media.geeksforgeeks.org/wp-content/uploads/20240402102643/Diagram-of-Alveoli.png.

8.3.3. Trachea and Bronchi

Trachea and bronchi are crucial in the conduction of air within the respiratory system. The trachea, or windpipe, is the chief airway that links the larynx to the bronchi and directs inhaled air from the upper respiratory system to the lungs effectively. Physiologically, the trachea is composed of C-shaped cartilaginous rings, which provide support so the airway will not collapse but is still pliable when one breathes. When the trachea bifurcates, it branches into the right and left bronchi and further into smaller bronchioles within the lungs. This rather elaborate system of branching is vital for air to be delivered throughout the lungs for effective gas exchange necessary for cellular respiration. The trachea and bronchi structural dynamics are essential to providing free passage for the flow of air, which is vital in maintaining homeostasis within the body. Apart from their structural components, the trachea and bronchi have various functions that are inherent to respiratory health. One of their primary functions is to act as a conduit for air, but they are also involved in air filtration and humidification before the air is inhaled. The inner lining of the trachea and bronchi has ciliated epithelial cells and goblet cells that secrete mucus that traps dust, pathogens, and other impurities. This mucociliary escalator system is an essential mechanism for protecting lung tissue from infection and inflammation and, therefore, enhancing respiratory efficiency. Moreover, the smooth muscle surrounding the bronchi supports bronchoconstriction and bronchodilation such that the airway governs airflow in accordance with physiological requirements. In so doing, the trachea and bronchi are not merely passive tubes but active players in preserving respiratory integrity and function in the respiratory system (Figure 8.10).

New advances in respiratory science have made it clear that new models must be designed to advance our understanding of bronchial and tracheal physiology. Because species variation in lung anatomy prevents the transfer of information from animal models to man, it has become increasingly important to develop in vitro systems.

Techniques such as three-dimensional organoids and organs-on-a-chip are being explored for their potential to replicate tracheal and bronchial epithelial function and responsiveness to stimuli within a controlled environment. Such models have the potential to aid in gaining an understanding of disease processes, mechanisms of regeneration, and consequences of environmental toxins on respiratory health. By facilitating the in vitro study of human lung physiology, these methods may complement standard research and further respiratory function and disease understanding, eventually guiding respiratory disease treatments (Thomas et al., 2018; Gkatzis et al., 2018) (Figure 8.11).

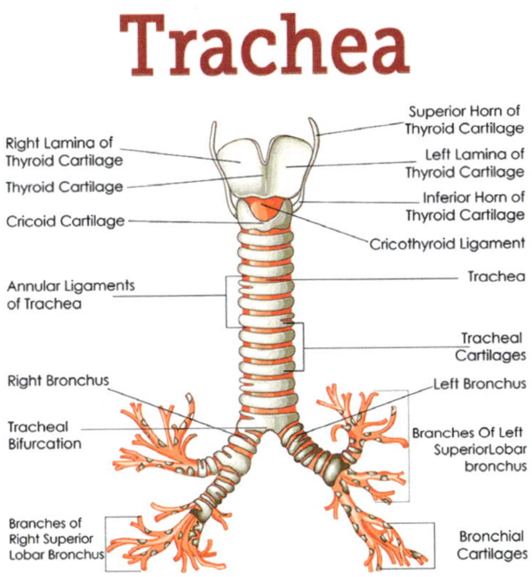

Figure 8.10. Trachea.

Source: https://assets.lybrate.com/imgs/tic/enadp/image-of-the-trachea.jpg.

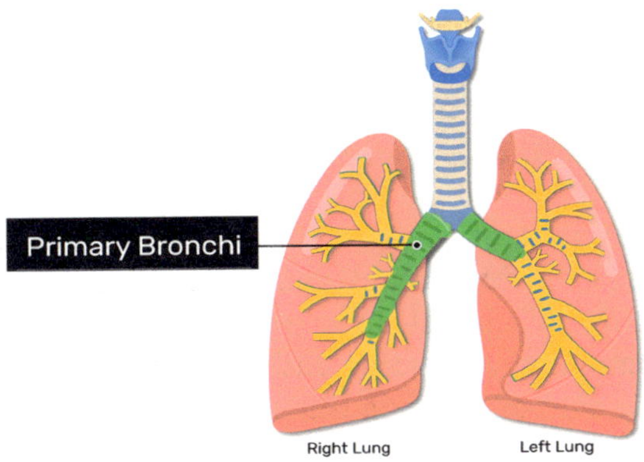

Figure 8.11. Primary bronchi.

Source: https://www.getbodysmart.com/wp-content/uploads/2017/10/Primary-Bronchi-1024x732.png.

Test Your Knowledge

1. What are the functions of the nose and nasal cavity in the respiratory system?
2. How do the lungs and alveoli work together to facilitate gas exchange?

8.4. Types of Respiration

Learning Outcome

1. Discuss the external respiration: gas exchange in the lungs
2. Explain the internal respiration: gas exchange at the cellular level
3. Define cellular respiration: energy production in cells

The respiratory system plays a vital role in sustaining life through various types of respiration, which can be broadly categorized into aerobic and anaerobic respiration. Aerobic respiration occurs with the assistance of oxygen and is the most efficient mechanism of energy production employed by most multicellular organisms. In this process, glucose is oxidized to produce carbon dioxide, water, and adenosine triphosphate (ATP), which is the cellular medium of energy. This type of respiration is much more efficient than anaerobic respiration, with a maximum of 36 ATP molecules yielded from a molecule of glucose. Anaerobic respiration occurs under situations where oxygen is lacking or absent, leading to the incomplete metabolism of glucose and byproducts such as lactic acid or ethanol. Understanding these two types of respiration provides information on how organisms manage to fit into their worlds, maximize energy return, and longevity (Breit et al., 2018). Another critical aspect of respiration is the distinction between external and internal respiration. External respiration entails gas exchange between the air and blood within the lungs. This occurs primarily through diffusion, where oxygen from the air is moved into the blood, and carbon dioxide is transferred from the blood to the air exhaled. Internal respiration is a gas exchange at the cellular level, where oxygen is utilized in cellular respiration and carbon dioxide is generated as a waste product of metabolism. These two processes are critical to maintaining homeostasis, allowing cells to perform vital metabolic processes. The efficiency of both external and internal respiration is essential for the overall operation of the respiratory system because interacting processes allow organisms to survive irrespective of the varying environmental conditions (Natalia et al., 2016). Metabolic status may also define the type of respiration employed by an organism. For instance, during heavy physical activity, muscle cells switch to anaerobic respiration when oxygen supply is low, resulting in the temporary buildup of lactic acid and causing fatigue. Under an adequate oxygen supply, aerobic respiration predominates with increased energy returns for muscle activity. Such flexibility in energy production is an evolutionary advantage for organisms that can cope with variable oxygen supply and energy demand. Besides that, certain organisms' species, such as yeast, switch between anaerobic and aerobic respiration depending on oxygen levels, thus demonstrating the adaptive respiration processes. With advancing studies, ever more intricate interactions of respiration processes with body conditions continue to surface, emphasizing their role in health and disease control (Breit et al., 2018).

8.4.1. External Respiration: Gas Exchange in the Lungs

The process of external respiration is crucial for homeostasis within the human system. The process entails the exchange of gases—oxygen and carbon dioxide—between the atmosphere and the circulatory system via pulmonary alveoli in the lungs. In inhalation, atmospheric air enters the respiratory pathway and extends to the alveoli, where the oxygen-rich air comes into contact with pulmonary capillaries. Such an interface enables oxygen to diffuse across the alveolar membrane into the bloodstream and carbon dioxide, which is a by-product of metabolism, to diffuse out of the blood into the alveoli to be eliminated. This process of gas exchange is efficient in cellular respiration because it allows sufficient oxygen supply and also eliminates carbon dioxide efficiently, hence enabling metabolic processes at the cellular level. The lung's structural design significantly affects the efficiency of outside respiration. The lungs are made up of countless tiny air sacs known as alveoli, which occur in clusters of grapes to yield maximum surface space for gas exchange. The thin walls of alveoli, often only one cell layer thick, facilitate the rapid diffusion of gases between the air in the alveoli and the blood in the capillaries surrounding them. Additionally, the presence of surfactant—a substance that reduces surface tension—within the alveoli is critical, as it prevents the collapse of these structures and enhances gas exchange. This structural adaptation, with an enormous surface area, makes the lungs extremely effective in oxygenating blood and removing carbon dioxide, thereby laying the groundwork for efficient external respiration during various physiological conditions (Beebe et al., 2019). Additionally, external respiration is controlled by several physiological processes like ventilation, diffusion, and perfusion. Ventilation is the mechanical entrance and exit of air by the respiratory system as a consequence of pressure gradients provided by the diaphragm and intercostal muscles. Diffusion occurs within the alveoli, where gases diffuse across the respiratory membrane based on partial pressure gradients, such that oxygen diffuses into the blood and carbon dioxide diffuses out. The third, perfusion, deals with the flow of blood through pulmonary capillaries that surround the alveoli, ensuring that the blood is well oxygenated and free from excess carbon dioxide. All these components need to function optimally for external respiration to be efficient, since any compromise in one or several of them can lead to loss of efficiency in gas exchange, causing the patient to breathe in distress or fail (Bekish et al., 2017) (Figure 8.12).

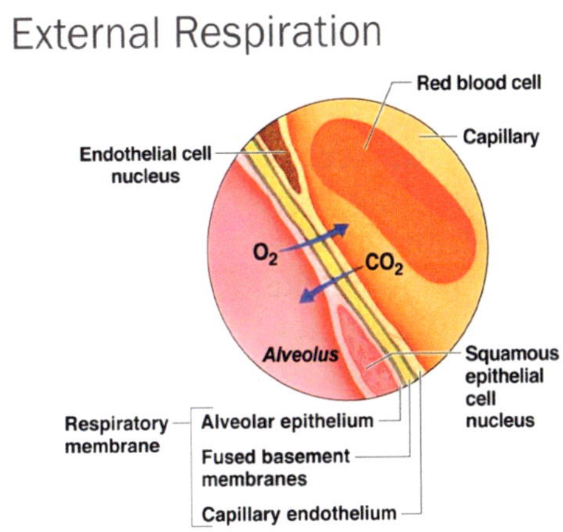

Figure 8.12. External respiration.

Source: https://image2.slideserve.com/5370082/external-respiration-l.jpg.

8.4.2. Internal Respiration: Gas Exchange at the Cellular Level

Internal respiration is a vital physiological process by which the interchange of gases between body cells and blood occurs. It is a form of respiration that appears at the cellular level, in which oxygen (O_2) is transported to the tissues from the blood and carbon dioxide (CO_2) is taken from the cells to the blood. The process is driven by the laws of diffusion, where gases diffuse from high concentration areas towards low concentration areas. The oxygen in the tissues gets used in cellular respiration to produce adenosine triphosphate (ATP), the energy currency of the cell, and it proves the interdependence of respiratory and metabolic processes. It is critical to sustaining cell processes and total metabolic equilibrium that such biochemical exchange occurs, specifically that cells require a constant supply of oxygen for aerobic respiration, which is more efficient than anaerobic alternatives. Various physiological variables, including circulation, the diffusion surface area, and partial pressures of O2 and CO2 in blood and tissue govern the internal respiration. For instance, when the body is more active, there is greater demand for O_2, leading to increased perfusion in active tissues. Increased perfusion increases oxygen delivery as well as carbon dioxide removal, thereby maintaining homeostatic balance. Further, the partial pressure of gases in the blood can also influence the rate of diffusion; higher oxygen levels in alveoli induce more uptake into the bloodstream, hence promoting higher internal respiration efficiency. All these processes highlight the need for controlling various physiological states to enhance gas exchange and cell respiration. Also, the function of internal respiration is not just about gas exchange since it has a direct connection to broader physiological and health implications. For example, diseases that interfere with circulation, such as cardiovascular ailments or shock, can significantly reduce the efficiency of internal respiration to the point of causing cellular hypoxia and, potentially, tissue damage. This has implications in numerous medical and health scenarios, where decreased oxygenation creates serious complications. Therefore, a full grasp of how internal respiration is conducted, as well as its control systems, is essential to clinicians and researchers who seek to treat respiratory and cardiovascular illness. Future studies may explore therapeutic interventions that can enhance internal respiration, particularly during pathological states, to enhance patient prognosis and tissue viability further (Bekish et al., 2014; Bekish et al., 2017) (Figure 8.13).

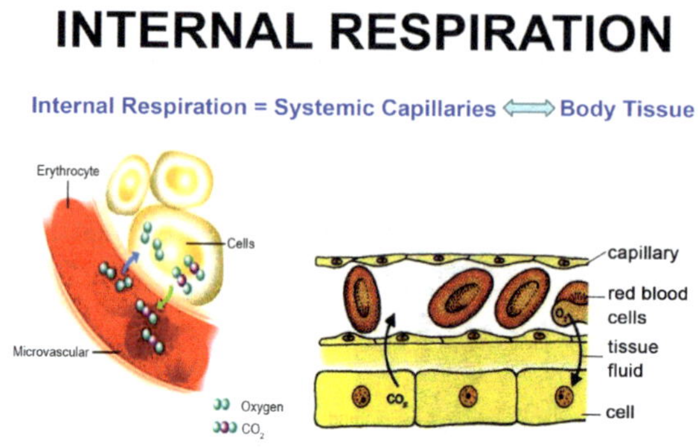

Figure 8.13. Internal respiration.

Source: https://image1.slideserve.com/3321367/internal-respiration-systemic-capillaries-body-tissue-l.jpg.

8.4.3. Cellular Respiration: Energy Production in Cells

Cellular respiration is an essential process of energy production in cells, wherein the biochemical energy of food is transferred to adenosine triphosphate (ATP), the primary energy currency of the cells. Cellular respiration is a complex process involving three primary stages: glycolysis, the Krebs cycle, and oxidative phosphorylation. Glycolysis occurs in the cytoplasm of the cell, where glucose is broken down into pyruvate, generating a net ATP gain of two molecules and two molecules of NADH. The subsequent Krebs cycle takes place in the mitochondria and produces additional NADH and flavin adenine dinucleotide (FADH2) and expels carbon dioxide as a byproduct. Finally, in oxidative phosphorylation, the electron transport chain generates most of the ATP by passing electrons from NADH and FADH2, ultimately reducing oxygen to form water. This beautiful coordination of biochemical processes emphasizes the importance of cellular respiration in sustaining life. The respiratory system supplements cellular respiration because it provides the means through which gases are exchanged to facilitate the production of ATP. When oxygen is inhaled into the body, it flows into the lungs and diffuses into the blood, which distributes it to cells throughout the body. The oxygen serves as the final electron acceptor in the electron transport chain, a key process in aerobic respiration by which cells can generate up to 34 molecules of ATP from a single molecule of glucose. In the absence of oxygen, anaerobic respiration occurs, which, although less efficient, enables cells to generate ATP through fermentation reactions, producing lactic acid or ethanol as waste products. The respiratory system, thus, not only supplies the necessary oxygen needed for maximal energy production but is also an essential function in carbon dioxide removal as a waste product of cell metabolism. Besides its primary purpose of energy production, cellular respiration is also involved in other metabolic processes in cells towards overall metabolic homeostasis. Not surprisingly, various energy substrates, such as fats and proteins, can be metabolized through the very same fundamental respiratory processes, testifying to the system's versatility. For instance, the ketogenic diet, under some conditions, can alter cellular respiration by promoting fat metabolism, with subsequent production of ketone bodies from fatty acids. This source of energy alternative is particularly significant under fasting or carbohydrate-restricted conditions, demonstrating the adaptability of cellular respiration to altered diet and metabolic demand. Lastly, the sophisticated relationship between cellular respiration and the respiratory system is essential to maintain energy balance and promote cellular function in various physiological conditions due to the complex interactions between different biological systems for sustaining life (Max et al., 2021; Zhu et al., 2022) (Figure 8.14).

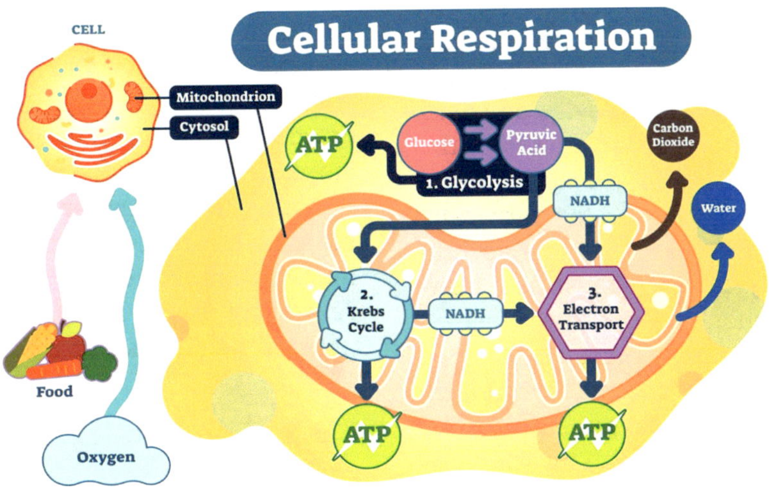

Figure 8.14. Cellular respiration.

Source: https://www.thoughtco.com/thmb/jZkrJoMIeDRpTxSMz_M-C2UJTfE=/1500x1000/filters:no_upscale():max_bytes(150000):strip_icc()/cellular_respiration-8fcc3f1ad3e54a828dabc02146ce4307.jpg.

Test Your Knowledge

1. What is external respiration, and how does gas exchange occur in the lungs?
2. How does internal respiration differ from external respiration, and where does it take place in the body?

8.5. Zones of the Respiratory System

Learning Outcome

1. Describe the conducting zone: pathways for air movement
2. Discuss the respiratory zone: sites of gas exchange
3. Explain the transitional zone: areas of mixed function

The respiratory system is broken down into distinct zones that maintain different functions essential for gas exchange and overall respiratory health. The conducting zone, composed primarily of the nasal cavity, pharynx, larynx, trachea, bronchi, and bronchioles, is the pathway through which air passes to the lungs. This region is also responsible for filtration, heating, and humidification of air inhaled into the body so that only the healthiest and best-conditioned air reaches the delicate alveolar structures. The intricate structural pattern of the conduits, including ciliated epithelium and mucous glands, is a testament to the system's ability to protect against pathogens and particulates, thus fulfilling a practical function in respiratory homeostasis (Bekish et al., 2014). In contrast, oxygen and carbon dioxide exchange occur in the respiratory zone. The respiratory zone consists of the respiratory bronchioles, the alveolar ducts, and numerous alveoli, the functional gas-exchange structures. The large surface area provided by the alveolar structure, together with the thin walls of the pulmonary capillaries, facilitates diffusion by which the oxygen is taken into the blood and carbon dioxide is removed from the blood. Understanding the physiology of the zones is essential to learn how to deal with numerous pathological conditions, such as COPD and pulmonary fibrosis, which can severely impair respiratory function and gas exchange (Bekish et al., 2017). Additionally, an understanding of the link between conducting and respiratory zones is essential to appreciate the effectiveness of the respiratory system. The transition from the conducting airways to the respiratory units also demonstrates the evolutionary modifications that make respiration successful. Lastly, the division between these regions is also valuable for clinical assessment and intervention strategies. For instance, understanding the applicability of conducting airways in the case of asthma emphasizes the use of both regions in treatment planning. With further investigation into these regions, effective treatment plans will become more and more reliant on detailed information regarding respiratory system anatomy and physiology (Bekish et al., 2014).

8.5.1. Conducting Zone: Pathways for Air Movement

The conducting portion of the respiratory system is vital in enabling airflow to the lungs, offering a passage for oxygen to be distributed to the alveoli for exchange. The conducting area comprises several anatomical structures that involve the nasal cavity, pharynx, larynx, trachea, bronchi, and bronchioles. Every structure is specialized to perform vital functions, which involve filtering, humidifying, and warming the air breathed in. For instance, the nasal tract has mucous membranes and cilia that trap particulate matter and microorganisms so that a purer air source enters the lower respiratory system. This preliminary filtration is crucial because it keeps the delicate lung tissues safe from damage that certain inhaled pollutants and germs are likely to cause. Deeper into the respiratory system, the trachea is a wide passage that brings air to the bronchi, which divide further into smaller bronchioles. These are conducting zone structures that taper progressively but maintain airflow to alveoli. Interestingly, the transition from the trachea to the main bronchi is a site of significant transition in the respiratory system; it illustrates the branching pattern that most efficiently disperses air. Furthermore, bronchial and bronchiole wall smooth muscle allows dynamic regulation of airway passage and allows for bronchoconstriction and bronchodilation in response to a wide range of stimuli. This versatility is necessary in ensuring adequate respiratory capacity with shifting physical requirements and environmental conditions. Throughout the conducting airway, the role of the mucociliary escalator functions is evident in maintaining respiratory health. This biological process relies on the coordinated movement of mucus and cilia to clear trash and bacteria from the airways, preventing inflammation and infection. Disruption of the process can lead to respiratory disease, emphasizing the significance of each component in the conducting zone. A greater understanding of these pathways leads to clinical strategies to improve respiratory function and target disorders such as asthma and chronic obstructive pulmonary disease. Thus, through the study of conducting zones pathways in entirety, we are taught valuable lessons regarding the respiratory system context, which is essential for sustaining life through effective gas exchange and homeostasis (Bekish et al., 2014; Beebe et al., 2019) (Figure 8.15).

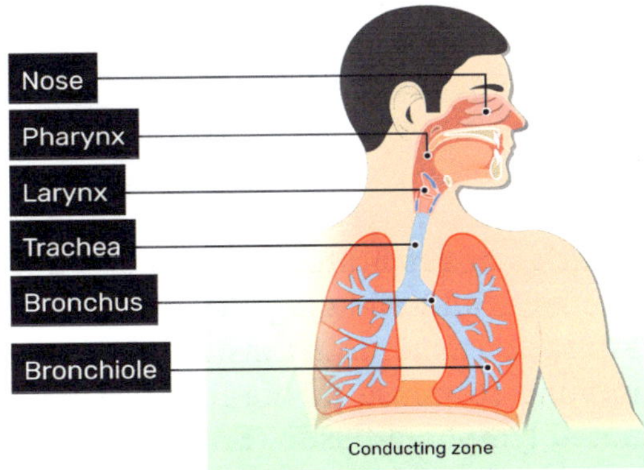

Figure 8.15. Conducting zone.

Source: https://www.getbodysmart.com/wp-content/uploads/2017/09/Respiratory-Conducting-Zone-1024x732.png.

8.5.2. Respiratory Zone: Sites of Gas Exchange

The lung's respiratory zone is crucial for the mechanism of gas exchange, whereby oxygen and carbon dioxide are traded between air and blood. The respiratory zone consists primarily of structures such as the alveoli, respiratory bronchioles, and alveolar ducts. Alveoli are small, sac-like structures that create a large surface area, approximately 70 square meters in the average adult lung. The walls of the alveoli are fragile, essentially a single layer of epithelial cells, to enable efficient diffusion of gases. This is an essential anatomical structure for the maintenance of steep concentration gradients necessary for gas exchange to allow the ingress of oxygen into the blood and the egress of carbon dioxide from the blood. In the respiratory zone, the alveoli are encompassed by capillaries in an extensive network to enable the exchange of gases. The proximity of the pulmonary capillaries and the walls of the alveoli is significant, as it allows for oxygen to diffuse from the air into the alveoli to the blood and carbon dioxide to diffuse in the opposite direction. This exchange process relies on the differences in partial pressure, a principle that describes the efficiency of the respiratory system. Alveolar macrophages are also essential to respiratory zone health through the elimination of extraneous material and bacteria, which can hamper gas exchange function. Understanding these dynamics is crucial for grasping the complexities of respiratory physiology and its impact on overall well-being. Besides, the role of the respiratory zones is intrinsically linked with the immune response in the lungs. Bronchus-associated lymphoid tissue (BALT) allows for a successful immune defense, particularly in birds, whose respiratory tract is exposed to pathogens continuously. BALT at bifurcations of the primary and secondary bronchi matures upon maturity in birds to provide a crucial interface for immune responses to respiratory infections. Research indicates that compartmentalization of immune responses in this tissue is to play a pivotal role in the manner in which the lungs respond to a variety of pathogens (Dalamani et al., 2006). This sophisticated connection between gas exchange and protection from disease indicates the respiratory zone's multifunctional nature in its role in maintaining not only respiratory health but also overall resilience and well-being and disease resistance (Beebe et al., 2019) (Figure 8.16).

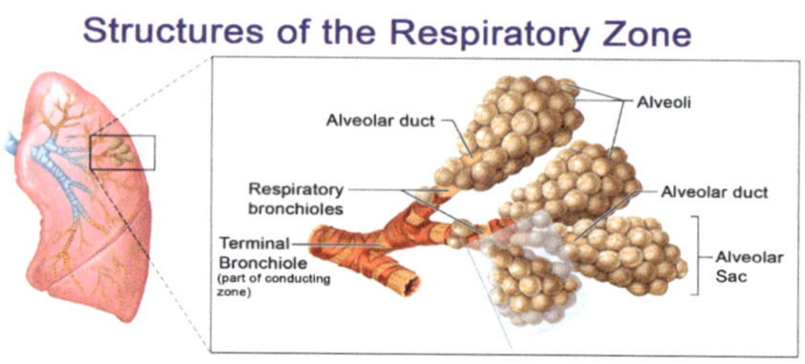

Figure 8.16. Structures of respiratory zone.

Source: https://antranik.org/wp-content/uploads/2024/10/structures-of-respiratory-zone-alveoli-alveolar-duct-alceolar-sac-alveolar-duct-respiratory-bronchioles-terminal-bronchiole.jpg.

8.5.3. Transitional Zone: Areas of Mixed Function

The transitional zone in the respiratory system covers zones with combined functions that are essential for air conduction and conditioning. The regions function to fill the gap between the upper and lower respiratory tracts and encompass structures such as the bronchi and bronchioles. The principal role of these areas is to ensure that inhaled air is adequately warmed, humidified, and filtered before it entered into sensitive alveoli, in which gas exchange occurs. This twofold role maintains the integrity of lung tissue as well as ensures maximum efficiency of oxygen absorption and carbon dioxide removal. Knowledge of the significance of transition zones makes sense of the intricate engineering of the respiratory pathway, highlighting how each structure helps in overall respiratory function. In addition to their role in air conditioning, transition zones are significant sites for respiratory defensive functions. The mucous-secreting cells and cilia lining the epithelial lining of bronchi and bronchioles trap and remove foreign matter, bacteria, and other pollutants from the airways. This protective function is vital, particularly in an era marked by overwhelming environmental pollution and respiratory illness. Coordination between ciliary movement and mucus secretion is essential to providing clear airways and preventing infection. As described in studies on the effectiveness of such defense mechanisms, the transitional zones represent a first line of defense against airborne pathogens and assist in resistance in the overall respiratory system (Beebe et al., 2019). The transitional zones function is also not restricted to processes of mere air processing and defense; it encompasses significant physiologic adjustments for the needs of different activities, such as exercise. During exercise, oxygen requirements are greater; accordingly, bronchi and bronchioles dilate to allow passage of air to the alveoli. Such a response is mediated by hormonal as well as neural signals, underscoring the adaptability of the respiratory system. The importance of adaptability is phenomenal, especially in sports training and rehabilitation, where understanding the functioning of transitional areas can predetermine therapeutic interventions. An understanding of such complexities reaffirms the necessity of such mixed-function spaces in the provision of respiratory efficiency and general physiological health (Bekish et al., 2014) (Figure 8.17).

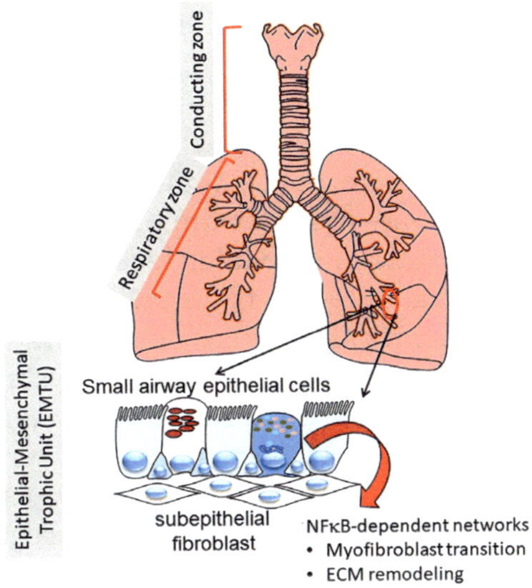

Figure 8.17. Transition zone in airway remodeling.

Source: https://www.researchgate.net/publication/357256227/figure/fig1/AS:11431281251855820@1718383194390/Role-of-the-transition-zone-in-airway-remodeling-Shown-is-a-schematic-view-of-the-human.tif.

Test Your Knowledge

1. What structures make up the conducting zone of the respiratory system, and what is their primary function?
2. Which parts of the respiratory system are included in the respiratory zone, and how do they facilitate gas exchange?

SUMMARY

The respiratory system is a delicate and vital aspect of human physiology, assigned the function of gas exchange to sustain life. The harmonious activities of its structural anatomy, from the nasal cavity all the way down to the alveoli, demonstrate the delicate efficiency of the system with respect to oxygenation and carbon dioxide elimination. Both of the organs, whether the trachea, bronchi, or lungs, play a specific and integral part, yet one which draws attention to the way their interrelation guarantees that respiration, far from being merely mechanical, is also a function inextricably involved with general well-being and homeostasis. Moreover, an appreciation of the numerous functions of the respiratory system draws attention to its significance in multiple body processes, including metabolic regulation and acid-base homeostasis, and thereby renders the respiratory physiology complex. Furthermore, the separation of respiration into distinct categories—such as external and internal respiration—provides the opportunity to structure the investigation of oxygen utilization at both the systemic and cellular levels. External respiration is the physical exchange of gases in the lungs, whereas internal respiration is the cellular uptake of oxygen and release of carbon dioxide. This divorce not only fortifies our understanding of respiratory mechanics but also suggests how disruption in either mode can lead to systemic complexities. For instance, pathophysiological conditions such as chronic obstructive pulmonary disease (COPD) are primarily about external respiration, thus impacting the effectiveness of internal respiration, referring to the interdependence of both processes. Both forms of respiration are essential building blocks for fully understanding how oxygen drives cellular respiration, thereby regulating metabolism and energy production. Finally, this examination of the respiratory system illustrates its structural areas—like the conducting and respiratory zones—and the specific functions they serve. The conducting zone, consisting of the upper and lower airways, is necessary for filtering, warming, and humidifying the incoming air. In contrast, the respiratory zone, primarily the alveolar regions, is where the most critical function of gas exchange occurs. Understanding these zones accounts for the physiological and anatomical adjustments that allow respiration to be adequate under a variety of circumstances. The emphasis on definitions and terminologies of the regions is significant in advancing quality communication within the medical fraternity, as reflected in the appeal for definite terminology that reflects scientific coherence and congruence. With the growth of literature, there is a need to offer terminological consistency to enhance academic discourse and clinical practice (Bekish et al., 2014; AlMehzaa et al., 2019).

The human body is maintained in homeostasis through the functions, structure, anatomy, and organs of the respiratory system. Essentially, the system facilitates gas exchange where oxygen gets into the bloodstream and carbon dioxide, which is a product of metabolism and a waste, is released. This critical process is enabled by sophisticated structures, such as the lungs, trachea, and bronchi, that create a maximum surface area for gas exchange. By understanding the architecture of the respiratory system collectively, it is apparent how pathological processes can interfere with these critical processes and result in diminished health. Research on the respiratory mechanisms that ensure respiratory functioning is ongoing, honing our comprehension of how intricate components interlock to uphold life (N/A, 2025). Moreover, the division of respiration into various types, external and internal respiration, highlights the multiple stages at which the respiratory system functions. External respiration is the exchange of gases between the external world and lungs, while internal respiration is the exchange of gases between tissue and blood. This is important for the understanding of the utilization of oxygen at the cellular level as well as the rise in the body's demand for oxygen while exercising or in disease processes. Besides, zoning of the regions within the respiratory system, such as the conducting and respiratory zones, highlights functional diversity typical of the system. Not only are the zones structurally diverse, but they also have disparate functions, which further highlight respiratory physiology complexity (Karolewski et al., 2013). A thorough description of the respiratory system shows a sophisticated interaction of its functions, structures, and varieties of respiration. Each organ and area within the system has a specific role in accomplishing the entire goal of gas exchange, demonstrating the importance of each part to overall respiratory health. These points not only serve to increase our knowledge of human physiology but also serve as a basis for future research in respiratory disease and therapy. The current study of this discipline holds the promise of guiding towards more effective therapeutic interventions that can enhance the quality of life in patients with respiratory disorders, deepening insight into complicated systems that sustain life (N/A, 2025).

KEY TERMS FROM THIS CHAPTER

- Nasal Cavity
- Larynx
- Bronchi
- Alveoli
- Pleura
- Intercostal Muscles
- External Respiration
- Gas Exchange
- Pharynx
- Trachea
- Bronchioles
- Lungs
- Diaphragm
- Pulmonary Ventilation
- Internal Respiration
- Oxygen Transport

CRITICAL THINKING QUESTIONS

1. **What is the main function of the respiratory system?**
   a. Pump blood throughout the body
   b. Break down food for energy
   c. Exchange oxygen and carbon dioxide between the body and environment
   d. Produce hormones
2. **Which of the following structures is the site of gas exchange in the lungs?**
   a. Trachea
   b. Bronchi
   c. Alveoli
   d. Larynx
3. **The diaphragm plays a key role in:**
   a. Circulating blood
   b. Digesting food
   c. Controlling vocal cords
   d. Breathing by contracting and expanding the lungs
4. **What is the pathway of air as it enters the respiratory system?**
   a. Pharynx → Larynx → Trachea → Bronchi → Alveoli
   b. Larynx → Pharynx → Bronchi → Trachea → Alveoli
   c. Bronchi → Trachea → Alveoli → Pharynx → Larynx
   d. Trachea → Pharynx → Larynx → Bronchi → Alveoli
5. **Which part of the respiratory system prevents food from entering the trachea?**
   a. Epiglottis
   b. Uvula
   c. Larynx
   d. Pharynx

Short Answer Questions

1. What are the main functions of the respiratory system?
2. How does the respiratory system help in gas exchange?
3. Name the major organs involved in the respiratory system.
4. What is the role of the diaphragm in respiration?
5. What are the two main types of respiration?
6. Differentiate between internal and external respiration.
7. What are the two zones of the respiratory system?
8. Which structures belong to the conducting zone and which to the respiratory zone?

Answer to Critical Thinking Questions

1. (c); 2. (c); 3. (d); 4. (a); 5. (a)

REFERENCES

1. Abdul, N., Sarwani, L., Fatima, A., James, H., Ebrahim, H., Almehzaa, A., & Chakravarty, M. (2019). Exploring use of incorrect terminology used in medical sciences: quest for scientific and academic verity. *Journal of Education and Practice*. https://doi.org/10.7176/jep/10-6-19Beebe, L., Hesse, D., & Massey, A. (2019). *UGA Anatomy and Physiology 2 Lab Manual* (3rd ed.). https://core.ac.uk/download/217306575.pdf (accessed on 14th June 2025).
2. Bekish, V. J., & Zorina, V. V. (2014). *Biology*. https://core.ac.uk/download/80152204.pdf (accessed on 14th June 2025).
3. Bekish, V. J., Logishinets, I. A., & Zorina, V. V. (2017). *Practical Book on Biology*. https://core.ac.uk/download/80152210.pdf (accessed on 14th June 2025).
4. Bhagirath, A. Y., Li, Y., Somayajula, D., Dadashi, M., Badr, S., & Duan, K. (2016). Cystic fibrosis lung environment and *Pseudomonas aeruginosa* infection. *BMC Pulmonary Medicine, 16*. https://doi.org/10.1186/s12890-016-0339-5 (accessed on 14th June 2025).
5. Breit, S., Kupferberg, A., Rogler, G., & Hasler, G. (2018). Vigus nerve as modulator of the brain–gut axis in psychiatric and inflammatory disorders. *Frontiers in Psychiatry, 9*. https://doi.org/10.3389/fpsyt.2018.00044 (accessed on 14th June 2025).
6. Cryan, S. A., Gilbert, J. L., O'Brien, F., O'Dea, S., et al. (2015). Respiratory tissue engineering: Current status and opportunities for the future. https://core.ac.uk/download/pdf/60777392.pdf (accessed on 14th June 2025).
7. Dalamani, G., Kaspers, B., & Reese, S. (2006). The avian lung-associated immune system. https://core.ac.uk/download/12174987.pdf (accessed on 14th June 2025).
8. Erdő, F., Bors, L. A., Farkas, D. L., Bajza, Á., & Gizurarson, S. (2018). Evaluation of intranasal delivery route of drug administration for brain targeting. *Brain Research Bulletin, 143*, 155–170. https://doi.org/10.1016/j.brainresbull.2018.10.009 (accessed on 14th June 2025).
9. Gkatzis, K., Taghizadeh, S., Huh, D., Stainier, D. Y. R., & Bellusci, S. (2018). Use of three-dimensional organoids and lung-on-a-chip methods to study lung development, regeneration and disease. *European Respiratory Journal, 52*, 1800876–1800876. https://doi.org/10.1183/13993003.00876-2018 (accessed on 14th June 2025).
10. Grigoriadis, K., Efstathiou, I., Petrianos, I., Bakalidou, D., Armaganidis, A., & Vasileiadis, G. (2009). Improvement of patient's ventilation by correcting the slid recumbent position in the ICU. https://www.semanticscholar.org/paper/d49a9494f68f75fe1b472ed2c19a5382c2fff31e (accessed on 14th June 2025).
11. Karolewski, P., Oleksyn, J., Schnitzer, S. A., Wyka, T., et al. (2013). Phenotypic correlates of the lianescent growth form: A review. https://core.ac.uk/download/237217373.pdf (accessed on 14th June 2025).
12. Keeley, T. P., & Mann, G. E. (2018). Defining physiological normoxia for improved translation of cell physiology to animal models and humans. *Physiological Reviews, 99*, 161–234. https://doi.org/10.1152/physrev.00041.2017 (accessed on 14th June 2025).
13. Keller, L. A., Merkel, O. M., & Popp, A. (2021). Intranasal drug delivery: Opportunities and toxicologic challenges during drug development. *Drug Delivery and Translational Research, 12*, 735–757. https://doi.org/10.1007/s13346-020-00891-5 (accessed on 14th June 2025).

14. Kulish, V., Lage, J. L., & Sourin, A. (2006). Fundamentals of alveolar gas diffusion: Mathematical modeling and visualization. *WIT Transactions on State-of-the-Art in Science and Engineering, 24.* https://www.semanticscholar.org/paper/b899714d0aba93a33ed2a36335f7d5b59134067e (accessed on 14th June 2025).
15. Møller, I. M., Rasmusson, A. G., & Van Aken, O. (2021). Plant mitochondria–past, present and future. *The Plant Journal, 108*, 912–959. https://doi.org/10.1111/tpj.15495 (accessed on 14th June 2025).
16. N/A. (2025). *Aerospace Medicine and Biology: A Continuing Bibliography with Indexes, Supplement 128, May 1974.* https://core.ac.uk/download/pdf/42893566.pdf (accessed on 14th June 2025).
17. N/A. (2025). *Aerospace Medicine and Biology: A Continuing Bibliography with Indexes (Supplement 309).* https://core.ac.uk/download/pdf/42832898.pdf (accessed on 14th June 2025).
18. Parlak Ak, T. (2021). Bronchus-associated lymphoid tissue (BALT) histology and its role in various pathologies. https://core.ac.uk/download/479934915.pdf (accessed on 14th June 2025).
19. Pérez Harguindeguy, N., Díaz, S., Garnier, É., Lavorel, S., Poorter, H., Jaureguiberry, P., Bret-Harte, M. S., et al. (2016). Corrigendum to: New handbook for standardized measurement of plant functional traits worldwide. *Australian Journal of Botany, 64*, 715–715. https://doi.org/10.1071/bt12225_co (accessed on 14th June 2025).
20. Sabuncuoğlu, S., Yalçınkaya, A., Zhou, X., Münch, G., Chang, D., Borrelli, E., Le, N. A., et al. (2022). Importance of oxidative stress and antioxidant system in health and disease. *Biochemistry.* https://doi.org/10.5772/intechopen.100949 (accessed on 14th June 2025).
21. Skoyles, J. R. (2008). Respiratory, postural and spatio-kinetic motor stabilization, internal models, top-down timed motor coordination and expanded cerebella-cerebral circuitry: A review. https://core.ac.uk/download/pdf/1569872.pdf (accessed on 14th June 2025).
22. Zhu, H., Bi, D., Zhang, Y., Kong, C., Du, J., Wu, X., Wei, Q., et al. (2022). Ketogenic diet for human diseases: The underlying mechanisms and potential for clinical implementations. *Signal Transduction and Targeted Therapy, 7.* https://doi.org/10.1038/s41392-021-00831-w (accessed on 14th June 2025).

THE DIGESTIVE SYSTEM

9

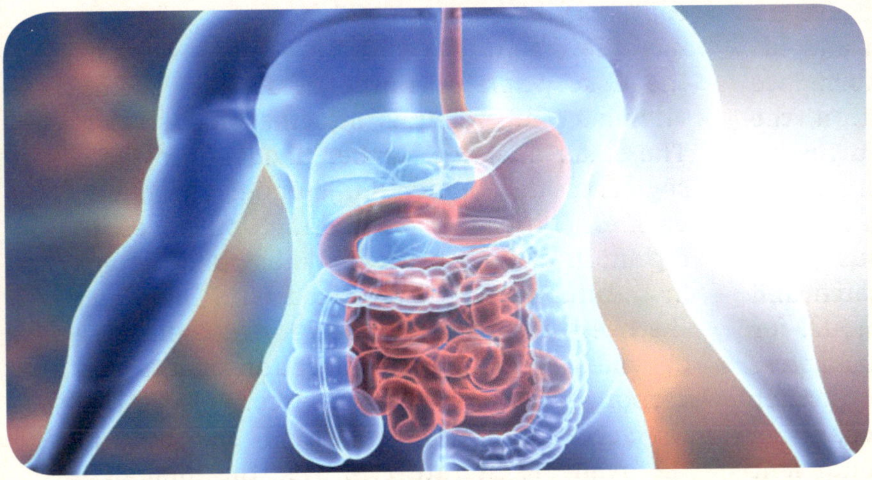

Introduction

The digestive system is a complex system that processes food, digests and absorbs nutrients and waste, and is generally responsible for the well-being of an organism. The complex system begins when food enters the organism and winds its way through the organism with numerous organs, including the stomach and intestines, where enzymatic reactions break down food into functional molecules. All components of the digestive system are specialized in a specific function that facilitates effective regulation of diverse food sources. Effectiveness is essential, especially with nutrients from foods that sustain cell processes and contribute to energy metabolism. Digestive system physiology encompasses not only its structure and function but also host-microbiota interaction, which significantly contributes to digestive health and overall health. The other essential element of the digestive system is the host organism-microbiota balance, the complex assembly of microbes residing in the gastrointestinal tract.

LEARNING OBJECTIVES

After studying this chapter, you will be able to:

1. Explain the anatomy and major organs involved in the digestive system
2. Explain the sequential process of digestion
3. Explain the role and function of enzymes to break down food in digestion
4. Describe common digestive disorders
5. Explain how different food habits influence the digestive system
6. Explain the role played by the gut microbiome in facilitating digestion

This symbiotic balance, or Eubiosis, centers on human physiology compatibility with microbial inhabitants of their body. Deteriorations in this compatibility can generate asymptomatic but deep ill health, such as dysbiosis. Recent evidence has described a link between altered gut microbiota and a range of conditions, most notably inflammatory bowel diseases, whose rising incidence has implications for gut health and physiology in general. Such dynamics become elementary when viewed against the broader context of digestive health because the symbiotic relationship between man and his microbiota is pivotal to the ideal performance of the digestive apparatus. In addition, the mention of organisms with specialist digestive specializations, such as *Nepenthes glandulifera*, serves to reveal interesting facts about other modes of digestion. This carnivorous plant employs modified pitcher traps to catch and digest insects and presents a single model for nutrient uptake via secretory and absorptive mechanisms. The digestive fluid of pitcher plants illustrates the evolutionary mechanisms through which it will thrive under subnutrient conditions, as opposed to human digestion. It has been found through studies that these plants have developed complex transport mechanisms for nutrient acquisition, and the investigation of these unusual digestive systems provides essential insights into human health that can inform treatment strategies for digestive diseases and optimal nutrient uptake in all organisms.

Definition of the Digestive System

The digestive system is a complex collection of glands and organs that cooperate to break down food, remove waste, and absorb nutrients. Essentially, the system begins in the mouth, where mechanical and chemical digestion begin. Saliva secreted from salivary glands contains enzymes that start the breakdown of carbohydrates, and chewing physically tears food. Food also undergoes greater chemical and mechanical digestion in transit from the esophagus to the stomach. The hydrochloric acid and protein-digestion-specific enzymes of the stomach mix into a liquid state called chyme, which is then passed on to the small intestine for further processing. Understanding early digestion is the basis of understanding how to absorb and use needed nutrients, as well as how digestive diseases would impact overall health. The majority of nutrient absorption occurs in the small intestine, following the stomach. It contains villi and microvilli, which significantly increase the surface area. These organs enable the absorption of amino acids, fatty acids, vitamins, and minerals into the bloodstream. The small intestine further divides into three segments: the duodenum, jejunum, and ileum, each of which serves distinct purposes in digestion and absorption. When food arrives in the duodenum, it is mixed with bile from the liver and pancreatic secretions containing enzymes crucial to the digestion of fats and carbohydrates. The intricate composition of the secretions during digestion, discussed in the available literature, proves the biological necessity of effective nutrient absorption towards health and wellness. This is proof of the high correlation between digestion and body metabolic processes necessary for sustaining human life (Edwards et al., 2020). Digestion is more than nutrient absorption; it includes the body's ability for waste product removal. Once the nutrients are absorbed in the small intestine, the remaining undigested residue enters the large intestine, where water and electrolytes are absorbed. There are healthy bacteria present in the colon that assist in the fermentation of indigestible fiber and, hence, assist in maintaining a healthy digestive process. Waste material then gets molded into feces, which is evacuated out of the body by the anus and rectum. Further, the digestive system is magnificent in that it accommodates various elements of diet, as certain foods affect the speed of digestion and overall well-being of the gut. Such information allows for knowledge regarding the function of the digestive system in human body physiology and how the system interfaces with habits of lifestyle and the etiology of gastrointestinal disease (Gaiseanu et al., 2018).

Importance of Digestion in Overall Health

To understand the function of digestion in overall health is to recognize its relationship with the nutrients necessary for proper body functioning. Digestion is not a mechanical function but rather one that relates most directly with biochemical processes that convert food into energy and materials for cellular development and maintenance. The digestive process breaks down complex food material into absorptive, digestible units through enzymatic processes, in which each step serves a unique role in homeostasis. As the literature explains, coordination among foods, metabolism, and overall health maintains active interchange between diet and body function. Lastly, digestion is the process of nutrient intake, which leads to boosted energy, enhanced immunity, and reduced susceptibility to disease, emphasizing the significance that health relies on what one consumes and how well our bodies can metabolize such substances (Sarmidi et al., 2012). Aside from mere nutrient uptake, the function of digestion also plays a significant role in preventing generalized metabolic disease. A healthy gut can ward off diseases such as obesity, which in today's modern world is increasingly prevalent. The relationship between digestion and long-term health outcomes is highlighted by the manner in which delivery of nutrients impacts metabolic health. Where the digestive process is flawed, as is mirrored in the majority of gastrointestinal diseases, the likelihood of acquiring long-term diseases like type 2 diabetes greatly increases. Personalized education interventions were reported to enhance nutritional knowledge and its impact on health, particularly among vulnerable populations (Belcourt et al., 2012) (Figure 9.1).

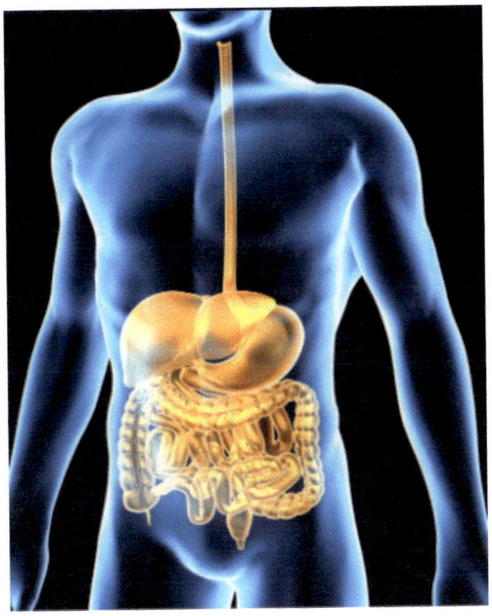

Figure 9.1. Illustration of the human digestive system, showing major organs involved in digestion.

Source: https://www.verywellhealth.com/thmb/8uwvIwgtVKuED83KkFL3juq4I7M=/1500x0/filters:no_upscale():max_bytes(150000):strip_icc()/human-digestive-system--artwork-136811327-599a0ae603f4020011c410a6.jpg.

This makes it essential to incorporate proper nutrition education in health systems because it encourages individuals to make informed decisions about their diet, thereby achieving complete well-being through enhanced digestion. Along with this, the function of digestion enters the field of mental wellness and health, aligning with the gut-brain axis that has gained extensive popularity over the past few years. There is emerging evidence that the gut microbiome, promoted by what we eat, modulates mood and intellectual function. High-fiber intake, probiotics, and prebiotics establish healthy gut microbiota, which has been demonstrated to reduce symptoms of depression and anxiety. In addition, the digestive processes can generate a sense of general well-being, as foods high in nutrients provide the materials for the building of neurotransmitters. With an understanding of the interdependence between digestion and emotional well-being, it is easy to understand that overall wellness must recognize diet and digestion as part of a larger matrix of overall health routines, affirming the necessity that these both have in achieving ultimate well-being (Sarmidi et al., 2012).

9.1. Anatomy of the Digestive System

Learning Outcome

1. Define the major organs involved in digestion
2. Analyze the accessory organs and their functions
3. Describe the role of the gastrointestinal tract

The anatomy of the digestive system is intricate, with many organs working in concert to break down food, absorb the nutrients, and eliminate waste. It begins in the mouth through mechanical digestion by chewing and enzymatic digestion with saliva. The food moves on down the esophagus, a muscular tube that employs peristalsis to propel the bolus into the stomach. In this, the food is further digested by gastric acids and enzymes into a semi-liquid food termed chyme. This indicates structural specialization of the digestive system, where every component is anatomically adapted to carry out specific functions, thus optimizing food processing as the food moves through the system. Understanding these body structures is key to research regarding how dysfunction can affect overall well-being and nutrition, so the study of the digestive tract is relevant. Chyme is drained from the stomach into the small intestine, a very specialized organ responsible for the absorption of nutrients. The small intestine is three separate segments: the duodenum, jejunum, and ileum, all involved in other phases of digestion and absorption. The duodenum is supported by the pancreas and liver secretions that contribute to neutralization of acid from the stomach and ongoing digestion of macronutrients. Jejunum and ileum are well supplied with villi and microvilli that offer excellent surface area for absorption, making vitamins, minerals, and other components to be significantly absorbed into the bloodstream. Besides, the relationship between the anatomy of the small intestine and its abundant supply of blood highlights its role in nutritional well-being and overall health.

Its disturbance at this level leads to malabsorption syndromes, highlighting the anatomy and function of its role. Not only is the anatomy of digestion limited to the gastrointestinal tract, but also to accessory organs like the liver and pancreas, playing an essential role in digestion as well as metabolic regulation. The liver provides bile for fat emulsification, whereas the pancreas delivers digestive enzymes and bicarbonate for neutralization of small intestine chyme. Coordination of these processes is essential, as highlighted in bariatric surgical patients, where anatomical changes in the body lead to complications such as pancreatic exocrine insufficiency (PEI) due to alterations in the secretion of digestive enzymes and gut anatomy. Presentation and symptoms of PEI are the same as other gastrointestinal diseases, hence making its diagnosis complicated; therefore, it is vital to have adequate knowledge of digestive anatomy. Also, management of these complications by using effective treatment options, including replacement therapy with pancreatic enzymes, is critical to digestive function and health recovery among affected patients (Arnelo et al., 2017) (Figure 9.2).

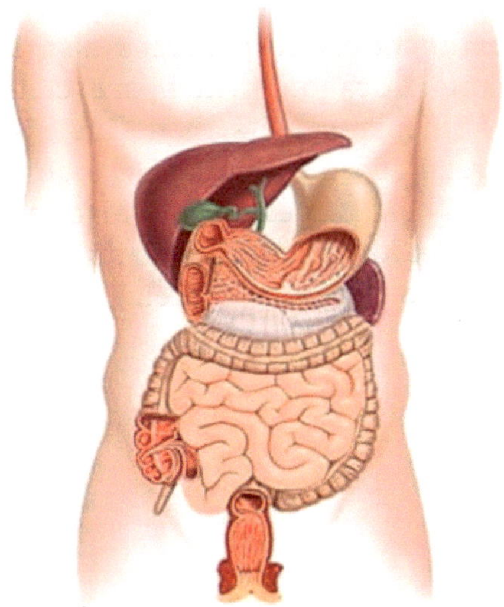

Figure 9.2. The digestive system.

Source: https://muschealth.org/-/sm/health/ddc/i/digestive-system-cutaway.jpg?h=333&w=300&hash=A7CB01ADCFA5AAB115AF7F458C30EFF8.

9.1.1. Major Organs Involved in Digestion

Digestion activities are performed via the services of several major organs that function in concert to ensure the body receives vital nutrients. Digestion begins in the mouth, where food undergoes mechanical breakdown via chewing. Salivary glands produce saliva and has enzymes like amylase that initiate the digestion of carbohydrates. As food is swallowed, it goes through the muscular tube, the esophagus, which forces it into the stomach. Inside the stomach, gastric juices composed of hydrochloric acid and pepsin further digest food, especially proteins, into a semiliquid state known as chyme. The stomach is not only a place where digestion occurs, but it is also tasked with regulating the release of chyme into the intestines so that digestion will proceed smoothly into the subsequent stage of nutrient absorption and utilization. Then comes the small intestine, which is the primary site where nutrients are absorbed. The three divisions of the small intestine are the duodenum, jejunum, and ileum, each with various roles in digestion and absorption. The duodenum, being the initial component, is where chyme is mixed with bile from the liver and pancreatic juices that have enzymes, further digesting carbohydrates, proteins, and fats. Jejunum and ileum are covered with villi and microvilli, which expand the surface area for absorption to let the nutrients reach the bloodstream efficiently (Figure 9.3).

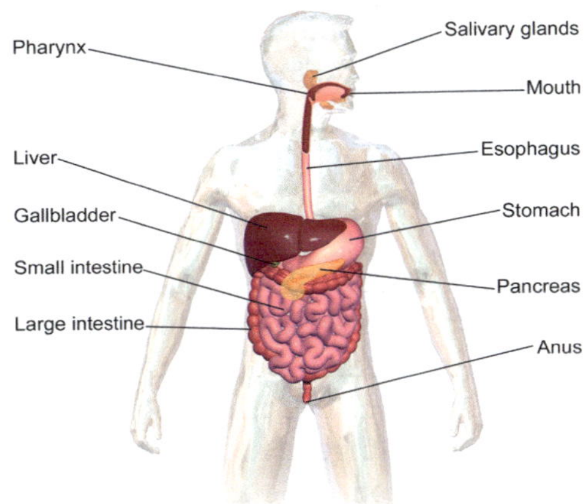

Figure 9.3. Organs of the human digestive system.

Source: https://dravinashtank.in/education/organs-of-the-human-digestive-system-an-in-depth-look/.

This intricate structure retains the primary function of the small intestine, which is to break down complex food components into fundamental molecules usable and processed by cells throughout the body. The efficiency of the process plays a huge role in overall health since nutrients provide fuel and material for physiological functions. Once the small intestine is done with it, the remaining undigested material is passed on to the large intestine, which performs several crucial roles. The primary role of the large intestine is the absorption of water and electrolytes, turning liquid waste into solid waste that can be expelled. Secondly, it has a complex microbiome, which is tasked with additional fermentation processes capable of extracting remaining nutrients from food. Large intestine walls have specialized cells that allow the large intestine to absorb vitamins such as vitamin K and part of the B vitamins, which are synthesized by bacteria in the gut. Lastly, the large intestine finishes digesting food by packing waste into the feces, which is prepared for expulsion. Large intestine well-being is vital to the body's fluid and electrolyte balance, placing it at the core of the entire digestive system and having an essential impact on overall health (Edwards et al., 2020; Patwardhan et al., 2008).

9.1.2. Accessory Organs and Their Functions

The accessory organs of the digestive tract include the liver, pancreas, and gallbladder, which are all responsible for breaking down and absorbing nutrients from food. The accessory organs are all included in the digestive processes together with the major components of the digestive tract, but not part of the gastrointestinal (GI) tract. The liver, for instance, is responsible for the secretion of bile, a compound essential in the emulsification of fats. This function enhances the absorption of lipids in the small intestine and thus the breakdown of fats. Moreover, the liver further processes other nutrients and removes toxins from the body, further emphasizing its diversified function in digestion (Rucker et al., 1901). Through breaking down and absorbing the nutrients to the best of its ability, the liver supplies the body with the pieces of the puzzle necessary to function at top capacity. The pancreas also complements the liver's function by secreting digestive enzymes and blood sugar-balancing hormones. It secretes proteases, amylases, and lipases into the duodenum to hydrolyze proteins, carbohydrates, and fats, respectively, during digestion. This enzymatic function is particularly significant as it allows the body to hydrolyze complex food molecules to simpler, absorbable entities. Apart from its digestive function, the pancreas also secretes insulin and glucagon, which are critical for glucose homeostasis. Its dual role highlights the pancreas as an essential accessory organ that not only aids digestion but also influences metabolic health, emphasizing its role in the context of the digestive system (Hideo et al., 2016) (Figure 9.4).

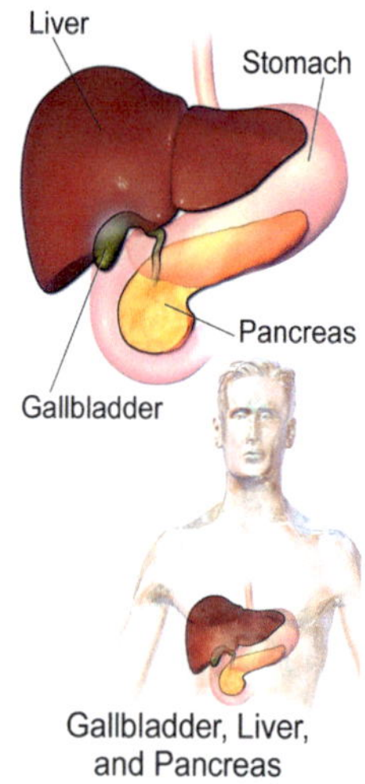

Figure 9.4. Accessory organs of digestion.

Source: https://humanbiology.pressbooks.tru.ca/wp-content/uploads/sites/6/2019/06/Blausen_0428_Gallbladder-Liver-Pancreas_Location-1.png.

Lacking the subtle regulating action of the pancreas, the efficiency of nutrient absorption would be significantly diminished. The gallbladder acts as a specialized unit that combines the action of the liver and pancreas. Its primary role is to sequester and concentrate bile produced by the liver until needed for digestion. Whenever food, particularly fatty food, reaches the small intestine, the gallbladder secretes bile to aid in fat emulsification. This is necessary in achieving maximum fat absorption and, by extension, adequate absorption of fat-soluble vitamins (A, D, E, and K). Bile concentration by the gallbladder enables the digestive system to act promptly when fatty substances are within the gut. These accessory organs work together to increase the process of digestion, ensuring nutrient breakdown and absorption are at their best, and thus overall body health and vigor are preserved. Taken all together, they show the complex relationship between the various digestive system elements and how essential they are to proper bodily function.

9.1.3. The Role of the Gastrointestinal Tract

The gastrointestinal system has a central role to play in the overall processes of digestion, being the main area for the breakdown and absorption of nutrients required by human health. Comprising a chain of organs ranging from the esophagus to the stomach, intestines, and rectum, this intricate system of organs is charged with the processing of the food we ingest, its conversion into energy, and the management of waste elimination. The intricate coordination of muscles along the gastrointestinal tract provides peristalsis, the rhythmic contraction and relaxation that propels food through the system. It is an essential motility for ensuring food is adequately digested and nutrients absorbed efficiently. Also, gastrointestinal motility disorders have the potential to disrupt daily life significantly, thus the significance of familiarizing oneself with the processes involved and the mechanisms thereof, such as the role of the enteric nervous system, which controls gastrointestinal function and can become compromised by viral infections (Chen et al., 2023). Also, the gut is not just a passive pipe for nutrients; it plays an active role in immune defense and overall wellness. The gastrointestinal mucous layer contains a rich variety of microbiota that is of utmost importance in maintaining the healthy status of the digestive system, metabolism of specific nutrients, and protection against pathogens. Research has indicated a connection between gut health and various systemic disorders, suggesting that disruptions in gut flora can lead to gastrointestinal disease, as well as autoimmune and metabolic syndrome. We can see that the gastrointestinal tract is a critical interface between the body's internal milieu and the external world, reinforcing the importance of maintaining a healthy gut for disease prevention and overall health. Furthermore, diet, lifestyle, and possibly microbe-targeted therapies have opened up new avenues for enhancing gastrointestinal wellness (Caragea et al., 2016) (Figure 9.5).

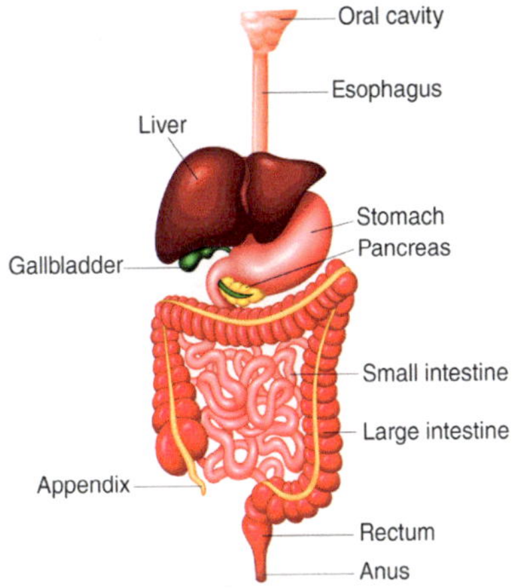

Figure 9.5. Gastrointestinal tract.

Source: https://cdn1.byjus.com/wp-content/uploads/2017/12/Gastrointestinal-Tract.png.

Applied to digestive diseases, the role of the digestive tract is extrapolated into its contribution toward more subtle disorders of health, such as gastrointestinal cancers. The multicentric nature of digestive cancers is one example of where gene, environmental, and psychosocial variables converge in this system. The heterogeneity of neurotransmitter signaling in the enteric nervous system is believed to modulate tumor growth and metastasis, offering one example of neural function as related to oncogenesis. Research shows that one can discover new targets and mechanisms of cancer treatment in the gastrointestinal tract by deciphering these connections. Furthermore, it also increasingly seems that psychological health and lifestyle factors may take significant roles in neoplasm prevention and management of the digestive tract, and thereby signal the need for an integrative approach to gastrointestinal wellness, considering the multi-faceted causes of such disorders (Caragea et al., 2016).

Test Your Knowledge

1. What are the major organs involved in digestion, and what roles do they play in breaking down food?
2. What are the accessory organs of the digestive system, and how do they support the digestive process?

9.2. The Process of Digestion

Learning Outcome

1. Define mechanical digestion: chewing and grinding
2. Explain the chemical digestion: enzymes and acids
3. Discuss the absorption of nutrients in the intestines

The intricate digestive process begins in the oral cavity, where mechanical and chemical processes concurrently begin to degrade food. When food is crushed in the mouth, saliva containing enzymes such as amylase initiates starch digestion, which actually reduces complex carbohydrates into simple sugars. This process of enzymatic activity plays a crucial role because it prepares food for digestion in the stomach and intestines. Once swallowed, food travels down the esophagus in a series of coordinated muscle contractions known as peristalsis and into the stomach, where it is subjected to violent acidic conditions and additional enzymatic action. The stomach's muscular walls churn food around and blend it with gastric juice, breaking down proteins some more and facilitating nutrients reaching the bloodstream. When the partially digested food, or chyme, is expelled from the stomach, it is sent into the small intestine, the primary site of nutrient absorption. The small intestine is remarkable in its vast surface area, immensely amplified by villi and microvilli that maximize the process of nutrient absorption. As chyme mixes with bile from the liver and pancreatic digestive enzymes, further digestion occurs. Amino acids, fatty acids, and simple sugars are picked up by the body from the walls of the intestines and transported to the body in the blood. Postprandial morphological changes in the intestinal epithelium demonstrate this adaptation to the absorption of nutrients, as in experiments with Burmese pythons, which reflect increases in enterocyte and microvilli length following ingestion, highlighting the dynamic nature of the gastrointestinal system and its capacity to adapt to food intake rapidly (Aldewachi et al., 2006). The final stage of digestion occurs in the large intestine, where electrolytes and water are reabsorbed and leftover indigestible food residues are prepared for expulsion. This segment of the digestive system plays a critical role in fluid balance and overall health. The composition of gut microbiota also significantly impacts processes in the large intestine, assisting in the fermentation of remaining nutrients as well as the production of short-chain fatty acids, which have numerous health benefits. In addition, the health of the digestive system can be impacted by environmental factors such as diet and environment. Identification of possible digestive disturbances, e.g., those suffered by dairy and livestock farming from waste management problems, is important in maximizing overall digestive well-being in farming systems, emphasizing the interdependence of digestion and broader ecological systems (Davis et al., 2025).

9.2.1. Mechanical Digestion: Chewing and Grinding

Mechanical digestion, as predominantly stimulated by the chewing and grinding mechanisms, is an essential part of the overall efficiency of the digestive system. Unlike most reptiles, which lack the capacity for successful mastication, mammals possess elaborate mechanisms for food breakdown so that higher metabolic potential is permitted. Not only does mastication reduce the particle size of food, but it also enhances the surface area for enzymatic action during chemical digestion. Mechanical action of teeth in herbivores allows for efficient grinding of plant food, which is usually complex and fibrous. It cannot be digestively broken down easily without physical breakdown before this. This remarkable disparity in mastication patterns between reptiles and mammals brings to the fore the evolutionary advancements that allow for nutrient recovery, testifying to the importance of mechanical digestion as a precursor to more advanced digestive processes (Barboza et al., 2010) (Figure 9.6).

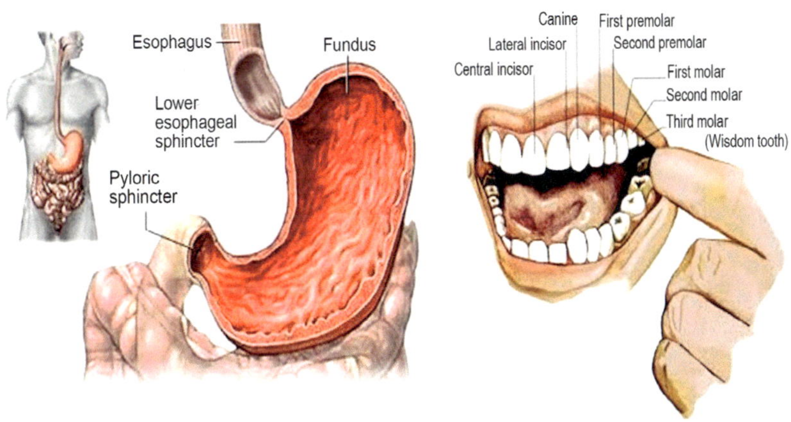

Figure 9.6. Mechanical digestion.

Source: https://i.ytimg.com/vi/Nws6SVDNqLs/sddefault.jpg.

The grinding and chewing mechanism employs many anatomical structures, of which jaw muscles and teeth are the most prominent. Mastication not only involves mechanics but also sensation, in that it is employed to feel food texture, which can influence food selection. In ruminants, chewing is more complex in that they initially consume material and then ruminate and regurgitate to chew. This sophisticated mechanism avoids the food from being inadequately processed prior to reaching the microbial-rich rumen environment in order to ferment. The efficiency of the two-stage digestion highlights the adaptive value of adapting mechanical digestion to suit dietary needs, particularly in herbivores, where cellulose diets necessitate further processing capacity (Astuti et al., 2018). In addition, the interaction between mechanical digestion and diet has significant implications for health and productivity. For example, feeding ruminants concentrate-rich diets can increase intake of energy; however, it can pose a greater threat of digestive diseases like ruminal acidosis if there is not enough fiber to provide regular stimulation to rumination. To minimize the above risks, mechanical stimulators and other means of fiber delivery have been used in place of traditional forage, providing healthier rumen activity while maintaining efficient production. Application of mechanical digestion tactics is therefore essential not only for optimal nutrient uptake but also to prevent metabolic issues caused by dietary imbalance (Astuti et al., 2018).

9.2.2. Chemical Digestion: Enzymes and Acids

Within the complex process of chemical digestion, enzymes and acids play a central role in breaking food into absorbable nutrients. The digestive system employs a variety of enzymes, with each one specializing in catalyzing the breakdown of macromolecules such as proteins, carbohydrates, and fats.

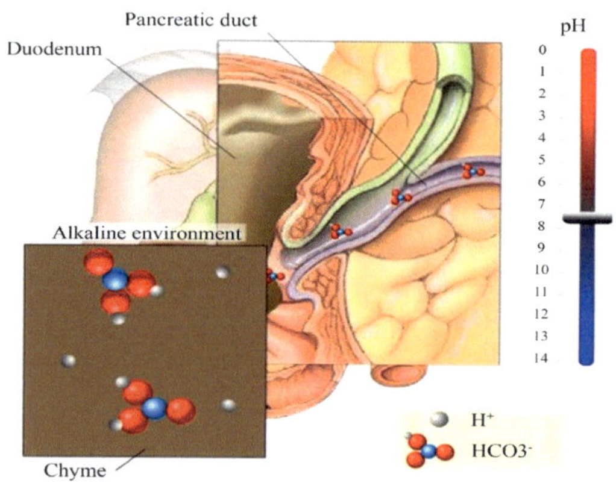

Figure 9.7. Digestive chemicals.

Source: https://biologynotesonline.com/mechanical-and-chemical-digestion-of-food-absorptions-of-differenet-molecules/.

For instance, amylase initiates carbohydrate breakdown in the mouth and continues within the small intestine. At the same time, pepsin, which is activated under acidic conditions within the stomach, is responsible for the breakdown of proteins. Not only do these enzymes cause breakdown, but they also enhance the bioavailability of nutrients to facilitate maximum absorption within the intestinal lining. The part played by pH in the process cannot be overstressed, as the acidic medium supplied by gastric acid prepares proteins for enzymic activity and prevents bacterial overgrowth (Figure 9.7).

The role of acids is not only to provide a favorable environment for enzymes; they are also required for the activation of proteins. Hydrochloric acid in the stomach not only denatures proteins but also activates pepsinogen into functional pepsin, an essential enzyme for protein digestion. The acidity of gastric juices is also vital for the solubilization of specific nutrients for their digestion by enzymes. In the small intestine, the acidic chyme of the stomach is neutralized by the pancreas's bicarbonate, which results in an equilibrated pH to allow for intestinal enzymes to function with the highest efficiency. Such delicate play of acids and enzymes makes digestion processes both effective and efficient, allowing for optimum intake of nutrients in the body. Recent studies have placed the significance of understanding chemical digestion into a broader context. As an example, research on *Nepenthes glandulifera*, which is a carnivorous plant, supplies details on digestive processes that are useful in the fields of agriculture and medicine. Digestive juices of the plant possess specific properties making them pertinent to the strategy of enzyme supplementation in human digestion, particularly in the case of celiac disease (Manuel et al., 2019). In addition, animal studies of the function of non-starch polysaccharides (NSP) and the supplementation of enzymes illustrate the complexity of gastrointestinal operation and nutrient uptake (Högberg et al., 2003). Through further research into these dynamics, scientists can develop techniques for optimizing digestion and improving health in livestock and human beings, illustrating the complex interdependencies of the digestive tract.

9.2.3. Absorption of Nutrients in the Intestines

The intestinal phase of digestion is an essential part of nutrient absorption, where the small intestine is the focal point of this activity. The physical form of the small intestine is blessed with specific adaptations to include microvilli, villi, and circular folds that give its surface a much larger area. These adaptations enable the efficient absorption of most nutrients, such as carbohydrates, proteins, fats, vitamins, and minerals. When food that has been digested passes from the stomach into the small intestine, pancreatic and intestinal lining enzymes assist in the molecular breakdown to a less complex state that facilitates their entry into the bloodstream. This tightly controlled process ensures that vital nutrients are absorbed in a manner that satisfies the body's metabolic requirements, underscoring the small intestine's role as both a channel and a crucial organ in nutrient absorption. Various mechanisms are required in absorption, such as passive diffusion, facilitated diffusion, osmosis, and active transport. The dynamics of these processes are controlled by forces such as concentration gradients and the presence of energy. For example, passive diffusion facilitates the uptake of small, nonpolar molecules through the intestinal membrane without the need for energy input. On the other hand, some nutrients, such as glucose and amino acids, are actively transported, needing energy to travel in the direction opposite to concentration gradients. The efficacy of such processes is critical; any compromise triggers malabsorption syndromes where the body cannot assimilate essential nutrients properly, triggering a host of health problems. Thus, the information regarding these pathways not only unwinds the intricacies of nutrient absorption but also hints at potential ramifications for disorders involving gastrointestinal function. In recent years, studies have shed light on the influence of diet on nutrient absorption. For example, utilization of specific additives such as charcoal in fishmeal has proven to enhance the growth rate of aquatic organisms such as catfish through histological improvement of the intestine and digestion of nutrients (Ekasari et al., 2025). These findings confirm the effect of dietary composition in improving the efficiency of absorption. Furthermore, modification of protein sources, for example, substitution of fishmeal by soybean meal in aquaculture diets, has demonstrated variable effects on protein digestibility and retention of nutrients (Muhammad et al., 2009). Such research enhances our understanding not only of the physiological mechanisms of absorption but also of applied uses in diet formulation and nutritional therapy, demonstrating the importance of nutrient absorption to human health as well as food production systems.

Test Your Knowledge

1. What is mechanical digestion, and how do chewing and grinding contribute to this process?
2. How do enzymes and acids facilitate chemical digestion in the digestive system?

9.3. The Role of Enzymes in Digestion

Learning Outcome

1. Explain the types of digestive enzymes
2. Define how enzymes facilitate digestion
3. Describe the factors affecting enzyme activity

The digestive system offers a home to a wide variety of enzymes, which are all significant in the digestion of food into nutrients that the body uses. Enzymes, as biocatalysts, catalyze biochemical reactions, which lead to the hydrolysis of macromolecules into simpler compounds, breaking complex carbohydrates, proteins, and lipids into their simpler counterparts. For example, amylases begin carbohydrate digestion in the mouth while proteases and lipases prolong protein and fat digestion in the small intestine and stomach. The specificity of each enzyme is to a particular substrate, ensuring a smooth digestion. Coordination of such enzymes not just promotes nutrient absorption but also metabolic balance, which demonstrates the pivotal nature of enzymes in overall health. Disruption of enzymatic activity may result in digestive illnesses, illustrating the importance of such biomolecules within digestion. Symbiotic relationships also enhance the process of digestion, showing the complexity of enzymatic activity in various organisms. For instance, certain sea creatures, including the shipworm, exploit enzymes produced by endosymbiotic bacteria to digest wood. The bacteria synthesize enzymes that facilitate the breakdown of lignocellulose and, therefore, nutrient acquisition in a specialist niche environment. Meta-transcriptomic and proteomic studies have shown that there exists an array of uncharacterized enzymes central to this digestive process and that the digestive tract of shipworms is dominated by its own enzymes and supplemented by those of symbiotic bacteria. These intricate processes illustrate how plants have evolved specialized digestive mechanisms to thrive in challenging conditions and highlight the adaptive function of enzymes during digestion and nutrient cycling through ecosystems (Bates et al., 2018) (Figure 9.8).

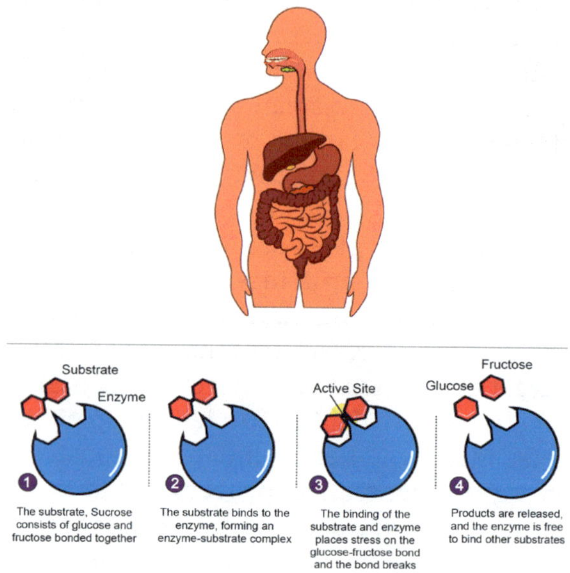

Figure 9.8. Digestive enzymes.

Source: https://cdn1.byjus.com/wp-content/uploads/2018/12/Digestive-Enzymes.png.

Similarly, the digestive machinery presented by plants such as *Nepenthes glandulifera* demonstrates the multifaceted role of enzymes in the intake of nutrients. Such plants secrete digestive fluids that contain a complex mixture of enzymes aimed at breaking down prey into its absorbable nutrient form. Later research focused on the unusual properties of these digestive fluids, with the potential that such applications beyond plant biology may have. Enzymes purified from Nepenthes species secretions have been studied for therapeutic medical applications, for instance, in the production of enzyme supplementation protocols for conditions such as celiac disease. Additionally, studies on the ultrastructural structure of digestive glands in Nepenthes plants provide information about nutrient absorption mechanisms and how enzymes and digestive processes have evolved to maximize the rate of nutrient acquisition from varying environments (Manuel et al., 2019).

9.3.1. Types of Digestive Enzymes

Digestive enzymes are proteins that facilitate the breaking down of macromolecules into small, absorbable units within the digestive system. The key groups of digestive enzymes are amylases, proteases, and lipases. Amylases perform the hydrolysis of carbohydrates, breaking down complex starches to simple sugars. These enzymes are synthesized primarily in the saliva by salivary glands, and secondarily by the pancreas, and are essential to carbohydrate digestion in the diet. Concentration and activity variations of enzymes can also influence digestive efficiency, demonstrating a pattern of enzyme type correlating with dietary needs, as observed in some species in the requirement for specific enzymes to meet their nutritional needs (Hollow et al., 1971). Knowledge of these pathways and enzymes is necessary to comprehend the process of digestion as a whole and how it influences health. Proteases or peptidases are specialized to break down proteins into peptides and amino acids. These enzymes are secreted in the inactive form by the stomach and pancreas so that autodigestion is not triggered. Activated proteases such as pepsin and trypsin ravage food proteins and make them bioavailable for absorption. The function of these enzymes varies across different regions of the digestive system, and some pH levels influence their effectiveness. For instance, pepsin is most effective at the acidic pH found in the stomach, while trypsin works best at the slightly alkaline pH of the small intestine. The effectiveness of proteases in digestion is also indicated by their binding to specific dietary proteins, accentuating the adaptive mechanisms of particular organisms (Hollow et al., 1971) (Figure 9.9).

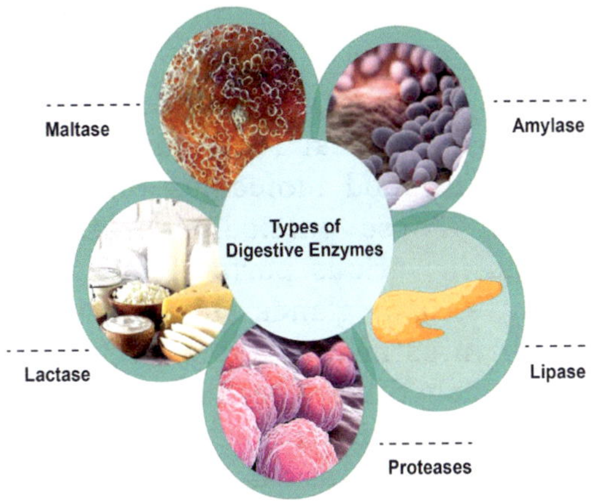

Figure 9.9. Types of digestive enzymes.

Source: https://advancedfoodintolerancelabs.com/blogs/news/what-are-digestive-enzymes.

This difference in protease structures is a reflection of the specificity and intricacy of protein digestion. Lipases are also significant digestive enzymes that act on lipids, hydrolyzing them into free fatty acids and glycerol. Lipases are primarily secreted by the pancreas but also occur in saliva and gastric juices to provide lipid digestion at several points in the digestion process.

The action of lipases is particularly critical in emulsifying fats, which are excluded from being absorbed by the body in the first place due to their hydrophobic nature. To facilitate effective lipid hydrolysis, bile salts are often involved, which support the activity of lipases through emulsification of fats into micelles, which are readily absorbed by the small intestine. Notably, the presence of specialized gut bacteria with the ability to synthesize enzyme complexes such as cellulases further aids in food constituent breakdown, illustrating an intricate web of relationships supporting digestion. Such a symbiotic relationship provides nutrients and maintains overall digestive health.

9.3.2. How Enzymes Facilitate Digestion

Enzymes play a key role in the digestive process, catalyzing biochemical reactions that break down complex food molecules into simpler compounds. These particular proteins are synthesized in various parts of the digestive system, e.g., salivary glands, stomach, pancreas, and small intestine. For instance, amylase initiates carbohydrate digestion in the mouth, while proteases initiate protein digestion in the stomach. Lipases are tasked with emulsification and further hydrolysis of fats in the small intestine. The efficiency of these enzymatic processes ensures nutrients are available for absorption into the body via the bloodstream. Without enzymes, the digestive system would be unable to break down vital vitamins, minerals, and macronutrients from food, which would cause malnutrition and impaired physiological processes. Therefore, understanding the particular mechanisms and roles of digestive enzymes is crucial for an overview of overall digestive health. Enzyme activity is particular, usually affecting particular substrates through a lock-and-key form of activity that is efficient and accurate. Each enzyme operates best in a specific pH and temperature, conditions that are maintained closely in the digestive system. For example, pepsin works best in the acidic conditions of the stomach and can therefore efficiently cleave peptide bonds within proteins. Conversely, pancreatic enzymes such as trypsin and lipase work best in the slightly alkaline condition of the small intestine. The specificity of such enzymes ensures that digestion processes occur in a logical and ordered manner, preventing early spoilage of food items before the arrival of the respective digestion stage. Such specificity is not only critical for effective uptake of nutrients but also for the overall integrity of the digestive process to ensure a reduced risk of digestive diseases. In addition, the role of enzymes in digestion is not limited to simple digestion; they are also instrumental in metabolic processes governed by the digestive functions. It is interesting to note the way research work on plant digestive systems, like that conducted with *Nepenthes glandulifera*, famous for having its distinctive digestive fluid, has revealed new facets of the functioning of enzymes and nutrient uptake (Manuel et al., 2019). These findings can have broader uses, including the development of enzyme supplementation protocols for conditions like celiac disease (Valls-Bellés et al., 2024). As such, studies into digestive enzymes not only expand our understanding of human digestion but also pave the way for the advancement of medical and nutritional treatment. Examining these intricate dynamics provides an integrated understanding of how enzymes facilitate not only digestion but also overall health and nutrient efficiency (Figure 9.10).

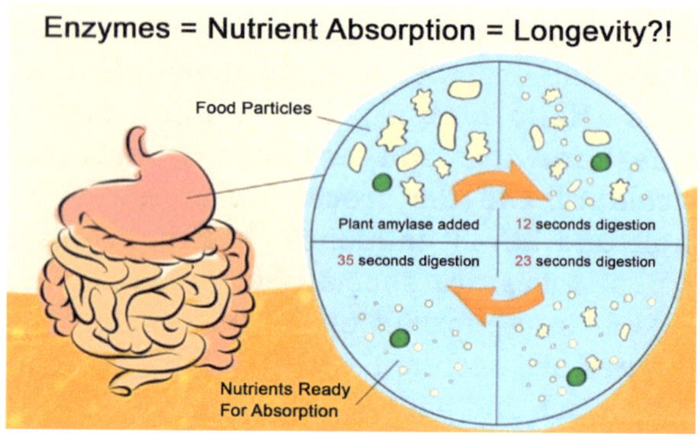

Figure 9.10. The mouth, pancreas, small intestine, and stomach create digestive enzymes, which speed up chemical reactions and break food into nutrients the body can absorb.

Source: https://thcksq.com/blog/index.php?post/31/What-Do-Digestive-Enzymes-Do.

9.3.3. Factors Affecting Enzyme Activity

Enzymes are vital catalysts of the digestive process, and their functioning depends on different factors like temperature, pH, and substrate concentration. Every enzyme has a specific temperature at which it works most efficiently. For instance, higher temperatures may raise the activity of enzymes to a point; beyond this point, enzyme denaturation can occur, leading to the dismantling of the active site essential for substrate binding. In addition, pH varies throughout the different regions of the digestive system such that enzymes must be adapted to their respective environments, i.e., the stomach's acidic environment in contrast to the alkaline environment of the small intestine. These differences in pH could affect enzyme conformation and, consequently, their catalytic efficiency as a whole, highlighting the importance of providing proper conditions for practical digestive function to occur. Apart from pH and temperature, substrate concentration is also significant in enzyme activity. As the substrate concentration increases, the rate of reaction tends to increase to a limit where all available active sites on the enzymes are occupied, with increments in substrate concentrations no longer increasing the rate of reaction (Figure 9.11).

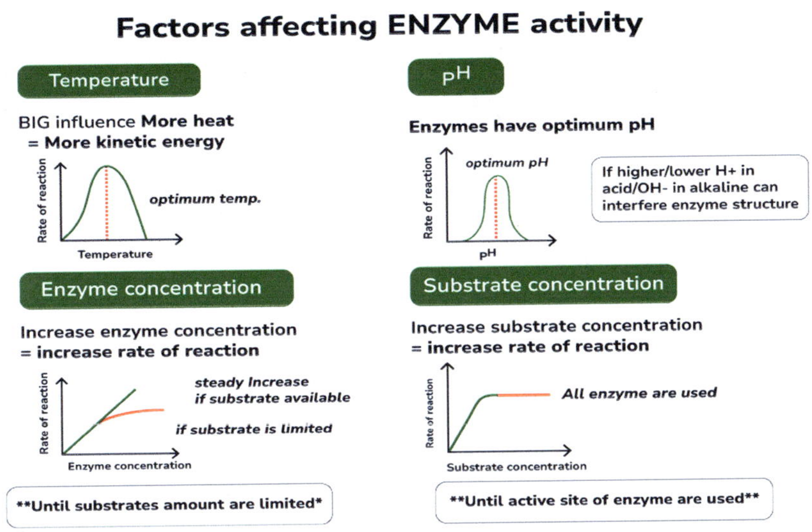

Figure 9.11. Factors affecting enzyme activity.

Source: https://media.geeksforgeeks.org/wp-content/uploads/20240328172456/Factors-affecting-ENZYME-activity.png.

This aspect shows how enzymes work optimally under a specific situation, where there is a need for a proper balance of substrates to ensure digestion is carried out efficiently. With these, the presence and the quantity of inhibitors or activators significantly affect enzyme operation. Inhibitors can bind to enzymes and hinder them from catalyzing a reaction, while activators can enhance their performance, indicating the regulatory aspect involved in digestive operations. The biochemistry of enzymes also intersects with exogenous variables such as the presence of organic contaminants in the gut, which has a strong influence on enzyme activity. For instance, exposure to certain environmental toxicants can induce the production of specific enzymes, for example, cytochrome P4501A (CYP1A), which is involved in the metabolism of ingested toxic substances. This induction can be considered a response to the increasing frequency of organic contaminants, since CYP1A protects cells from oxidative damage by catalyzing the degradation of these contaminants.

Furthermore, as per research on numerous organisms, it is essential to achieve a balance between production and antioxidant defense in reactive oxygen species (ROS). Reactive oxygen species will interfere with enzymes, but a well-controlled antioxidant response will reduce this, thereby maintaining the delicate balance needed for maximum functioning of digestive enzymes (Förlin et al., 1994; Högberg et al., 2003).

Test Your Knowledge

1. What are the different types of digestive enzymes, and what specific nutrients do they target?
2. How do digestive enzymes facilitate the breakdown of food during digestion?

9.4. Common Digestive Disorders

Learning Outcome

1. Discuss the gastroesophageal reflux disease (GERD)
2. Understand the irritable bowel syndrome (IBS)
3. Define celiac disease and gluten intolerance

Gastrointestinal diseases are highly heterogeneous conditions that can cause the quality of life and overall health of an individual to decline significantly. These disorders include gastroesophageal reflux disease (GERD), irritable bowel syndrome (IBS), and celiac disease, with very characteristic symptoms and pathophysiology. GERD is characterized by the backflow of acid from the stomach into the esophagus, where it produces heartburn and induces esophageal mucosal damage if left untreated. Both disorders are typically long-standing in duration, requiring diet modification and drugs to reduce pain and prevent complications. IBS is a functional bowel disorder characterized by alterations in bowel function and abdominal pain. While not harmful, its symptoms can render normal daily activities an actual hardship for patients who suffer from them. Becoming aware of these common gastrointestinal illnesses is necessary to manage and prevent them properly. In addition to IBS and GERD, celiac disease is a commonly diagnosed gastrointestinal illness based on an autoimmune response to gluten, a protein found in grains. When individuals with celiac disease consume gluten, the immune system responds by damaging the lining of the small intestines, leading to malabsorption of nutrients and other systemic manifestations. The variety of possible presentations ranges from gastrointestinal complaints, such as bloating and diarrhea, to extra-intestinal presentations of fatigue and neurological complaints. Celiac disease diagnosis might involve serological tests and intestinal biopsies, as proper diagnosis of the condition is essential. Even though a strict gluten-free diet is the primary therapy, knowledge and education about food labeling are also essential for patients who wish to avoid gluten and alleviate their symptoms accordingly. The rising incidence of gastrointestinal conditions has been of significant interest to researchers and practitioners alike. As technology improves and methods of data collection become more efficient, an increasing number of studies are being conducted and reported that identify the causative factors of such conditions. For example, a recent infodemiological study reviewed over 41,000 online forum posts. It revealed an array of evidence on electronic cigarette use-related symptomatology and disorders that predominantly involved various organ systems, with the gastrointestinal tract being among them (Hristidis et al., 2020). Similarly, pedigree dog and their hereditary disorder research demonstrates the benefits of summarizing and accessing information about the prevalence of disease even in non-human samples (Evans et al., 2017). This general focus on data gathering and assessment, as well as the furtherance of knowledge of common digestive illnesses, also directs public health policy towards prevention and education, enhancing outcomes for those so affected.

9.4.1. Gastroesophageal Reflux Disease (GERD)

GERD is a chronic illness where the contents of the stomach reflux into the esophagus, leading to inflammation and pain. This pathologic retrograde movement occurs when the lower esophageal sphincter fails to close properly, leading to the development of heartburn, regurgitation, and dysphagia. While occasional attacks of reflux are common to the general public, GERD is distinguished by the chronic and severe nature of these attacks that result in a damaging effect on quality of life. Chronic reflux might also lead to more serious complications such as stricture of the esophagus, Barrett's esophagus, and even esophageal carcinoma, which denotes the disease's potential to not only undermine the function of the digestive system but also overall health outcomes. In the treatment of GERD, a holistic approach is required, as lifestyle modifications, pharmacotherapy, and surgery all play a role in management. Patients are typically advised to change their diet, reducing intake of known offenders like caffeine and high-fat meals, and adopting the practices of smaller portion sizes and upright position postprandially. Proton pump inhibitor use is frequent in the management of this condition and efficiently lowers gastric acid production and provides symptom relief. The surgical approach, such as laparoscopic sleeve gastrectomy (LSG) with cruroplasty, is efficacious, especially in those with concomitant hiatal hernia. Evidence indicates that obese patients undergoing this procedure experience worthwhile postoperative improvement in reflux symptoms when absorbable mesh crura buttressing is added, demonstrating how surgical procedures to address GERD are evolving (Badiali et al., 2017) (Figure 9.12).

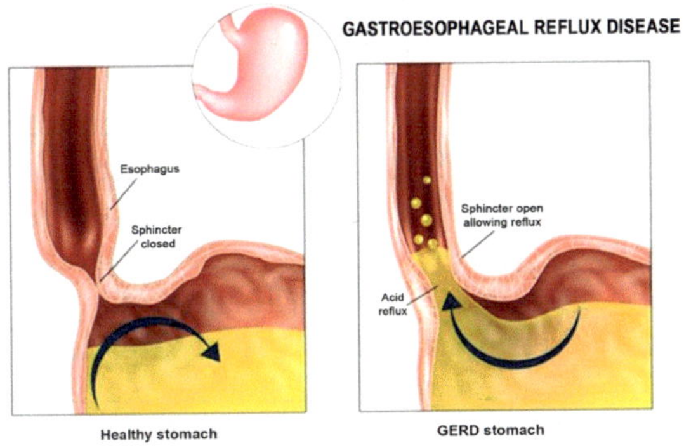

Figure 9.12. Gastroesophageal reflux disease (GERD).

Source: https://www.gleneagles.com.sg/conditions-diseases/gastro-oesophageal-reflux-disease/symptoms-causes.

The connection with other conditions of GERD necessitates a deep understanding of its mechanisms and course, particularly in patients with concomitant comorbidities such as ischemic heart disease. The connection between GERD and chronic diseases can complicate treatment, as symptoms are similar and often aggravated. For instance, the development of inflammation as a result of GERD may cause significant discomfort to the patient, thereby making the presentation clinical for sufferers of cardiovascular disease. Besides, treatment of one of these conditions might have the effect of influencing treatment of another. It is essential to acknowledge these associations to create effective, individualized treatment patterns that consider both GERD and other existing conditions, thus ensuring the best care for patients in response to the complexities of medical conditions (Drozd et al., 2016).

9.4.2. Irritable Bowel Syndrome (IBS)

IBS is a functional gastrointestinal disorder that significantly affects an individual's quality of life. The illness entails recurrent abdominal pain and bowel habit modification, and manifests as diarrhea, constipation, or both. Remarkably, the symptoms appear intermittently, which leads to severe distress for the patient. The variable nature of IBS can be attributed to varied physiological and psychological factors since it changes with emotional stressors as well as dietary variety. Such variegation necessitates a complete understanding of the disorder within the context of the digestive system because it involves multiple systems of physiology that have a significant impact on gut function and patient experience. Recent research has been more inclined towards the interaction between hormonal change and stress as etiological factors for the pathophysiology of IBS. Evidence suggests that hormonal change may induce symptoms of IBS, like cramping and constipation, particularly with fluctuating levels of progesterone. Evaluation of the role of hormones, such as progesterone, with the gastrointestinal tract will help identify the options of therapy available for the treatment of IBS, apart from symptomatic relief (Linson et al., 2013). In addition, as demonstrated in more recent studies, stress also has a key part in generating and sustaining IBS symptoms, influencing visceral sensitivity and brain-gut axis response. This holds the promise of more subtle treatment regimens to target both hormonal and psychological factors of the disorder. The role of stressors in the causation and exacerbation of IBS symptoms is of special importance, suggesting a biopsychosocial model of the illness. Experimental models attest to the possibility of various psychological and physical stressors eliciting or aggravating symptoms of IBS, emphasizing the brain-gut axis's critical function (Larauche et al., 2011). These stressors play a role in visceral hypersensitivity, rendering the clinical presentation and response to treatment of IBS complicated. By exploring the mechanisms of stress-induced modulation of visceral pain, scientists can identify new therapeutic targets aimed at enhancing the action of stress on IBS patients. Consequently, treatment with a multimodal strategy combining stress management techniques along with dietary and hormonal therapy could be incredibly advantageous in managing the complex nature of this prevalent gastrointestinal disorder (Figure 9.13).

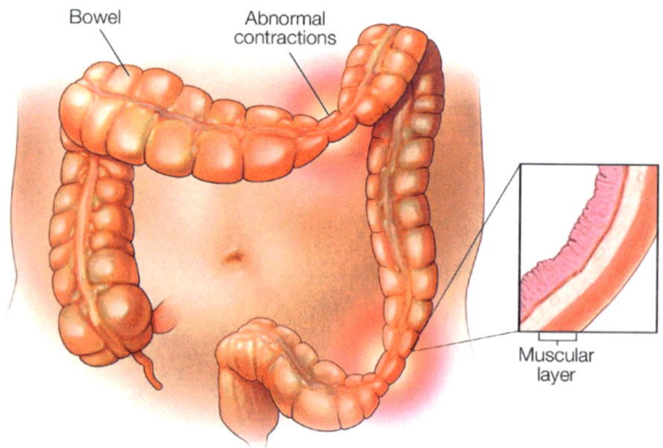

Figure 9.13. Irritable bowel syndrome (IBS).

Source: https://drrohitgoyalgastro.com/wp-content/uploads/2024/06/Untitled-design-1170x684.png.

9.4.3. Celiac Disease and Gluten Intolerance

Gluten intolerance and celiac disease are two disparate yet comparable disorders of the gastrointestinal system, revealing the complex relationship between diet and gastrointestinal health. CD is an autoimmune disease with a misplaced immune response to gluten, a wheat, barley, and rye protein, leading to widespread villous atrophy of the small intestine. Such damage not only warps nutrient absorption but also triggers a range of systemic symptoms, including gastrointestinal distress and neurological manifestations. The differential diagnosis between celiac disease and non-celiac gluten sensitivity (NCGS) is crucial because NCGS does not necessarily correlate with the same level of intestinal damage, with symptoms residing mainly in varying levels of discomfort and psychological comorbidities. Understanding the differences is essential to accurate diagnosis and management, since both conditions require a gluten-free diet to alleviate symptoms and improve general health. Still, the level of restriction and awareness can be worlds apart between them (Thomas et al., 2020). Education and understanding of gluten-related disorders, including celiac disease and gluten intolerance, have increased significantly over the past few years, particularly among college-aged individuals. Research conducted at Southern New Hampshire University aimed to establish awareness and occurrence of such conditions among the students, with a focus on education regarding dietary limitations and health consequences. The research entailed the determination of gluten occurrence in foods commonly taken and elucidating symptoms and effects of gluten intolerance compared to celiac disease. Understanding the population most affected by these disorders is crucial, as certain populations, such as women and individuals with a family history of autoimmune disorders, show higher prevalence rates. This awareness enhances the ability of schools to provide appropriate accommodations and support to those individuals, incorporating dietary needs and creating a healthier school environment (Thomas et al., 2014). The increasing rates of diagnosis of celiac disease and gluten intolerance necessitate serious scrutiny of their repercussions on public health policy and the food industry. The reasons for the increased reported cases include better diagnostic techniques, heightened awareness, and perhaps environmental cause factors such as changes in eating practices and how wheat is being processed. These trends require research and review to assess the evidence supporting the increase in both conditions. The consequences of untreated celiac disease may have severe complications, and thus, early and correct diagnosis and gluten-free diet counseling become a necessity. Moreover, by learning about higher prevalence and social impacts of gluten-related disorders, stakeholders, including health care professionals and policy makers, can make efforts to accommodate the affected individuals, ensuring their well-being and welfare in spite of the complexities of contemporary diets (Thomas et al., 2020) (Figure 9.14).

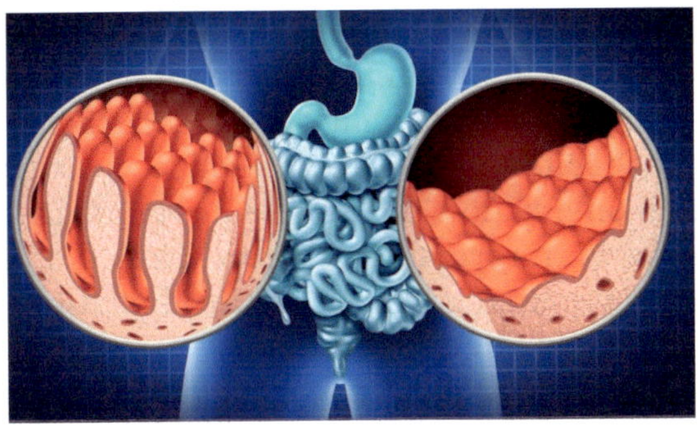

Figure 9.14. Celiac Disease.

Source: https://bgapc.com/wp-content/uploads/2021/04/image1-1024x635.jpg.

Test Your Knowledge

1. What are the main characteristics of irritable bowel syndrome (IBS), and how does it affect digestive health?
2. How does celiac disease differ from gluten intolerance, and what impact do they have on the digestive system?

9.5. The Impact of Diet on Digestive Health

Learning Outcome

1. Understand the importance of fiber in digestion
2. Define effects of processed foods on the digestive system
3. Explain the role of hydration in digestive health

The intricate relationship between diet and digestive health is supported by the manner in which the composition of the diet influences the functioning of the gut. It requires a healthy diet that consists of high fiber, whole grains, and adequate hydration to guarantee digestive motility and the gut's general health. Fiber, in particular, is significant because it guarantees regular bowel movement and helps maintain a healthy microbiota. The breakdown of dietary fiber in the colon yields short-chain fatty acids (SCFAs) that are required for cellular function and gut homeostasis. Conversely, low-fiber intake can lead to dysbiosis of the gut microbiota, constipation, and gastrointestinal distress, which can trigger inflammatory responses. Comprehending the intricacies of how specific nutrients influence intestinal health offers knowledge of dietary adjustments that can improve digestion and prevent gastrointestinal disease, reaffirming the role of educated dietary decisions in preserving digestive health. Dietary lifestyle has direct effects on the content and function of the gut microbiota, which plays a relevant role in digestive performance. The metabolic function of colonic microbiota, as proven in research, is heavily determined by one's diet, thereby suggesting that the type of food one consumes may lead to varying microbial communities and gastrointestinal effects. Experiments have indicated that high-residue diets lead to greater fecal output and frequency of bowel movements, enhancing overall gastrointestinal function and comfort (Garaventa et al., 2017). On the contrary, residue-depleted diets can result in reduced fecal volume and even gastrointestinal disturbances. This highlights the importance of incorporating varied, fiber-rich foods into daily diets to foster a healthy microbiome, which in turn supports digestion, nutrient absorption, and immune protection. The convergence of dietary patterns and gut microbiota is thus an essential factor in promoting optimal digestive well-being. Additionally, the impacts of diet change on digestive health are particularly evident at critical life points, such as weaning in young children or dietary modification in adults.

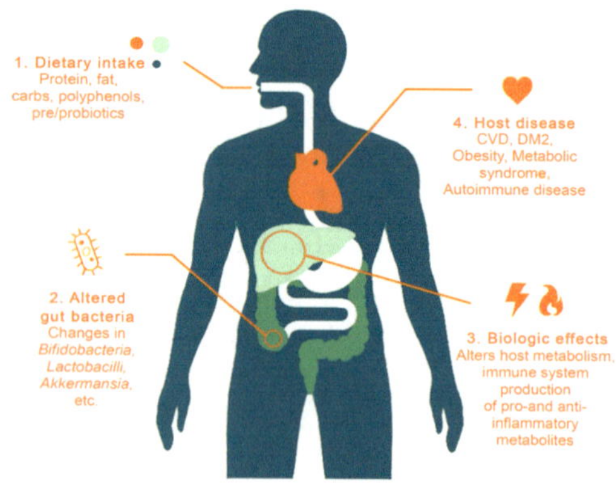

Figure 9.15. Impact of diet on the human health.

Source: https://external-content.duckduckgo.com/iu/?u=https%3A%2F%2Fwww.researchgate.net%2Fpublication%2F315978151%2Ffigure%2Ffig1%2FAS%3A963516475383820%401606731637652%2FImpact-of-diet-on-the-gut-microbiome-and-human-health.gif&f=1&nofb=1&ipt=1b5a1ff224fb1c464afd1b59ef064c4b0b160d224b29f77b4600e3e48c37c923.

The weaning phase is a time of significant physiological alteration in the gut that could potentially lead to gastrointestinal disorders if it is not managed through a nutrient-dense diet (Bauer et al., 2011). Transitional diets consisting of high levels of specific nutrients can aid in the necessary adaptation of the digestive system, alleviating such nuances as diarrhea or constipation. In adults, diet modification, such as being placed on a high-fiber diet, can also aid in the adaptation to the changed needs of the digestive system, depending on aging or health factors. With the change in diets, knowing the interaction between food intake and gut health is essential, emphasizing the role of specific foods in maintaining gut stability, recovery, and health (Figure 9.15).

9.5.1. Importance of Fiber in Digestion

The intricate digestive processes are heavily reliant on dietary fiber, which is essential for maintaining overall gastrointestinal health. Fiber, predominantly in plant foods, is a non-digestible carbohydrates that facilitate digestion in various ways. By providing bulk to stool, fiber maintains regular bowel movements and prevents constipation, thereby maximizing the digestive process. Moreover, soluble fiber, such as that found in oats and legumes, can hold water and form a gel-like substance that slows down gastric emptying. The slow release of nutrients not only maintains stable blood sugar levels but also ensures enhanced nutrient absorption, a critical metabolic process. The high complexity of the fiber affects its interaction with the digestive tract, emphasizing its importance in diet control (Edwards et al., 2020). Plant cell wall structural cells also contribute significantly to the power of digestibility of fiber. The cell walls consist of a range of polysaccharides, including cellulose, hemicellulose, and pectin, contributing to the overall efficiency of the fibers. The composition and structure of these elements determine how bioaccessible they are and how they are metabolized within the gastrointestinal tract. The inclusion of insoluble fiber, for example, can increase stool bulk, promote the transit of waste through the colon, and potentially reduce the risk of colorectal disease. Since fiber content in diets enhances gut microbiome, fermentation of certain soluble fibers by beneficial bacteria results in short-chain fatty acids, which further improve colonic health and enhance nutrient absorption (Högberg et al., 2003) (Figure 9.16).

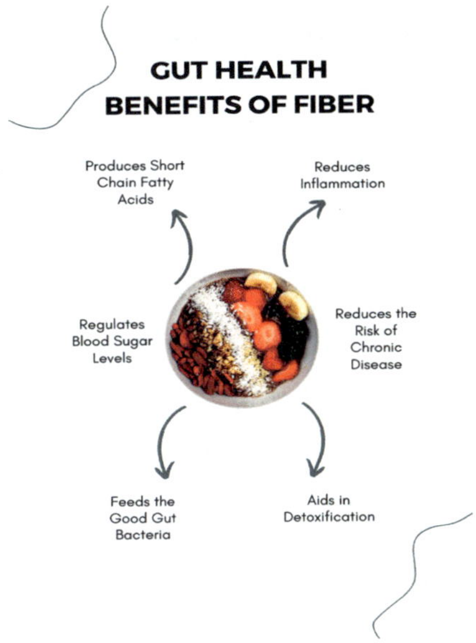

Figure 9.16. The benefits of fiber for gut health.

Source: https://external-content.duckduckgo.com/iu/?u=https%3A%2F%2Fi0.wp.com%2Fnikkiyeltonrd.com%2Fwp-content%2Fuploads%2F2021%2F12%2FNikki-Yelton-RD-leaky-gut-functional-medicine-fiber-for-gut-health-fiber-rich-foods-gut-health-fiber-benefits-health8.png%3Fresize%3D960%252C1440%26ssl%3D1&f=1&nofb=1&ipt=51da183e5f52c578dcc04863313ff11fb35dbd7ac468224f71849827cd4b875a.

Ensuring one has the right amount of fiber in their diet, particularly during periods of necessary growing time or adjustment to new eating patterns, is essential to attain optimal digestive health. Experimental evidence indicates that high non-starch polysaccharide (NSP) diets affect gastrointestinal function, as has been demonstrated in experiments with developing pigs. Findings suggested that higher NSP content resulted in alteration of the digestive environment that had a detrimental effect on organic matter digestibility. These findings depict the flexibility and adaptability of the digestive system to the changing forms of fiber, yet at the same time underscore the importance of balanced consumption to optimize nutrient release and uptake. Therefore, recognizing the multifaceted functions of fiber in digestion is paramount to human health and meal preparation (Edwards et al., 2020).

9.5.2. Effects of Processed Foods on the Digestive System

Digestion is an essential process for nutrient processing and extraction from food, and the intake of processed foods very much influences it. Processed foods contain a high level of additives and lack natural fiber, hence failing to support proper digestive health. Food processing may weaken structural cell wall properties in plant foods, thus making them less bioaccessible and less rich in available nutrients. As noted in previous literature, the intricate organization and structure of polysaccharides such as cellulose and hemicellulose in cell walls dictate their role in the gastrointestinal tract. With degradation of the structures by processing, the digestive system is compromised in its ability to decompose nutrients to an optimal extent, leading to decreased overall nutrient absorption and potentially contributing to gastrointestinal disorders and gut microbiota dysbalance, compromising long-term health. Furthermore, the chemical preservatives contained in most processed foods provide an additional burden for the digestive system. The majority of these additives, including artificial sweeteners and preservatives, can cause interference with the normal functioning of the gut microbiome—a mixture of microbes crucial to digestion and nutrient synthesis. Maintaining the proper balance by these microbes is essential for homeostasis, as they facilitate the breakdown of complex carbohydrates and synthesize vitamins. As outlined in recent studies, such disruption has the potential to induce states like dysbiosis, a form of imbalance capable of causing gastrointestinal upset, bloating, and inflammation. The chronic consumption of such foods thus not only exacerbates gut upset but also can have implications for metabolic health, emphasizing the importance of a balanced, minimally processed diet facilitating gastrointestinal function and general health (Sarmidi et al., 2012). Further, long-term consequences of a diet with high levels of processed foods have implications beyond transient gastrointestinal discomfort, possibly influencing systemic health outcomes. The loss of dietary fiber—a principal constituent found in abundance in whole foods—impairs gut motility and regulates stool consistency, leading to complications such as constipation and prolonged gastrointestinal transit time. High-fiber intake is required to regulate digestion and produce regular bowel movements. To the contrary, reliance on processed food for dieting is most likely to lead to decreased intake of dietary fibers and essential nutrients, with the capacity to initiate a cascade of metabolic issues with time. Food composition, metabolic control, and gut health interact in an intricate but key manner to maintain human health and cellular homeostasis, a fact that translates to making food evaluations according to their gastrointestinal consequences worthwhile (Edwards et al., 2020).

9.5.3. Role of Hydration in Digestive Health

Hydration plays a core role in sustaining optimal digestive health and influences several physiological functions to promote the efficient breakdown and absorption of nutrients. Water is required for the production of saliva, which not only aids the mechanical breakdown of food but also contains enzymes that start carbohydrate digestion. Moreover, hydration also provides for the optimal functioning of mucosal membranes along the gastrointestinal tract to foster an environment that is favorable for nutrient uptake. With a well-hydrated body, one can regulate the consistency of stool satisfactorily such that constipation is avoided, and intestinal transit becomes smoother. In general, water plays a lubricating and solvent function throughout digestion, highlighting its essential contribution in the digestive functions of the body as noted in the literature on nutritional science and gastrointestinal physiology. Also, there is a direct correlation between hydration and balance within the gut microbiota, an imperative aspect of overall digestive health. The gut microbiome, consisting of trillions of microorganisms, stays healthy in an optimally hydrated environment with its prolific diversity of activities like fermentation and production of nutrients. A study reveals that dehydration will result in an undesirable shift in microbial populations, weakening the gut's ability to perform its required functions, such as immune function and metabolism. Furthermore, in the absence of sufficient water intake, the digestive system will have additional pressure, resulting in potential inflammatory responses and disorders. These results highlight the intricate interaction between hydration and microbial wellness, with emphasis on hydration as a critical component of achieving balanced gut flora for maximum digestive outcomes, supplementing results of the current body of research. Dietary fiber in combination with hydration also remains a pivotal player in the promotion of digestive well-being. Fiber is a bulking agent of the intestines that requires sufficient water to effectively transit through the intestines and facilitate the expulsion of waste. Inadequate fluid intake with a meal high in fiber content may result in gastrointestinal distress and obstruction of the bowel. Recent studies suggest that eating should be supported by foods rich in fiber and adequate water intake to enhance their impacts. To this end, synergistic interaction between dietary fiber and water intake is such that both elements synergize to improve gut function. Consequently, maintaining proper hydration matters not only for the immediate digestive process but also for long-term prevention of gastrointestinal disease, supporting the relevance of holistic dietary interventions in gut health as indicated in the literature (Figure 9.17).

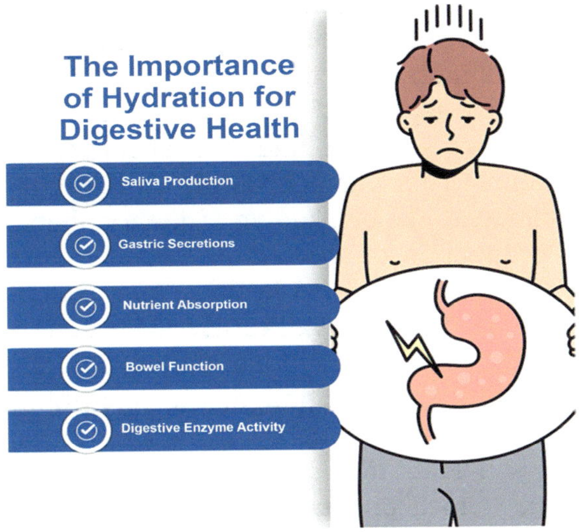

Figure 9.17. The importance of hydration for digestive health.

Source: https://external-content.duckduckgo.com/iu/?u=http%3A%2F%2Fgastro-doc.co.za%2Fwp-content%2Fuploads%2F2024%2F05%2Fimage1.png&f=1&nofb=1&ipt=137cef7a6b081c3f6afed379eb13df64b1c645c4b797332cee297c15e9ba7ec0.

Test Your Knowledge

1. Why is dietary fiber important for healthy digestion, and what benefits does it provide?
2. How can processed foods negatively affect the digestive system?

9.6. The Microbiome and Digestion

Learning Outcome

1. Explain the definition and significance of the gut microbiome
2. Define how microbiota influence digestion
3. Discuss the probiotics and their benefits for digestive health

The role of the microbiome in digestion is increasingly being recognized as a critical aspect of the digestive system's function. In the human gut, a highly complex community of microbes interacts with the host to contribute to various aspects of digestion, including the breakdown of food and the absorption of nutrients. This gut microbiota is thought to contribute to the breakdown of dietary fiber and the production of short-chain fatty acids that are important for colon health. Their existence increases the bioavailability of nutrients, thereby affecting nutritional status. Evidences show that dysregulation of the microbiome, usually brought about by antibiotics or poor diet, will lead to disorders of the digestive system, which emphasizes the importance of having a balanced gut flora. This balance not only facilitates digestion but is also able to suppress gastrointestinal disease and display the microbiome's dual role as a digestion mediator and a gut health protector. Having specific microorganisms, such as Giardia, within the gut can offer insight into intricate relationships between digestion and microbiota. Giardia, a protozoan traditionally seen as pathogenic, is a complex interaction with the gut microbiome. Even though it causes dysfunction in digestion in some circumstances, it could be creating a symbiotic system under other circumstances and aiding digestion in certain wildlife and possibly the human microbiome. Giardia, for instance, is thought to influence the gut environment by altering the proportion of bacteria, which can shift from anaerobic to aerobic regimes, which improves digestive function. The evolving vision of such an encounter calls for a greater insight into how various microorganisms can simultaneously be pathogenic and symbiotic in nature. This contradiction of Giardia's nature is vital to the quality of the microbiome, which governs the health of the human digestive system as well as other organisms, and thus a key area to be explored in the future (Gillen et al., 2017). Aside from human digestion, the study of ocean ecosystems identifies how microbiomes influence digestion among sea animals. Scientists have discovered that external pressures, such as ocean acidification, can alter an ocean animal's microbiome, influencing digestive efficiency. Seaweed chemistry and associated microbiome, for example, can change in terms of herbivorous grazers' gut microbiome. This shows that microbiomes respond actively to environmental stresses, which may have effects on the digestion of food by the host. Interestingly, some bacterial genera, such as Planctomycota, were found to increase in abundance in isopods that consumed acidified seaweed, which suggests that changes in the microbiome fine-tune food digestion under such altered conditions. This image not only highlights the pivotal roles of microbiomes in digestion across varied ecosystems but also invokes interest in how human-induced environmental transformation could influence our own digestive microbiome in the future (Aires et al., 2018).

9.6.1. Definition and Significance of the Gut Microbiome

The gut microbiome is a diverse ecosystem with trillions of microorganisms, including bacteria, viruses, fungi, and archaea, that colonize the host's gastrointestinal tract. Microbiota is an essential element in the performance of most body functions, particularly digestion and absorption of nutrients. The symbiotic process between humans and the gut microbiota enables the breakdown of complex carbohydrates and the synthesis of necessary vitamins, highlighting its role in metabolic health. Some studies have suggested that the gut microbiome structure likely contributes significantly to how an individual responds to diet, drugs, and environmental factors, implying that variations in microbial populations are not random but central to overall well-being. Furthermore, education on the gut microbiome is key to elucidating its position in metabolic disease, inflammatory disorders, and other gastrointestinal disease processes, bringing attention to its role in the gastrointestinal tract. Research shows that the gut microbiome is dynamic and influenced by a very large array of factors, including diet, lifestyle, and even genetic predisposition. What's interesting is that a diverse microbiome is associated with better health outcomes. Conversely, dysbiosis or imbalance of microbiota has been associated with a variety of diseases. This correlation highlights the need to have a healthy gut microbiota to maintain normal digestive function and general well-being. Besides, conferences like the one held by the North American branch of the International Life Sciences Institute have aimed at determining quantifiable characteristics of a healthy gut microbiome that signify health. Such gatherings have tried to develop a scientific framework for understanding microbiome-host interactions, moving toward the development of targeted therapies and preventative measures for health concerns in the gut (Antonopoulos et al., 2019). Recent research in microbiome science, including the use of model organisms like rattlesnakes, illustrates how distinct microbial communities are established by environmental influences and specific digestive processes. Particular species of snakes, for example, possess special gut microbiota that align with their respective kinds of venom, suggesting a process of microbial diversity selection through evolution (Stiers et al., 2020) (Figure 9.18).

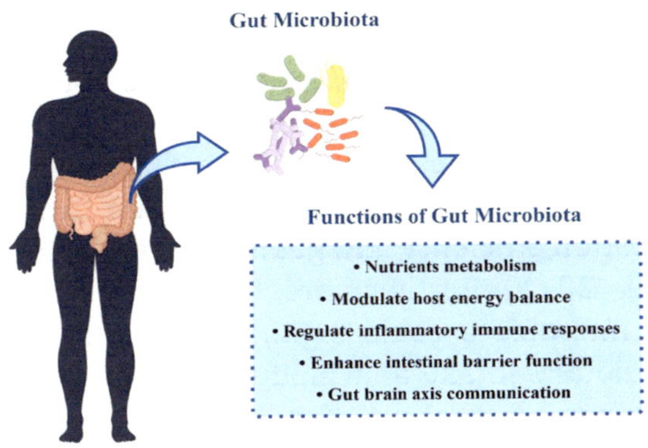

Figure 9.18. Functions of the gut microbiota.

Source: https://www.mdpi.com/microorganisms/microorganisms-12-00323/article_deploy/html/images/microorganisms-12-00323-g001.png.

Such discoveries enlighten the evolutionary significance and potential for adaptation of microbiomes, which, in addition to their role in digestion, provide immunological benefits and regulate metabolic processes. As research continues, understanding the intricate interactions between gut microbiota and their hosts will prove significant in preventing various health problems. Thus, studying the gut microbiome's role within the gut emphasizes not just its significance but also reveals potential for new therapies to rebalance the microbiome and maximize health outcomes.

9.6.2. How Microbiota Influence Digestion

The intricate dynamic between digestion and microbiota is key to maintaining the entire gut healthy and operational. Microbiota, made up primarily of bacteria in the intestines, are required to digest complex carbohydrates that enzymes in the body itself cannot dissolve. This enzymic action produces fermentable indigestible fiber, which yields short-chain fatty acids (SCFAs) that not only are absorbed and used as a source of energy but also play a part in having beneficial gut health. Recent research indicates the existence of evidence showing that SCFAs derived from such bacteria can regulate gene expression in the intestine, impacting functions such as nutrient absorption and immune function, both of which position the microbiota's impact in achieving optimization of digestion efficiency and gut homeostasis (Bauer et al., 2011). Furthermore, the composition of gut microbiota could significantly shift based on dietary intake and modulate digestion and nutrient absorption. For example, probiotic supplementation with lactic acid bacteria (LAB) and yeast was reported to alter the gut microbiota manner, enhancing the digestibility and health condition of such animal models as growing pigs. In a few studies, the performance and health of piglets were supported by some strains of LAB by altering gut environments and facilitating nutrient uptake soon after weaning. This highlights the potential for changing microbiota content by specially designed nutritional intervention to optimize digestive functions (Giang et al., 2010) (Figure 9.19).

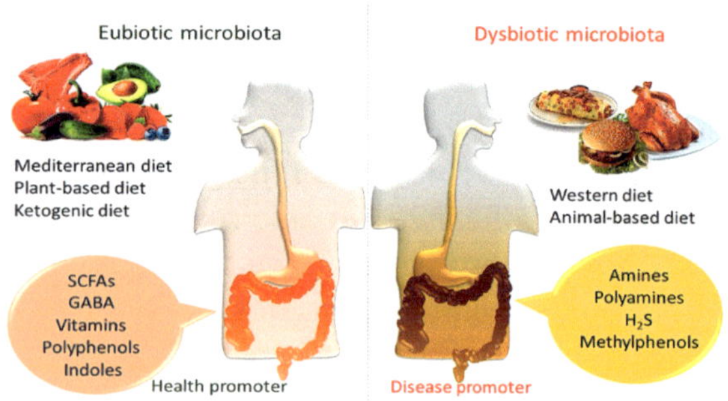

Figure 9.19. Dietary effect on gut microbiota and health. The gut microbiota takes part in the digestion of food ingredients and in the regulation of host metabolic functions.

Source: https://www.mdpi.com/1422-0067/21/10/3688.

As researchers probe further into these correlations, the message becomes apparent: for successful digestion and prevention of gastrointestinal disease, a balanced microbiota is paramount. Aside from their function in digestion, microbiota also interact with the host immune system, providing light on their intricate role in gut health. The microbiome of the gut acts as a defense barrier against pathogenic microorganisms, consequently reducing the rate of infection that can disrupt digestion. Furthermore, metabolites produced by the gut microbiota, like SCFAs, not only nourish intestinal cells but also play anti-inflammatory roles that cascade throughout the intestines, promoting balance in immune response. Dysbiosis, an imbalance, can be caused by a change in microbiota and can lead to gastrointestinal issues such as diarrhea or inflammatory bowel disease. Thus, understanding the mechanisms by which microbiota influence digestion highlights the need for a stable and diverse microbial community to avoid disease as much as it supports optimal health and digestion within the gastrointestinal tract (Bauer et al., 2011).

9.6.3. Probiotics and Their Benefits for Digestive Health

The function of probiotics in gut health has gained much interest over the past ten years as research continues to unearthing their varied roles in the intestinal tract. Probiotics are live microorganisms that have beneficial health effects when consumed in typical quantities, and they are involved in gut balance by augmenting the development of good bacteria and inhibiting harmful pathogens. An equilibrium of healthy microbiota is accountable for effective digestion, as it aids in food degradation, nutrient absorption, and digestive system homeostasis. Moreover, probiotic interaction with gut epithelial cells can strengthen the intestinal barrier, which prevents diseases like leaky gut syndrome, recognized as an etiology of assorted gastrointestinal disorders. This dynamic relationship highlights the need to incorporate probiotics into diets to promote gastrointestinal health and enhance quality of life. Specific advantages of probiotics in gastrointestinal health have been elucidated by scientific studies, notably in the management of gastrointestinal disorders such as irritable bowel syndrome (IBS) and antibiotic-associated diarrhea. Probiotics may enhance IBS symptoms by modulating gastrointestinal motility and promoting microbial diversity, which usually is depleted in patients with IBS. Additionally, probiotics must be taken together with antibiotics because antibiotics possess the ability to destroy both pathogenic and beneficial bacteria indiscriminately. With the use of probiotics, gut microbiota may be replenished, and the incidence and severity of antibiotic-associated diarrhea may be reduced. The findings of ongoing research emphasize pharmacists' critical role in educating patients on probiotics and their potential applications other than for gastrointestinal health, including immune system function and mental health, with the necessity of a holistic comprehension of probiotic benefits (Abbas et al., 2024). Despite the growing awareness of the advantages of probiotics for the gut, there remain considerable knowledge gaps for healthcare professionals, and particularly pharmacists. A study of pharmacists' knowledge and attitudes towards probiotics revealed that the majority were well aware of their role in supporting digestive health. In contrast, their role in cardiovascular health and mental health was less well known. For instance, less than 30% of participants identified probiotics' impact on cardiovascular health, and this shows the need for targeted educational initiatives to cover these shortfalls. With the continued advancement of the gut microbiome's complexity, keeping up with evidence-based practice for probiotics becomes of greatest importance among health care professionals. Fostering ongoing professional development among pharmacists is crucial in improving their patient counseling role, thus the promise of probiotics toward delivering holistic health outcomes to the population (Antonopoulos et al., 2019).

Test Your Knowledge

1. How do probiotics contribute to maintaining or improving digestive health?
2. In what ways can an imbalance in gut microbiota affect overall digestive function?

SUMMARY

In studying the digestive system, it is essential to recognize its simplicity and fundamental role in maintaining a human being's health. The digestive system facilitates digestion through the fragmentation of food, rendering the absorption of nutrients essential for physiological activities. The digestive system comprises various organs that extend from the mouth, stomach, and intestines, each contributing its share to the intricate digestive process. An understanding of physiological and anatomical factors reveals how these factors interact to produce maximum digestion and metabolism. As Ayurvedic works emphasize the significance of detailed knowledge regarding human physiology so one can relish the factors of health, modern science continues to find nuances in the digestive system (Patwardhan et al., 2008). This worldwide outlook is fostering increased awareness of how eating habits and food choices can impact digestive health tremendously, and hence overall well-being. Moreover, researchers are continuously discovering the molecular and physiological bases of the digestive system, which explain its systems of regulation. Rates of growth and digestive capacity are linked with gene expressions within the system. For instance, the interpretation of differential gene expression in mollusks not only provides information on growth but also provides analogies with human physiology. Such research illustrates the role of specific genes in managing digestive processes, energy metabolism, and nutrient uptake (Saavedra et al., 2017). Knowing such associations allows one to make informed dietary choices, thus impacting digestive health. As we become more aware of these genetic factors, we can better grasp the numerous forces operating on the efficacy of the digestive system and our general health. The digestive system is actually an active, vital network with far-reaching impacts on human health. Controlling issues such as gut microbiota and diet is a key factor in digestive equilibrium and avoiding disorders. By combining traditional Ayurvedic methods with modern scientific insights, we have developed a balanced understanding of digestion that emphasizes balance and harmony within the body. With ongoing research illuminating the complexities of this process, it is increasingly evident that it is imperative to take care of our digestive health. Through education, awareness, and preventive measures, we can build better functioning digestion, leading to increased quality of life and well-being. With any health problems that come up, knowing all about the digestive system gives people the knowledge to make informed decisions about their health journeys.

A detailed study of the digestive system picks up staggering nuances behind its complex workings. Primarily, digestion is separated into mechanical and chemical stages, initiated in the oral cavity, where food is mechanically treated in chewing. Subsequently, salivary enzymes initiate the biochemical process, paving the way for the food bolus to travel down the esophagus and into the stomach. Here, enzymes and acids of the stomach further break down food particles, eventually producing the chyme sent to the small intestine. The small intestine is a central site of nutrient absorption, so structural specializations here, such as villi and microvilli, are crucial to attaining maximum efficiency of digestion. These processes demonstrate the cooperative interdependence of mechanical and chemical digestion to maximize the utilization of nutrients in the human body. Besides that, the digestive process operates through an integrated system of organs and enzymatic reactions that collectively ensure the digestion of macronutrients into forms that can be absorbed. The pancreas also contributes by secreting digestive enzymes into the small intestine that assist in hydrolyzing carbohydrates, proteins, and fats. In addition, liver-secreted bile stored in the gallbladder helps emulsify fats, rendering them more soluble and absorbable. The brush border enzymes of the small intestine are especially relevant as they carry out terminal digestion, breaking down oligosaccharides and peptides into monosaccharides and amino acids. As noted in key research, such as that recognized by Hooton et al., the exclusion of such a key stage in in vitro models can have the effect of leading to misrepresentations of digestive efficiency; therefore, there is a need for proper knowledge of the digestive environment in vivo (Hooton et al., 2018). Alongside this, financial interdependence between various sources of research funding, as illustrated by research by Cancer Research UK and the Office of Health Economics, places the activity of medical research alongside understanding physiological processes like digestion into broader health advance narratives. The mutual co-operation among the public, charitable, and private sectors ensures the continuous enhancement and development of medical information, which subsequently offers evidence in support of clinical practice for digestion and nutrition. A robust underpinning framework of financing medical research is necessary; the cuts can be detrimental to advancements in our understanding of digestive biology and associated disorders (Crane et al., 2014). Thus, the collective knowledge is not only from the biological accounts of the digestive system, but from socio-economic models on which forthcoming research within this crucial field of medicine will be based.

KEY TERMS FROM THIS CHAPTER

- Mouth
- Esophagus
- Small Intestine
- Jejunum
- Large Intestine
- Colon
- Anus
- Gallbladder
- Salivary Glands
- Stomach
- Duodenum
- Ileum
- Cecum
- Rectum
- Liver
- Pancreas

CRITICAL THINKING QUESTIONS

1. **What is the primary function of the digestive system?**
   a. Transport oxygen
   b. Regulate hormones
   c. Break down food and absorb nutrients
   d. Filter blood
2. **Which organ is responsible for producing bile?**
   a. Stomach
   b. Pancreas
   c. Liver
   d. Small intestine
3. **Where does most nutrient absorption occur in the digestive system?**
   a. Stomach
   b. Large intestine
   c. Esophagus
   d. Small intestine
4. **What is the role of the enzyme amylase in digestion?**
   a. Breaks down proteins
   b. Breaks down fats
   c. Breaks down carbohydrates
   d. Breaks down fiber
5. **Which part of the digestive system stores waste before it is eliminated?**
   a. Stomach
   b. Small intestine
   c. Rectum
   d. Pancreas

Short Answer Questions

1. What are the main organs involved in the digestive system?
2. What is the primary function of the small intestine in digestion?
3. Describe the process of digestion from ingestion to elimination.
4. Name two enzymes involved in digestion and their specific roles.
5. What are common symptoms of digestive disorders such as GERD or IBS?
6. How can diet influence the health of the digestive system?
7. What is the gut microbiome, and why is it important for digestion?
8. How do probiotics support digestive health?

Answer to Critical Thinking Questions

1. (c); 2. (c); 3. (d); 4. (c); 5. (c)

REFERENCES

1. Abbas, M. O., Ahmed, H., Hamid, E., Padayachee, D., Abdulbadia, M. T., Khalid, S., Abuelhana, A., & Rasool, B. K. A. (2024). Pharmacists' Knowledge, Perception, and Prescribing Practice of probiotics in the UAE: A Cross-Sectional Study. *Antibiotics*, *13*(10), 967. https://doi.org/10.3390/antibiotics13100967
2. Accarino Garaventa, A. M., Azpiroz Vidaur, F., Bendezú García, Á., Malagelada Benapres, J. R., et al. (2017). Colonic content: Effect of diet, meals, and defecation. https://core.ac.uk/download/81582130.pdf (accessed on 14th June 2025).
3. Aires, M., Asnaghi, V., Asplund, M., Mary, A., Barbieri, E., et al. (2018). Acidification increases abundances of *Vibrionales* and *Planctomycetia* associated to a seaweed-grazer system: Potential consequences for disease and prey digestion efficiency. https://core.ac.uk/download/187434287.pdf (accessed on 14th June 2025).
4. Akamine, D. T. M., Brienzo, M., Kronemberger, G. S., Terrone, C., et al. (2021). Diversity and bioprospecting of filamentous fungi isolated from *Nausitora fusticulus* (Bivalvia: Teredinidae) digestive organs for lignocellulolytic enzymes / Diversidade e bioprospecção de fungos filamentosos isolados dos órgãos digestivos de *Nausitora fusticulus* (Bivalvia: Teredinidae) para obtenção de enzimas lignocelulolíticas. https://core.ac.uk/download/597559122.pdf (accessed on 14th June 2025).
5. Akiyoshi, H., Kudoh, S., Tanabe, Y., Yamamoto, T., et al. (2016). Comparative morpho-functional study in the digestive organs of the Antarctic rock cod, *Trematomus bernacchii*, in relation to phylogeny. https://core.ac.uk/download/51492563.pdf (accessed on 14th June 2025).
6. Aldewachi, H., Carey, M., Cramp, C., Helmstetter, C., Diamond, J., Diaz, J., et al. (2006). Postprandial morphological response of the intestinal epithelium of the Burmese python (*Python molurus*). http://arxiv.org/abs/q-bio/0611019 (accessed on 14th June 2025).
7. Andrada, D., Ioan Sergiu, M., Manea, M. E., Marilena, D., et al. (2020). Microbiota: The missing link in the etiology of inflammatory bowel disease. https://core.ac.uk/download/304672907.pdf (accessed on 14th June 2025).
8. Antonopoulos, D., Armitage, A., Singapore, A. V. A., Azad, M., Bäckhed, F., Schneeman, B. O., et al. (2019). Establishing what constitutes a healthy human gut microbiome: State of the science, regulatory considerations, and future directions. https://core.ac.uk/download/323068488.pdf (accessed on 14th June 2025).
9. Arnelo, U., Haas, S. L., Löhr, J. M., Martin, J., et al. (2017). Pancreatic exocrine insufficiency after bariatric surgery. https://core.ac.uk/download/188827229.pdf (accessed on 14th June 2025).
10. Astuti, D. A., Nurmeiliasari, N., Priyanto, R., Salundik, S., et al. (2018). Utilization of rumen mechanical stimulator as pseudo fiber in ruminant to minimize metabolic problem. https://core.ac.uk/download/236128858.pdf (accessed on 14th June 2025).
11. Badiali, D., Balla, A., Paganini, A. M., Palmieri, L., et al. (2017). Hiatoplasty with crura buttressing versus hiatoplasty alone during laparoscopic sleeve gastrectomy. https://core.ac.uk/download/153370704.pdf (accessed on 14th June 2025).
12. Barboza, P. S., Bjorndal, K. A., Bolten, A. B., Dierenfeld, E. S., et al. (2010). To chew or not to chew: Fecal particle size in herbivorous reptiles and mammals. http://www.zora.uzh.

ch/36242/5/JF_reptile_particles_REVIEW_100419.pdf (accessed on 14th June 2025).

13. Bates, R., Besser, K., Bruce, N. C., Cragg, S., et al. (2018). Uncovering the molecular mechanisms of lignocellulose digestion in shipworms. https://core.ac.uk/download/146491146.pdf (accessed on 14th June 2025).

14. Bauer, E., Metzler-Zebeli, B. U., Mosenthin, R., Verstegen, M. W. A., et al. (2011). Intestinal gene expression in pigs: Effects of reduced feed intake during weaning and potential impact of dietary components. https://core.ac.uk/download/pdf/29230036.pdf (accessed on 14th June 2025).

15. Belcourt, J., Coulson, D., DeBruyn, L., Francis, H., et al. (2012). The significance of a K-12 diabetes-based science education program for tribal populations: Evaluating cognitive learning, cultural context, and attitudinal components. https://digitalscholarship.unlv.edu/cgi/viewcontent.cgi?article=1045&context=jhdrp (accessed on 14th June 2025).

16. Caragea, D., Florescu, C., Pirici, D., Târtea, C., et al. (2016). The substrate of the biopsychosocial influences in the carcinogenesis of the digestive tract. https://core.ac.uk/download/144552990.pdf (accessed on 14th June 2025).

17. Chen, Q., Chen, X., Li, Y., Wang, L., et al. (2023). The mechanisms of nerve injury caused by viral infection in the occurrence of gastrointestinal motility disorder-related diseases. https://core.ac.uk/download/619411820.pdf (accessed on 14th June 2025).

18. Crane, P., Farrell, C., Garau, M., Grassano, N., et al. (2014). Exploring the interdependencies of research funders in the UK. https://core.ac.uk/download/30608686.pdf (accessed on 14th June 2025).

19. Davis, B. L. (2025). An economic analysis of a dairy anaerobic digestion (A.D.) system: Will dairy producers invest in A.D. technology to reduce potential litigation suits? https://core.ac.uk/download/pdf/6756822.pdf (accessed on 14th June 2025).

20. Drozd, V. Y., Hryniuk, O. E., Khukhlina, O. S., Mandryk, O., et al. (2016). Certain unsolved questions of pathogenetic interrelation between gastroesophageal reflux disease and chronic forms of ischemic heart disease (review of the references). https://core.ac.uk/download/144960609.pdf (accessed on 14th June 2025).

21. Edwards, C. H., Grundy, M. M. L., Holland, C., Ryden, P., et al. (2020). Plant cell walls: Impact on nutrient bio accessibility and digestibility. https://core.ac.uk/download/287579488.pdf (accessed on 14th June 2025).

22. Ekasari, J., Fardila Putri, R., Jusadi, D., Setiawati, M., et al. (2025). Utilization of fish bone charcoal in feed on growth and physiological responses of catfish fry *Clarias gariepinus*. https://core.ac.uk/download/639373533.pdf (accessed on 14th June 2025).

23. Evans, K. M., Lewis, T. W., Llewellyn-Zaidi, A. M., O'Neill, D. G., et al. (2017). Large-scale survey to estimate the prevalence of disorders for 192 Kennel Club registered breeds. https://core.ac.uk/download/141439117.pdf (accessed on 14th June 2025).

24. Förlin, L., George, S. G., & Livingston, D. R. (1994). Molecular biomarkers and toxic consequences of impact by organic pollution in aquatic organisms. https://core.ac.uk/download/11020749.pdf (accessed on 14th June 2025).

25. Gaiseanu, F. (2018). Destiny or free will decision? A life overview from the perspective of an informational modeling of consciousness. Part II: Attitude and decision criteria, free will

and destiny. https://core.ac.uk/download/186331556.pdf (accessed on 14th June 2025).

26. Giang, H. H. (2010). Impact of bacteria and yeast with probiotic properties on performance, digestibility, health status and gut environment of growing pigs in Vietnam. https://core.ac.uk/download/11695542.pdf (accessed on 14th June 2025).

27. Gillen, A. L., & Sherwin, F. (2017). The design of *Giardia* and the genesis of giardiasis. https://core.ac.uk/download/213464355.pdf (accessed on 14th June 2025).

28. Högberg, A. (2003). Cereal non-starch polysaccharides in pig diets. https://core.ac.uk/download/11694626.pdf (accessed on 14th June 2025).

29. Hollow, W. B. (1971). Histochemical investigation on the distribution and localization of digestive enzymes in the alimentary canal of the caddis fly larvae, *Brachy Centrus occidentalis* Banks. https://core.ac.uk/download/481531315.pdf (accessed on 14th June 2025).

30. Hooton, D. F. (2018). Brush border digestion: Development of a physiologically relevant *in vitro* model (Doctoral dissertation, Massey University, Manawatū, New Zealand). https://core.ac.uk/download/162617434.pdf (accessed on 14th June 2025).

31. Hristidis, V., Hua, M., Sadah, S., Talbot, P., et al. (2020). Health effects associated with electronic cigarette use: Automated mining of online forums. https://core.ac.uk/download/286729292.pdf (accessed on 14th June 2025).

32. Larauche, M., Mulak, A., & Taché, Y. (2011). Stress-related alterations of visceral sensation: Animal models for irritable bowel syndrome study. https://core.ac.uk/download/323080393.pdf (accessed on 14th June 2025).

33. Linson, E. A. (2013). The interplay between hormones and irritable bowel disease. https://open.bu.edu/bitstream/2144/12149/6/Linson_Elyse_2013_nosig_nocv.pdf (accessed on 14th June 2025).

34. Manuel, S. (2019). Ultrastructural analysis of the digestive gland secretory and absorptive processes in *Nepenthes glandulifera*. https://core.ac.uk/download/212887700.pdf (accessed on 14th June 2025).

35. Öpik, A. A., Öpik, A. A., Klann, A. E., Lee, A. P., Chatterton, B. D. E., Felgenhauer, B. E., et al. (2012). Controls on gut phosphitylation: The trilobites from the Weeks Formation Lagerstätte (Cambrian; Utah). https://core.ac.uk/download/14524908.pdf (accessed on 14th June 2025).

36. Patwardhan, K. (2008). Concepts of human physiology in Ayurveda. https://core.ac.uk/download/pdf/87482.pdf (accessed on 14th June 2025).

37. Petrovskiy, K. S. (2025). Alimentary hypokinesia. https://core.ac.uk/download/pdf/42865789.pdf (accessed on 14th June 2025).

38. Rucker, A. (1901). The Texan *Koenenia*. https://core.ac.uk/download/211338452.pdf (accessed on 14th June 2025).

39. Saavedra, C., Cordero, D., Bargelloni, L., Cancela, M. L., Milan, M., Leite, R. B., et al. (2017). A microarray study of carpet-shell clam (*Ruditapes decussatus*) shows common and organ-specific growth-related gene expression differences in gills and digestive gland. https://core.ac.uk/download/225163051.pdf (accessed on 14th June 2025).

40. Sarmidi, M. R. (2012). Food is our medicine. https://core.ac.uk/download/11801185.pdf (accessed on 14th June 2025).

41. Stiers, E. (2020). The microbiome of southwestern rattlesnakes. https://core.ac.uk/download/354492794.pdf (accessed on 14th June 2025).

42. Syed Muhammad, S. R. (2009). Comparative study of *in vivo* and *in vitro* methods in determining protein digestibility of feeds for bagrid catfish, *Mystus nemurus*. https://core.ac.uk/download/32600184.pdf (accessed on 14th June 2025).

43. Thomas, M. (2014). Celiac disease and gluten intolerance at Southern New Hampshire University. https://core.ac.uk/download/71369254.pdf (accessed on 14th June 2025).

44. Thomas, V. (2020). Comparisons of celiac disease and non-celiac gluten sensitivity. https://core.ac.uk/download/322851056.pdf (accessed on 14th June 2025).

45. Valls-Bellés, V. (2024). The biochemistry of digestion. https://core.ac.uk/download/614526814.pdf (accessed on 14th June 2025).

THE URINARY SYSTEM

10

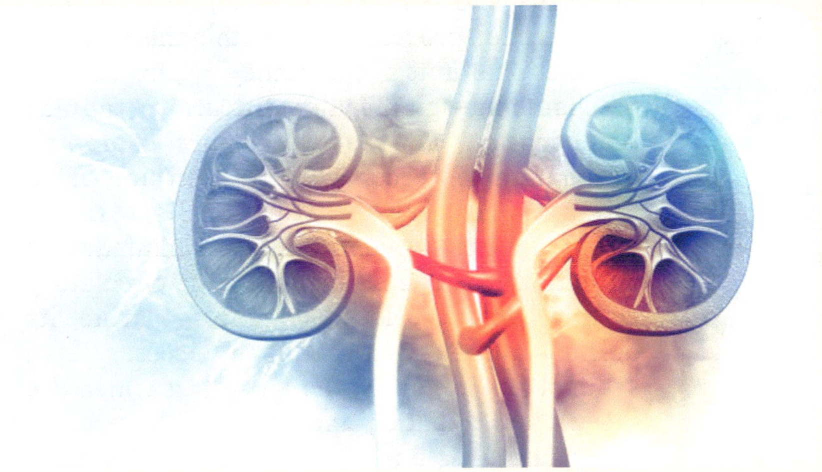

LEARNING OBJECTIVES

After studying this chapter, you will be able to:

1. Define anatomy of the urinary system
2. Describe the functions of the urinary system
3. Explain the urine formation process
4. Understand the hormonal regulation
5. Identify the common disorders of the urinary system
6. Define the Diagnostic Techniques of the Urinary System

Introduction

The urinary system plays a crucial role in maintaining the body's homeostasis through the regulation of the balance of electrolytes, water, and waste products. The complex system includes the kidneys, ureters, bladder, and urethra, with each playing a specific role in the entire process of urine formation and elimination. The kidneys, colloquially referred to as the body's natural filters, cleanse toxins and metabolic wastes from the blood. Their intricate structure comprises nephrons, which are the functional units responsible for the process of filtration. During the time that the system is active, not only does it eliminate wastes, but it also regulates significant functions such as the regulation of blood pressure and acid-base balance, showing the interdependence of human physiology. Understanding these processes is essential, as urinary system dysfunction has significant health complications and highlights the importance of awareness and research in this life-saving field of medicine. The latest developments in medical technology and research have further informed us about the urinary system and its pathology. Use of –omics technology, including proteomics, has now become a revolutionary system in the personalization of medicine, and particularly in urinary diseases. Such developments allow for a comprehensive analysis of biomarkers for diseases like bladder cancer, which high rates of heterogeneity and recurrence have defined. Precision medicine advancements aim to improve outcomes for patients through the application of such molecular insights to guide therapeutic interventions. For instance, the measurement of urinary energy excretion can offer significant information regarding the metabolic status of an individual and can prove to be useful in controlling urinary tract disorders. The amalgamation of these new methods with traditional medical practices serves as a basis for establishing a robust understanding of urinary system illness and its impact on overall well-being and calls for constant research and integration of these findings into practice. Despite the advances, the urinary system is plagued with various challenges that necessitate ongoing research and public education. Urinary incontinence, kidney stones, and urinary tract infections are prevalent chronic ailments with profound impacts on patients' quality of life. Moreover, awareness campaigns regarding preventive measures and the importance of lifestyle are needed to promote urinary well-being. Although certain dietary behaviors may influence urinary function, the accurate assessment of dietary metabolizable energy intake is crucial in the prescription of appropriate diet modification for urinary dysfunctions. Current methodologies used in estimating dietary metabolizable energy may not be ideal, particularly in the event of special diets. Results indicate that calculated and determined values may vary significantly, hinting at more accurate dietary recommendations to support urinary health. Addressing these subtleties within the grand scheme of the urinary system will continue to be of prime importance in medical school and public health curricula.

Definition of the Urinary System

Urinary system, which is a part of human anatomy, involves a system of organs that participate in fluid balance, electrolyte balance, and excretion of waste products from the body. Central to the system are the kidneys that filter blood to form urine, eliminating toxic metabolites and excess materials and conserving essential nutrients. This filtration process occurs within the nephron, or functional unit of the kidney, where various mechanisms—glomerular filtration, tubular reabsorption, and secretion—are combined to maintain homeostasis. Excretion and urine formation are primary ways of disposing of waste, thereby preventing the accumulation of potentially toxic material within the circulatory system. Once the kidneys generate urine, its delivery and ejection are made necessary by a sequence of conduits, the largest of which are the ureters, bladder, and urethra. Ureters are muscular tubes employed to move urine from the kidneys to the bladder, where it is stored until expelled from the body. Bladders' elasticity allows them to expand as they fill and signals the urge to urinate through sensory nerves. When an eventual capacity is achieved, the tension to urinate triggers a complex interaction of neural impulses that inform the sphincter muscles to relax, resulting in the voluntary emission of urine through the urethra. The apparatus is not only a demonstration of a vital route of waste elimination, but also a complex mechanism of balancing fluids and electrolytes in the body. While the urinary system serves to excrete waste, it also plays a vital role in many physiological processes, such as the regulation of blood pressure and acid-base balance. The kidneys determine how systemic blood pressure is influenced by the renin-angiotensin-aldosterone mechanism, regulating fluid and sodium retention. Also, parts of the urinary system have played an essential role in medical research; e.g., studies have revealed how urinary composition analysis is utilized to ascertain nutritional health and metabolic status. Research based on animal models, e.g., those studying age-related changes through urinary proteomics, has opened up cross-species comparison opportunities, as evidenced by typified changes in urinary peptide profiles with increasing age in mice and humans (Bajwa et al., 2017). These findings underscore the systemic function of the urinary system beyond the elimination of fluid, affecting systemic homeostasis and control over health (Zou et al., 2007).

Importance of the Urinary System in Human Physiology

The urinary system is crucial in the human organism for homeostasis. The intricate system has the primary responsibility of regulating blood pressure, blood volume, and the balance of electrolytes, all elements crucial for a healthy state. The removal of harmful chemicals detrimental to physiological function is ensured through the filtration of waste products, excess salt, and poisons from the blood by the kidneys, which is done by the urinary system. Besides, it assists in acid-base balance through the secretion of hydrogen ions and the reabsorption of bicarbonate ions, thereby controlling the pH levels necessary for most enzymatic processes in the body. The functioning of this system demonstrates the integrative nature of various physiological functions, making its significance in the sustenance of life and promotion of health valid. Specifically, the nephron, or functional unit of the kidney, is the core of the urinary system's function. Nephrons provide a sophisticated process of filtration, reabsorption, and secretion. Intracellular mechanisms for sodium chloride (NaCl) transport in the nephron, particularly in the cortical collecting duct, have been described by recent research as flexible. Investigations have shown that several types of duct cells have been proven to regulate NaCl balance and acid-base homeostasis collectively. This groundbreaking understanding not only portrays nephrons' versatility but also accentuates the need for such processes in maintaining electrolyte balance and sufficient levels of fluids, both essential for cardiovascular stability and overall body function (Crambert et al., 2017). Additionally, the function of the urinary system does not end at eliminating waste but extends to endocrine functions, highlighting its multifaceted importance in human physiology. The kidneys secrete hormones such as erythropoietin, which acts to stimulate bone marrow to produce more red blood cells, and renin, whose action is to control blood pressure by the renin-angiotensin-aldosterone system. This endocrine signaling role illustrates the function of the urinary system in overall physiological functions, including respiration and metabolism. Thus, understanding the entire function of the urinary system enlightens its importance in homeostatic regulation and lays down its importance in health and disease management, particularly with its interconnectedness to other body systems, as in the case of traditional understanding of physiology (Patwardhan et al., 2008).

10.1. Anatomy of the Urinary System

Learning Outcome

1. Describe the structure and function of the kidneys
2. Explain the role of the ureters
3. Describe the anatomy and functions of the bladder and urethra

The urinary system anatomy is a harmonious union of structures and organs that synergistically regulate the body's fluids, electrolytes, and waste. The main organ of the system is the kidney, a pair of bean-shaped retroperitoneal organs located in the abdominal cavity. The kidney consists of roughly one million nephrons, functional units that cleanse blood and produce urine. When blood passes through the kidneys, waste and excess substances are filtered out, and essential molecules like glucose and amino acids are taken up. Urine formed in this way passes through the ureters to the bladder, illustrating the importance of structural organization in the urinary system. learn about these anatomical associations since they provide them with an understanding of potential health issues and their symptomatic presentation. The narrow tubes, about 25-30 centimeters long, called ureters, convey urine from every kidney to the bladder and are responsible for the flow of urine. This body structure is characterized by its muscular walls that provide the peristaltic movement to propel urine at all times. The ureters pierce the bladder at an oblique angle, a configuration that prevents backpressure of urine when the bladder contracts. Within the bladder, a highly elastic muscular bag contains vast volumes of urine, exemplifying the structure and function relationship within the urinary system. The trigone, a triangular area on the floor of the bladder, signifies the area where the ureters enter and the urethra exits, embodying the vital relationship that renders voiding efficient and harmonized. This architectural arrangement ensures that processes of urine storage and secretion are maximally controlled, thereby providing fluid homeostasis. The final component of the urinary system is the urethra, the urine exit tract from the bladder. This aspect is significantly different in both length and purpose between men and women, with the male urethra approximately 20 centimeters long and serving the dual purpose of transporting both urine and semen. On the other hand, the urethra of women is about 4 centimeters, accentuating anatomical distinctions that affect urinary health. Urinary tract infections (UTIs) are likely to happen more often based on anatomical distinctions, which is why it is essential to learn about the anatomy of the urinary tract. Similarly, advances in technology in the medical field, as observed in recent studies, have raised our visualization of anatomy, with the resultant enhanced surgical technique and health outcomes, further reinforcing the necessity for an integrated understanding of the urinary system (Moro et al., 2017) (Figure 10.1).

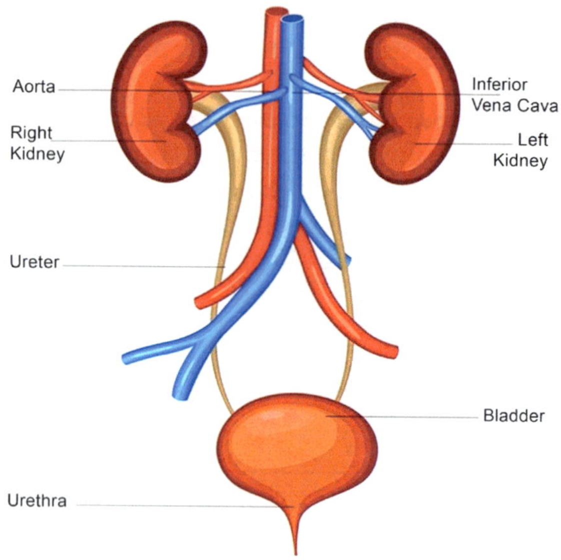

Figure 10.1. Anatomy of the urinary system.

Source: https://www.news-medical.net/image-handler/picture/2018/9/shutterstock_638539345.jpg.

10.1.1. Kidneys: Structure and Function

The kidneys, which are essential components of the urinary system, are complex organs that play a central role in maintaining homeostasis within the body. One kidney consists of millions of nephrons, which are the functional units responsible for filtering blood and producing urine. Nephrons consist of a renal corpuscle, in which plasma is separated, and a renal tubule, which further processes the filtrate to reclaim water, electrolytes, and nutrients. The design of the kidneys accommodates their multi-tasking functions, including elimination of wastes, regulation of electrolytes, and acid-base balance. The kidneys also function in the endocrine system by producing hormones such as erythropoietin, which initiates red blood cell production when the body is low on oxygen, and renin, which regulates blood pressure. Understanding the complex structure of the kidneys is critical to comprehending their whole function in the urinary system (Figure 10.2).

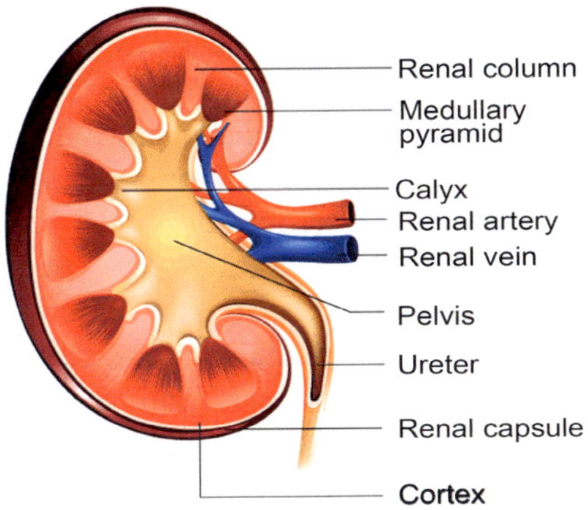

Figure 10.2. Structure and Function of the kidneys.

Source: https://cdn1.byjus.com/wp-content/uploads/2022/06/kidney-diagram.png.

Microscopically, the architecture of the nephrons is intricately designed to optimize its functions to a maximum extent. The renal corpuscle is made up of the glomerulus, a network of spongy capillaries that do the filtering of blood, within Bowman's capsule, which captures the filtrate. The filtration is followed by the tubular portion of the nephron—comprising the proximal tubule, loop of Henle, distal tubule, and collecting duct—that fine-tunes the process of urine formation. Every segment of the nephron performs distinctive tasks, namely in reabsorbing vital materials, such as water and sodium, to be utilized in maintaining fluid balance. The loop of Henle helps in the concentration of urine through a countercurrent multiplication mechanism that optimizes the kidneys' ability to conserve water and eject very concentrated urine. Therefore, the intricate structural complexity of the kidneys is directly linked to their functional ability to regulate body fluids, salts, and waste. Recent studies have begun to unravel some of the other functions carried out by kidney-specific proteins such as the Tamm-horsfall protein (THP) also known as uromodulin. This secreted protein, found in the thick ascending limb of Henle's loop, possesses roles that go beyond filtration, to include immunomodulation in the renal interstitium. Remarkably, THP has been shown to regulate the activity and density of renal mononuclear phagocytes (MPCs), which are crucial for immune function in the kidney. Research has revealed that THP can activate macrophage growth and regulate phagocytic activity, particularly in the context of AKI. Furthermore, loss of THP leads to decreased MPC numbers and impaired repair following injury, suggesting a protective role for this protein in the context of stress. These findings emphasize the complex dynamic interrelationship between structural components and functional mechanisms in the kidneys, making them a critical part of the broader urinary system (Dagher et al., 2017; Takahashi et al., 2018).

10.1.2. Ureters: Role in Urine Transport

The ureters play a vital function in the urinary system by serving as tubes for transporting urine from the kidneys to the urinary bladder. This is accomplished with a series of coordinated muscular contractions known as peristalsis, which propel the urine downward in the tubular channels. Each ureter, approximately 10 to 12 inches long, is lined with transitional epithelium so that it can be stretched and carry varying amounts of urine without damage. Anatomical alignment matters; the ureters descend retroperitoneally and are angled towards the bladder so that there is no back flow of urine, and hence the transport mechanism becomes one-way. This top-level structure emphasizes the importance of the ureters for ensuring the smooth flow of urine and reflects their role as part of the overarching system of the urinary system. Additionally, the ureters are very flexible in their functioning, which is adjusted based on the changes in pressure and volume of the urine (Figure 10.3).

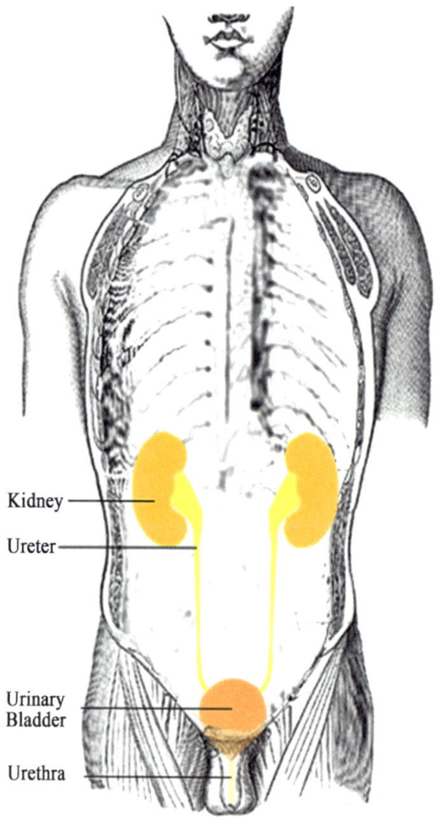

Figure 10.3. Urinary tract: The transport and removal of urine from the body follows the urinary tract.

Source: https://university.pressbooks.pub/test456/chapter/urine-transport-storage-and-elimination/.

Urine, produced in the kidneys, is collected in the renal pelvis before entering into the ureters. Transition from the renal pelvis to the ureters is necessary in maintaining the flow and pressure needed for effective transport. During filling of the renal pelvis, the increasing pressure results in the peristaltic movement of the ureters, thus urine is constantly pushed into the bladder. Also, the presence of ureteral valves at the junction level with the bladder adds to this dynamic further, as these inhibit reflux. This condition can lead to infections and other complications. An awareness of such mechanisms is crucial for the understanding of urinary physiology and how disorders, such as kidney stones, which interfere with this critical transport function have an impact. several pathological conditions can effectively compromise their function. For instance, kidney stones may occlude the ureters, leading to hydronephrosis and pain. These obstructions, in addition to impeding urine flow, also have the potential to lead to damage to the kidneys if left untreated. The ureters are also controlled by systemic factors associated with more generalized diseases, like metabolic disease and environmental agents that can impair urinary system performance (Gupta et al., 2020). In classical medical traditions, such as Ayurveda, urine production and function are seen as part of health. The Ayurvedic system of understanding the urinary system emphasizes healthy production and elimination of urine as a requirement, reflecting an awareness of the ureters' delicate balance being maintained (Gupta et al., 2020). Thus, the ureters are more than mere urinary transport tubes but are part of preserving homeostasis along with kidney health within the urinary system.

10.1.3. Bladder and Urethra: Storage and Excretion

The urethra and bladder play a significant role in urine excretion and storage, and are central urinary system parts. The bladder is a storage organ that holds urine temporarily until it is voluntarily ejected. The bladder contains a muscular wall known as the detrusor muscle, which relaxes during storage but contracts to expel urine during micturition. The coordinated action of the sphincters, both internal and external urethral sphincters, controls the flow of urine from the bladder through the urethra. An elaborate mechanism emphasizes neurological and muscular integrity in the event of intact urinary function, pointing out that pathologies may give rise to anomalies such as incontinence, overactive bladder, or urinary retention.

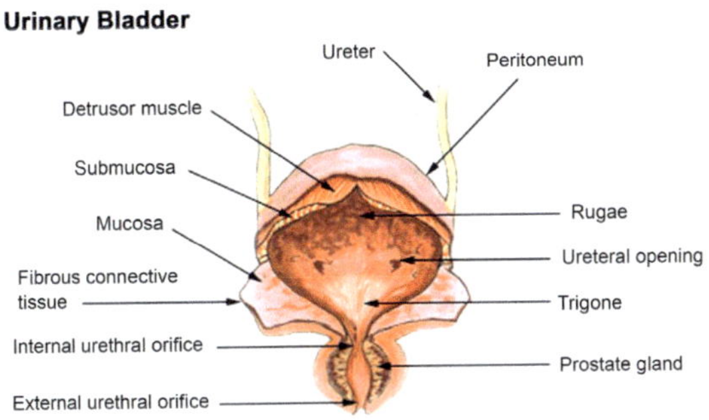

Figure 10.4. The urinary bladder is composed of several layers of tissue that facilitate urine storage and expulsion. The associated structures of the urinary and male reproductive tract are labelled.

Source: https://s3-us-west-2.amazonaws.com/courses-images/wp-content/uploads/sites/1940/2017/05/31172709/illu-bladder.jpeg.

Micturition, the process of urination, is a highly organized reflex having both voluntary and involuntary components. It is activated upon filling of the bladder, which stretches its walls and tells the nervous system to initiate contraction of the detrusor muscle. This results in a complex interaction between the central and peripheral nervous system, with brainstem and higher centers sending signals for coordination of the micturition reflex (Figure 10.4).

The role of neurotransmitters, serotonin and noradrenaline, has been advocated in recent research, suggesting that their modulation would have an extensive effect on urinary control and, consequently, a profound impact on social behavior associated with urinary activity (Antonio et al., 2015). Understanding these neurological determinants can open new therapeutic avenues in managing urinary dysfunctions, which offers hope for improving the quality of life of those afflicted by it. Anatomically, the urethra is the final conduit of urine excretion of the bladder into the world outside. The length and anatomy of the urethra vary significantly between men and women. In men, it is longer and transports urine along with semen, whereas in women, it is shorter and used only for urine excretion. The anatomical difference emphasizes the importance of understanding gender-specific urinary states of diseases. Aside from that, Ayurveda's historical knowledge, among others, reveals the physiological function of the urinary system, emphasizing how urination and excretion are crucial in human well-being and harmony (Gupta et al., 2020). Interconnected knowledge of the systems not only benefits enhanced medical intelligence, but it also promotes the development of culturally capable health practice that upholds traditional knowledge as well as contemporary science.

Test Your Knowledge

1. How do the kidneys function in filtering blood and producing urine?
2. What is the role of the ureters in the urinary system?
3. How do the ureters transport urine from the kidneys to the bladder?

10.2. Functions of the Urinary System

Learning Outcome

1. Discuss the filtration of blood and waste removal
2. Define the regulation of electrolyte balance
3. Discuss the maintenance of fluid homeostasis

The urinary system assists in the establishment of homeostasis in the human body by regulating the quantity and composition of fluids. One of the primary functions is the removal of metabolic waste products. These wastes, particularly urea, creatinine, and uric acid, must be excreted from the blood to prevent their buildup, which, if uncontrolled, is poisonous. Kidneys are equipped with extremely delicate structures in the form of nephrons that filter out the blood, a process that is crucial for eliminating these wastes. Not only is this filtration responsible for the purification of the blood, but it also regulates electrolyte levels and pH so that the body operates at an optimum range for systemic functions. Thus, through efficient removal of wastes, the urinary system has a crucial role to play in the body's overall health and equilibrium. The other significant function of the urinary system is in blood pressure regulation via the renin-angiotensin-aldosterone system (RAAS). During decreased blood volume or sodium concentration, the kidneys release an enzyme called renin, which catalyzes the production of angiotensin II. This peptide not only induces vasoconstriction, raising blood pressure, but also induces secretion of aldosterone, which causes the kidneys to reabsorb water and sodium back into circulation. Through such an indirect mechanism, the urinary system plays a vital role in the regulation of blood pressure by maintaining fluids and vascular resistance within normal limits. Because fluctuations in blood pressure can have an extreme impact on cardiovascular condition, the kidneys' regulatory mechanisms in this system identify the dynamic functions of the urinary system in ensuring body operations and supporting overall physiological balance. In addition, the urinary system contributes vitally to acid-base balance in the body. The kidneys regulate the excretion or retention of hydrogen ions and bicarbonate, which are substances required to maintain the level of pH for the blood and body fluids. Enzyme function, metabolic processes within the cells, and overall health require proper pH. During periods of acidosis, the kidneys initiate mechanisms to excrete excess hydrogen ions and reabsorb bicarbonate, which subsequently neutralize acidity. On the contrary, in alkalosis, the excretory process can also adapt to make sure there is an appropriate acidic environment. This responsive process indicates the ability of the kidneys to respond to various physiological challenges. Moreover, it describes an essential element of homeostasis that depicts the urinary system's critical role in supporting life through effective physiological regulation and response mechanisms (Valparaiso University, 1916; Dorsher, 2009).

10.2.1. Filtration of Blood and Waste Removal

The elimination of waste and blood filtration are critical functions of the urinary system, primarily supplied by the kidneys. As the body's internal filter, the kidneys actively work to remove waste products and excess materials from the blood for the purpose of maintaining homeostasis. This intricate process begins within the nephrons, which are the functional nephrons of the kidney and are comprised of a glomerulus and renal tubule. Pressure blood is introduced into the glomerulus, allowing water, ions, and other small molecules to pass through to Bowman's capsule while excluding large proteins and blood cells. The resulting filtrate is then selectively reabsorbed and secreted along the renal tubule to finally form final urine. This sophisticated system not only eliminates metabolic waste but also regulates the body's fluid and electrolyte balance, and this serves to highlight the kidney's important role in maintaining overall wellness and health. The recent advances in filtration technologies, such as the development of acoustofluidic systems, are just some of the current research efforts looking to improve blood filtration procedures.

These devices utilize ultrasound waves within microfluidic systems to isolate exosomes from blood without chemical tagging or invasive processes. A cell-removal module is incorporated to successfully isolate exosomes from other larger blood components with an incredibly high purity rate of over 98.4% (Chen et al., 2017) (Figure 10.5).

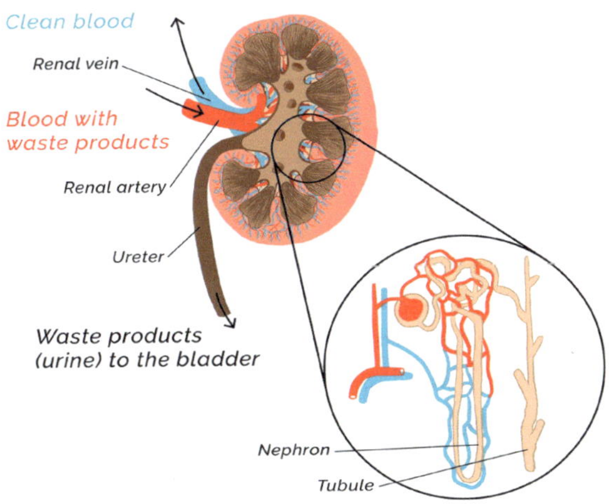

Figure 10.5. The role of the kidneys in waste removal.

Source: https://ckdexplained.co.uk/functions-of-kidney-waste-removal/.

These technologies offer promising opportunities for advancing both diagnostic capabilities and therapeutic treatments in medicine, particularly the health of the kidneys. By examining the exosomal content that is derived from blood, researchers can gain information on various physiological and disease states, creating opportunities for personalized medicine strategies that can lead to improved outcomes for patients with kidney disease. Moreover, residual kidney function plays a pivotal role when considering blood filtration and its effects on waste removal in patients with end-stage kidney disease. RKF refers to residual kidney function that persists despite the institution of renal replacement therapies like dialysis. Identification of the effectiveness of RKF is crucial as it could easily enhance homeostatic equilibrium, facilitating an optimal reduction of waste compared to dialysis alone (Kalantar-Zadeh et al., 2024). Preservation of RKF has been shown to influence morbidity and mortality outcomes in dialyzed patients, thus necessitating maintenance of kidney function where possible. Therefore, the natural and artificial blood filtration process identifies the ever-growing body of knowledge regarding renal health and the need for more specific intervention to optimize processes of waste removal in those suffering from renal challenges (Figure 10.6).

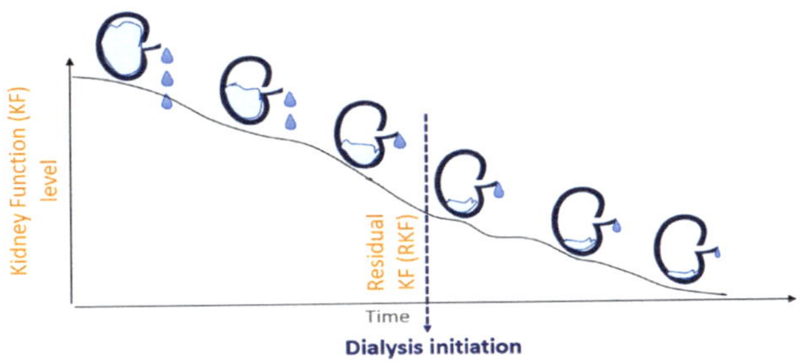

Figure 10.6. Kidney function before and after dialysis initiation. Residual kidney function (RKF) denotes the level of kidney function present at the time and after dialysis initiation.

Source: https://www.researchgate.net/figure/Kidney-function-before-and-after-dialysis-initiation-Residual-kidney-function-RKF_fig1_381905828.

10.2.2. Regulation of Electrolyte Balance

The regulation of electrolyte balance is a significant function of the urinary system to maintain homeostasis in the human body. Electrolytes such as sodium, potassium, and calcium are engaged in critical physiological processes like muscle contraction, transmission through nerves, and fluid regulation. Kidneys, primarily through nephrons, filter blood, reabsorb vital electrolytes, and eliminate excess amounts in the urine. This intricate process keeps blood electrolytic levels stable, again illustrating the function of the kidneys in general health. Dysregulation of electrolytes can lead to severe illness, highlighting the need for normal kidney function to control homeostasis. An understanding of the mechanisms controlling the balance of electrolytes might be applied to guide clinical intervention and therapeutic management for the treatment of conditions like hypertension and heart failure. The kidneys accomplish this one way through having several hormonal effects, in this instance through the action of aldosterone and atrial natriuretic peptide (ANP). Aldosterone, which is secreted from the adrenal cortex, causes reabsorption of sodium from the distal convoluted tubule and collecting ducts and excretion of potassium simultaneously. This sodium reabsorption keeps blood volume and blood pressure in check as a consequence. Conversely, ANP is a hormone that acts as a diuretic to promote the excretion of sodium, lowering blood volume and pressure in response to increased cardiac atrial stretch. The delicate balance among these hormones reflects the body's need for delicate control of the fluid and electrolytes. As time passes, control of these processes becomes significant when evaluating the effect of pharmacologic agents on the urinary system and overall electrolyte homeostasis, particularly in patients with fluid overload or dehydration disorder (Figure 10.7).

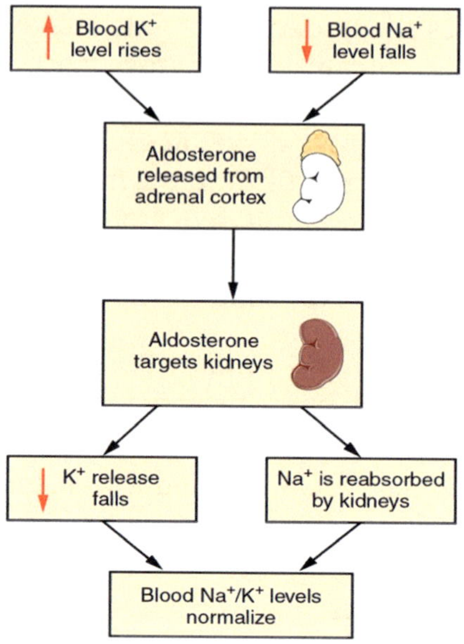

Figure 10.7. Aldosterone, which is released by the adrenal gland, facilitates reabsorption of Na^+ and thus the reabsorption of water.

Source: https://courses.lumenlearning.com/suny-ap2/chapter/electrolyte-balance-no-content/.

Subsequent studies examining newer pharmacologic strategies, such as the sodium glucose cotransporter 2 inhibitors (SGLT2i), have found putative mechanisms for better fluid and electrolyte balance regulation. SGLT2i is a cause of osmotic diuresis leading to increased clearance of free water and electrolytes from the interstitial fluid, resulting in decongestion in heart failure patients. This effect, distinct from traditional diuretics, makes SGLT2i symptom-reducing without significantly influencing blood volume or arterial perfusion and, therefore, capable of addressing one of the most significant issues in treating heart failure. This finding indicates that what is learned about electrolyte regulation not only imparts elementary physiological principles but also has tremendous significance in clinical therapies. With the evolving field, ongoing research in the regulation of electrolyte balance and its relationship with many drugs will result in optimal treatment approaches to numerous renal and cardiovascular pathologies (Vecchis et al., 2017; Leonard, 2025).

10.2.3. Maintenance of Fluid Homeostasis

Fluid homeostasis is perhaps the most vital of the many functions performed by the urinary system, mainly through the kidneys. Such organs are responsible for filtering blood, regulating the amount of water, electrolytes, and other solutes for physiological balance. In periods of fluctuations of fluid intake, the kidneys react through mechanisms such as changing glomerular filtration rates and modifying tubular reabsorption mechanisms. Specifically, as the hydration level increases, the kidneys stimulate diuresis, which allows the excess water to be expelled. When they are dehydrated, however, they step up the process of reabsorption, reclaiming vast amounts of water back into circulation in a bid to prevent the ill effects of hypovolemia. Essentially, the kidneys are not just filters but also volume and concentration controllers of body fluids, ensuring homeostatic conditions at all times. Besides filtration, the kidneys employ a variety of tubular processes to further modulate fluid homeostasis, primarily in nephron segments such as the proximal tubule and distal convoluted tubule. For instance, the intricate sodium-potassium balance of reabsorption is vital in terms of water retention and overall fluid equilibrium. The regulation of remaining nephrons following renal loss, i.e., following nephrectomy, illustrates the kidneys' capability to enhance functional performance. Under these conditions, SNGFR increments are required to compensate for the demands of overfiltered loads. Nevertheless, findings show that, in some situations, an increase in SNGFR is not sufficient to fully normalize sodium balance, which confirms the complexity of the regulating mechanisms in maintaining homeostasis upon renal adaptation (Edwards et al., 2017). Additionally, the cortical collecting duct (CCD) is also involved in the final steps of sodium and water reabsorption, and these processes are vital in maintaining fluid balance and acid-base homeostasis. The recent studies show that the CCD principal and intercalated cells are highly versatile in NaCl transport mechanisms. This allows them to respond adaptively to alterations in the body's physiological state, such as shifting levels of hydration and electrolyte composition. The mutual dependence of sodium and acid-base transport processes in the CCD highlights the integrated character of fluid homeostasis. The urinary system thus exemplifies an integrated interplay of physiological processes for establishing equilibrium, a function which is required to keep the whole organism healthy (Crambert et al., 2017) (Figure 10.8).

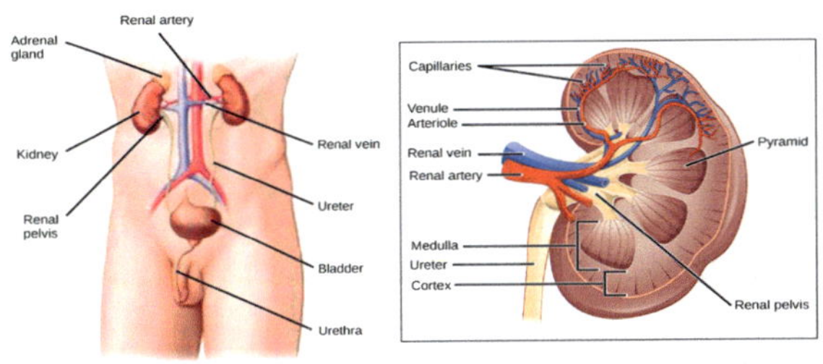

Figure 10.8. Homeostatic role of kidneys.

Source: https://opentextbc.ca/biology/wp-content/uploads/sites/96/2015/02/Figure_16_01_02.jpg.

Test Your Knowledge

1. How do the kidneys filter blood and remove metabolic waste products?
2. What role do the kidneys play in regulating electrolyte balance in the body?

10.3. Urine Formation Process

Learning Outcome

1. Define glomerular filtration
2. Discuss the tubular reabsorption
3. Explain the tubular secretion

Urine formation is an essential function of the urinary system, and most of it occurs in the kidneys in three tightly linked processes: filtration, reabsorption, and secretion. Initially, during filtration, blood plasma enters the glomerulus, and water, ions, and small molecules pass through the semipermeable membrane to the Bowman's capsule, thus separating the filtrate from the larger elements of blood such as proteins and cells. This ultrafiltration is essential because it gives a filtrate that closely mimics plasma but lacks the large solutes. This filter also relies on the efficacy of blood pressure and the permeability of the glomerular membrane, and therefore, impacts on these elements may result in alterations in urine content and renal function altogether, and thus highlighting the importance of maintaining homeostasis within the renal system. The second stage of urine formation is reabsorption, during which the required nutrients and water are reabsorbed from the renal tubule and returned to the bloodstream. This is facilitated by the presence of specialized transport mechanisms and channels allowing selective permeability. The majority of the water, ions, glucose, and amino acids are reabsorbed primarily in the proximal convoluted tubule through passive as well as active transport processes to avoid the loss of crucial substances in the urine. The loop of Henle plays a vital part in creating osmotic gradients that make adequate reabsorption of water possible. Disorders of reabsorption have unfavorable consequences, such as the loss of glucose in the urine characteristic of diabetic mellitus. Hormones that govern, including antidiuretic hormone (ADH) and aldosterone, tightly control the reabsorption process to maintain fluid balance and the body's electrolyte status. The final exam stage of urine formation is termed secretion, where the kidneys create an active transport of additional waste materials and excess ions from blood into the tubular fluid. It's not only an enhancement of the removal of harmful materials but also assists in pH balance through the secretion of hydrogen ions or reabsorption of bicarbonate as necessary. Throughout this time, specific transporters and enzymatic activities are essential in removing unwanted metabolic waste products and excess minerals. Further, the secretory phase is also crucial in infection-related conditions such as those caused by Proteus species, the causative agents of urinary tract infections (UTIs) and sequelae related thereto, such as stone formation from alkaline urine resulting from urease activity. This interplay of filtration, reabsorption, and secretion serves to underscore the sophisticated mechanism of regulation of the urinary apparatus in an effort to maintain maximum health and homeostasis.

10.3.1. Glomerular Filtration

Glomerular filtration is a critical physiological process that has significant effects on renal function and overall homeostasis in the urinary system. It occurs in the nephron, the functional unit structure of the kidney, i.e., in the glomerulus. In this case, blood is pumped through the afferent arterioles and filtered as its plasma is pushed by the glomerular membrane, a highly specialized one that can selectively remove waste products and excess material but not vital blood elements like proteins and cells. Glomerular filtration rate (GFR), which quantitatively measures the kidneys' filtration capacity, is an essential parameter to assess renal function. It is crucial to maintain GFR within the optimal level because variations from it can be a sign of underlying diseases, e.g., glomerular disease or systemic disease affecting kidney function. Glomerular filtration integrity can be compromised in various types of kidney disease with severe implications for overall health (Figure 10.9).

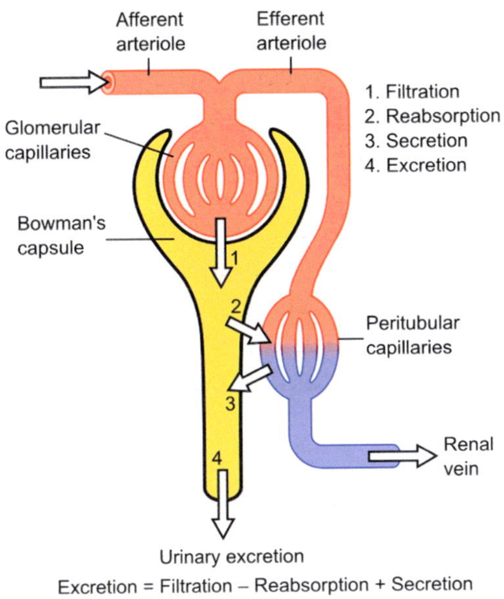

Figure 10.9. Glomerular filtration rate.

Source: https://upload.wikimedia.org/wikipedia/commons/thumb/2/2b/Physiology_of_Nephron.png/800px-Physiology_of_Nephron.png.

For instance, the state of Fabry disease, involving globotriaosylceramide (GL-3) accumulation, has been shown to cause cellular and vascular injury in renal tissue early on. It may result in reduced GFR and can further result in clinically significant renal events. A study of a group of patients with Fabry disease in childhood revealed that histologic proof for GL-3 accumulation was present before the onset of microalbuminuria, emphasizing the importance of early diagnosis and treatment in preserving renal function. The results are significant in pointing to the extent of further research into the glomerular filtration mechanisms and their relationship to systemic disease for enhanced early diagnosis and therapeutic strategies (Haack et al., 2015). Furthermore, glomerular filtration is intimately related to mechanisms underlying several glomerular diseases, including the most prevalent primary glomerular disease, IgA nephropathy (IgAN). Advances in -omics technologies have allowed researchers to identify new findings on new molecular signatures of IgAN that affect glomerular filtration and overall kidney function. Through urinary proteomics analysis and putting this information into pathways, IgAN key proteins can be identified. These studies reveal the intricacy of the pathophysiology of glomerular diseases and aid in the identification of possible therapeutic targets. The association of deranged glomerular filtration with IgAN verifies the preeminence of early and precise molecular examinations in improving therapy and understanding the multi-factorial nature of glomerular function within the urinary system (Cisek et al., 2017).

10.3.2. Tubular Reabsorption

The mechanism of tubular reabsorption is critical in understanding how the urinary system operates, particularly in the kidneys' capacity to recover valuable materials from the resultant filtrate during glomerular filtration. Tubular reabsorption primarily occurs in the proximal convoluted tubule, where approximately 65-70% of water filtered, sodium, and the majority of solutes such as glucose and amino acids are reabsorbed into circulation. The system is very selective and depends on active and passive transport mechanisms for the reabsorption of essential nutrients and the elimination of waste products. Disturbance in the reabsorption mechanism could lead to severe health issues, either as excessive elimination of nutrients or accumulation of wastes in the blood. Tubular reabsorption plays a vital role in elucidating kidney function in homeostasis and emphasizes the key role played by the kidney in various metabolic processes. In diabetic nephropathy and other diseases, tubular reabsorption can be significantly impaired. A case in point is the decrease in transporter expression such as megalin and cubilin and diabetic nephropathy. As shown by studies, some initial alterations in tubulointerstitial damage will disrupt the kidneys' capability to effectively reabsorb proteins, leading to increased urinary excretion of albumin and vitamin D-binding proteins (Bahamonde et al., 2017) (Figure 10.10).

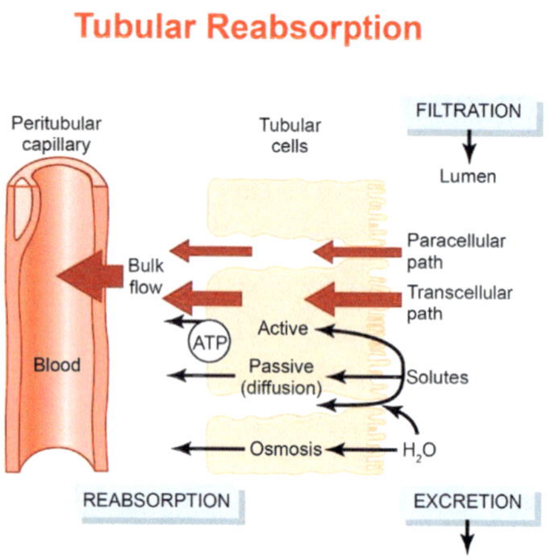

Figure 10.10. Tubular reabsorption.

Source: https://external-content.duckduckgo.com/iu/?u=https%3A%2F%2Fimage1.slideserve.com%2F2569204%2Fslide3-l.jpg&f=1&nofb=1&ipt=417fd78d5b5ad44ddb6aa2891399cb475890fe63eb41e8117f7d35fbf2ef8fa4.

This dysfunction is not only a deviation in the normal function of the proximal tubule but also indicates the interconnection between systemic disease processes and renal function. Tubular reabsorption, once successfully accomplished, is more than a local renal function; it determines the kidneys' function as an integrative organ, reacting to fluctuating metabolites in the body. Additionally, blood pressure and salt homeostasis regulate tubular reabsorption, which has a delicate balance that is essential to general health. The thick ascending limb of the loop of Henle is significant in sodium reabsorption, and higher sodium reabsorption may lead to hypertension or high blood pressure. This is an indicator of the significance of proper functioning of tubules in preventing salt-sensitive hypertension, a condition that is exacerbated by excess dietary intake of salt (Dominiczak et al., 2017). As research continues to demystify the mechanisms of such interventions, a possibility emerges of the development of specific treatments aimed at enhancing tubular reabsorption or lowering blood pressure, with the significance of understanding the urinary system as an integral regulator of maintaining physiological balance at large.

10.3.3. Tubular Secretion

The urinary system is a highly complex network that is responsible for the regulation of body fluids, electrolytes, and waste excretion. Tubular secretion forms part of the key elements of such a system, and it constitutes the movement of selected substances from the blood into the renal tubules.

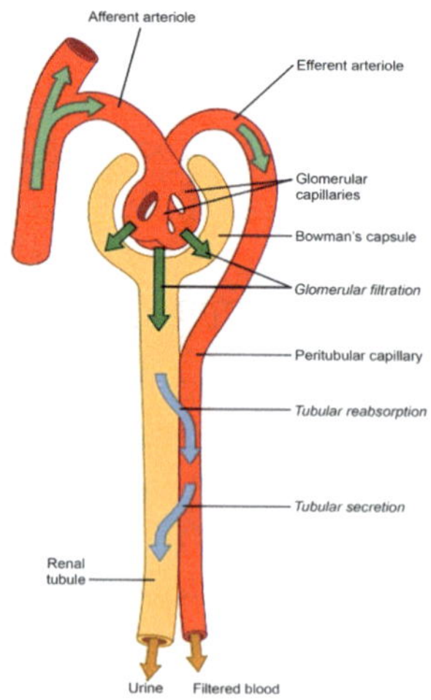

Figure 10.11. Tubular secretion.

Source: https://www.pharmacy180.com/article/tubular-secretion-3673/.

This is the cornerstone of ensuring homeostasis by facilitating the excretion of excess ions, toxins, and metabolites formed as a result of cellular metabolism. Tubular secretion is the most common occurrence in the proximal convoluted tubule, where drugs such as hydrogen ions, potassium, and other organic anions are secreted. Not only does this process contribute to blood pH and electrolyte balance, but also to the body's capacity for drug and toxin excretion, showcasing the kidneys' crucial role in detoxifying the blood and ensuring overall health. For the context of kidney disease, an understanding of tubular secretion is vital, particularly in the context of diabetic kidney disease (DKD). There is growing evidence to suggest a connection between proximal tubular function and the initial pathogenesis of DKD, demonstrating how disturbances of tubular secretion could contribute to the progression of kidney disease. Research on the mercapturate pathway, which is a metabolic detoxification pathway, emphasizes the role of the tubular cell in avoiding oxidative stress and inflammation. As tubular function decreases, so does the ability to effectively secrete and clear harmful substances, further complicating diabetes. Therefore, studying the mechanisms of tubular secretion and their relevance to kidney health could yield new paths for the prevention and treatment of diseases like DKD, now identified as more prevalent within modern society (Antunes et al., 2019) (Figure 10.11).

Tubular secretion also points out the importance of biomarker discovery in kidney disease treatment. As found in studies, urinary biomarkers can uncover tubular function and the body's response to metabolic derangement. Such biomarkers are essential to consider when assessing diseases such as DKD since they are intervening pathophysiological processes that may go undetected until late in the disease course (Gutiérrez et al., 2019). The capacity of tubular cells to secrete certain compounds not only indicates their functional integrity but also constitutes a critical line of defense against the accumulation of harmful metabolites. Greater awareness of these biomarkers and their potential Applications in the clinical setting can serve to significantly improve early detection, leading to timely interventions that improve the long-term prognosis of renal disease patients. Hence, further research into tubular secretion and its effects will remain critical in advancing renal physiology knowledge and therapeutic interventions.

Test Your Knowledge

1. What is glomerular filtration, and where does it occur in the nephron?
2. How does tubular reabsorption contribute to conserving essential substances in the body?

10.4. Hormonal Regulation

Learning Outcome

1. Describe the role of antidiuretic hormone (ADH)
2. Explain the influence of aldosterone
3. Identify the impact of atrial natriuretic peptide (ANP)

Hormonal regulation is fundamental to the functioning of the urinary system, influencing filtration, reabsorption, and excretion. The kidneys, the primary organs responsible for urine production, are controlled by various hormones, which regulate their function based on the body's internal status. For instance, antidiuretic hormone (ADH), or vasopressin, is secreted by the posterior pituitary gland when the body is dehydrated, enhancing the ability of the kidneys to reabsorb water from urine, thereby concentrating and conserving body fluids. When the body is fluid-replete, ADH release is inhibited, and dilute urine is produced. This homeostatic process underscores the vital role played by hormones in maintaining balance and overall homeostasis in human physiology. Another key hormone involved in the regulation of urination is aldosterone, which is secreted by the adrenal cortex. Aldosterone plays explicitly the role of regulating sodium reabsorption in the distal convoluted tubule and the collecting ducts of the nephron. Through sodium retention, this hormone indirectly controls water retention via osmotic effects and thereby elevates blood volume and blood pressure. The release of aldosterone is also commonly stimulated by the renin-angiotensin-aldosterone system (RAAS), which is triggered by low blood pressure or low sodium. This feedback mechanism through a systemic hormone not only ensures the homeostasis of blood pressure but also the optimal function of the urinary system. Dysregulation of aldosterone can lead to conditions such as hypertension and electrolyte imbalance, which mark the protective role played by hormonal control of renal function. Apart from ADH and aldosterone, other hormones such as atrial natriuretic peptide (ANP) play crucial regulatory roles in the urinary system. ANP, which is released by the cardiac atria when blood pressure and volume rise, acts on the kidneys to excrete sodium and water, reducing blood pressure. ANP counteracts the action of ADH as well as aldosterone, another instance of the delicate balance attained by counteracting hormonal pressures for kidney activity regulation. The dynamic interaction between these hormones depicts a sophisticated regulatory system that ensures the urinary system reacts to fluctuating physiological status. Understanding of these hormonal interactions is central to the comprehension of how the body integrates fluid homeostasis and overall physiological health, both in states of health and disease (Lopez M-T et al., 2011; Chen et al., 2015).

10.4.1. Role of Antidiuretic Hormone (ADH)

The ADH, also known as vasopressin, plays a key role in the regulation of water balance in the urinary system. The ADH is produced in the hypothalamus and released by the posterior pituitary gland. ADH functions to control the reabsorption of renal water by binding to specific receptors in the kidney. Whenever plasma osmolality increases, suggesting dehydration or increased solute concentration, ADH is secreted to increase water reabsorption in collecting ducts, thereby concentrating the urine and decreasing loss of water. This helps in homeostasis, especially in fluid imbalance conditions. The impaired function or secretion of ADH can lead to conditions such as diabetes insipidus, wherein there is an inappropriate excess of urine produced with increased thirst, reflecting the hormone's central role in body fluid balance and overall well-being (Crocker et al., 2006). ADH serves its role primarily by its action on aquaporins, water channel proteins of the renal tubules. On binding of ADH with its receptor, it triggers a cascade that activates the insertion of aquaporin-2 channels into the apical membrane of collecting duct cells, which markedly increases the permeability to water. This enhances greater reabsorption of water from the tubular fluid into the blood, which condenses the urine and reduces the volume of urine. Further, research reveals the intricate interplay between protein kinase signaling pathways and ADH activity and suggests that the mechanisms of signaling could modulate aquaporin density and function within cell membranes (Shi et al., 1990) (Figure 10.12).

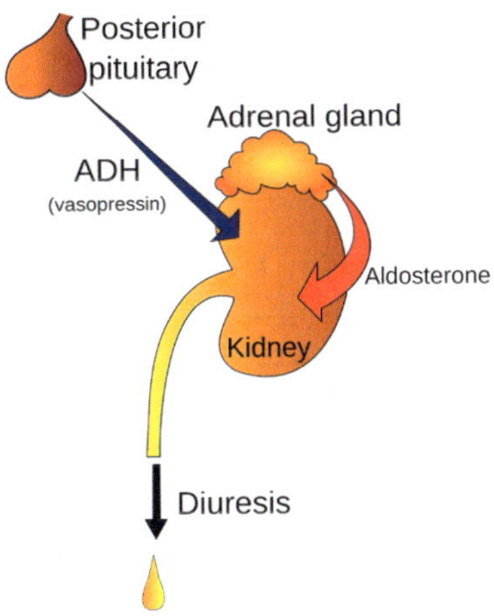

Figure 10.12. Antidiuretic hormone (ADH) axis.

Source: https://teachmephysiology.com/urinary-system/regulation/antidiuretic-hormone/.

Through regulation of aquaporin activity and quantity, ADH ensures the kidneys' effective management of the body's hydration status, responding to environmental variations and maintaining homeostatic balance. In addition to its role in water reabsorption, ADH is involved in blood pressure regulation, thus introducing its multifaceted nature within the urinary system. Through the promotion of water reabsorption, ADH indirectly elevates blood volume and therefore blood pressure. Moreover, ADH also initiates vasoconstriction in peripheral arteries, a function that increases its role as a blood pressure regulator. The relationship of ADH with the other body systems reflects its primary role beyond fluid regulation; dysregulation of its release can lead to complications seen in a variety of clinical disorders. Understanding the complex function of ADH in the urinary system not only emphasizes its physiological importance but also begs for further research into disorders that have to do with its abnormal dynamics (Crocker et al., 2006).

10.4.2. Influence of Aldosterone

Aldosterone, the principal mineralocorticoid hormone produced by the adrenal cortex, is crucial in the regulation of the urinary system, particularly in its action on the sodium and potassium balance. The hormone primarily acts on the distal nephron with effects on renal collecting ducts and the distal convoluted tubule. By causing stimulation of sodium reabsorption and potassium secretion, aldosterone directly affects the volume of fluid retained in the body and, therefore, blood pressure and fluid balance. Biochemical mechanisms triggered by aldosterone action are activation of epithelial sodium channels (ENaC) and sodium-potassium ATPases, leading to greater sodium reabsorption and potassium excretion. This intricate regulatory process serves to illustrate the hormone's role in regulating electrolytes, particularly in states of dehydration or hypovolemia, which basically affects the urinary system's function of efficiency in waste elimination and fluid balance. The interaction between aldosterone and renal mechanisms is not just confined to electrolyte balance but entails more extended measures for the health and disease of the kidney. For instance, prolonged exposure to aldosterone excess can trigger maladaptive processes in the kidney interstitium, causing renal fibrosis—a disease characterized by erroneous extracellular matrix deposition, which may cause CKD. Studies indicate that renal fibrosis is a central pathological endpoint of a variety of kidney disease states, justifying an understanding of aldosterone's role in fibrotic development. Aldosterone has been theorized in feline models to have a function in the induction of renal tubulointerstitial fibrosis, consistent with findings reported in human research. With renal fibrosis being well established as an ideal parameter correlated with kidney function, future treatments directed towards aldosterone's effect may offer promising avenues for CKD control and prevention of fibrotic processes (Elliott et al., 2015) (Figure 10.13).

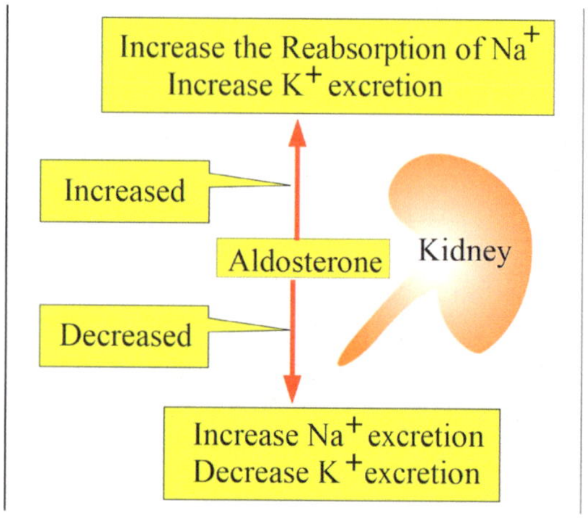

Figure 10.13. Role of aldosterone on kidney.

Source: https://external-content.duckduckgo.com/iu/?u=https%3A%2F%2Fwww.labpedia.net%2Fwp-content%2Fuploads%2F2020%2F01%2FAldosterone-effect-on-kidney.jpg&f=1&nofb=1&ipt=a9949d7b6ca09d26d776e08138802d9e15c7438d8dc38caedba29d01cccdf85a.

Furthermore, the control of water reabsorption by aldosterone by way of its action in the collecting duct underscores its function as a central agent in volume status regulation within the urinary system. The collecting duct is a significant site for tuning of urine composition, and regulation of aldosterone directly affects electrolyte homeostasis as well as osmoregulation. Aldosterone binds to mineralocorticoid receptors (MR) in collecting duct principal cells, facilitating the deployment of tight junction proteins such as claudins, which are responsible for membrane permeability. Specifically, studies highlight how various claudin proteins maintain overall tight junction integrity and function, which in turn influences the collecting duct's functionality to regulate blood pressure and fluid homeostasis. Functionally disturbed tight junctions may bring about significant disruption in renal fluid management, demonstrating aldosterone's far-reaching influence on the urinary apparatus and its regulation of systemic blood pressure and fluid balance (Leiz et al., 2019).

10.4.3. Impact of Atrial Natriuretic Peptide (ANP)

ANP plays a critical role in kidney function regulation, with implications for renal fluid and electrolyte balance. The heart's atrial cells secrete and release this peptide as a response to the increase in blood volume and pressure. ANP's primary action is to trigger natriuresis, or the excretion of sodium in urine, hence lowering blood volume and pressure. Through the direct inhibition of sodium reabsorption within the renal tubules, ANP directly reduces fluid retention, proper in such disorders as hypertension and heart failure. In doing so, ANP's effects lead to maintaining homeostasis in the urinary system and total cardiovascular system, which makes it of considerable importance as a counter-regulatory hormone for the action of other systems leading to fluid retention, including the renin-angiotensin-aldosterone system. Current research illuminates pathophysiologic expressions of dysregulated ANP levels in various renal disorders. Experimental results indicate that reduced plasma levels of ANP potentially precede the onset of advanced renal insufficiency and hypertension, as evidenced in fructose excess models of metabolic syndrome. In these settings, reduced renal sodium excretion is linked to increased insulin levels and systolic blood pressure, suggesting an essential correlation between hormonal modulation and renal function. Specifically, modification of natriuretic mechanisms can play a role in renal dysfunction, expressed as changes in sodium homeostasis and increased microalbuminuria, thus adding difficulty to cardiovascular disease management. This forms the basis of the realization that best control of ANP function is essential not only for cardiovascular stability but also for renal function maintenance, and this demonstrates a complex interplay between these two organ systems. In addition, species variability in ANPs role has essential implications for veterinary medicine, as is evident from initial research on equine biomarkers. In equines, research is starting to make connections between ANP concentrations and cardiac measurements, which could potentially affect the assessment of renal function and overall cardiovascular health in these species. Recognizing the implications of ANP in animals and in humans can potentially form the basis of targeted therapies aimed at treating conditions caused by atrial dysfunction. For example, assessing ANP as a marker for renal disease progression could be helpful in both veterinary and human medicine. This implies that further investigation into the regulatory functions of ANPs within the urinary system can open up diagnostic and therapeutic strategies across different species, subsequently resulting in better knowledge of its impact on kidney health.

Test Your Knowledge

1. How does antidiuretic hormone (ADH) regulate water balance in the body?
2. How does atrial natriuretic peptide (ANP) affect blood volume and pressure?

10.5. Common Disorders of the Urinary System

Learning Outcome

1. Explain the causes and symptoms of urinary tract infections (UTIs).
2. Identify the causes and symptoms of kidney stones, and describe their effects on the urinary system
3. Describe the stages of chronic kidney disease (CKD)

The urinary system is prone to several disorders, all of which impact its functioning and general health differently. UTIs is most prevalent, owing mainly to bacteria entering the urinary system and leading to inflammation and a wide range of symptoms, such as painful urination, frequency and urgency to urinate. UTIs are possible in any part of the urinary system, including the kidneys, the bladder, and the urethra, ultimately causing immense pain and complications when left untreated. Surprisingly, recurrent UTIs are a significant problem, particularly for women, that needs effective treatment measures and prevention to lower their occurrence and manage their symptoms effectively. Kidney stones are another frequent disorder in humans that involves the development of mineral deposits, which are painful and can lead to urinary obstruction. Kidney stone disease (KSD) has been increasing in prevalence worldwide in both children and adults. One interesting finding is that genetic factors can be involved in the formation of stones, with monogenic mutations linked to the presence of KSD in about 30% of children and 1-5% of adults, indicating a genetic factor in some cases (Spasiano et al., 2024). Diagnosis generally involves imaging studies and metabolic testing for stone composition and urinary chemistries, which may guide treatment as well as prevention. As knowledge of genetic factors grows, clinical practice will have to adapt to earlier treatment and treatment selection to reduce recurrence and improve patient outcomes. Current bedrock bladder conditions, including overactive bladder (OAB) and interstitial cystitis (IC), add additional complexity to the urinary system health picture. OAB is characterized by a sudden urge to void that is typically associated with frequency and, in some individuals, urge incontinence. This disorder may have a significant impact on quality of life and needs a multifaceted treatment strategy, which may include lifestyle modification, pharmacologic treatment, and methods of bladder training. Interstitial cystitis, however, is associated with chronic pelvic pain and discomfort, which can obstruct diagnosis and care based on the lack of clarity of its cause (Gremyr et al., 2019). Comprehending the complexity of the conditions is critical in planning therapeutic strategies, making the need for ongoing research and development imperative in the field of urology and urinary health sciences.

10.5.1. Urinary Tract Infections (UTIs)

UTIs are a serious and ubiquitous health issue that infects millions of people worldwide yearly. UTIs are mainly brought about by uropathogenic *Escherichia coli* (UPEC), which are strains of *E. coli* with adapted virulence factors that enhance their ability to colonize and endure in the urinary tract. The symptoms and presentation of UTIs could be varied, ranging from trivial dysuria to more severe renal involvement, based on the severity and site of infection. UTIs are highest in women and have been primarily blamed on anatomical and hormonal predisposing factors. It is basic to identify the prevalence and risk factors for UTIs to adequately design prevention and management strategies because the impact of UTIs can be beyond the urinary tract, sometimes escalating healthcare costs and substantial burden on patients' quality of life (Amos et al., 2018) (Figure 10.14).

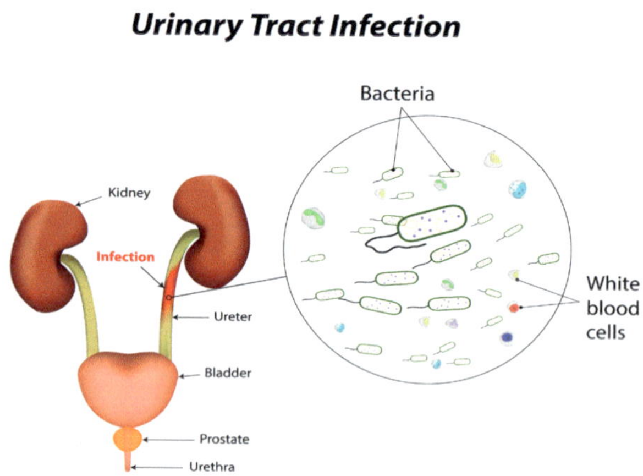

Figure 10.14. Urinary tract infection.

Source: https://www.uturology.com/wp-content/uploads/2015/06/UTI-in-TN.jpg.

UTI treatment is frequently with antibiotics, but it is complicated by the growing instances of antibiotic-resistant UPEC strains, posing the most significant challenge to date. Studies indicate that the majority of strains of UPEC are resistant to most prescribed antibiotics, hence challenging UTI treatment and demanding alternative treatment strategies. Elucidation of virulence factors present in such strains will be critical to establishing their pathogenicity and formulation of targeted therapies. Studies with model organisms such as Caenorhabditis elegans have proven incredibly insightful in terms of the virulence mechanism of UPEC. Such research supports the necessity to conduct further studies aimed at examining the complex relationship between host defense and pathogenic bacteria with the end goal of reducing antibiotic resistance as well as enhancing treatment effectiveness (Amos et al., 2018). In addition to antibiotic resistance, lifestyle and behavior also have significant roles in UTI susceptibility. These habits can exacerbate one's susceptibility to these infections. Women, in particular, run the risk of recurrent UTIs because of the anatomy and hormonal changes, making education regarding prevention strategies a necessity. Prevention against UTIs may include increased fluid intake, personal hygiene, and administration of specific probiotics to enhance urinary function. Public health interventions that promote education on UTIs and prevention are needed, especially in vulnerable populations. Given that UTIs are such a common health problem, education on the underlying cause and risk factors can assist with improved management practices and improved patient outcomes (Amos et al., 2018).

10.5.2. Kidney Stones: Causes and Symptoms

Kidney stone, or calculi, pathogenesis occurs as a result of the complex interaction of genetic, metabolic, and dietary factors. The chief constituents of these stones are calcium, oxalate, uric acid, and cystine, which precipitate in the urinary tract when their concentrations exceed the solubility limits. Excessive intakes of dietary oxalate, found in vegetables and nuts, and inadequate fluid intake can cause stone formation. Metabolic disorders like hyperparathyroidism and renal tubular acidosis can also increase calcium or uric acid in the urine, predisposing a person to stone formation. Awareness of these etiological factors facilitates the recognition of vulnerable subjects and prevention, hence emphasizing diet's and lifestyle's contributions to renal safety as well as lowering the risk of stone formation (Figure 10.15).

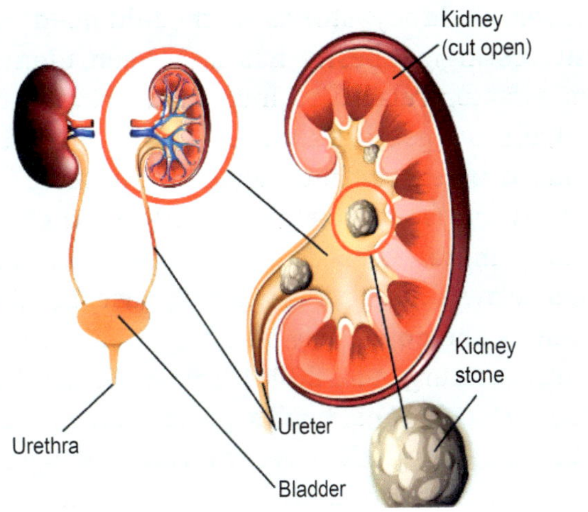

Figure 10.15. Kidney stones.

Source: https://www.westminsterclinic.ae/wp-content/uploads/2022/04/Kidney-and-Ureteral-Stones.jpg.

Symptomatically, kidney stones present with severe pain and a multitude of clinical presentations that depend on the size and location of the stone in the urinary tract. Commonly reported symptomatic features include painfulness, which is usually a cramping, sharp pain in the abdomen or lower back, and hematuria or urine containing blood. Other presenting symptoms might be frequent urination, urgency, and, in a few cases, nausea or vomiting. The sudden onset of the pain—characteristically occurring when the stone occludes the urinary tract—is crippling and can necessitate immediate treatment. Recognition of these signs is critical to early intervention, as untreated stones can lead to complications such as urinary tract infection and irreversible kidney damage, underscoring the crucial connection between effective relief of symptoms and long-term kidney well-being. The link between kidney stones and other renal conditions further illustrates why understanding the underlying risk factors is essential. For instance, studies have determined that patients with chronic illnesses such as diabetes mellitus and hypertension may develop kidney stones with enhanced risks. Interestingly, obesity has also been identified as a factor related to increased prevalence of calculi, suggesting that metabolic alterations caused by excess body weight may drive renal overwork (Astuti et al., 2017). Furthermore, heavy metal exposure, particularly cadmium, has drawn interest toward its use in kidney toxicity and potentially inducing stone formation (Brandenburg et al., 2006). Through establishing such associations, health professionals will be able to better guide prevention and management strategies for patients who come with risk factors, thus promoting a preventive culture of optimal urinary system function (Figure 10.16).

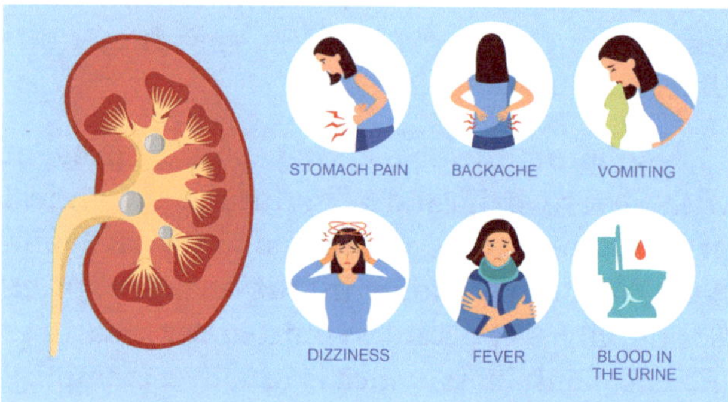

Figure 10.16. Symptoms of kidney stones.

Source: https://wp04-media.cdn.ihealthspot.com/wp-content/uploads/sites/342/2023/02/iStock-1344192779.jpg.

10.5.3. Chronic Kidney Disease (CKD): Stages and Implications

CKD is a chronic condition where the kidney function declines progressively, categorized into five stages based on the glomerular filtration rate (GFR). Stages 1 to 3 are typically symptom-free with minimal or no symptoms, whereas patients are still enduring normal kidney function with minor damage (stage 1) and mild reduction of GFR (stage 2). During stage 3, renal function further deteriorates, whereby patients may start to develop symptoms such as fatigue and water retention, which is why it is essential to monitor vulnerable groups constantly. Importantly, when CKD advances to stages 4 and 5, patients face progressively worse complications, including cardiovascular disease and the requirement for dialysis or kidney transplantation, underscoring the extreme importance of early diagnosis and treatment to improve long-term results and quality of life, reiterating a thorough grasp of the stages and consequences of the condition (Figure 10.17).

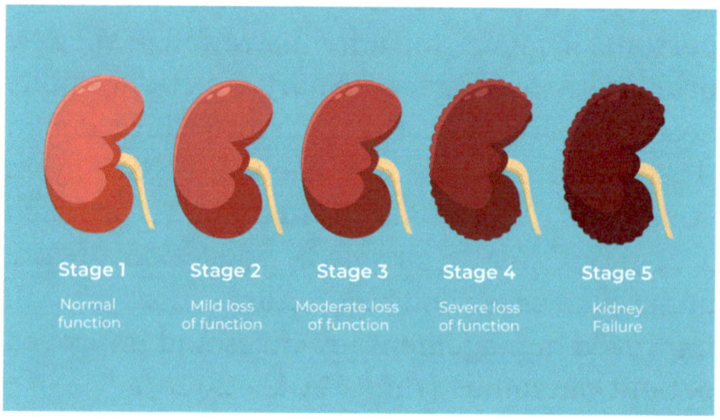

Figure 10.17. The five stages of kidney disease.

Source: https://images.ctfassets.net/pxcfulgsd9e2/1oDUtkU1aPBSW8L9v96G88/22e22e765ef229e633481563480 84ba1/The_5_Stages_of_Chronic_Kidney_Disease_HN3600_Cover_Sized.png.

The pathophysiologic consequences of CKD are significant, as the kidneys are central to many body functions, including the removal of waste, regulation of fluid and electrolyte balance, and blood pressure control. As kidney function declines, toxic uremic substances build up in the blood, resulting in toxic effects that profoundly disrupt health and quality of life. One such uremic toxin, p-Cresyl sulfate (pCS), is particularly challenging since it is protein-bound and toxic to several biological systems, among them the cardiovascular system. High levels of pCS in patients with CKD have been linked with adverse outcomes, thereby making it essential to delineate the metabolic origins and pathways of the toxins to guide the design of targeted therapeutic interventions. Interaction between kidney disease and gut microbiota might also be involved, with scope for interventional strategies to decrease levels of pCS to override toxicity, and highlighting the complex interaction in the treatment of CKD. Biochemical evolution in CKD stages is crucial in planning therapeutic interventions. Metabolomic and proteomic profiling have been recent research efforts towards expanding our understanding of the disease process. For instance, science has proven to create a significant correlation between several urinary and plasma biomarkers and kidney function, enabling physicians to predict disease progression better and individualize care plans. Through the examination of samples in several CKD patients, scientists found a group of metabolites and peptides that have excellent predictive value about the impairment of kidney function in both short- and long-term. Such an approach would be in the position to revolutionize the management of CKD by making early interventions that are tailored to the specific biochemistry of the individual patient, and thereby improve patient outcomes and restrict the toll of end-stage kidney disease, particularly in those at higher risk, as noted by studies in the field (Argilés et al., 2014; Glorieux et al., 2017).

Test Your Knowledge

1. What are the common causes and symptoms of urinary tract infections (UTIs)?
2. What factors contribute to the formation of kidney stones, and what symptoms do they cause?

10.6. Diagnostic Techniques

Learning Outcome

1. Explain the purpose and basic procedures of urinalysis
2. Describe common imaging studies such as ultrasound and CT
3. Interpret key blood tests used to assess kidney function

The urinary tract diagnostic complexities make early, accurate diagnosis of various bladder abnormalities, particularly bladder cancer (BCa), a priority. Over the years, conventional imaging techniques have been employed for this purpose, with cystoscopy remaining the cornerstone of the initial diagnosis. While helpful for identifying visible tumors, cystoscopy is poor at the detection of carcinoma in situ (CIS) and cannot definitively differentiate between benign and malignant lesions. Computed tomography (CT) and computed tomographic urography (CTU) are also consistently recommended to enhance the sensitivity and specificity of diagnosis. While helpful, they are also problematic, particularly when differentiating T1 and T2 BCa. New imaging modalities with increased specificity and sensitivity are required to allow the improved control of BCa, emphasizing the ongoing need to develop innovative diagnostic measures across the urinary system (Halpern et al., 2018). In the urinary tract infection arena, diagnostic procedures have emerged as key in managing renal transplant recipients (RTR). Due to heightened vulnerability to UTIs, over 50% of RTRs experience at least one infection annually, a reality that is fueled by the limitations of conventional urinalysis methods. Research has shown that the routine tests, such as leukocyte esterase and nitrite dipstick tests, possess high insensitivity and present false negatives for the majority of true infections. Less complex approaches, for example, adenosine triphosphate (ATP) concentration measurement and intracellular bacteria detection in shed urothelial cells, are more efficient in identifying UTIs in RTRs. Other approaches can potentially surpass the shortcomings of daily bedside tests, illustrating that conventional tests often fail to identify subclinical infection, which can cause graft loss and increased morbidity (Contreras-Sanz et al., 2014). The addition of advanced diagnostic techniques within the urinary system not only enhances pathogen identification but also affects treatment and management approaches towards patients. For example, combining conventional bacterial culture with cutting-edge approaches based on ATP levels and cell examination can provide a deeper understanding of the urinary system's state, enabling interventions to be activated at an earlier stage. As the medical field works to streamline these methods, it becomes apparent that the combination of conventional and new diagnostic techniques can improve patient results. This changing scene is part of a larger movement within medicine toward personalized medicine, where diagnoses are both precise and customized to meet the individual needs of the patient. The establishment of these diagnostic techniques serves the purpose of ensuring that researchers and medical practitioners continue to carry out research and innovation so that they can effectively manage urinary system disorders (Contreras-Sanz et al., 2014).

10.6.1. Urinalysis: Purpose and Procedures

Urinalysis is a valuable diagnostic aid in urinary system research, which provides information on numerous physiological and pathological conditions. The initial and primary purpose of urinalysis is to examine the physical, chemical, and microscopic properties of urine. With urine examination, doctors are able to assess renal function, diagnose metabolic diseases, diagnose urinary tract infections, and monitor the effects of some treatments. This painless and relatively simple test enables clinicians to obtain important information about a patient's health. Moreover, urinalysis can identify deviations such as the presence of glucose in diabetes, blood in other kidney diseases, or protein indicating damage to the kidneys. Thus it is a very useful component of standard medical examinations (Figure 10.18).

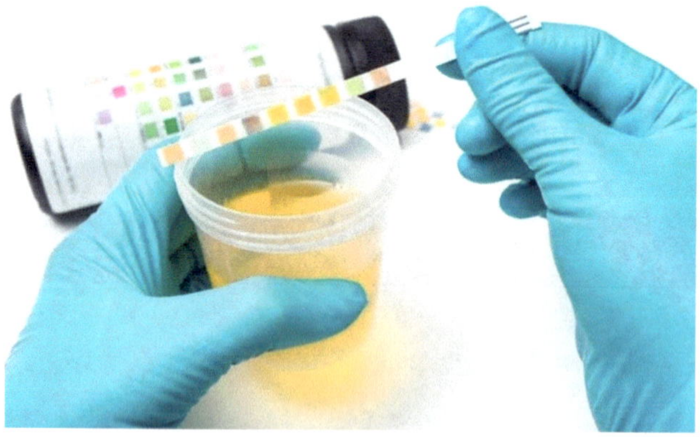

Figure 10.18. Urinalysis test.

Source: https://www.news-medical.net/image-handler/picture/2016/6/Urine_analysis_shutterstock_146356910.jpg.

The urinalysis process typically has three major phases: the macroscopic examination, chemical analysis, and microscopic examination. During the macroscopic phase, color, clarity, and odor are evaluated, providing a preliminary hint about a patient's condition. Chemical analysis via reagent strips examines various constituents like pH, specific gravity, protein, glucose, and ketones, each parameter providing varying information about kidney and metabolic function. The microscopic phase is where the centrifuged urine is checked for cellular components, such as red and white blood cells and crystals, that may be indicative of underlying health issues. These two phases combined give complete insight into the health of the urinary system, allowing practitioners to create accurate diagnoses and treatment options. The urinalysis continues to evolve with new techniques, supported by advancements in medical science and technology. For instance, it has been highlighted that the differentiation of asymptomatic bacteriuria (ASB) from urinary tract infections (UTIs) is important as this has the potential to affect treatment in a setting like nursing homes significantly. Missed diagnosis of ASB as UTI usually leads to inappropriate overtreatment, which results in adverse patient outcomes like antibiotic resistance and morbidities like Clostridium difficile infections (Olson et al., 2012). To counteract this, evidence-based policies and procedures for the evaluation of clinical status change have been developed that give much emphasis to accurate urinalysis interpretation in these risk groups. In such a manner, not only does urinalysis find diagnostic uses but also plays an equally important role as a determinant in shaping clinical practice, thereby contributing towards better patient care in terms of the urinary system.

10.6.2. Imaging Studies: Ultrasound and CT Scans

Imaging tests play a critical role in diagnosing many conditions that affect the urinary system, and the most common of these imaging modalities used are ultrasound and computed tomography (CT) scans. The most commonly utilized is ultrasound because it is non-invasive, low in cost, and does not utilize ionizing radiation. It is used to obtain real-time images that can identify the size, shape, and structure of the kidneys, bladder, and surrounding tissues. It is therefore instrumental in identifying abnormalities such as cysts, tumors, or blockages. It is also frequently the imaging modality of initial choice in children due to its safety. Its utility in allowing further diagnostic interventions and procedures also reflects its significance in urinary tract assessments. CT scans, however, have greater resolution and are particularly worthwhile under emergency circumstances where speed of diagnosis is a factor. They are also effective in identifying urolithiasis complications, like the correct position and size of renal calculi. According to research, CT scans have become routinely used in the emergency department, especially among patients with flank pain or a strong suspicion of kidney stones (Afonso et al., 2020) (Figure 10.19).

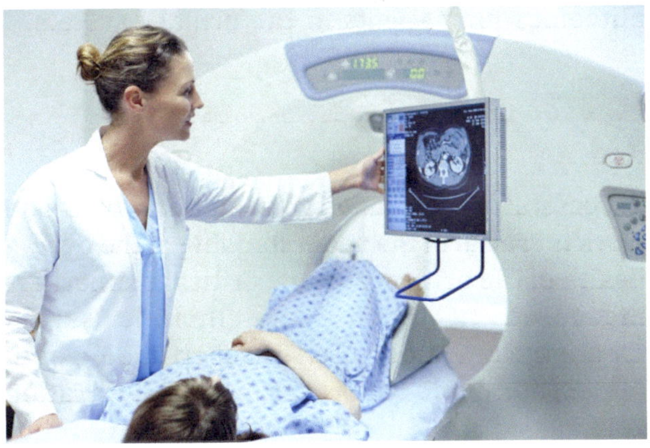

Figure 10.19. Imaging tests for detecting kidney stones.

Source: https://www.healthimages.com/content/uploads/sites/2/2019/12/mri-procedure.jpg.

The modality has high sensitivity and specificity, which makes it more diagnostic with the ability to evaluate renal and extrarenal structures critically. Furthermore, advances in CT technology such as the introduction of low-dose schemes minimize anxiety concerning radiation exposure while maximizing the quality of images. This development underscores the pivotal role of CT in modern urological practice. Ultrasound and CT scanning complement each other in urinary tract disease diagnosis. Clinical indications and patient-related criteria typically determine the choice between these imaging modalities. For instance, while ultrasound may be adequate for follow-ups and routine evaluations, CT scans are employed in more complex situations that require precise anatomical information. Existing literature suggests that an integration of these imaging modalities can add a significant contribution to clinical management, particularly in nephrolithiasis, where stone composition information is a critical component in planning treatment (Bove et al., 2013). By exploiting the complementary power of both modalities, clinicians can optimize diagnosis and tailor therapy to specific needs, eventually improving outcomes for patients in the urinary system.

10.6.3. Blood Tests: Assessing Kidney Function

Successful kidney function evaluation by blood work is crucial in the understanding of the overall health of the urinary system. Critical biomarkers measured in blood work include serum creatinine and blood urea nitrogen (BUN), both of which provide data regarding renal filtration function. Increased levels of these substances suggest potential kidney malfunction, and further investigation is needed. Although serum creatinine is a reliable predictor of glomerular filtration rate (GFR), it should be remembered that hydration status and muscle mass may influence its validity. For instance, patients with reduced muscle mass might have spuriously low serum creatinine even in the presence of impaired kidney function. Hence, for an original diagnosis and therapy of kidney conditions, a comprehensive assessment consisting of several tests and clinical examinations must be carried out. Other than routine blood tests, recent advances in urinary proteomics have offered new directions in the assessment of kidney disease. Such an innovative method employs mass spectrometry to quantify proteins in urine, thereby generating a vast amount of data about the kidney condition. For example, urinary biomarkers such as collagen peptides and uromodulin have been shown not only to diagnose established kidney diseases but also to predict disease progression. The sensitivity and specificity of such biomarkers are greater than those of conventional blood tests, offering improved diagnostic and prognostic markers. Available evidence suggests that integration of urinary proteomics into clinical practice can significantly enhance our ability to follow patients with chronic kidney disease, enabling early intervention that decreases patient morbidity, thus enhancing the potential of this avenue regarding the urinary system as a whole (Magalhães et al., 2016). The demand for kidney transplantations underlines the necessity for personalized medicine.

Test Your Knowledge

1. How are ultrasound and CT scans used in diagnosing urinary system conditions?
2. Which blood tests are commonly used to evaluate kidney function, and what do they measure?

SUMMARY

The intricate workings of the urinary system are a key element in waste excretion, as well as the body's overall homeostasis. The relationship between its various components, i.e., the kidneys, ureters, bladder, and urethra, makes for a very effective process that is critical to being healthy. How well this system works can have profound implications for well-being, as evidenced in studies that have identified many individuals, particularly postpartum women, who may experience urinary system problems. As seen in recent studies, research has shown that out of 16 postpartum women, only one was diagnosed with urinary retention, which indicates the necessity of continuous observation and treatment during this vulnerable time (et al., 2018). Therefore, understanding the functioning of the urinary systems and management of likely disorders are most significant to improve health outcomes. Proper care by nurses is essential in cases of patients afflicted by disorders of the urinary system. By employing theories such as Orem's Self Care Deficit Theory, health professionals can quantify and augment patients' abilities to meet their self-care needs. The practice of this theory underscores the importance of personalized care in managing urinary disorders appropriately. Evidently, most patients have urinary elimination disorders, which call for specific nursing interventions (Hidayati et al., 2018). Additionally, education interventions to address gaps in knowledge among patients can encourage independence and reduce risks of urinary complications. Therefore, nursing practice founded on evidence-based theoretical supports is needed to enhance recovery and quality of life. Finally, greater awareness of the complexity of the urinary system and augmented nursing practices can improve patient outcomes and healthcare delivery. As highlighted in the various studies, the burden of urinary disorders calls for an active response in clinical practice and community health initiatives. Awareness among healthcare providers and patients of urinary health can help avoid the effects of prevalent disorders, such as urinary retention and incontinence, so that individuals are provided with early interventions. Besides, since complications arising from urinary issues have a broader impact on overall health, a combined plan that brings together education, assessment, and individualized care is necessary. Treating such issues holistically can enhance the quality of care and empower patients to manage their own health, thereby positively impacting society.

The urinary system plays a crucial role in maintaining homeostasis in the human body by regulating the excretion of waste products, electrolyte balance, and blood pressure. The focal point of the system is the kidneys, which filter the blood and excrete urine. It is crucial to understand the various stages of kidney disease, particularly diabetic nephropathy, because of its commonality among type 1 diabetic individuals. The role of microRNA in kidney disease development and gene regulation has been of notable interest. Research has shown that urinary microRNA signatures differ significantly between stages of diabetic nephropathy and potentially are of paramount significance in early diagnosis and effective risk stratification for complications such as end-stage renal disease (Krupa et al., 2013). This highlights the need for further research in disease and metabolic regulation to establish practical therapeutic approaches in nephrology. Apart from functional kidney dynamics, vulnerability of the urinary system to infection also highlights the need for practical treatment approaches. Urinary tract infections (UTIs), often caused by uropathogenic Escherichia coli (UPEC), can contribute to severe impairment of an individual's health. UPEC employs a set of virulence factors, including targetable adhesins such as those that render it capable of surviving in urinary tissues. Development of therapies against such infections, particularly in the light of growing antibiotic resistance, is now a matter of high priority. Emerging progress in structural biology and synthetic chemistry identifies compelling strategies for designing antivirulence therapeutics, for example, glycomimetic inhibitors targeting UPEC adhesins. These inhibitors successfully inhibited UPEC adhesion in vitro and in vivo and showed promise for novel therapeutic options in the treatment of UTIs and blocking the transmission of multidrug-resistant infections (Chugani et al., 2018). The interdependency of kidney function and urinary tract health is an essential field of research interest, especially given the increasing global incidence of diabetes and antibiotic resistance. The findings of urinary microRNAs and their potential for utilization offer promise for the enhancement of diagnostic tools and therapeutic agents in diabetic nephropathy. Similarly, the development of antivirulence agents provides a promising track towards the treatment of UTIs by resistant pathogens. As research goes on to delve into the intricacy of the urinary tract, the confluence of molecular biomarkers and new pharmacological strategies will likely prove to impact clinical outcomes significantly. As such, understanding the urinary system's intricate role in health and disease can contribute considerably to the formation of disease-specific treatments and patient management approaches, leading ultimately to better health in affected individuals.

KEY TERMS FROM THIS CHAPTER

- Kidneys
- Renal Cortex
- Ureters
- Urethra
- Bowman's Capsule
- Loop of Henle
- Collecting Duct
- Reabsorption
- Nephrons
- Renal Pelvis
- Urinary Bladder
- Glomerulus
- Proximal Convoluted Tubule
- Distal Convoluted Tubule
- Filtration
- Secretion

CRITICAL THINKING QUESTIONS

1. **Which of the following is the primary function of the kidneys?**
   a. Produce digestive enzymes
   b. Regulate blood sugar levels
   c. Filter waste products from the blood
   d. Store urine until excretion
2. **What is the tube that carries urine from the kidneys to the bladder called?**
   a. Urethra
   b. Nephron
   c. Ureter
   d. Loop of Henle
3. **What structure in the nephron is responsible for the filtration of blood?**
   a. Loop of Henle
   b. Glomerulus
   c. Collecting duct
   d. Renal pelvis
4. **Which hormone regulates the amount of water reabsorbed by the kidneys?**
   a. Insulin
   b. Estrogen
   c. Antidiuretic hormone (ADH)
   d. Glucagon
5. **Where is urine stored before it is excreted from the body?**
   a. Kidney
   b. Ureter
   c. Urethra
   d. Bladder

Short Answer Questions

1. What are the main anatomical components of the urinary system?
2. What are the primary functions of the urinary system?
3. How is urine formed within the kidneys?
4. Which hormones regulate the function of the urinary system?
5. What are some common disorders that affect the urinary system?
6. What diagnostic techniques are used to assess urinary system health?

Answer to Critical Thinking Questions

1.(c) 2.(c) 3.(b) 4.(c) 5.(d)

REFERENCES

1. Afonso, G., Alves, P., Gomes, A., et al. (2020). Adequação dos exames de radiologia solicitados por um departamento de emergência: Um estudo retrospetivo. https://core.ac.uk/download/288958467.pdf (accessed on 14th June 2025).
2. Schifano, E., Marazzato, M., Ammendolia, M. G., Zanni, E., Ricci, M., Comanducci, A., Goldoni, P., Conte, M. P., Uccelletti, D., & Longhi, C. (2018). Virulence behavior of uropathogenic Escherichia colistrains in the host model Caenorhabditis elegans. *MicrobiologyOpen*, *8*(6). https://doi.org/10.1002/mbo3.756Antonio, C., Claus, M., Jimena, M., Ricatti, M., et al. (2015). Serotonin and noradrenaline reuptake inhibitors improve micturition control in mice. https://core.ac.uk/download/53519469.pdf (accessed on 14th June 2025).
3. Antunes, A., Coelho, N., Correia, M. J., Gonçalves-Dias, C., et al. (2019). Mercapturate pathway in the tubulocentric perspective of diabetic kidney disease. https://core.ac.uk/download/188486500.pdf (accessed on 14th June 2025).
4. Argilés, À., Dakna, M., Delles, C., Duranton, F., et al. (2014). Assessment of metabolomic and proteomic biomarkers in detection and prognosis of progression of renal function in chronic kidney disease. https://core.ac.uk/download/42354001.pdf (accessed on 14th June 2025).
5. Astuti, A. Y., & Mohammad, A. M. (2017). Gender-based health disorders in end-stage renal disease patients in the hospital Elmarj city of Libya. https://media.neliti.com/media/publications/164690-EN-gender-based-health-disorders-in-end-sta.pdf (accessed on 14th June 2025).
6. Babu, P. V. V., Balaji, Bhukya, & Subrahmanyam, C. V. S. (2019). Nephrolithiasis–Most debilitating renal disorder. https://core.ac.uk/download/230499548.pdf (accessed on 14th June 2025).
7. Bahamonde, J., Ezquer, F., Ezquer, M., Giraud Billoud, B., et al. (2017). Tubulointerstitial injury and proximal tubule albumin transport in early diabetic nephropathy induced by type 1 diabetes mellitus. https://core.ac.uk/download/159301014.pdf (accessed on 14th June 2025).
8. Bajwa, S., Bascands, J. L., Bechtel-Walz, W., Borries, M., et al. (2017). The use of urinary proteomics in the assessment of suitability of mouse models for ageing. https://core.ac.uk/download/78838013.pdf (accessed on 14th June 2025).
9. Bove, P., Finazzi Agrò, E., Kim, F. J., Miano, R., Micali, S., Rosa, M., & Usai, P. (2013). Recent finding and new technologies in nephrolithiasis: A review of the recent literature. https://core.ac.uk/download/pdf/54580708.pdf (accessed on 14th June 2025).
10. Brandenburg, P., Esche, V., Godt, J., Groneberg, D., et al. (2006). The toxicity of cadmium and resulting hazards for human health. https://core.ac.uk/download/14524906.pdf (accessed on 14th June 2025).
11. Chen, C., Dao, M., Huang, P. H., Huang, K., et al. (2017). Isolation of exosomes from whole blood by integrating acoustics and microfluidics. https://core.ac.uk/download/156872780.pdf (accessed on 14th June 2025).
12. Chen, L., Delville, C., Derous, D., Douglas, P., et al. (2015). The effects of graded levels of calorie restriction: II. Impact of short-term calorie and protein restriction on circulating hormone levels, glucose homeostasis and oxidative stress in male C57BL/6 mice. https://core.ac.uk/download/30435896.pdf (accessed on 14th June 2025).

13. Choi, M. R., del Mauro, J. S., Fernandez, B. E., Gironacci, M., et al. (2018). La alteración de sistemas natriuréticos renales se asocia con el desarrollo de hipertensión arterial y precede en el tiempo a la aparición de daño renal en un modelo de síndrome metabólico. https://core.ac.uk/download/288803470.pdf (accessed on 14th June 2025).

14. Chugani, R., Conover, M. S., Hibbing, M. E., Hultgren, S., et al. (2018). Structure-based discovery of glycomimetic FmlH ligands as inhibitors of bacterial adhesion during urinary tract infection. https://core.ac.uk/download/212863647.pdf (accessed on 14th June 2025).

15. Cisek, K., Delles, C., Filip, S., Gakiopoulou, M., et al. (2017). Identification of novel molecular signatures of IgA nephropathy through an integrative -omics analysis. https://core.ac.uk/download/96883268.pdf (accessed on 14th June 2025).

16. Contreras-Sanz, A., Farmer, C. K., Peppiatt-Wildman, C. M., Courtneidge, H. R., Malone-Lee, J., Durodie, J., Kelley, et al. (2014). Urinary ATP and visualization of intracellular bacteria: A superior diagnostic marker for recurrent UTI in renal transplant recipients? https://core.ac.uk/download/30706795.pdf (accessed on 14th June 2025).

17. Crambert, G., & Edwards, A. (2017). Versatility of NaCl transport mechanisms in the cortical collecting duct. https://open.bu.edu/bitstream/2144/39547/1/Edwards%20AJP%20Renal%202017%20Versatility%20of%20NaCl%20transport%20mechanisms.pdf (accessed on 14th June 2025).

18. Crocker, M., Smith, M., Tisdall, M., Watkiss, J., et al. (2006). Disturbances of sodium in critically ill adult neurologic patients: A clinical review. https://core.ac.uk/download/1671042.pdf (accessed on 14th June 2025).

19. Dagher, P. C., El-Achkar, T. M., Ghosh, J., Hato, T., et al. (2017). Tamm-Horsfall protein regulates mononuclear phagocytes in the kidney. https://core.ac.uk/download/228066343.pdf (accessed on 14th June 2025).

20. Dal Moro, F. (2017). How robotic surgery is changing our understanding of anatomy. https://core.ac.uk/download/141698977.pdf (accessed on 14th June 2025).

21. De Clercq, D., Decloedt, A., Van Der Vekens, N., van Loon, G., et al. (2012). The use of cardiac biomarkers in veterinary medicine: The equine perspective. https://core.ac.uk/download/55801182.pdf (accessed on 14th June 2025).

22. De Sadeleer, C., Dobbeleir, A., Ham, H., Peremans, K., et al. (2011). Nuclear medicine: Investigation of renal function in small animal medicine. https://core.ac.uk/download/55842771.pdf (accessed on 14th June 2025).

23. De Vecchis, F., Ferrannini, E., Fitchett, A., Greenberg, B., Heise, M., et al. (2017). Why do SGLT2 inhibitors reduce heart failure hospitalization? A differential volume regulation hypothesis. https://core.ac.uk/download/96885768.pdf (accessed on 14th June 2025).

24. Dominiczak, A., Ferreri, N. R., & Graham, L. A. (2017). The role of renal transporters and novel regulatory interactions in the TAL that control blood pressure. https://core.ac.uk/download/82893296.pdf (accessed on 14th June 2025).

25. Dorsher, P. (2009). The neuroanatomic basis of the acupuncture principal meridians. https://core.ac.uk/download/pdf/288827.pdf (accessed on 14th June 2025).

26. Drzewiecka, D., Kwil, I., Maszewska, A., Moryl, M., Ostrowska, K., et al. (2013). *Proteus* sp.–An opportunistic bacterial pathogen–classification, swarming growth, clinical significance and virulence factors. https://core.ac.uk/download/71976791.pdf (accessed on 14th June 2025).

27. Edwards, A., Layton, A. T., & Vallon, V. (2017). Adaptive changes in GFR, tubular morphology, and transport in subtotal nephrectomies kidneys: Modeling and analysis. https://open.bu.edu/bitstream/2144/39539/1/Layton%20AJP%20Renal%202017%20Adaptive%20changes%20in%20UNX.pdf (accessed on 14th June 2025).

28. Elliott, J., Jepson, R. E., Lawson, J. S., Syme, H. M., et al. (2015). Renal fibrosis in feline chronic kidney disease: Known mediators and mechanisms of injury. https://core.ac.uk/download/36777966.pdf (accessed on 14th June 2025).

29. Fonteh, A. L. (2018). Erotic aciduria. https://core.ac.uk/download/213462592.pdf (accessed on 14th June 2025).

30. Frantzi, M., Latosinska, A., Merseburger, A. S., Mischak, H., et al. (2017). Clinical proteomics for precision medicine: The bladder cancer case. https://core.ac.uk/download/111557480.pdf (accessed on 14th June 2025).

31. Glorieux, G., Gryp, T., Vaneechoutte, M., Vanholder, R., et al. (2017). p-Cresyl sulfate. https://core.ac.uk/download/84045396.pdf (accessed on 14th June 2025).

32. Gremyr, A., Andersson Gäre, B., Greenhalgh, T., Malm, U., Thor, J., & Andersson, A. C. (2019). Using complexity assessment to inform the development and deployment of a digital dashboard for schizophrenia care: Case study. *Journal of Medical Internet Research, 22*. https://www.semanticscholar.org/paper/eec0afa693f313ee6a1b52233a7162695b81e5cb (accessed on 14th June 2025).

33. Gupta, R., & Sharma, T. (2020). Review of urine formation in Ayurveda. https://core.ac.uk/download/478521600.pdf (accessed on 14th June 2025).

34. Gutiérrez Rodríguez, A. (2019). Diagnosis of some diseases through biomarkers. https://core.ac.uk/download/288157992.pdf (accessed on 14th June 2025).

35. Haack, A., Bichet, D. G., Bénichou, B., Clarke, J., et al. (2015). Characterization of early disease status in treatment-naive male pediatric patients with Fabry disease enrolled in a randomized clinical trial. https://core.ac.uk/download/323068429.pdf (accessed on 14th June 2025).

36. Halpern, E. J., Kim, S., Salmanoglu, E., Thakur, M., et al. (2018). A glance at imaging bladder cancer. https://core.ac.uk/download/227055407.pdf (accessed on 14th June 2025).

37. Hamid, R., & Losco, G. (2014). Pelvic organ prolapse-associated cystitis. https://core.ac.uk/download/29410932.pdf (accessed on 14th June 2025).

38. Hidayati, W., & Kusuma, H. (2018). Analysis of nursing care based on self-care Orem's theory among patients with urinary elimination disorders. https://core.ac.uk/download/186474452.pdf (accessed on 14th June 2025).

39. Horridge, M., Iannone, L., Jupp, S., Klein, M., et al. (2010). Populous: A tool for populating ontology templates. http://arxiv.org/abs/1012.1745 (accessed on 14th June 2025).

40. Kalantar-Zadeh, K., Murea, M., Obi, Y., Raimann, J. G., et al. (2024). Residual kidney function in hemodialysis: Its importance and contribution to improved patient outcomes. https://core.ac.uk/download/614876515.pdf (accessed on 14th June 2025).

41. Khatri, P., Roedder, S., Sarwal, M. M., Vitalone, M., et al. (2011). Biomarkers in solid organ transplantation: Establishing personalized transplantation medicine. https://core.ac.uk/download/323074810.pdf (accessed on 14th June 2025).

42. Krupa, A., Micera, A., Phillips, A. O., John, B., Argyropoulos, C., Lunn, D., et al. (2013). Urinary MicroRNA profiling in the nephropathy of type 1 diabetes. https://core.ac.uk/download/12214608.pdf (accessed on 14th June 2025).

43. Leiz, J., & Schmitt-Ott, K. M. (2019). Claudins in the renal collecting duct. https://core.ac.uk/download/286097290.pdf (accessed on 14th June 2025).

44. Leonard, J. I. (2025). Fluid-electrolyte responses during prolonged space flight: A review and interpretation of significant findings. https://core.ac.uk/download/pdf/42845533.pdf (accessed on 14th June 2025).

45. Magalhães, P., Mischak, H., & Zürbig, P. (2016). Urinary proteomics using capillary electrophoresis coupled to mass spectrometry for diagnosis and prognosis in kidney diseases. https://core.ac.uk/download/74362547.pdf (accessed on 14th June 2025).

46. Martin-Tereso Lopez, J., & Verstegen, M. W. A. (2011). A novel model to explain dietary factors affecting hypocalcemia in dairy cattle. https://core.ac.uk/download/pdf/29230002.pdf (accessed on 14th June 2025).

47. Olson, A. R. (2012). Evidence-based policy for asymptomatic bacteriuria in the institutionalized elderly. https://core.ac.uk/download/217307227.pdf (accessed on 14th June 2025).

48. Patwardhan, K. (2008). Concepts of human physiology in Ayurveda. https://core.ac.uk/download/pdf/87482.pdf (accessed on 14th June 2025).

49. Shi, L. B., Verkman, A. S., & Wang, Y. X. (1990). Regulation of the formation and water permeability of endosomes from toad bladder granular cells. https://core.ac.uk/download/323072161.pdf (accessed on 14th June 2025).

50. Spasiano, A., Treccani, M., De Tomi, E., Malerba, G., Gambaro, G., & Ferraro, P. M. (2024). Characteristics and yield of modern approaches for the diagnosis of genetic causes of kidney stone disease. *Genes, 15*. https://www.semanticscholar.org/paper/2defeca0934a2ff22e6bfa5618ef7c1226872f13 (accessed on 14th June 2025).

51. Takahashi, S. (2018). Identification of urinary Activin A as a novel biomarker reflecting the severity of acute kidney injury. https://core.ac.uk/download/249372123.pdf (accessed on 14th June 2025).

52. Valparaiso University. (1916). *Old School Catalog 1916–17, Chicago College of Medicine and Surgery*. https://core.ac.uk/download/216810822.pdf (accessed on 14th June 2025).

53. Zou, M. L. (2007). Variation in the apparent fecal digestibility of macronutrients and urinary energy excretion for three diets varying in fat and fiber content—Assessment of the Atwater factors and related energy conversion factors: A thesis presented in partial fulfillment of the requirements for the degree of Master of Science in Nutritional Science at Massey University, Palmerston North, New Zealand. https://core.ac.uk/download/162617248.pdf (accessed on 14th June 2025).

THE REPRODUCTIVE SYSTEM

11

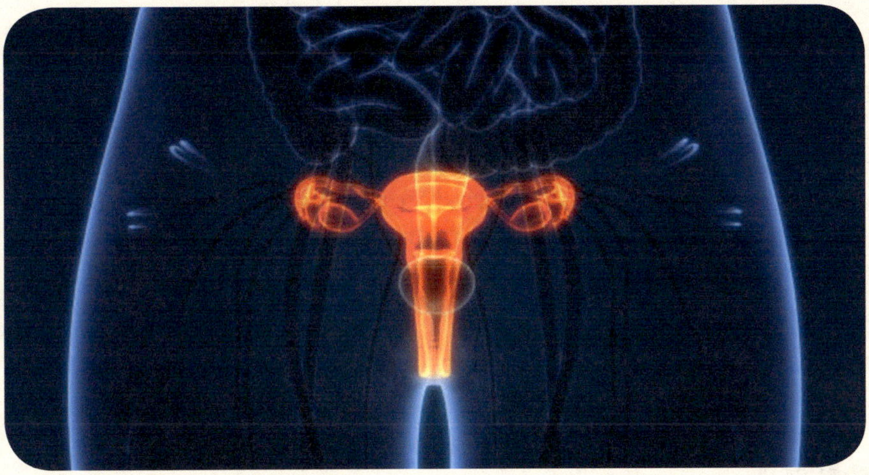

LEARNING OBJECTIVES

After studying this chapter, you will be able to:

1. Describe the anatomy of the female and male reproductive system
2. Explain the process of gametogenesis
3. Describe the process of fertilization
4. Describe the pregnancy and development stages
5. Talk about the major points of reproductive health

Introduction

The reproductive system is a fundamental aspect of the human system, and it plays a vitally significant role in ensuring species survival and genetic diversity maintenance. Its elaboration includes a cascade of structures and functions that distinguish between the male and the female to a very substantial degree. Identifying such differentiation is of the utmost significance to understand how thc rcproductive system constructs human development, health, and society. The educational role in this regard cannot be overestimated; sexual education for adults can rationalize and legitimate the complex reproduction processes. However, most students do not have the correct information regarding these matters, as the report Birds, Bees and Bias: How Absent Sex Ed Standards Fail New York's Students confirms that the sex education in most public-school districts is within the wrong, missing, and biased category (Yager et al., 2012). This sort of lack of proper education can be blamed for making false assumptions and stopping proper development. The impact of external environmental elements upon the reproductive system again deserves the passion and urgency with which this topic needs to be approached.

The initial candidate for one of these elements is Bisphenol A (BPA), an endocrine disruptor, causing serious reproductive health problems. BPA exposure has, according to studies, been found to exert adverse impacts on key reproductive hormones, especially Luteinizing Hormone. This hormone plays an essential role in spermatogenesis and reproductive well-being. One study conducted with Wistar rats confirmed that the low doses of BPA led to decreased levels of Luteinizing Hormone, hence possibly suppressing steroidogenesis by the testicular Leydig cells (Agha et al., 2006). Results of experiments of this kind are the intricate synthesis of environmental agents and reproductive health as a reflection of the degree of need for regulation against exposure to dangerous substances.

A more extensive vision of the reproductive system needs to be incorporated into school curricula to provide better chances for health and decision-making based on informed choices. Sound education not only eradicates prejudicial myths and bias, but also prepares people to confront advanced arguments on issues of reproductive health, including family planning, sexually transmitted diseases, and reproductive rights. By incorporating the most current studies on scientific issues, such as environmental chemicals like BPA, into curricula, people can be equipped with the facts they need to make more informed reproductive health-promoting decisions. Further, by bridging gaps of current curriculum needs, artists can advocate for changes, offering students more comprehensive and equal sexual education. All this work ultimately will lead to healthier communities and more educated citizens.

Definition of the Reproductive System

The reproductive system is an organ of the body that plays a significant role in the perpetuation of the species through reproductive processes. It consists of a series of organs and glands that work in unison to facilitate the production of gametes, males as sperms and females as ova, and the ensuing process required for fertilization and development of offspring. In man, and in the majority of other mammals, the reproductive system is characterized by sharply differentiated anatomical structures and physiologic processes that are enormously different between males and females. For instance, while male reproductive anatomy emphasizes outer body structures such as the penis and scrotum and inner structures such as the prostate gland and testes, the female system is primarily internal. It comprises structures such as the ovaries, fallopian tubes, uterus, and vagina. The variations indicate the evolutionary adjustments that optimize reproduction in varying environments. Alongside, the reproductive system is also intimately associated with endocrine control that governs its activity throughout the life of an organism. Hormones are individually accountable for both the growth and aging of reproductive organs as well as the coordination of reproductive processes in males and females. Testosterone plays a central role in primary and secondary sex feature development in men and governs sperm numbers and desire. They undergo a cyclical hormonal variation led by estrogen and progesterone that controls the menstrual cycle and prepares the uterine cavity for potential implantation of a fertilized ovum. The activity of these hormones on the reproductive system not only facilitates reproduction but also reacts to social and environmental stimuli, exhibiting a level of evolutionary flexibility at the center of human development and reproduction strategy as envisioned by contemporary science of evolutionary development biology (Templeton et al., 2013). The role of the reproductive system holds a significance greater than mere biological purpose; sociocultural influences also influence it and represents more universal human experience. For instance, gender roles are commonly defined by societal norms and play pivotal roles in the manner in which individuals view their reproductive options and well-being. This struggle between personal identity and societal norms can be staged in various ways, most notably in the arenas of reproductive rights, sex education, sexual health, and gender roles in the workplace and as a form of self-expression. As constructed in recent controversy about the law, the construction of sex and gender works to define how individuals experience their reproductive rights and responsibilities within a societal system that will probably uphold traditional gender roles (Seaman et al., 2007). Airing the reproductive system, therefore, is about multidisciplinary inquiry not only of biological processes but also the role that social construction and policy play in reproductive self-determination and health.

Importance of Studying the Reproductive System

Research on the reproductive system encompasses an increasingly diverse array of biological, medical, and ecological determinants, all of which are the foundations for understanding human health and its impact on society as a whole. Through examining the nuances of reproduction, researchers can identify key elements that impact fertility, reproductive health, and prevention of sexually transmitted disease (STIs). It is necessary for not only medical staff but also for students and teachers of life sciences to learn the terminological and conceptual language of the reproductive system. According to new pedagogical trends, the development of professional and terminological competence in biology provides students with background information that encompasses biodiversity and sustainable development goals topics (Britchenko et al., 2020). This information provides the avenue for health improvement and public welfare through reproductive decision-making knowledge. In addition, knowledge of the reproductive system provides insights regarding environmental influences and reproductive welfare. Environmental conditions may impact reproductive processes, hence the need for designing effective public health interventions. For example, amphibians are ecological indicators that play a significant role in determining the reproductive welfare of an ecosystem. Biodiversity loss, coupled with the reduction in amphibian population, actually increases the urgency of creating reproductive mechanisms that have central roles in guaranteeing overall ecosystem services (Babbitt et al., 2014).

By examining such interdependencies, researchers and policy-makers can create very valuable insights on population dynamics and the environmental stability role of the reproductive systems and ultimately the route to ecological resilience and human health. Lastly, knowledge about the reproductive system adds to an understanding of social life and cultural beliefs regarding reproduction. Solutions to such problems as reproductive rights, access to reproductive health services, and ethically using new reproductive technologies must be based on biological science. Discussion of reproduction's intricacies not only improves individual health but also illuminates public policy and cultural perception discourse. Overlooking these issues in proper measures can generate colossal disparities in access to reproductive health, education, and advocacy within the health sector. The emphasis of research on the reproductive system can allow society to aim for equitable health solutions and a brighter future for everyone based on interdependence between reproductive health, social well-being, and environmental health.

11.1. Anatomy of the Male Reproductive System

Learning Outcome

1. Identify the key organs involved in male reproduction
2. Discuss the function of the male reproductive system
3. Define hormonal regulation in males

The male reproductive anatomy is a highly developed structure with sperm generation and transportation functions for sexual reproduction. The system's center is the testes, which possess the critical function of spermatogenesis, the process for sperm cell generation. The testes are housed in the scrotum, an external pouch that offers the optimal temperature for sperm maturation as temperatures slightly less than body temperature enhance fertility. Next to the testes are the epididymis, where the sperm mature and are stored until ejaculation. The sophistication of the system illustrates the biological requirement of temperature regulation and spatial organization necessary for effective sperm development and motility. Following maturation in the epididymis, sperm move via a system of ducts, including the vas deferens and the ejaculatory duct. The vas deferens is a duct that conveys sperm from the epididymis to the ejaculatory duct, to which seminal fluid secreted by the seminal vesicles and the prostate gland is added. The fluid not only nourishes the sperm but also provides a medium through which they are carried during ejaculation. The interaction between sperm and seminal fluid is significant, as it affects both the health of the sperm and the overall success of fertilization. Thus, the constructional composition of such ducts and associated glands is significant in achieving maximum reproductive potential (Figure 11.1).

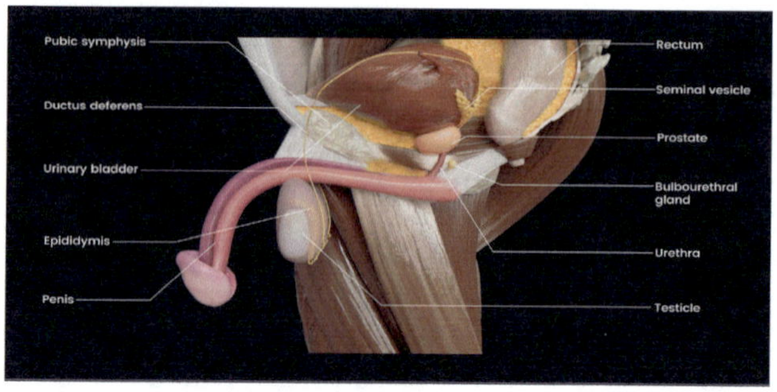

Figure 11.1. Male reproductive system.

Source: https://admin.anatomy.app/Media/images/418b8bcc-f46e-4eea-b1d0-2b3c02b47afd_large.jpg.

Aside from the principal structures, some accessory glands are also involved in the function of the male reproductive system. The seminal vesicles produce a majority of seminal fluid, which contains fructose as a source of energy for the sperm. The prostate gland plays a critical role in secreting fluid to aid in sperm mobility and protecting the sperm from the acidic environment of the female reproductive system. Besides, the bulbourethral glands also produce pre-ejaculatory fluid that lubricates the urethra and neutralizes any acidity. Synergistically, the glands ensure that sperm not only survive but also maintain high functioning, demonstrating the subtle anatomical and physiological relationships in the male reproductive system that ensure reproduction is a successful venture (Chatdarong et al., 2003; Gebre et al., 2007).

11.1.1. Key Organs Involved in Male Reproduction

The male reproductive system consists of several significant organs that work in harmony to allow reproduction. The focus of the system is the testes, which are responsible for producing sperm and testosterone, the principal male sex hormone. The testes are located in the scrotum, which is a superficial pouch maintained at slightly below the body's core temperature, which plays a crucial role in effective spermatogenesis. Adjacent to the testes is the epididymis, a tube-like structure where sperm develop and get stored before their journey through the vas deferens. It is the coordinated function of these organs that is of utmost importance, not just in sperm production but also in maintaining male secondary sexual characteristics and reproductive behavior, which underscores their significance to overall male reproductive health. Following production and maturation of sperm in the testes and epididymis, the journey of sperm then continues to the vas deferens, a muscular tube. The duct conveys the sperm from the epididymis to the ejaculatory duct, where it merges with seminal fluid from accessory glands, i.e., the seminal vesicles, prostate gland, and bulbourethral glands. These fluids not only provide nourishment to the sperm but also constitute an alkaline environment required for neutralization of the female reproductive tract's acidity. The prostate gland also makes its contribution by providing a secretion that helps in sperm motility and sperm survival. Combined, these accessory structures and secretions enhance sperm viability at ejaculation and thereby ensure maximum opportunities for successful fertilization. Finally, the urethra also plays a vital role in the male reproductive system as it is a channel for both urine and semen, albeit distinctly (Figure 11.2).

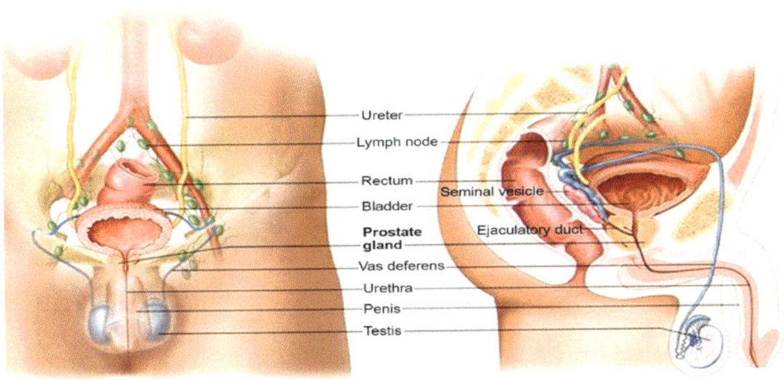

Figure 11.2. Male reproductive organs.

Source: https://nci-media.cancer.gov/pdq/media/images/766188-571.jpg.

During ejaculation, the internal sphincter of the bladder contracts to shut off the flow of urine into the urethra so that only semen is released. This is all regulated by complex neurological and hormonal feedbacks, which enable the reproductive and the urinary systems to coordinate perfectly. Besides, the penis, as an extrinsic organ, provides for the delivery of semen into the female reproductive system through erection and ejaculation, steps made possible by filling erectile tissues with blood. The knowledge of these key organs and their concerted operation is crucial not only for the understanding of male reproductive biology but also for the overcoming of reproductive disorders that may arise under various contexts (Barcaccia et al., 2015; Echenique et al., 2017).

11.1.2. Function of the Male Reproductive System

The male reproductive system exists mainly for the purpose of producing, maintaining, and moving spermatozoa, the male gametes utilized in sexual reproduction. This intricate system travels through several significant structures, including the testes, epididymis, vas deferens, and accessory glands. The scrotum houses the testes, which manufacture the sperm and testosterone. Testosterone creates male secondary sexual traits and libido. In addition, the epididymis matures and stores sperm, preparing them for ejaculation. Sperm transport involves muscular contractions of the vas deferens, highlighting the synergy between various components of the male reproductive system to enable successful reproduction. Apart from sperm production, the male reproductive system has intimate relationships with hormonal regulation, particularly the impact of growth hormone (GH). GH is critical to the physiological development of male reproductive organs and the maintenance of reproductive function. GH has been found to affect cellular proliferation and differentiation in the testes, with actions on

Leydig and Sertoli cells of particular importance to the production and maturation of sperm. GH also acts through both autocrine and paracrine mechanisms as well as endocrine effects that modulate systemic physiological responses. This triple-functioning function of GH thus underscores its significance in the maintenance of male reproductive health, further affirming the interdependent relationship between reproductive function and hormonal regulation. The accessory organs, such as the prostate gland and seminal vesicles, have a significant role to play in the reproductive process by secreting seminal fluid, which nourishes and transports the sperm. The prostate gland, for instance, secretes fluids containing enzymes, citric acid, and prostaglandins necessary for sperm motility and viability. Furthermore, the coagulating gland has mechanisms that improve fertility, implying it has a neglected role to play in reproductive physiology. Though long-neglected in scientific studies, its role as a local renin-angiotensin system demonstrates its significance in the preservation of reproductive homeostasis. By mixing seminal fluid and affecting localized hormonal regulation, these glands not only make the sperm's environment better but also become a central point for furthering the understanding of male reproductive health and fertility, as highlighted by ongoing research in reproductive physiology (Sengupta et al., 2017). Knowing these functions elucidates how the male reproductive system ensures continuity in the species by effective sperm production and delivery, accompanied by critical hormonal impact (Choubey et al., 2020).

11.1.3. Hormonal Regulation in Males

The endocrine system plays a significant role in controlling male reproductive processes by way of the intricate interaction of hormones. Testosterone, a steroid hormone, is the key hormone involved in the control and is secreted mainly by the testes. Testosterone is responsible for the development of masculine secondary sex characteristics like enhanced muscular growth, body hair, and a deeper voice. Testosterone is also significantly responsible for spermatogenesis, sperm formation. Synthesis and release of testosterone are regulated by the hypothalamic-pituitary-gonadal axis, where release of the hypothalamic gonadotropin-releasing hormone (GnRH) leads to release of luteinizing hormone (LH) and follicle-stimulating hormone (FSH) from the pituitary gland.

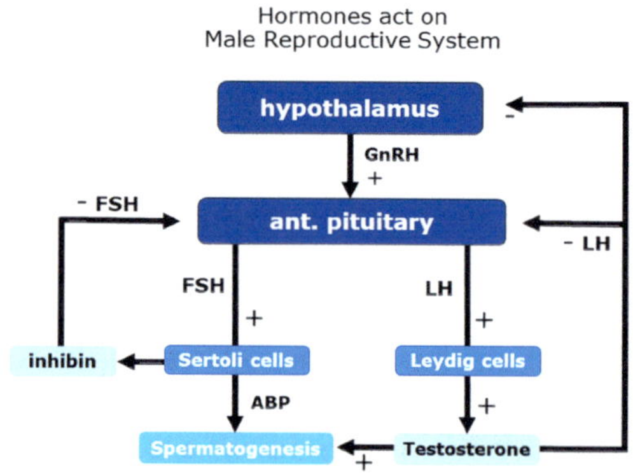

Figure 11.3. Hormonal control of the male reproductive system is mediated by the hypothalamus, anterior pituitary and testes.

Source: https://iastate.pressbooks.pub/humanreproduction/chapter/new/.

These subsequently lead to stimulation of the production of testosterone and enable maturation of the sperm, thus demonstrating the complex hormonal orchestration to help male fertility as well as reproduction in general. Furthermore, the interaction between testosterone and estrogen, although dwarfed by their discussion within the realm of male reproductive health, is significant. Testosterone is convertible to estrogen via aromatization, and its influence reaches beyond the level of physiological processes of reproduction. Estrogen receptor alpha (ER-α) mediates testosterone's action on physiology and behaviors, particularly in the limbic system and hypothalamus. Research confirms that ER-α signaling is crucial to maintaining basal reproductive function, stress response regulation, and cycling sleep, and that testosterone and estrogen play dual roles in male reproductive health. Hence, the balance between testosterone and estrogen hormones is of the highest importance, with imbalance having the potential to create not only reproductive issues but also remote effects on emotional and bodily well-being (Barakat et al., 2017) (Figure 11.3).Additionally, hormonal regulation in men can be impacted by several extrinsic factors like caloric intake and lifestyle. For example, caloric restriction has been shown to affect hormone signaling pathways, particularly those mediated by ER-α in the hypothalamus. It would have long-term effects on reproductive health and lifespan. The interaction between energy balance and hormonal regulation highlights the importance of a holistic strategy to male reproductive health, with consideration of environmental as well as biological factors. Stress or alterations in body composition can have a direct impact on the release of GnRH, thus impacting testosterone secretion and fertility. Therefore, the identification of mechanisms in hormonal control in men becomes necessary, not only for their fertility but for general health and well-being in the context of the reproductive system (Deniselle et al., 2016).

Test Your Knowledge

1. What are the key organs involved in the male reproductive system?
2. What is the primary function of the male reproductive system?

11.2. Anatomy of the Female Reproductive System

Learning Outcome

1. Identify the key organs involved in female reproduction
2. Explain the function of the female reproductive system
3. Discuss the hormonal regulation in females

The female reproductive anatomy is a multicentric relationship between structures that are designed for reproduction, hormonal balance, and overall reproductive well-being. The system consists of several key structures: the ovaries, fallopian tubes, uterus, and vagina, each with various but complementary functions. The ovaries are the primary reproductive organs and are responsible for secreting both eggs and hormones such as estrogen and progesterone, which have significant roles in regulating the menstrual cycle and getting the body ready for the prospect of pregnancy. The fallopian tubes enable the passage of the egg from the ovaries to the uterus, where fertilization typically occurs. Understanding the spatial interactions and physiological processes of these parts is significant to female reproductive health and associated disorders. The uterus is also a focal point in the female reproductive system in that it provides a setting that is conducive to embryo implantation and fetal development. The uterine lining, or endometrium, experiences cyclic change during the menstrual cycle as it thickens in preparation for implantation of a fertilized ovum and is shed when fertilization fails to occur. The vagina is both the birth canal and the route for menstrual fluid, a dual role that emphasizes its multifaceted place in the reproductive tract. Since research employs a variety of models to study reproductive health, including mouse models, it considers variability across species for developmental and anatomical characteristics.

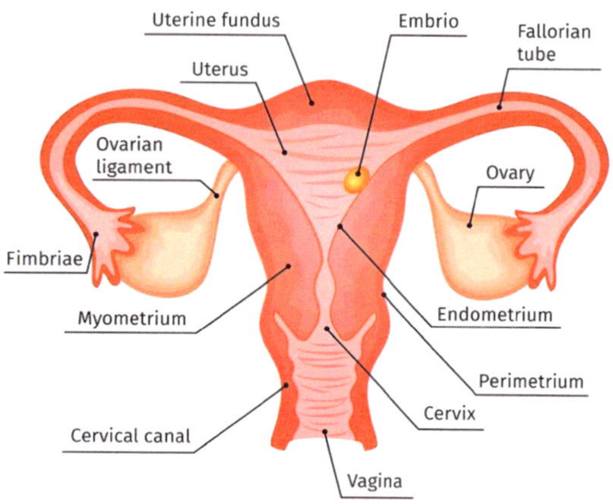

Figure 11.4. Female reproductive system.

Source: https://media.geeksforgeeks.org/wp-content/uploads/20240302131037/Female-Reproductive-System.jpg.

According to research, while there are deep similarities in mammalian reproductive tract development, each species also possesses unique characteristics that must be considered within translational research (Baskin et al., 2019). Furthermore, understanding perceptions of the female reproductive anatomy can also shed light on the educational needs that exist with populations. Studies have indicated that students' understanding of their internal organs, including reproductive organs, alters qualitatively with age and education level. Gender differences in representations of reproductive organs, though restricted, imply that educational intervention can be effective in being specific to address unusual interests and knowledge gaps of male and female students (Reiss et al., 2001). By utilizing proper teaching practices that emphasize anatomy and physiology, we can progress toward greater health literacy regarding the female reproductive system. This knowledge is not merely significant to those who want to study their own bodies, but also valuable in order to ensure informed discussion in societal and health settings (Figure 11.4).

11.2.1. Key Organs Involved in Female Reproduction

About the female reproductive system, there are several key organs with essential functions to perform in the complex processes of reproduction. Ovaries, for instance, play a pivotal role in the formation and secretion of oocytes (eggs) and the secretion of hormones such as estrogen and progesterone. These hormones regulate a great many physiological functions, including the menstrual cycle and pregnancy. Fallopian tubes, which connect the ovary to the uterus, are the site of fertilization where sperm and an ovum meet. Once fertilized, the zygote travels down the fallopian tube and embeds into the uterine lining to begin embryonic growth. Knowledge of the intricate function and interrelationship between these organs is essential to understanding of female reproductive health and associated disorders, leading to improvements in reproductive medicine. The uterus, also known as the womb, is a muscular organ that provides support to the developing fetus. It includes the endometrium, myometrium, and perimetrium, each of which plays a significant role in its operation during pregnancy and menstruation. The endometrium's lining experiences cycles with shifting hormone levels in anticipation of the potential implantation of an egg that has been fertilized. When implantation is unsuccessful, the endometrium is lost during menstruation, demonstrating the organ's ability to regenerate.

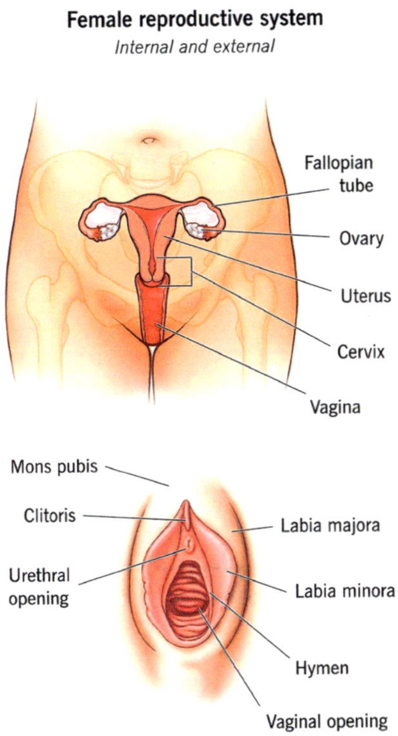

Figure 11.5. Internal and external organs of the female reproductive system.

Source: https://my.clevelandclinic.org/-/scassets/images/org/health/articles/9118-female-reproductive-system.

The cervix, which is the lower part of the uterus, also has a vital role during giving birth and menstruation. The cervix opens to facilitate passing menstrual flow and opens later to allow the process of giving birth. This dynamic organization of the reproductive system highlights the uterus's significance to female fertility and reproductive health. Finally, the accessory structures like the vagina and vulva belong to the female reproductive system. Vagina is the birth canal and the penis sheath during intercourse, providing a conduit through which sperm have access to the reproductive system. Its acidic environment plays a key role in protecting against pathogens as well as sperm viability. The vulva, including the external genitalia, plays a significant role in sexual arousal and the protection of the internal structure. Coordination between the organs is central to reproductive success, and its failure can lead to complications like infertility or infection of the reproductive tract. As our knowledge of reproductive anatomy advances, research using sophisticated imaging methods such as those outlined in (Behringer et al., 2024) informs our understanding of relationships between organs in the reproductive system. Additionally, research into reproductive strategies, such as those uncovered in (Barcaccia et al., 2015), increases our knowledge of the intricacies of female reproduction (Figure 11.5).

11.2.2. Function of the Female Reproductive System

The intricate function of the female reproductive system is essential to the success of reproductive health and the upkeep of the species. Essentially, this system revolves around several elementary structures that comprise the ovaries, the fallopian tubes, the uterus, and the vagina. The ovaries are the primary reproductive organs, which produce essential hormones such as estrogen and progesterone and ovulate (discharge) ova (eggs). Hormones play a crucial role in managing the menstrual cycle, ovulation induction, and pregnancy. The fallopian tubes provide conduits for the ova, providing the site of fertilization when sperm unite with an egg. This complex interrelation of the structures and hormonal regulation highlights the function of the female reproductive system in reproduction and overall health. Hormonal regulation in the female reproductive system is particularly regulated by external and internal regulators that modulate its functions. Environmental alterations, including light and photoperiod, have significant influences on reproductive well-being. The normal circadian rhythm of melatonin as it relates to exposure to light has been reported to play a role in regulating the menstrual cycle and the ovulatory process. Disruptions in melatonin levels due to extended periods of exposure to artificial light or disrupted sleep cycles can negatively affect reproductive hormone levels, leading to irregular cycles and even infertility. Coordinating body rhythms with external stimuli is thus needed for reproductive health, highlighting the presence of a connection between environmental stimuli and the function of the female reproductive system as presented in (Szlafrok et al., 2012) (Figure 11.6).

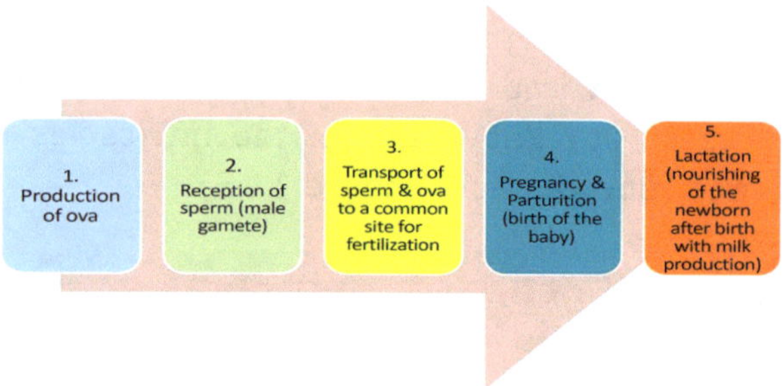

Figure 11.6. Function of the female reproductive system.

Source: https://external-content.duckduckgo.com/iu/?u=https%3A%2F%2Fimage1.slideserve.com%2F2130991%2Ffunctions-of-the-female-reproductive-system-l.jpg&f=1&nofb=1&ipt=e5c0666393a7cac5c687c72813db20445c6d65ef773694d7d7f0b63756d428de.

Moreover, circadian biology's complexities also reveal mechanisms involved in female fertility and sexual function. Emerging research identifies that disruptions to circadian rhythms, whether by life events like shift work or jet lag, negatively impact reproductive health. This dysregulation has the potential to lead to hormonal imbalance, affecting ovulation and overall female fertility, as evidenced in studies indicating that desynchronization of biological rhythms compromises fertility. The identification of the neural circuits that control such rhythms in the hypothalamus provides promising leads to enhancing reproductive well-being. It is hence the identification of the intertwined function between circadian timing and reproductive hormone regulation that is essential to the design of the proper measures to reverse fertility-related problems in women, as stated in (Vieth et al., 2025).

11.2.3. Hormonal Regulation in Females

The control of the female reproductive cycle is through hormones, which coordinate a series of intricate physiological processes resulting in reproduction.

The menstrual cycle, which comprises well-differentiated phases, is controlled by a sophisticated interplay of hormones like estrogen, progesterone, luteinizing hormone (LH), and follicle-stimulating hormone (FSH). During the follicular phase, rising estrogen levels induce the growth of ovarian follicles, leading to a surge in LH that ultimately causes ovulation. Following ovulation, the luteal phase is defined by high production of progesterone, preparing the lining of the endometrium for potential implantation. Disruptions of these hormonal signals can lead to menstrual anomalies, and thus, hormonal balance is essential in guaranteeing reproductive health (Asadova et al., 2025). In addition to the menstrual cycle, hormonal regulation is also crucial in reproductive senescence, a significant period in the life of a female when reproductive function declines. Characterized by specific endocrine changes in the hypothalamus, pituitary gland, and ovaries resulting in decreased gonadal hormone secretion, this stage has been found to occur with altered expressions of neuropeptides such as RFamide-related peptide-3 (RFRP3) in middle-aged females before any apparent alterations in their estrous cycles. Increased RFRP3 mRNA in the hypothalamus is a signal preceding the final reproductive decline, marked by declining kisspeptin and gonadotropin-releasing hormone (GnRH) expression (Figure 11.7).

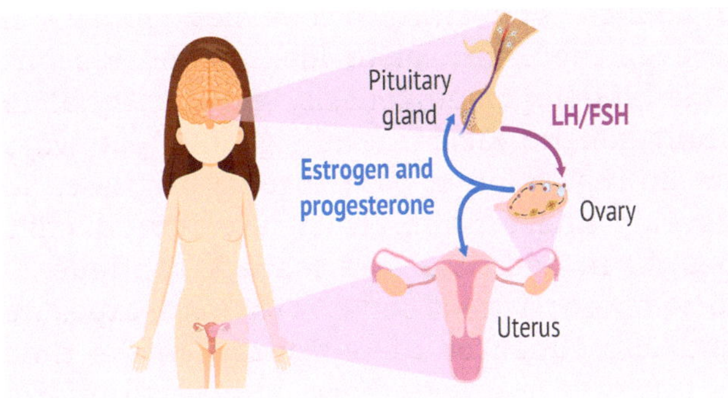

Figure 11.7. Hormonal regulation of the menstrual cycle.

Source: https://www.invitra.com/en/female-hormone-check/hormonal-regulation-of-the-menstrual-cycle/.

These hormonal fluctuations account for the neuroendocrine changes associated with aging that have far-reaching implications on reproductive function and general well-being (Bentley et al., 2016). Hormonal regulation in females extends beyond reproductive capabilities and includes more widespread concerns regarding disease and health. Endocrine disturbances may result in some reproductive disorders such as PCOS, endometriosis, and infertility. The interaction between progesterone and estrogen plays an essential dynamic role in not only affecting menstrual health but also mental and physical health. Further, the development of reproductive endocrinology has emphasized the value of hormone-targeted therapy to rectify hormonal imbalance, maximizing fertility treatment, and enhancing the quality of life among women with symptoms of hormonal imbalance. Hence, a proper understanding of hormone control is crucial in addressing both reproductive ailments and overall female health issues (Asadova et al., 2025).

Test Your Knowledge

1. What is the primary function of the female reproductive system?
2. How do hormones regulate the female reproductive system?

11.3. Gametogenesis

Learning Outcome

1. Explain the process of sperm production in males and females
2. Define the comparison of gametogenesis in both sexes

Gametogenesis is a crucial role in the reproductive system that describes the process by which gametes—sperm in the male and oocytes in the female—are produced. It is a highly controlled process involving a sequence of mitotic and meiotic cell divisions, which are responsible for genetic heterogeneity and species constancy. During spermatogenesis, testicular stem cells follow a precisely coordinated pathway to give rise to mature sperm cells. In the same manner, oogenesis is comprised of the maturation of ovarian stem cells into viable oocytes, essential for fertilization. Interestingly, gametogenesis is not only a biological process but one controlled by multiple intracellular signaling pathways, such as the Jak/Stat pathway. This pathway has been shown to play a significant role in maintaining reproductive homeostasis. It could be an essential factor in explaining fertility complications as they are related to aging and environmental stress (Giedt et al., 2018). The integrity of gametogenesis is more and more under attack by environmental conditions that assail reproductive health. Chemicals in the environment, particularly synthetic and industrial chemicals, have been a cause for concern because of the risk of their toxicity. It has been revealed by studies that some chemicals, such as bisphenol A (BPA) and phthalates, disrupt normal gametogenesis and result in adverse reproductive effects. Recently, an assay with the yeast Saccharomyces cerevisiae was developed, enabling screening of extensive collections of such chemicals, enabling a high-throughput method for reproductive toxicity testing. The findings identify numerous chemicals that pose a negative effect on gametogenesis, making it vital to prioritize their evaluation for reproductive damage to humans. Data that can be obtained through such research is critical in protecting generations to come and involves an intersectoral collaboration between environmental science and reproductive biology (Abrahamsson et al., 2024). Furthermore, consequences of deranged gametogenesis extend beyond immediate reproductive effects, reaching ecological stability and population dynamics. As fertility diminishes globally, it is even more crucial to identify the reasons that hinder gametogenesis. It is essential to study genetic variants and signaling pathways in the regulation of gametogenic processes to develop interventions to ensure reproductive health. In addition, as scientists continue to look for associations between chemical exposure and consequences to reproduction, the time is pressing to utilize these findings to inform regulatory policy that safeguards human health. By generating synergies across disciplines such as toxicology, endocrinology, and reproductive biology, a multi-dimensional approach can be developed that not only helps promote healthy gametogenesis but also overall reproductive health in the subsequent generation (Giedt et al., 2018).

11.3.1. Process of Sperm Production in Males

Spermatogenesis, which is the process of sperm formation in males, is a complex physiological process occurring primarily in the testes. The process begins with differentiation of spermatogonia, which are undifferentiated germ cells of the seminiferous tubules. On undergoing a series of mitosis and meiosis divisions, these cells finally form haploid spermatozoa. The process is also categorized into three steps: spermatogonial stage, meiotic stage, and spermiogenesis (Figure 11.8).

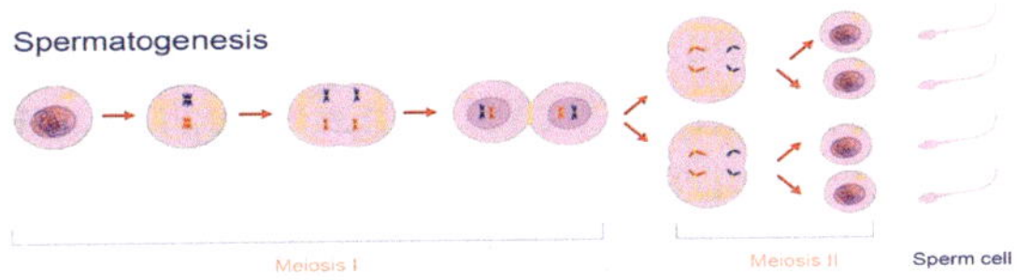

Figure 11.8. Spermatogenesis.

Source: https://d2uvynux30dg3.cloudfront.net/theturekclinic.com/wp-content/uploads/20231122003322/spermatogenesis.jpg.

At all these phases, it is crucial to have hormonal regulation, particularly by testosterone and follicle-stimulating hormone (FSH), to achieve the delicate balance necessary for the production of optimal sperm. It is essential to learn all these intricate mechanisms so that male fertility can be understood, since any loss of this subtlety leads to fertility issues. Spermatogenesis is not a unidirectional process but is accompanied by massive cellular transitions and a controlled microenvironment inside the testes. At the meiotic stage, spermatogonia undergo meiosis, halving the chromosome number to produce secondary spermatocytes that develop into spermatids and then spermatozoa. This is accompanied by radical morphological transformation as cells shed excess cytoplasm and gain flagella, which are crucial for movement. Sertoli cells also provide vital support, nutrition, and protection to cells developing into sperm at this stage.

The sophisticated interaction among these cells is revealing a fundamental property of reproductive biology, emphasizing the need for an adequately functioning testicular environment for the sustenance of sperm viability and quality. The spermatozoa produced are characterized by their morphology, which is optimally adjusted to their reproductive role. Each sperm contains a head, which contains genetic material, a midpiece packed with mitochondria that supply energy, and a tail that provides movement (Figure 11.9).

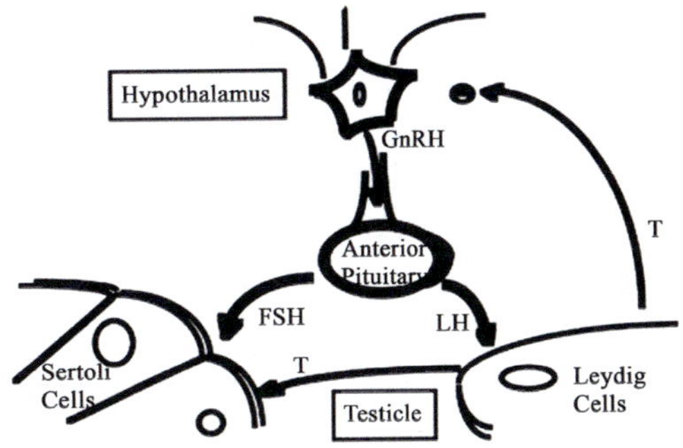

Figure 11.9. The hormone axis that controls sperm production. T=Testosterone.

Source: https://www.theturekclinic.com/male-spermatogenesis/.

Successful fertilization and egg transport also depend on various factors, including sperm motility and viability, which are influenced by factors such as the environment, nutrition, and genetics. The female reproductive system is also part of the sperm selection process through its role in facilitating competition among various male sperm as they compete to penetrate the egg. This dynamic process highlights the complexity of reproduction by demonstrating how male and female reproductive strategies converge to facilitate effective fertilization, thereby illustrating the postcopulatory sexual selection theory as presented in current biological studies (Civetta et al., 2002). Thus, the understanding of sperm development extends far beyond the simplistic cellular mechanisms and reaches as far as an intricate game of coevolutionary strategy that emphasizes the function of the male reproductive system in the broader landscape of human anatomy.

11.3.2. Process of Egg Production in Females

The process of egg production in females, or oogenesis, is a highly developed and well-controlled biological process that occurs to ensure reproduction. It begins with the differentiation of primordial germ cells into primary oocytes in the ovaries during fetal life. Throughout fetal life, each primary oocyte initiates meiosis but remains arrested at the prophase stage until puberty, when hormonal signals stimulate maturation. The menstrual cycle starts every month with the release of luteinizing hormone (LH) and follicle-stimulating hormone (FSH), which promote the development of ovarian follicles. As the dominant follicle grows, it releases estrogen, which causes the thickening of the uterine lining in expectation of possible fertilization. This synchronization between hormonal action and ovarian function is essential to successful reproduction. Within the context of environmental factors affecting oogenesis, studies have set out the deleterious effects of estrogenic pollutants on mechanisms of egg formation (Figure 11.10).

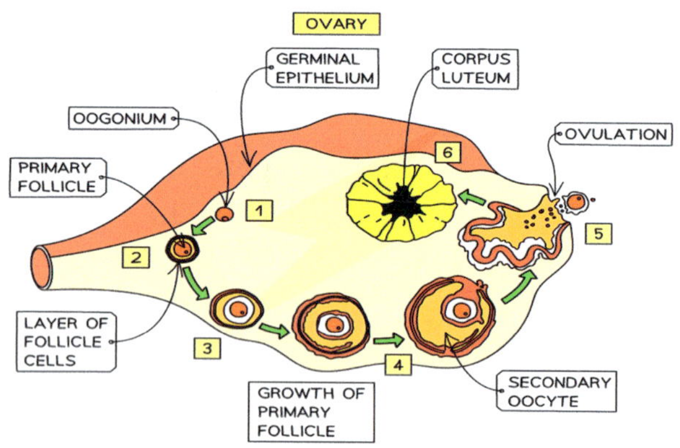

Figure 11.10 Oogenesis.

Source: https://www.tutoroot.com/blog/wp-content/uploads/2022/10/oogenesis-1.png

For instance, exposure to 17 alpha-ethynyloestradiol and o,p-DDD has been observed to disrupt eggshell formation in birds such as domestic hens. Domestic hens exposed to such pollutants laid eggs with thinner shells, which is a consequence of disruption of their shell gland function, which is enzyme-dependent mainly, such as carbonic anhydrase. This disruption is noteworthy in that it illustrates the vulnerability of the female reproductive system to environmental contaminants, with potential for precipitous declines in reproductive success and population viability. These results underscore the interconnectedness of ecological health and reproductive biology, particularly in birds. Other effects of exposure to endocrine disruptors involve not only egg production but a myriad of reproductive health problems. In addition to abnormally sized eggshells, the physical morphology of reproductive organs can be impacted as well. Experiments indicate that exposure to certain pollutants during embryogenesis leads to infundibulum and oviduct malformations that prevent mature birds from laying eggs. Such alterations indirectly impact fertility because affected structures significantly impair the process of egg laying. Moreover, such research has broader implications in wildlife conservation and wildlife management processes. Understanding the mechanisms involved in environmental effects on reproductive health is crucial for planning effective interventions to protect species affected by industrial pollutants and for maintaining the sustainability of bird populations in changing environments (Arnold et al., 2001; Hermansson et al., 2007).

11.3.3. Comparison of Gametogenesis in Both Sexes

Gametogenesis is the critical process of the reproductive system that separates into distinct sexes. In animals that are male or males, spermatogenesis will typically occur in testes, where the diploid germ cells multiply twice to become haploid spermatozoa. Ongoing production characterizes this kind of production, whereby the males can reproduce at various ages, commonly in response to external stimuli such as weather and food availability. Most notably, the processes of gene expression in gametogenesis have been extensively studied and demonstrate that aspects such as temperature will affect sperm development and quality. Female gametogenesis or oogenesis, on the other hand, occurs in the ovaries and is a more complex process with follicular growth and choreographing of hormonal signals. This cyclical pattern of female gametogenesis leads to a low number of oocytes, thereby varying reproductive strategies that focus on the exclusive functions of males and females within the reproductive system. Molecular signaling that plays a critical role in regulating such processes is a significant aspect of gametogenesis. Experiments conducted on other species, for instance, Mytilus edulis, confirm that molecular markers with a sex-specific character, such as vitelline coat lysin (VCL) and vitelline envelope receptor for lysin (VERL), play significant roles in determining male and female reproductive cycles. Research has established that the expression of the transcripts could be a forecaster of the reproductive cycle, at specific times in a year, for instance, February and July-August (Gorbman et al., 2012). This illustrates not only the physiological needs of each sex but also environmental stimuli that can impact reproduction. These findings underscore the need for data on the synchrony of gametogenesis and hormonal regulation, as the variance can lead to a reduced yield from reproduction, based on whether gamete maturation and availability have occurred. Additionally, the roles of estrogen receptors in gametogenesis expose the complexity of mechanisms for reproduction in each sex. Estrogen has been found to have several effects once it interacts with some receptors, such as the G protein-coupled estrogen receptor (Gper) and nuclear estrogen receptors. Research in the European sea bass indicates that these receptors' patterns of expression fluctuate across the reproductive cycle, and this has a significant influence on male and female gametogenesis (Alvarado et al., 2018). For instance, in females, GPERa levels are heightened during vitellogenesis, while GPERb is kept constant, highlighting the differential role these receptors may play in hormonal control. This complex interaction of genetic and environmental factors in gametogenesis highlights the need for future research on gender-specific reproductive strategies, which can inform conservation efforts and aquaculture management of aquatic stocks exposed to environmental stressors (Figure 11.11).

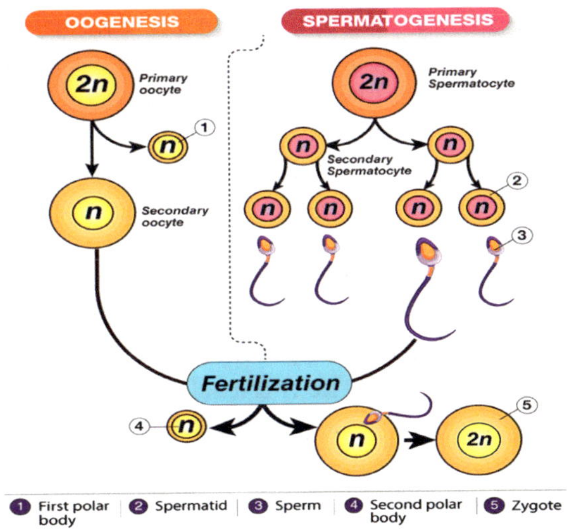

Figure 11.11. Spermatogenesis vs oogenesis.

Source: https://byjus.com/biology/gametogenesis-spermatogenesis-oogenesis/.

Test Your Knowledge

1. What is the process of sperm production in males called, and where does it occur?
2. How are gametes (sperm and eggs) produced in males and females?

11.4. Fertilization

Learning Outcome

1. Define the mechanism of sperm meeting egg
2. Describe the role of the fallopian tubes
3. Understand the factors affecting fertilization success

Fertilization is a critical moment in the reproductive process, where male and female gametes meet to initiate the establishment of a new organism. This biological event is realized upon the successful penetration of the oocyte by a sperm cell, a process that is intricate and demanding. The successful completion of fertilization initiates a series of cellular activities to develop a zygote. After union, the zygote grows and splits into an embryo that later becomes a complete organism. Various factors, including genetic compatibility and environmental conditions control fertilization. Interference in the process will lead to infertility or abortion, underscoring the susceptibility of the process for successful reproduction. Attunement to the nuances of fertilization provides vital data about reproductive health and potential hardship for individuals seeking to become pregnant. The intricacies of fertilization are more than simple gamete combination; they are a series of biochemical signals facilitating healthy sperm migration to the oocyte. The female reproductive tract is paramount in sperm guidance and maintenance through multiple physiological barriers. Following deposition of the sperm, these require capacitation, an occurrence that enhances their motility and allows them to penetrate the oocytes' protective coats. This demonstrates the sophisticated interaction between the male and female reproductive systems, as it emphasizes that fertilization is not only a physical process but a highly choreographed biological occurrence depending on numerous factors. Disruptions to this extremely well-coordinated process have significant consequences, including reduced fertility and issues with assisted reproduction. As science advances further, information regarding these processes offers potential methods for the alleviation of infertility and improved reproductive success. Along with the biology of fertilization, the effect of environmental and chemical substances on the reproductive system is being revealed through new studies. For example, research points to the effects of some toxins on gamete viability and early embryo development, creating concern over the long-term impact on fertility. The significance of learning about these effects is realized by thinking of global fertility trends, where decreasing fertility has been noted in many populations. New technology in the form of in vitro culture systems is being developed to assess the impact of such environmental factors on human reproductive biology. Through these advanced methods of study, scientists can gain valuable knowledge on how to enhance reproductive health by examining the fertilization process along with toxicological action. Conquering the barriers imposed by external factors will ultimately be crucial to understand and aid the mechanisms propelling successful fertilization and, consequently, healthier reproductive outcomes (Nishimura et al., 2025; Franklin-Hall et al., 2020).

11.4.1. Mechanism of Sperm Meeting Egg

The intricate mechanism of sperm meeting egg is a key part of the reproductive mechanism, offering varying evolutionary solutions across species. In most terrestrial animals, including mammals, sperm must navigate several anatomical barriers to meet the egg and require both chemotactic and motility movement to track molecules released by oocytes. This process is also made more complex by physical obstacles within the female reproductive tract, where sperm are under selective pressures that can permit only the most promising to fertilize the egg. It is believed that the female reproductive tract environment is an active agent in this selection process, and can enhance chances for successful fertilization and maintain genetic diversity within a population (Arnold et al., 2001). Unlike terrestrial mechanisms, aquatic organisms exhibit distinct fertilization mechanisms, particularly evident in spermcast mating. In this, spermatozoa are ejaculated into the water column where they can survive for extended periods before they reach the eggs. This method allows for several males to be involved in donating sperm, thereby offering higher genetic diversity among offspring. The role of maternal tissue in fertilization underscores contact-based sperm-egg interactions that are capable of driving compatibility and success in fertilization. Comparative analyses of the phenomenon show the benefits of sperm cast mating, particularly when egg and sperm dispersal can make fertilization occur at enhanced levels while minimizing the costs of copulation (Bishop et al., 2016) (Figure 11.12).

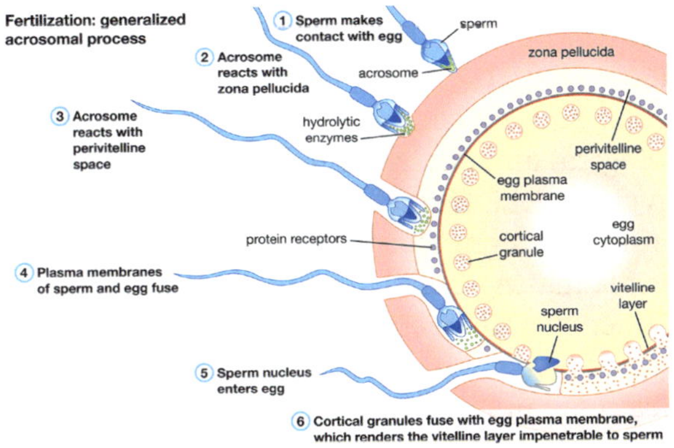

Figure 11.12. After a sperm cell comes in contact with the outer layers of an egg cell, the acrosome, which is a prominence at the anterior tip of the spermatozoa, undergoes a series of well-defined structural changes that opens a path for the sperm nucleus.

Source: https://www.britannica.com/science/fertilization-reproduction/Events-of-fertilization.

Research on the mechanism of sperm-egg interaction also indicates the significance of signaling pathways activated during fertilization. Sperm produce vital stimuli that trigger a series of biochemical processes in the oocyte, leading to successful fusion and activation of developmental processes. In addition, the interaction is often controlled by external factors, such as environmental conditions, which can play a significant role in the success of fertilization. Understanding such mechanisms gives not just insight into reproductive strategy across different species but to broader concerns of evolutionary biology and adaptation that have evolved in response to shifting ecological pressures in an effort to accomplish successful reproduction (Arnold et al., 2001).

11.4.2. Role of the Fallopian Tubes

The fallopian tubes play a vital role in the female reproductive system as the site of essential processes, including gamete transport, fertilization, and early embryonic development. The tube is composed structurally of smooth muscle cells and ciliated epithelial cells, which work in concert to provide a suitable environment for these functions. The smooth muscle's contractile capacity helps in egg movement from the ovary to the uterus, while ciliated cells help in the movement of sperm towards the egg. These physiological processes highlight the tube's crucial role in conception, underscoring the importance of maintaining health and functionality to achieve pregnancy and carry it to term (Habib et al., 2007). In addition, cooperation between the hormonal regulation and the immunological environment within the fallopian tubes is essential. Hormones such as estrogen and progesterone induce changes in the morphology of the tubal epithelium, enhancing its function. Current studies emphasize the function of immune cells, i.e., macrophages and lymphocytes, in establishing an optimal transport and possible fertilization environment.

The presence of macrophages, which are linked to anti-inflammatory roles, suggests an intricate balance at play, enabling gamete interaction without inducing unwarranted immune responses. This interaction sheds more light on how the fallopian tubes perform reproductive functions while achieving immune tolerance, supporting their double role in reproduction and immunity (Habib et al., 2007) (Figure 11.13).

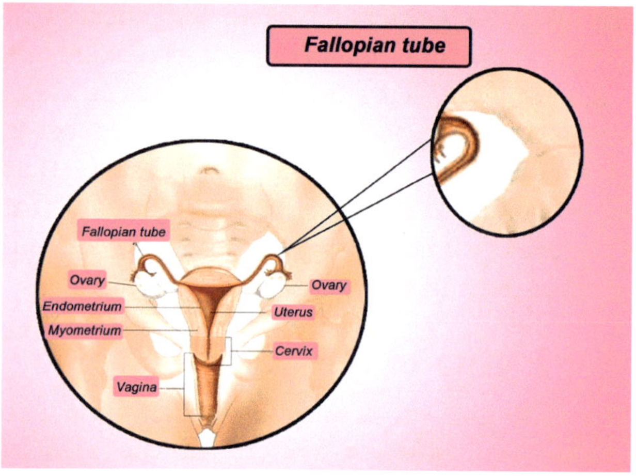

Figure 11.13. State the function of the fallopian tube.

Source: https://www.vedantu.com/question-sets/a056f7df-40db-4207-b05b-34e9e77ccbd3822806378911767 4552.png.

Experiments have also revealed the immune defense processes in the fallopian tubes, such as those involving Toll-like receptors (TLRs) on the epithelial cells. These are responsible for the recognition of the pathogens and mediating the inflammation, which confirms that the fallopian tubes are not passive gamete channels but are actively engaged in the protection against infection. Studies have revealed that different cell types of the epithelium react differently to TLRs, where ciliated cells play a more significant role in immune responses. The production of proinflammatory cytokines like IL-6 and IL-8 in response to stimulation of TLRs indicates that there is an active equilibrium between reproductive function and innate immunity in the fallopian tubes. This underscores the significance of maintaining the structural and functional integrity of fallopian tubes for optimal reproductive health.

11.4.3. Factors Affecting Fertilization Success

The success of fertilization relies many factors that interact dynamically in the reproductive system. The most crucial factor, initially, is the physiological health of the male and female gametes. In females, age, endocrine balance, and overall health can go a long way towards influencing ovulation and the quality of the oocyte. For the male, motility, morphology, and density of sperm are determinant factors of successful fertilization. Furthermore, both environmental factors, such as temperature and toxin exposure, can negatively influence gamete viability. Sexual intercourse timing in reference to ovulation is also of paramount importance since it influences the possibility that sperm will meet the egg during the fertile period. The intricate interplay between these variables highlights that adequate fertilization is not a matter of luck but an equally complex process determined by biological and environmental forces. Other than physiological factors, behavioral factors also contribute significantly to fertilization success. Couple mating behavior, e.g., sexual intercourse frequency and availability of appropriate sexual conduct, is necessary. In some species, e.g., particular mating rituals, reproductive success is enhanced through enhanced pair bonding or peak ovulation timing. Moreover, stress levels in partners can affect reproductive hormones and, ultimately, fertility. Hormonal imbalances caused by stress also interfere with the ovulation of women and reduce sperm production in men. Such behavioral conditions, as well as bodily conditions, give an overall image of reproductive success that considers, beyond biological compatibility, individuals' emotional and psychological states within the procreative relationship. Socioeconomic status also significantly influences success in fertilization. In some cases, access to reproductive health education and fertility care can be dramatically different for different populations and can often determine the reproductive outcome. For other situations, reproductive rights and the health of women are undermined to a great extent due to policy frameworks that curtail their autonomy. As suggested by research that examines the interactions between socioeconomic status and reproductive health, poorly designed policies of health sector reforms may have adverse effects on women's reproductive rights and health (Evers et al., 2001). Globalization has also introduced diverse degrees of reproductive health issues, with economic and cultural conditions potentially influencing attitudes and the availability of family planning services. Then, fighting these socioeconomic determinants is crucial in the context of understanding fertilization success as well as employing successful reproductive health interventions.

Test Your Knowledge

1. What is the mechanism by which a sperm meets and fertilizes an egg?
2. What role do the fallopian tubes play in the process of fertilization?

11.5. Pregnancy and Development

Learning Outcome

1. Define the stages of pregnancy
2. Understand the changes in the female body during pregnancy
3. Explain the importance of prenatal care

The intricate pregnancy process is a pivotal stage in human development where profound physiological changes occur, enabling fetal development. The well-being of the mother and environmental conditions outside during this period will significantly influence not only the fate of pregnancy but also the future well-being of the child. Research indicates that early gestation window exposure to environmental chemicals (ECs) disrupts developmental processes, with specific effects on neuroendocrine systems. Most notably, exposure of the mother to ECs before conception or pregnancy alters gene expression relevant to reproductive function with evident sensitivity of the developing neuroendocrine system. Such disruption is likely to predispose the male and female fetus to adult-onset reproductive dysfunction and highlights the pivotal mechanism through which environmental conditions impact development and health outcomes (Bellingham et al., 2016). Also, an encouraging recent teratogenic study using stevia, an increasingly used sweetener, demonstrates the importance of testing the safety of numerous substances during pregnancy. Pregnant Wistar rats received stevia in the organogenesis stage, which is a critical period for fetal growth in this experiment. Stevia did not adversely affect the mother's health or the morphology of the fetuses, demonstrating that it may be administered during pregnancy without ill effects. This finding is exciting in the context of pregnant women who often seek alternatives to aspartame. Such studies point towards the need to study food habits and exposure during pregnancy, as even innocuous substances can be crucial in terms of both maternal and fetal health outcomes (Kusumadewi et al., 2011). The engagement of maternal factors and fetal development underscores the need for complete prenatal care that accounts for both bodily and environmental welfare. Pregnant individuals must be made aware of the potential danger of certain substances, including drugs and foods, to the embryo and fetal development.

Medical professionals must also make sure that AppComponent screening of socio-environmental and biological factors is the priority. Enhanced understanding of the effects of environmental exposures on reproductive health can be empowering to pregnant women to make informed decisions, ultimately resulting in healthier pregnancies and fewer complications for both the mother and baby. As research continues, the public relevance of this type of research reinforces the urgency of prevention policy efforts aimed at avoiding harmful exposures during this vulnerable period of development.

11.5.1. Stages of Pregnancy

The pregnancy periods, a critical aspect of the reproductive system, develop through three critical trimesters. They each possess specific physiological changes that not only influence the growing fetus but also the well-being and health of the mothers. The first trimester, weeks one to 12, sees critical developments occurring, including the formation of key organs and systems. This is a phase of cellular growth, differentiation, and proliferation, setting the foundation for future development. The physiological changes in the mother, such as hormonal fluctuations and an increase in blood volume, also play key roles in facilitating fetal development. These are dynamics that need to be appreciated, particularly because the phase also poses dangers, such as miscarriage and maternal complications, which require observation and informed medical intervention (Paxton et al., 2008). Following the first trimester, the second trimester, weeks 13-26, brings a tide of changes in both the mother and fetus. During this time, the fetus grows quite rapidly, with increased movement as muscle and skeletal components are established. The mother also finds that early indications of pregnancy, such as nausea, decrease, and she begins to adapt to pregnancy's physical demands. Interestingly, this trimester is a determining time to evaluate fetal health by various prenatal examinations. Most healthcare providers will observe fetal development and maternal indicators of health to determine that both are progressing as well as can be expected. Furthermore, this time highlights the importance of knowing environmental factors that might affect fetal health because exposure to some chemicals in the mother could be detrimental and necessitate appropriate precautions (Mattison et al., 1991).

The third trimester, weeks 27 to 40, marks the climax of the pregnancy process. This is characterized by the final rapid growth of the fetus in preparation for delivery. The mother's body prepares for labor through a series of physiological changes, including the opening of the cervix and the onset of uterine contractions. Around the due date, prenatal care has an increasingly significant function, with fetal position and maternal health under close monitoring from health practitioners. The emphasis here is on having a safe delivery, and also in treating any potential complications, such as gestational diabetes or preeclampsia, that may arise. Understanding the complexities of the stages is the foundation of comprehending the complexities of human reproduction and the significance of the mother's health in ensuring positive outcomes for the mother and child (Paxton et al., 2008) (Figure 11.14).

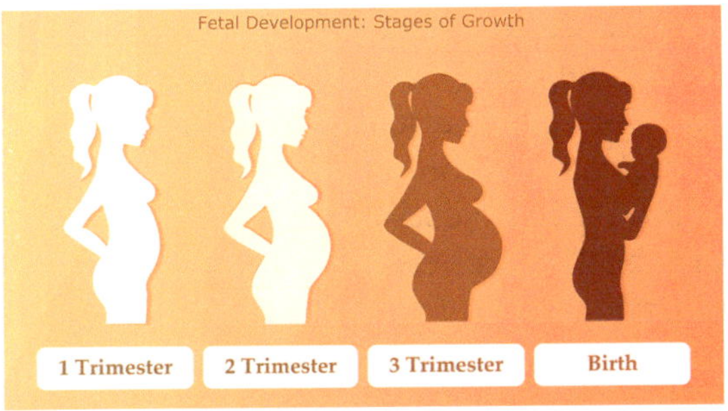

Figure 11.14. The 4 stages of the pregnancy.

Source: https://healthbanks.us/wp-content/uploads/2022/03/Pregnancy-Stages-Infographic-copy.jpg.

11.5.2. Changes in the Female Body During Pregnancy

During pregnancy, some profound physiological changes in the female body take place, reflecting the complex processes needed to maintain the growing fetus. The reproductive system adapts significantly, with a change in hormonal profile that suits the progression of pregnancy. Increased levels of progesterone and estrogenic hormones are required because these stimulate the development of the uterus and maintain pregnancy. These changes also enhance the blood flow to the uterus, a critical adjustment that ensures adequate nutrition and oxygen to the fetus. The body also modifies its metabolic processes to meet increased energy requirements, showing the delicate balance of systems at work. This hormonal and bodily shift serves to emphasize the female body's remarkable ability to prepare for and sustain new life, in terms of the reproductive system's active role during this shifting experience. Gastrointestinal shifts also serve to emphasize pregnancy, due to hormonal alterations that affect appetite and nutrient absorption. Research indicates changes in gut hormones such as ghrelin, peptide-YY (PYY), and glucagon-like peptide-1 (GLP-1) in pregnancy that regulate hunger and satiety. For instance, increased levels of ghrelin may be the cause for increased caloric intake commonly seen in pregnant women, reflecting a biological imperative to nourish both mother and developing fetus. Additionally, alterations in gut size reflect the body's preparedness to accommodate increased nutritional demands, illustrating the interrelatedness of gastrointestinal function with reproductive health. These adaptations underline the dynamic interplay between hormonal regulation and physiological change that collectively support successful pregnancy and the complexity of women's reproductive biology (Johnson et al., 2015) (Figure 11.15).

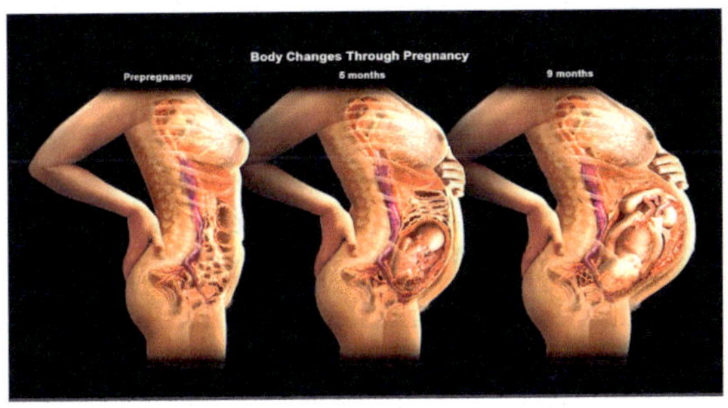

Figure 11.15. Changes in organ systems during pregnancy.

Source: https://cdn.storymd.com/optimized/RA845aH9A9/thumbnail.webp.

Further, there are structural changes made to the reproductive organs as pregnancy progresses. As a point of illustration, the uterus undergoes massive enlargement and remodeling to accommodate the developing fetus. Both the lining epithelium and the mucosal organization change in ways that optimize fetal growth and implantation conditions. During early pregnancy, the endometrium lining thickens to provide an environment for the support of the fertilized ovum. As gestation progresses, these alterations to the functional adjustments are necessary for placental expansion and fetal growth. The ovaries themselves undergo structural and activity changes within the follicles due to their central role in maintaining pregnancy. All these alterations are critical in understanding the complex reproductive system's operation during one of the most significant moments in a woman's life (Ali et al., 2020).

11.5.3. Importance of Prenatal Care

The contribution made by prenatal care to the reproductive system cannot be overstated, since it lays the foundation of fetal and maternal health. As a means of allowing healthcare practitioners to monitor pregnancy development and to make sure that the mother receives the appropriate medical examinations and counsel throughout this critical phase, comprehensive prenatal care is imperative. Routine check-ups may also be able to detect early signs of possible complications, such as gestational diabetes or preeclampsia, both of which can be seriously problematic to the mother as well as the developing fetus. Further, prenatal checks typically include counseling about nutritional intake, lifestyle choices, and vaccinations required, all of which play a fundamental role in establishing a healthy pregnancy and reducing the risk for adverse outcomes. Identifying the groundbreaking role of prenatal care underscores its worth not only to foster the mother's health but also to prepare for a healthy delivery and establish strong foundations for future child health. In addition to the immediate health effects, prenatal care also plays a significant role in overcoming the social determinants of health that impact pregnancy. The conditions surrounding the pregnant woman can significantly influence their health trajectories and the well-being of the offspring. The research has shown that the circumstances and situations encountered by parents before conception can affect the phenotypes and the resilience of the offspring through various epigenetic mechanisms (Berretta et al., 2018). These interactions raise the necessity of providing parents with supportive information and education so that they can have healthy pregnancies and child development. By establishing an environment where both parents are educated about the ramifications of their lifestyle and potential risks, prenatal care allows for healthier generations, thereby eliminating systemic health disparities in medical care. The psychological aspect of prenatal care must also take precedence, as it exerts significant influences on the mental well-being of the mother and the emotional health of the child. In addition to emphasis on physical health, prenatal care emphasizes the emotional health of pregnant mothers, with the provision for discussion of any concerns or problems they may experience during pregnancy. This kind of support is essential in the case of complexities resulting from ethical and legal issues, for example, wrongful birth actions, which can create inappropriate psychological pressure for mothers to operate in a pervasively stigmatized societal context (Yakren et al., 2018). Holistic prenatal care guarantees that pregnant women are treated with dignity and given empowerment, establishing the foundation for a healthy environment of healthy familial relationships. By integrating mental health services into prenatal care, healthcare systems can significantly enhance the quality of care for both children and their mothers, ultimately establishing a stronger reproductive health system.

Test Your Knowledge

1. What are the main stages of pregnancy, and what occurs in each stage?
2. What are some physical and hormonal changes that occur in the female body during pregnancy?

11.6. Reproductive Health

Learning Outcome

1. Discuss the common reproductive health issues
2. Understand the importance of regular check-ups
3. Identify the impact of lifestyle on reproductive health

The term reproductive health is used to signify a comprehensive set of variables that guarantee that people are physically, emotionally, and socially healthy in relation to their reproductive systems. It should be appreciated that reproductive health extends beyond disease prevention, but also the protection of people's rights over informed choice in matters relating to their reproductive lives. These are decisions such as family planning, availability of safe contraceptives, and education on STIs. At the center of reproductive health is integrating services addressing maternal and reproductive health needs at once, as seen in sub-Saharan Africa, where concurrent HIV prevention and maternal health means addressing the need comprehensively and holistically. Without an integrated healthcare system prioritizing these needs, numerous women are left underserved and at risk of adverse health outcomes that might otherwise be prevented by concerted healthcare interventions (Bärnighausen et al., 2015). Over the last decade, research has increasingly highlighted the importance of environmental determinants in reproductive health. Notably, the advent of mobile telephony, while facilitating communication, has been a cause for concern with respect to its potential to cause damage to human health. Studies indicate that exposure to mobile phone EMR might affect male reproductive processes, with studies pointing towards alterations in semen quality. The controversy surrounding the topic is sharply divided, with some researchers arguing that there is no data available in support of a causal relationship between mobile telephony and reproductive dysfunction. Still, this debate underscores the necessity for more research to demarcate the potential dangers emanating from exposure to EMR, especially as the expansion of mobile phone usage is poised to accelerate globally. Addressing such concerns is critical to ensuring reproductive health, particularly as lifestyle factors increasingly become intertwined with technology (Jayram et al., 2024). Finally, advancing reproductive health programs necessitates a complex intervention that involves education, policy reform, and community action.

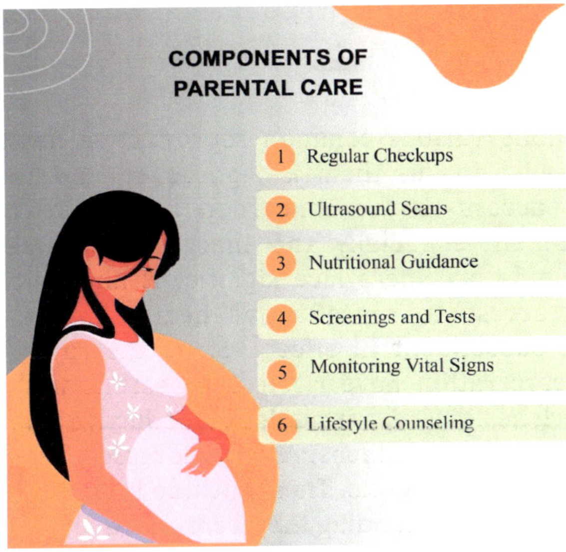

Figure 11.16. The components of prenatal care.

Source: https://continentalhospitals.com/uploads/mceu_71808782611723102235013.jpg.

Reproductive health programs for priority must promote access to information and sexuality education specifically tailored to meet demographic needs. In the context of reproductive rights and healthcare, community involvement can promote cultural shifts that enable individuals to place a higher priority on their reproductive health. Furthermore, policies must enable the integration of reproductive health services into broader health management systems, particularly in low-resource settings where disparities in access to healthcare are most pronounced. Through ensuring a conducive and informed setting, reproductive health programs can lower stigmas associated with issues like HIV and unintended pregnancy, leading eventually to improved health outcomes for individuals and families. The implementation of comprehensive strategies that bridge gaps between community sensitization and health care services is the solution to achieving sustainable improvement in reproductive well-being (Bärnighausen et al., 2015) (Figure 11.16).

11.6.1. Common Reproductive Health Issues

Among various common reproductive health issues, one of them is significant, and that is, access to the concerned healthcare for women, especially the marginalized ones. Female prisoners face significant hindrances to access to reproductive health care and its subsequent ill effects. Since the rates of incarceration have risen, it is essential that such health issues, including reproductive health issues, are commensurately addressed within incarceration units. These include being aware of and understanding their reproductive rights. These health systems are punitive rather than supportive and lead to inequalities in access to such fundamental services as prenatal care and preventive screening. As settled in the literature, there is an absolute requirement for models of leadership with a focus on collaboration and ethical practice that have the capacity to bridge such gaps and ensure women receive proper reproductive healthcare while in custody. Curing such imbalances not only improves the health of individuals but also the societies from which these women originate once their sentence has been completed (N/A, 2008). Another reproductive health critical condition is the extent to which chronic diseases, in this case diabetes, contribute to women's reproductive health. Diabetes has the potential to cause several reproductive complications like delayed puberty, amenorrhea, and infertility. These are encountered at various stages, ranging from puberty complications to conception complications in the reproductive age to menopause complications. What is notable is that with improvements in the management of diabetes, some of the problems of the past with type 1 diabetes and reproduction have been overcome; nevertheless, polycystic ovarian syndrome continues to be a complication in most women. Even though a greater number of teenagers are at risk for type 2 diabetes development, health practitioners must gain an understanding of the multifaceted interface of reproductive health and diabetes as well as the ability to provide individual interventions specific to the specific women's needs throughout the course of their lives (Dakshayini et al., 2023). Finally, psychosocial well-being is a greatly underappreciated aspect of reproductive health, contributing significantly to overall well-being. Women's reproductive health issues are also typically linked with psychological distress, and this in turn exacerbates the physical expression of illnesses such as polycystic ovarian syndrome or infertility. The interplay between mental and reproductive health can also create a vicious cycle of harm where one harms the other, making treatment and management even more complex.

For instance, stress and anxiety in dealing with fertility issues can prolong the women's struggle to conceive. To address such concerns, a need arises for health professionals to apply an integrated strategy that recognizes the role of mental well-being and encompasses psychological care within reproductive medicine. By a thorough analysis and management of all these interconnected aspects of women's health, improved outcomes can be anticipated towards a healthier and more conducive reproductive health climate.

11.6.2. Importance of Regular Check-Ups

The need for regular reproductive health check-ups cannot be overstated because the checks are key to early detection and prevention of other health complications. Regular checks help medical professionals monitor reproductive organs and diagnose sexually transmitted infections, polycystic ovary syndrome, and fibroids. Through early detection of complications as stated above, patients can be treated with interventions that can prevent complications and enhance long-term reproductive outcomes. Apart from this, these check-ups provide a continuous dialogue between patients and health care providers, hence guaranteeing education on reproductive health, menstrual cycle, and contraception. This gives people the capacity to act proactively in managing their reproductive health, leading to healthy life choices overall. Regular check-ups also contribute significantly towards controlling reproductive health at pivotal points in life, for instance, puberty, pregnancy, and menopause. Each of these advances has specific issues and possible health challenges to contend with. As a particular example, when a woman is pregnant, routine tests can monitor fetal development and detect complications at an early stage, protecting mother and baby. Maternal programs tend to highlight the value of routine prenatal care. The finding of Anganwadi Centers confirms that check-ups not only influence individuals but also have broader effects on community health outcomes, indicating larger reproductive health care effects (Chourasiya et al., 2010). Therefore, the value of routine check-ups extends beyond the individual to influence family and social health processes. Again, the relationship between reproductive health and socio-economic status indicates how regular check-ups can be an effective tool in the war against health inequalities. Evidence suggests that socio-economic barriers are most probably going to prevent the utilization of reproductive health care significantly, and this leaves vulnerable populations with unchanged health. Regular check-ups serve as both a prevention intervention and a means of addressing these differences. By extending these interventions to the remotest points, allied health systems can assess and respond to diverse needs, thereby addressing poverty-related and inequality-related health issues (Aldaz-Carroll et al., 2025). This system lens once again confirms that investment in frequent reproductive health check-ups is not only good for personal health but can also result in healthier communities, emphasizing once more the importance of universal access to quality health care services (Figure 11.17).

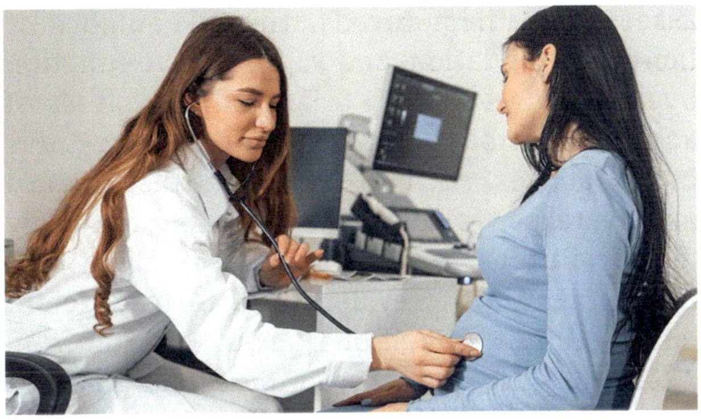

Figure 11.17. Routine gynecological check-up during pregnancy to monitor maternal and fetal health.

Source: https://drbiplabdeb.com/wp-content/uploads/2024/08/Importance-of-Regular-Gynaecological-Check-ups.jpg.

11.6.3. Impact of Lifestyle on Reproductive Health

Regular habits also have a core function in the development of reproductive health because many of the variables, like nutrition, physical activity, and exposure to environmental pollutants, directly affect fertility. Diet is the central point of this entire formula, and studies have shown that certain dietary habits can be used to facilitate or impair reproductive function. Intake of processed foods, trans fatty acids, and sugars has also been linked to adverse effects like endocrine disturbance and disorders of ovulation in women. Conversely, a balanced diet consisting of fruits, vegetables, and whole grains will protect overall fertility. Endocrine disruptors, which are in profusion in processed foods, are most harmful since they interfere with hormone balance, leading to reproductive issues. The position of nutrition in reproductive health places emphasis on the significance of the interaction between lifestyle and physiological mechanisms controlling fertility (Younes et al., 2024). Physical conditioning also has a significant impact on dictating reproductive health consequences. Exercise has been associated with improved hormonal equilibrium, increased ovulation, and reproductive function overall. However, both a lack of and excess of activity have been shown to result in negative consequences, such as menstrual disturbance and decreased fertility. As an example, low body fat female athletes with irregular menstrual cycles are quite prevalent due to insufficient energy. Obesity conditions, however, result from a sedentary life, and sedentariness is a significant danger in females and males. Regular moderate exercise not only preserves reproductive well-being but also mental well-being, which is no less essential to individuals attempting successful conception. As such, promoting exercise as a lifestyle intervention to reproductive well-being becomes paramount (Mills et al., 2013). Environmental factors also complicate lifestyle interaction with reproductive health. Exposure to heavy metals and pollutants poses a high risk because these chemicals can interfere with both male and female reproductive functions. Direct involvement in ovulatory dysfunction and semen quality issues has been implicated in some heavy metals, such as mercury and lead. Moreover, the modern environment contains endocrine disruptors that can alter hormone processes, thus affecting menstrual cycles and fertility. Such contaminants are typically attributed to industrial processes, agrochemicals, and plastics, which also carry additional health risks. Through increased awareness of lifestyles and the contribution made by the environment to reproductive health, it is essential to combat such extrinsic factors. Efforts at reducing these risks can assist in enabling individuals to make lifestyle choices that increase their reproductive virility (Younes et al., 2024).

Test Your Knowledge

1. What are some common reproductive health issues in males and females?
2. Why are regular reproductive health check-ups important?

SUMMARY

While explaining the intricate functioning of the reproductive system, it is evident that understanding its various components and functioning is essential for studying biology as a whole. The reproductive system itself is pivotal to species reproduction as well as the intricate play of genetics and environment. The chapter has explored various facets of hormonal control to physiological adaptation in various organisms. The insights acquired through model organism research, like Neurospora crassa, are indicative of the importance of genomic study in unfolding reproductive mechanisms. The insights necessitate putting reproductive biology in larger ecological as well as evolutionary contexts, requiring future research to continue adapting and revising these models in a manner to keep pace with discoveries (Menkis et al., 2020). Also, the study of reproductive strategies among and within species indicates the adaptive significance of these systems in response to environmental stress. The reproductive ecology of common dolphins, for instance, illustrates how behavioral variation based on calf age can significantly influence maternal investment and survival of offspring. These results highlight the need for reproductive behaviors to be studied in the field, since they have the potential to disclose adaptive strategies vital to the success of populations in varied ecological environments. The patterns between maternal activities and calf health are a good example of how reproductive strategy are influenced by both biological needs and environmental interactions, again demonstrating the intricate link between environment and reproduction (Schaffar-Delaney et al., 2004). Lastly, learning about the reproductive system is intended to emphasize the dependence of biological systems and their evolutionary significance. As science evolves, it is essential to integrate data from various biological models and natural observations to enhance our understanding of reproduction. This multi-faceted approach not only improves our understanding of reproductive functions but also informs conservation programs for endangered species and ecosystems. Future research directions should aim to elucidate further how various reproductive strategies adapt to changing environments, and therefore offer scientists and policymakers the information they need to manage biodiversity in an increasingly unpredictable world properly. Through ongoing exploration of these questions, we can come to appreciate the rich tapestry of life and the reproductive strategies by which it is sustained.

The system of reproduction is the basis for biological continuity among species, guaranteeing the reproductive process, development, and growth. To comprehend its multifunctional nature, one needs to study in depth both the male and female systems, as well as the multifunctional hormonal control of their systems. The male system of reproduction is primarily sperm production, which is facilitated by organs such as the testes and seminal vesicles. Alternatively, the female reproductive system has evolved to support ovum growth, conception, and gestation, just like in the case of the ovaries, the fallopian tubes, and the uterus. Coordination among these systems is nevertheless regulated by hormonal signals, which dictate reproductive activity and accompanying behavior. In-depth knowledge of these fundamental elements testifies to the complexities associated with reproductive health and directs clinical processes to address fertility issues. In addition, any disruption in the reproductive pathway can lead to various health issues, impacting the health of an individual and extending into public health. PCOS, endometriosis, and infertility are significant diagnostic and treatment complexities. Understanding the physiological and biochemical processes of these conditions is essential as they are typically the outcome of a complex interaction of genetic, environmental, and hormonal factors. Moreover, assisted reproductive technologies (ART) and in vitro fertilization (IVF) offer significant options for individuals with issues of infertility. Analyzing these developments not only provides better understanding of reproductive biology but also raises ethical concerns about reproductive autonomy as well as access to the technologies (Dennis, 2009). Moreover, recent studies highlight the need to research endocrine-disrupting chemicals and lifestyle issues affecting reproductive health. Research has shown that exposure to certain chemicals, including those found in various environmental toxins, can have an adverse effect on reproductive physiology, leading to long-term health effects. For instance, research on wastewater treatment effluent-exposed fish has evidenced alteration in reproductive biomarkers, evidently demonstrating the material impacts of endocrine disruptors (Abel et al., 2009). Hence, further study on these extrinsic factors is instrumental to determining ways through which their consequences could be minimized on reproductive health. Overall, current research on the reproductive system across different environments speaks volumes about its significance in individual health and broader ecological systems.

KEY TERMS FROM THIS CHAPTER

Testes
Vas Deferens
Prostate Gland
Ovaries
Uterus
Cervix
Mammary Glands
Spermatogenesis
Epididymis
Seminal Vesicles
Penis
Fallopian Tubes
Endometrium
Vagina
Gametogenesis
Oogenesis

CRITICAL THINKING QUESTIONS

1. **Which hormone is primarily responsible for the development of female secondary sexual characteristics?**
   a. Testosterone
   b. Progesterone
   c. Estrogen
   d. Oxytocin
2. **What is the site of fertilization in the female reproductive system?**
   a. Uterus
   b. Ovary
   c. Vagina
   d. Fallopian tube
3. **Which of the following is a function of the testes?**
   a. Store sperm
   b. Produce testosterone
   c. Produce estrogen
   d. Transport sperm
4. **Which structure carries sperm from the testes to the urethra?**
   a. Epididymis
   b. Vas deferens
   c. Prostate gland
   d. Seminal vesicle
5. **What is the function of the uterus?**
   a. Produce eggs
   b. Site of fertilization
   c. Protect and nourish the developing fetus
   d. Store sperm

Short Answer Questions

1. What are the major structures of the male reproductive system and their functions?
2. What are the main components of the female reproductive system and their roles in reproduction?
3. What is gametogenesis, and how does it differ between males and females?
4. Where and how does fertilization typically occur in the human body?
5. What are the key stages of pregnancy and embryonic development?
6. How does the placenta support fetal development during pregnancy?
7. What are some common reproductive health issues in males and females?
8. Why is regular reproductive health screening important for both men and women?

Answer to Critical Thinking Questions

1. (c) 2.(d) 3.(b) 4.(b) 5.(c)

REFERENCES

1. Abel, D., Cook, A., Juergens, M. D., Katsiadaki, I., et al. (2009). A catchment-based study of endocrine disruption in surface waters: Multivariate evaluation of the health of a sentinel fish species exposed to sewage treatment works effluent. https://core.ac.uk/download/60806.pdf (accessed on 14th June 2025).
2. Kumar, R., Oke, A., Rockmill, B., De Cruz, M., Verduzco, R., Shodhan, A., Woodruff-Madeira, X., Abrahamsson, D. P., Varshavsky, J., Lam, J., Robinson, J. F., Allard, P., Woodruff, T. J., & Fung, J. C. (2024). Rapid identification of reproductive toxicants among environmental chemicals using an in vivo evaluation of gametogenesis in budding yeast Saccharomyces cerevisiae. *Reproductive Toxicology, 128*, 108630. https://doi.org/10.1016/j.reprotox.2024.108630Aflatoonian, A., Aflatoonian, R., Amjadi, F., Fazeli, M. R., et al. (2018). Variable localization of Toll-like receptors in human fallopian tube epithelial cells. https://core.ac.uk/download/157863281.pdf (accessed on 14th June 2025).
3. Al Agha, M., Gharravi, A. M., Ghasemi, J., Ghorbani, R., et al. (2006). Altered pituitary hormone secretion in male rats exposed to Bisphenol A. https://core.ac.uk/download/52205141.pdf (accessed on 14th June 2025).
4. Aldaz-Carroll, E., & Castañeda, T. (2025). The intergenerational transmission of poverty: Some causes and policy implications. https://core.ac.uk/download/pdf/6295049.pdf (accessed on 14th June 2025).
5. Ali, M., & Sikandar, A. (2020). Micro-architecture of the female reproductive system. https://core.ac.uk/download/322580266.pdf (accessed on 14th June 2025).
6. Alvarado, M. V., Andrade, A., Estêvão, M. D., Felip, A., et al. (2018). Duplicated membrane estrogen receptors in the European sea bass (*Dicentrarchus labrax*): Phylogeny, expression and regulation throughout the reproductive cycle. https://core.ac.uk/download/288958632.pdf (accessed on 14th June 2025).
7. Arnold, B. S., Gross, T. S., McDonald, K., Spulveda, M. S., et al. (2001). Relations of environmental contaminants, algal toxins, and diet with the reproductive success of American alligators on Florida lakes. https://core.ac.uk/download/11016994.pdf (accessed on 14th June 2025).
8. Asadova, F., & Temirova, N. (2025). The mechanism of hormonal regulation of the sexual cycle. https://core.ac.uk/download/651277458.pdf (accessed on 14th June 2025).
9. Babbitt, K. J., & Hocking, D. J. (2014). Amphibian contributions to ecosystem services. https://core.ac.uk/download/84123792.pdf (accessed on 14th June 2025).
10. Barakat, R., Brooks, G. A., Efe, G., Garan, M., et al. (2017). Roles of estrogen receptor-alpha in mediating life span: The hypothalamic deregulation hypothesis. https://core.ac.uk/download/305124015.pdf (accessed on 14th June 2025).
11. Barcaccia, G., Sharbel, T. F., Galla, G., Heiko, K., et al. (2015). *De novo* sequencing of the *Hypericum perforatum* L. flower transcriptome to identify potential genes that are related to plant reproduction *sensu lato*. https://core.ac.uk/download/53524393.pdf (accessed on 14th June 2025).
12. Bärnighausen, T., Fawzi, W. W., Kendall, T., Langer, A., et al. (2015). Towards comprehensive women's healthcare in Sub-Saharan Africa: Addressing intersections between HIV, reproductive and maternal health. https://core.ac.uk/download/28952453.pdf (accessed on 14th June 2025).

13. Baskin, L. S., Cao, M., Cunha, G. R., Ricke, W. A., et al. (2019). Reproductive tract biology: Of mice and men. https://core.ac.uk/download/323311356.pdf (accessed on 14th June 2025).

14. Behringer, R. R., Kircher, B. K., Larina, I. V., McCown, B., et al. (2024). Structural analysis of the female reptile reproductive system by micro-computed tomography and optical coherence tomography†. https://core.ac.uk/download/619412835.pdf (accessed on 14th June 2025).

15. Bellingham, M., Cotinot, C., Evans, N. P., Fowler, P. A., et al. (2016). Timing of maternal exposure and fetal sex determine the effects of low-level chemical mixture exposure on the fetal neuroendocrine system in sheep. https://core.ac.uk/download/74230048.pdf (accessed on 14th June 2025).

16. Bentley, G. E., Geraghty, A. C., Kaufer, D., Kriegsfeld, L. J., et al. (2016). The role of RFamide-related peptide-3 in age-related reproductive decline in female rats. https://core.ac.uk/download/323063128.pdf (accessed on 14th June 2025).

17. Berretta, E., Caporali, P., Cutuli, D., Gelfo, F., et al. (2018). Pre-reproductive parental enriching experiences influence progeny's developmental trajectories. https://core.ac.uk/download/188827871.pdf (accessed on 14th June 2025).

18. Bishop, J. D. D., & Pemberton, A. J. (2016). The third way: Sperm cast mating in sessile marine invertebrates. https://core.ac.uk/download/85218741.pdf (accessed on 14th June 2025).

19. Britchenko, I., Krupskyi, O., Lavrentieva, O., Pererva, P., et al. (2020). Issues of shaping the students' professional and terminological competence in science area of expertise in the sustainable development era. https://core.ac.uk/download/305120659.pdf (accessed on 14th June 2025).

20. Chatdarong, K. (2003). Reproductive physiology of the female cat. https://core.ac.uk/download/11694645.pdf (accessed on 14th June 2025).

21. Choubey, M. (2020). Growth hormone and insulin-like growth factor-I: Novel insights into the male reproductive health. https://core.ac.uk/download/322445876.pdf (accessed on 14th June 2025).

22. Chourasiya, S., Dixit, S., Patel, G. S., Sakalle, A., et al. (2010). Evaluation of functioning of ICDS project areas under Indore and Ujjain divisions of the state of Madhya Pradesh. https://core.ac.uk/download/pdf/87445.pdf (accessed on 14th June 2025).

23. Civetta, A., Singson, A., Carvalho, A. B., Bateman, A. J., Chippindale, A. K., et al. (2002). Postcopulatory sexual selection. https://core.ac.uk/download/59809.pdf (accessed on 14th June 2025).

24. Dakshayini, P. N., Kolgi, R. R., Shrivastava, R., Sharma, S., Singh, S. R., Patil, S. J., & Roy, U. B. (2023). Efficacy of phytoextracts on female reproduction and impact on diabetes mellitus. https://core.ac.uk/download/603897353.pdf (accessed on 14th June 2025).

25. Dennis, S. (2009). Making aid effectiveness work for family planning and reproductive health. https://core.ac.uk/download/71342625.pdf (accessed on 14th June 2025).

26. Echenique, C. V., Garbus, I., Leblanc, O., Ortiz, J. P., et al. (2017). Temporal and spatial expression of genes involved in DNA methylation during reproductive development of sexual and apomictic *Eragrostis curvula*. https://core.ac.uk/download/159296903.pdf (accessed on 14th June 2025).

27. Evers, B., Juarez, M., Nanda, P., Cook, R., Petchesky, R., & Ramachandran, V. (2001). Globalization, health sector reform, gender and reproductive health. https://core.ac.uk/download/71347768.pdf (accessed on 14th June 2025).

28. Franklin-Hall, L. (2020). The animal sexes as historical explanatory kinds. https://core.ac.uk/download/199234750.pdf (accessed on 14th June 2025).

29. Giedt, M. S. (2018). *JAK/STAT Signaling Regulates Gametogenesis and Age-Related Reproductive Maintenance*. https://core.ac.uk/download/232582944.pdf (accessed on 14th June 2025).

30. Gonzalez Deniselle, M. C., Lara, H. E., Recabarren, S. E., Roselli, C. E., et al. (2016). Developmental and functional effects of steroid hormones on the neuroendocrine axis and spinal cord. https://core.ac.uk/download/159294623.pdf (accessed on 14th June 2025).

31. Gorbman, A., Hines, A., Scarpato, A., Tanguy, A., Viarengo, A., Wacker, A., et al. (2012). Annual variation in the levels of transcripts of sex-specific genes in the mantle of the common mussel, *Mytilus edulis*. https://core.ac.uk/download/293850885.pdf (accessed on 14th June 2025).

32. Habib, F. A., Oweiss, N. Y., & Safwat, M. D. (2007). Distribution of macrophages in the human fallopian tubes: An immunohistochemical and electron microscopic study. https://core.ac.uk/download/268450551.pdf (accessed on 14th June 2025).

33. Hermansson, A. (2007). Effects on the reproductive system in domestic fowl (*Gallus domesticus*) after embryonic exposure to estrogenic substances. https://core.ac.uk/download/11695140.pdf (accessed on 14th June 2025).

34. Jayram, K., & Srinivasa, M. S. (2024). Effect of mobile telephony on male reproduction: A review. https://core.ac.uk/download/620836149.pdf (accessed on 14th June 2025).

35. Johnson, M. L. (2015). Gastrointestinal appetite hormones change with maternal adaptations to pregnancy and lactation in the rat. https://core.ac.uk/download/200248118.pdf (accessed on 14th June 2025).

36. Kiik, K. (2017). *Ohustatud Euroopa naaritsa (Mustela lutreola) sigimine ja käitumine tehiskeskkonnas*. https://core.ac.uk/download/143642945.pdf (accessed on 14th June 2025).

37. Kusumadewi, A. P. (A.), Murhandini, S. (S.), & Widowati, L. (L.). (2011). *Keamanan Stevia Hasil Budidaya B2P2TO2T Dalam Aspek Teratogenitas*. https://media.neliti.com/media/publications/150670-ID-none.pdf (accessed on 14th June 2025).

38. Mattison, D. R. (1991). Risk assessment for developmental toxicity: Airborne occupational exposure to ethanol and iodine. https://core.ac.uk/download/72056985.pdf (accessed on 14th June 2025).

39. Mekasha Gebre, Y. (2007). *Reproductive Traits in Ethiopian Male Goats*. https://core.ac.uk/download/11695178.pdf (accessed on 14th June 2025).

40. Mills, W. (2013). *Grandma's Pill*. https://core.ac.uk/download/215536284.pdf (accessed on 14th June 2025).

41. N/A. (2008). Improving the provision of reproductive health services to incarcerated women. https://core.ac.uk/download/213906525.pdf (accessed on 14th June 2025).

42. Nishimura, T., & Takebe, T. (2025). Synthetic human gonadal tissues for toxicology. https://core.ac.uk/download/613888917.pdf (accessed on 14th June 2025).

43. Paxton, A., MacKay, A. P., AbouZahr, C., Chandra-Sekar, C., Hunger, C., Ronsmans, C., et al. (2008). Measuring maternal mortality: An overview of opportunities and options for developing countries. https://core.ac.uk/download/177066.pdf (accessed on 14th June 2025).

44. Reiss, M., & Tunnicliffe, S. D. (2001). Students' understandings of human organs and organ systems. https://core.ac.uk/download/pdf/82146.pdf (accessed on 14th June 2025).

45. Schaffar-Delaney, A. (2004). *Female Reproductive Strategies and Mother-Calf Relationships of Common Dolphins (Delphinus delphis) in the Hauraki Gulf, New Zealand: A Thesis Presented in Partial Fulfilment of The Requirements for The Degree of Master of Science in Zoology at Massey University, Albany, New Zealand.* https://core.ac.uk/download/148645668.pdf (accessed on 14th June 2025).

46. Seaman, J. A. (2007). The peahen's tale, or dressing our parts at work. https://core.ac.uk/download/62548124.pdf (accessed on 14th June 2025).

47. Sengupta, P. (2017). An update on coagulating gland renin-angiotensin-prostaglandin system: A new hypothesis on its renin function. https://core.ac.uk/download/477852823.pdf (accessed on 14th June 2025).

48. Szlafrok, R. (2012). Do photoperiodic changes in melatonin secretion detrimentally affect the female reproductive cycle? https://core.ac.uk/download/217329241.pdf (accessed on 14th June 2025).

49. Templeton, A., Arquitt, A. B., Migliano, A. B., Pesonen, A. K., Parent, A. S., Bogin, B., Campbell, B., et al. (2013). Evo-devo of human adolescence: Beyond disease models of early puberty. https://core.ac.uk/download/18528095.pdf (accessed on 14th June 2025).

50. Vieth, A., Zarghani-Shiraz, A., Appo, A., Palmer, B., et al. (2025). A time for sex: Circadian regulation of mammalian sexual and reproductive function. https://core.ac.uk/download/648141197.pdf (accessed on 14th June 2025).

51. Yager, A., Lok, E., Miller, J., Noel, K., Goodman, M., & Santamaria-Schwartz, R. (2012). Birds, bees and bias: How absent sex ed standards fail New York's students. https://core.ac.uk/download/71361426.pdf (accessed on 14th June 2025).

52. Yakren, S. (2018). Wrongful birth claims and the paradox of parenting a child with a disability. https://core.ac.uk/download/216958966.pdf (accessed on 14th June 2025).

53. Younes, V. (2024). The role of specific nutrients and pollutants with endocrine activity on fertility in women. https://core.ac.uk/download/620848711.pdf (accessed on 14th June 2025).

THE ENDOCRINE SYSTEM

12

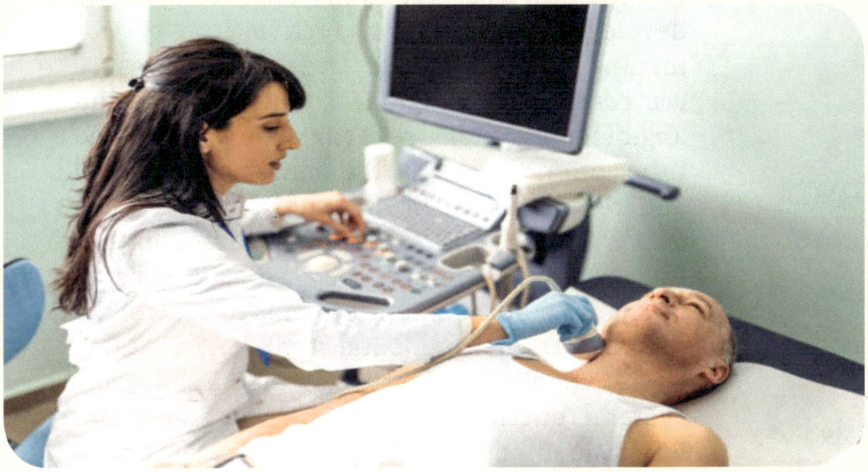

LEARNING OBJECTIVES

After studying this chapter, you will be able to:

1. Identify the primary glands of the endocrine system
2. Define hormones and Their Functions
3. Discuss disorders of the endocrine system
4. Describe the role of the endocrine system in homeostasis

Introduction

The delicate ballet of biological processes that govern human physiology is choreographed, most notably, by a system of glands that secrete hormones, the endocrine system. The endocrine system regulates many body functions, including growth, metabolism, and mood. The endocrine system operates through a system of feedback processes, which keeps hormone levels in equilibrium, a parameter required for the achievement of homeostasis. Disruptions to this highly organized system can have a range of negative impacts on our well-being, from diabetes to thyroid disorder, which underscores the need to understand its glands and functions. By looking at the key glands, hormones, and processes at work, we can gain valuable insight into how the endocrine system influences our overall well-being and health. Lastly, grasping these fundamental principles not only enhances our biological literacy but also allows us to make informed choices about our health.

Definition of the Endocrine System

The endocrine system is a complex system of glands that controls and secretes hormones, which are necessary chemical messengers within the body. Unlike the nervous system, which utilizes electrical impulses for quick communication, the endocrine system uses the bloodstream to communicate, allowing for hormones to affect distant organs and tissues over long spans of time.

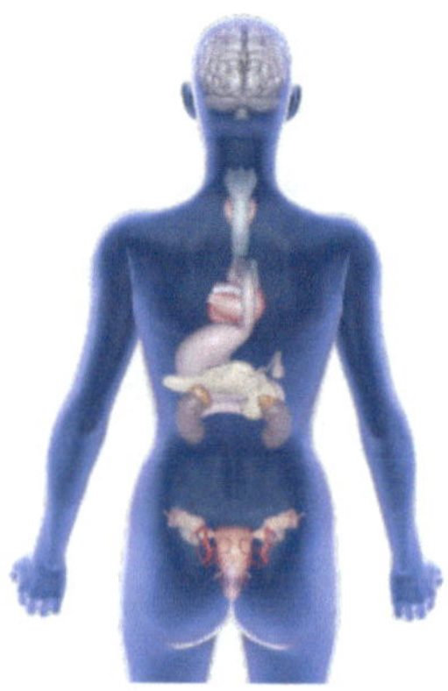

Figure 12.1. Posterior view of the female body highlighting key organs of the endocrine system.

Source: https://giastewartdietitian.com.au/wp-content/uploads/2023/08/Endocrine-.svg.

This is a system comprising various glands such as the pituitary, thyroid, adrenal, and pancreas, each with its own function in homeostatic regulation and coordination of the physiological functions, all the way from metabolism and growth to mood. The complexity of the interaction between hormones and feedback mechanisms only increases the importance of this system for general health. Knowing about the endocrine system is imperative, as conditions can cause serious health problems, supporting the necessity of expert-level knowledge in treating and diagnosing (Almar et al., 2019). By looking into the manner in which these glands operate and with whom they work together, one can see the vital role they have in maintaining life (Figure 12.1).

Importance of the Endocrine System in Human Physiology

Endocrine glands maintain the human body in a state of homeostasis, influencing everything from metabolism to stress. The chemical messengers released by endocrine glands, known as hormones, influence target organs to regulate body functions such as growth, development, and reproductive activity. For instance, fluid balance and blood pressure are controlled to a great extent by the renin-angiotensin system, reflecting the complicated interaction between the endocrine system and renal and cardiovascular function (Baan et al., 2020). The system also has complex interaction with other body systems such as the nervous and immune systems to control the response to environmental stimuli. As a leading health condition, obesity has made endocrine system function in metabolic disorders not an issue of doubt anymore, with deranged hormone signaling being a causative factor in increased cardiovascular risks, primarily through perivascular adipose tissue-engaged mechanisms (Costa et al., 2018). Appreciating these interactions reminds us of the sheer importance of the endocrine system in human physiology.

Overview of Hormones and Their Functions

Hormones are essential biochemical messengers that regulate many of the body's physiological processes. These substances, manufactured and discharged from a variety of glands in the endocrine system, travel through the bloodstream to influence target organs, where specific reactions result in functions such as metabolism, growth, and reproduction being regulated. A subtle understanding reveals their diverse origins and activities; e.g., peptide hormones such as insulin play a critical role in glucose homeostasis, whereas steroid hormones such as cortisol control stress responses and immune functions. Moreover, the complexity of hormonal interaction emphasizes the delicacy required for homeostasis, as illustrated by intricate feedback regulation maintaining stable internal states. While research continues to advance, the role of hormones goes beyond classical function, showing potential for implications of treatment in numerous disorders.

Comparison with the Nervous System

Both the endocrine and nervous systems regulate body function, but they do this by employing mechanisms essentially different from each other. The endocrine system uses the mechanism of hormones, chemical messengers released into the bloodstream, to exert systemic influences over a longer duration. The nervous system employs electrical impulses to transmit signals and produce quick responses in a localized area. This is illustrated through the mortality profile analysis, where subtle alterations in cortisol metabolism can be influenced by external factors, e.g., alcohol intake. These kinds of multifaceted interactions imply a different operational tempo; e.g., while cortisol levels have variability to alcohol as suggested by (Evans et al., 1979), quick reflex responses from the nervous system do not allow the same metabolic accommodations. Lastly, understanding both systems' complementary functions is imperative in learning about the intricacies of human physiology and health outcomes, like mortality trends as quoted in comparative analyses (Aline Desesquelles et al., 2010).

Historical Background of Endocrine Research

The exploration of endocrine research has a rich historical tapestry that reflects a growing understanding of biological systems and their complexities. Initial investigations in the late 19th and early 20th centuries unveiled the role of hormones in regulating various physiological processes, laying the foundational principles of endocrinology. Initial work focused on the identification of specific glands, such as the thyroid and adrenal glands, and their hormone secretion, which promoted interest in the function of these chemicals in terms of behavior and health. Leaders in the discipline used observation and experimentation techniques, oftentimes producing results that linked social behavior and endocrine activity. For example, information on the physiological mechanisms involved in controlling social conduct reveals the relationship between behavior and hormone, as documented in modern integrative models emphasizing the environmental context role (Adam et al., 2010). It is through such advances in history that modern endocrine research has been able to employ more complex methods to differentiate the relationship between hormone and behavior further.

Key Components of the Endocrine System

The endocrine system is made up of a complex network of glands that produce and release hormones, regulating varied physiological processes within the body. Key features are the pituitary gland, popularly referred to as the master gland, because it regulates the activity of other endocrine glands through hormonal stimulation. Other glands, such as the thyroid, adrenal, and pancreas, also play key roles in metabolism, stress, and blood glucose regulation. Recent studies illuminate the similarities in endocrine and neuronal signaling, and it is hypothesized that the exact calcium-dependent mechanisms regulate exocytosis, the mode of hormone secretion (Ahnert-Hilger et al., 1994). Moreover, understanding the interaction between the hormones and the environmental pressures illustrates the importance of considering exogenous chemicals that can interfere with hormone function, particularly in cases like breast cancer, where oestrogenic-like chemicals pose a significant risk (Plant et al., 2016). All of these contribute to the intricate role that the endocrine system has in health and disease prevention in general.

Scope of the Endocrine System

The endocrine system is essential in regulating many body functions through the secretion of hormones, which are chemical messengers that influence almost every cell, organ, and function in the body. The regulation includes growth, metabolism, reproduction, and mood, which reflect the broad impact of endocrine communication. For instance, the intricate dynamic relationship between oviduct fluid and hormones signifies how the environment can make fundamental reproductive operations such as fertilization and embryo development possible, yielding excellent information on subfertility and fertility (Arnold et al., 2016). Further, the adaptability of biophysical systems with the endocrine setting highlights the sensitivity of the system to physiological and pathophysiological situations (Cardon et al.). By understanding these dynamics, researchers can study means of improving clinical outcomes and develop therapeutic strategies. Thus, the scope of the endocrine system is broad, including not just the synthesis of hormones but their widespread importance in health and disease.

Brief Overview of Subsequent Topics

As we delve deeper into understanding the secrets of the endocrine system, a discussion of the components—hormones, glands, and their regulatory roles—will serve better to explain the overall significance of this complex system. The subsequent sections will explore the roles of prominent glands such as the pituitary, thyroid, and adrenal glands, each with its unique respective hormones that control metabolism, growth, and stress reaction. Clarification of these interactions not only sheds light on normal physiological functions but also underscores the effects of hormonal imbalance that can lead to serious health issues. In addition, current trends in endocrinology research will be considered, including new applications for technology and personalized medicine. This will reflect the advancements seen in fields like music performance manipulation, where technology increases user engagement, as illustrated in applications like PerMORFer and MoodifierLive (Marco Fabiani et al., 2011; Of et al., 2018). Overall, this carefully prepared overview will provide the basis for an elaborate discussion of the endocrine system's vital role in human health.

12.1. Major Glands of the Endocrine System

Learning Outcome

1. Describe the structure and function of the pituitary gland
2. Explain the role of the thyroid gland in regulating metabolism
3. Identify the functions of the adrenal glands
4. Describe the function of the pancreas in blood sugar regulation through insulin
5. Explain the role of the gonads (ovaries and testes)
6. Describe the function of the pineal gland
7. Explain the role of the thymus gland in immune system development
8. Describe the functions of the hypothalamus in maintaining homeostasis
9. Explain the function of the parathyroid glands

The endocrine system is a collection of several major glands that are tasked with playing significant roles in the sustenance of various physiological processes. The major glands include the pituitary, thyroid, adrenal, and pancreas, all of which secrete hormones that impact metabolism, growth, and stress. The pituitary gland, or master gland, controls other glands and governs the workings of the body through the release of its hormones. Ironically, the adrenal glands also play a significant role in the body's stress response, releasing corticosteroids and catecholamines to ensure homeostasis during trying times. Also, as has been signaled by recent research, the skin is found to be a principal endocrine organ with its own HPA-like axis that influences local hormone activity and is capable of influencing skin diseases such as acne and rosacea (Clark et al., 2020). Grasping these interrelated systems indicates the way hormonal regulation is essential to health, a reflection of the complexity of endocrine interaction within the human body (Steinhart et al., 2001) (Figure 12.2).

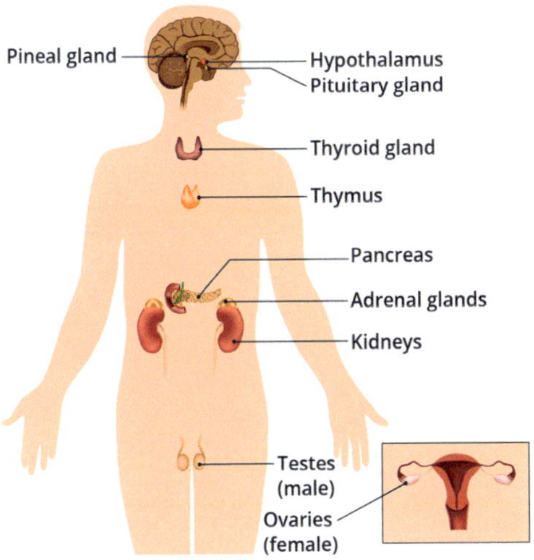

Figure 12.2. Endocrine glands and their hormones.

Source: https://media.healthdirect.org.au/images/inline/original/endocrine-glands-and-their-hormones-85e01a.png.

12.1.1. The Pituitary Gland: The Master Gland

Better referred to as the master gland, the pituitary gland plays a central role in regulating many physiological functions by coordinating the activity of other endocrine glands. Located at the base of the brain, it is divided into the anterior and posterior lobes, each with a distinct, separate function. The anterior lobe secretes essential hormones, such as growth hormone and adrenocorticotropic hormone, that cause growth and influence stress responses, respectively.

The hypothalamus shares a close connection with the pituitary, sending information that regulates the gland's hormone release, thus generating an integrated response to varying body demands. Interestingly, the pituitary gland regulation of cortisol levels demonstrates its critical function in stress management; long-term dysregulation results in undesirable health consequences, as emphasized in recent literature by the correlation between stress and mood disorders (Georgina Russell et al., 2019; William H. Walker et al., 2020). As a result, the pituitary gland serves an essential function in balancing hormones and overall homeostasis within the body (Figure 12.3).

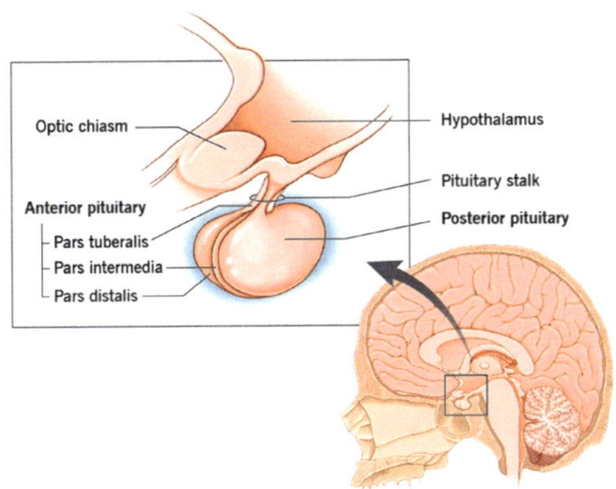

Figure 12.3. Anatomy of the pituitary gland.

Source: https://my.clevelandclinic.org/-/scassets/images/org/health/articles/23150-posterior-pituitary-final.

12.1.2. The Thyroid Gland: Metabolism Regulation

The primary regulator of metabolism is centered in the thyroid gland, which regulates most functions of the body through the release of hormones such as thyroxine (T4) and triiodothyronine (T3). Thyroid hormones are involved in carbohydrate, fat, and protein metabolism and therefore influence energy and metabolic rate.

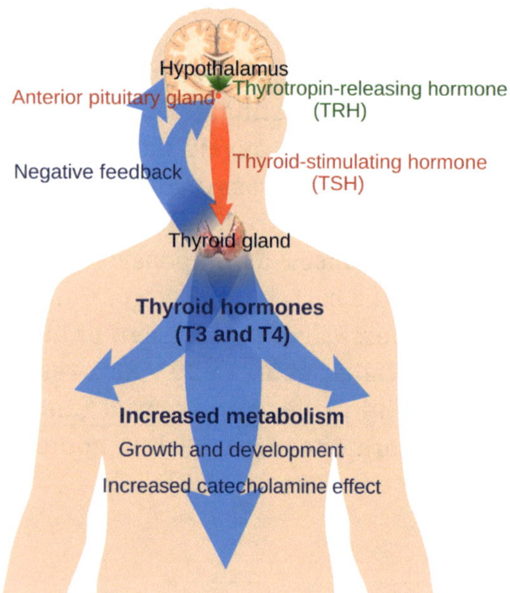

Figure 12.4. The thyroid gland.

Source: https://upload.wikimedia.org/wikipedia/commons/d/d1/Thyroid_system.svg.

Abnormal thyroid function leads to severe endocrine disorders, including hypothyroidism, where metabolic processes decrease, and hyperthyroidism, whereby metabolism increases abnormally. Thyroid disease patients often demonstrate altered rheological properties of the blood, which can serve as diagnostic markers. For example, erythrocyte aggregation has been described as altered in thyrotoxicosis and thyroid tumors, reflecting that these factors play a role in metabolic regulation (Javakhishvili et al., 2024). Furthermore, novel treatments that incorporate homeopathic agents have been recommended to possess the capability to enhance thyroid function and metabolic outcomes in patients with cancer, demonstrating the gland's complex role in disease and health (2021) (Figure 12.4).

12.1.3. The Adrenal Glands: Stress Response

One of the body's chief players in stress response, the adrenal glands, guide a complex cascade of hormones that help organisms survive stressors. When detecting stress, the hypothalamus causes the pituitary gland to release adrenocorticotropic hormone (ACTH), which in turn stimulates the adrenal cortex to release cortisol, a hormone instrumental in the regulation of stress (cite24).

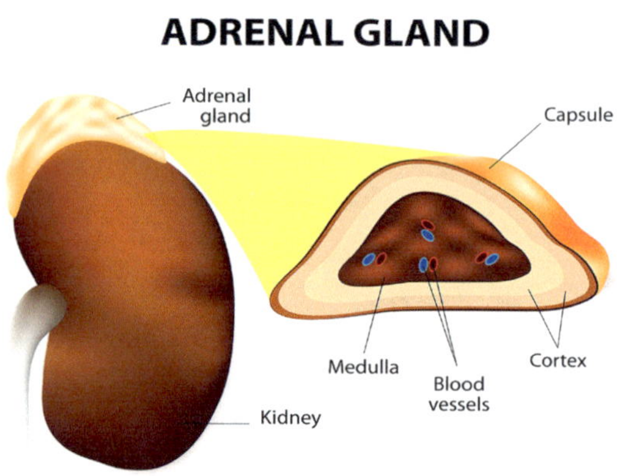

Figure 12.5. Adrenal glands.

Source: https://www.hopkinsmedicine.org/health/conditions-and-diseases/-/media/ksw-images/adrenalglanddiagram.ashx?h=&w=&hash=BB7406B83D322CE01DCB0CF18F65F8DC.

This response is systemic not only in nature but also localized in function within peripheral endocrine organs, including the skin. The existence of a cutaneous hypothalamic-pituitary-adrenal (HPA) axis provides the skin with the ability to react on its own to stress, synthesizing and breaking down hormones like cortisol, which modulates inflammatory diseases like acne and rosacea further (Clark et al., 2020). Thus, the identification of the adrenal glands' function goes beyond mere organ activity to highlight their pivotal position in both systemic health and local regulation of hormones in response to stress (Figure 12.5).

12.1.4. The Pancreas: Blood Sugar Control

Its residence in the abdomen, the pancreas is a central controller of blood sugar, primarily through the hormones that it secretes, such as insulin and glucagon. Insulin, secreted when blood glucose is elevated after a meal, permits cells to absorb glucose for energy or storage, averting hyperglycemia.

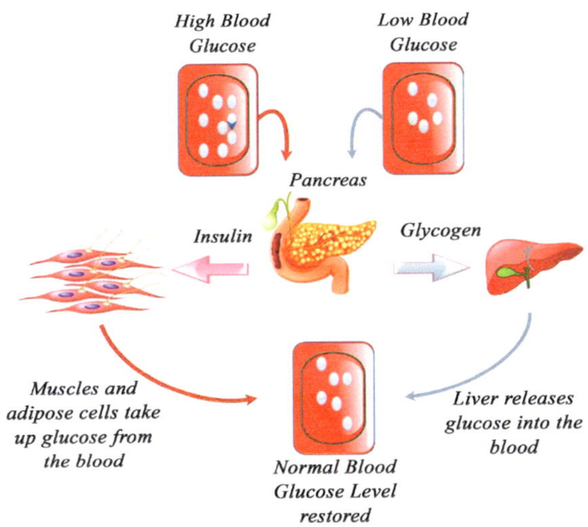

Figure 12.6. Pancreas controlling blood glucose level in the human body.

Source: https://www.researchgate.net/figure/Pancreas-controlling-blood-glucose-level-in-the-human-body_fig1_348649285.

On the other hand, glucagon assists in bringing blood sugar levels up during fasting by triggering the release of glucose by the liver. Since variations from normal glucose levels can result in major health problems, including diabetes, the pancreas' careful balance is essential. Organizational forms, such as the closure of restrictions, provide a multi-angled approach to regulation; they highlight how various modes of interaction between hormones promote the upkeep of homeostasis in glucose metabolism (Bich et al., 2020). The pancreas, therefore, is the essence of the intricate processes within the endocrine system that are necessary for maintaining body balance and overall health (Mujtahid et al., 2020) (Figure 12.6).

12.1.5. The Gonads: Reproductive Hormones

The gonad-sectored hormone complex, i.e., testosterone in men and estrogen and progesterone in women, plays a crucial role in regulating reproduction and secondary sexual characteristics. These hormones regulate several physiological events ranging from gamete formation to the menstrual cycle and sexual behavior. Also, exposure to endocrine-disrupting chemicals (EDCs) such as bisphenol

A (BPA) and phthalates can adversely impact gonadal function and result in reproductive disorders. This influence is strengthened by lifestyle choices, including the use of alcohol and the smoking of tobacco, which have been shown to interfere with the activity of hormones and the hypothalamus-pituitary-gonadal (HPG) axis (Czarnywojtek et al., 2023). In addition, thyroid hormones can influence the migration and function of gonadotropin-releasing hormone (GnRH) neurons, demonstrating the delicate equilibrium within the endocrine system (Clarisse et al., 2023). Understanding these complex interactions emphasizes the importance of protecting both environmental and individual elements to ensure reproductive health.

12.1.6. The Pineal Gland: Sleep Regulation

Concealed deep within the brain, the pineal gland plays a vital role in regulating sleep by means of its production of melatonin, a hormone that heralds the start of night. This small but significant structure reacts to messages from the outside world through light, primarily influencing circadian rhythms and ensuring that various physiological processes coincide with day and night. Researchers recognize the detrimental effects of artificial light exposure at night (ALAN) on the endocrine function in the way of melatonin production disturbance resulting in sleep disorders and other diseases (Arendt et al., 2018). Additionally, sheep experiments have confirmed that the pineal gland's melatonin secretory capacity could decrease following neural changes, such as superior cervical ganglionectomy, before eventually regaining with the mechanism of re-innervation (Prangley et al., 1993). Thus, the pineal gland's integrity and functioning need to be ensured to extend effective sleep control and overall well-being, highlighting the gland's important role in the endocrine system (Figure 12.7).

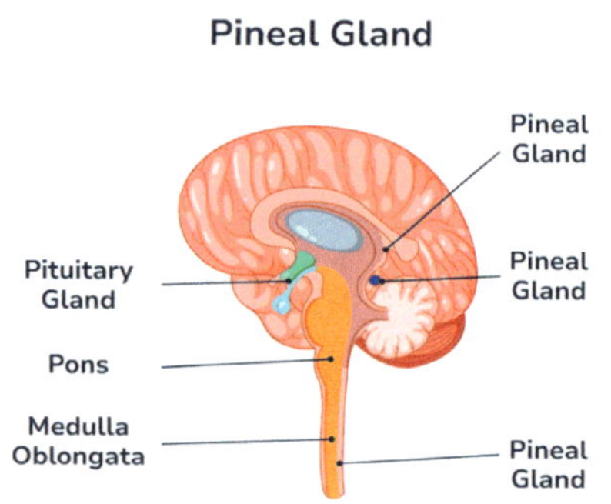

Figure 12.7. Pineal gland.

Source: https://media.geeksforgeeks.org/wp-content/uploads/20240606160923/pineal-gland.png.

12.1.7. The Thymus: Immune Function

Among the significant organs of the immune system, the thymus plays a primary role in the maturation of T lymphocytes, which are crucial for adaptive immunity. The gland, apart from the production of thymulin, a peptide that influences T cell proliferation and differentiation, is also a site of mature immune cell selection, thus inducing self-tolerance and preventing autoimmune attacks. Various other factors, including hormonal influences, contribute to the function of the thymus. For instance, sex steroids and progesterone have been known to induce instantaneous physiological changes in thymic epithelial cells that can affect the secretion of thymulin and consequently the immune response (Brucker et al., 1999). In addition, photoperiod-dependent seasonality in immune ability places stress on the thymus ability to withstand environmental stimulation, suggesting a subtle interaction between endocrine cues and immune function (Demas et al., 1995). The interaction emphasizes the importance of the thymus not just in the maturation of the immune system but also in modulating overall homeostasis of the endocrine system.

12.1.8. The Hypothalamus: Hormonal Control Center

Situated below the brain, the hypothalamus is an essential hormonal control center that controls a wide range of functions in the body through the regulation of the endocrine system. This small but complex piece of tissue is vital to maintaining the body in homeostasis because it links the nervous system with the endocrine system via the pituitary gland. By secreting, releasing, and inhibiting hormones, the hypothalamus controls processes such as growth, metabolism, and responses to stress. For instance, it interacts with the pituitary gland to manage adrenal activity and indirectly influence the body's response to stress (Clark et al., 2020).

Further, it is essential to value the intricate physiology of male reproductive endocrinology, such as the hypothalamic-pituitary-gonadal axis, to achieve successful hormonal treatment of male reproductive medicine (Clavijo et al., 2018). Thus, the hypothalamus is not just a master regulator of hormone release but also symbolizes the intricate interplay of various body systems.

12.1.9. The Parathyroid Glands: Calcium Homeostasis

The parathyroid glands, in maintaining calcium homeostasis, are significant via the secretion of parathyroid hormone (PTH), the immediate influence of which is on blood levels of calcium. With a fall in serum calcium, the glands secrete PTH, with subsequent mobilization of calcium from bone, augmented renal reabsorption of calcium, and increased conversion of vitamin D to its active form. This total response keeps calcium levels in a very tight range that is required for necessary physiological processes. Furthermore, the intricate interaction between parathyroid function and such factors as fibroblast growth factor-23 (FGF23) and Klotho signaling highlights the complexity of control of mineral metabolism. Reduced expression of Klotho in diseases like chronic kidney disease has been implicated in changes in calcium balance and illustrates the parathyroid glands' contribution to the body's overall homeostasis (Parker et al., 1972; Olauson et al., 2013). These mechanisms are and essential in understanding the more general functioning of the endocrine system.

Test Your Knowledge

1. How do the thyroid and adrenal glands contribute to metabolism and the body's stress response?
2. What roles do the pancreas and gonads play in regulating blood sugar and reproductive hormones?

12.2. Hormones and Their Functions

Learning Outcome

1. Define hormones and distinguish between different types
2. Explain the mechanisms of hormone action
3. Describe how hormones regulate metabolism
4. Identify key hormones involved in growth and development
5. Explain the hormonal response to stress
6. Describe the roles of reproductive hormones
7. Explain how hormones regulate fluid and electrolyte balance in the body
8. Describe feedback mechanisms that control hormonal secretion and maintain homeostasis
9. Identify common disorders caused by hormonal imbalances

Hormones are biochemical messengers that have a profound influence on much of the body's physiology. They are produced by glands in the endocrine system and transported in the blood to target organs, where they bind to specific receptors to elicit their effects. The range of hormones, including insulin to regulate glucose levels and adrenaline to prepare the body for fight-or-flight responses, underscores their role in homeostasis. These signaling compounds not only regulate metabolic functions but also play highly significant roles in growth, development, and mood regulation. The intricacies of hormone functions are further evident when examining such diseases as diabetes, where defective insulins lead to severe health issues. A good understanding of hormones is thus required for comprehending how they regulate themselves in the body and how illnesses may occur as a result of an imbalance of such systems (Kling et al., 1939; Arnold et al., 2001) (Figure 12.8).

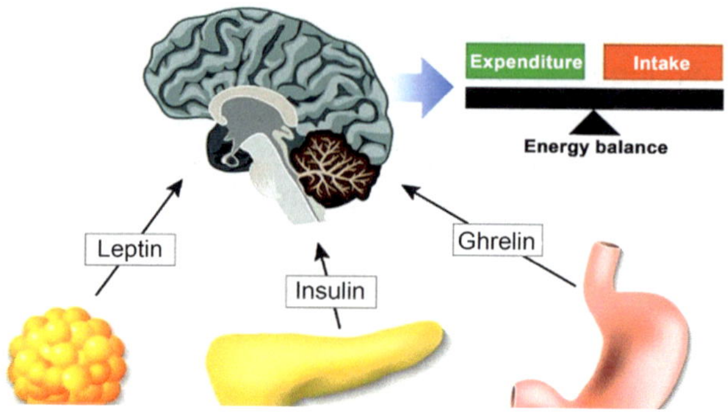

Figure 12.8. Hormones and their functions.

Source: https://img.jagranjosh.com/imported/images/E/Articles/List-of-hormones-in-human-body.webp.

12.2.1. Definition and Types of Hormones

Hormones are biochemical messengers that take part in the regulation of some of the body's physiological processes. They are generally classified into various types based on their chemical structures: peptide hormones, steroid hormones, and amine hormones, among others. Peptide hormones, which are composed of amino acids, include insulin and growth hormone, and they primarily function by binding with cell surface receptors to produce their effects. By way of contrast, steroid hormones, which include cholesterol-derived hormones such as cortisol and estrogen, pass through cell membranes to bind with intracellular receptors and directly influence gene expression. Amine hormones, on the other hand, such as adrenaline, are derived from single amino acids and can have different effects depending on the target tissue. Understanding these various types of hormones and mechanisms of action is important in appreciating the complexity of the endocrine system and how it maintains homeostasis in the human body (Mathias Uhlén et al., 2015; Omer et al., 2016) (Figure 12.9).

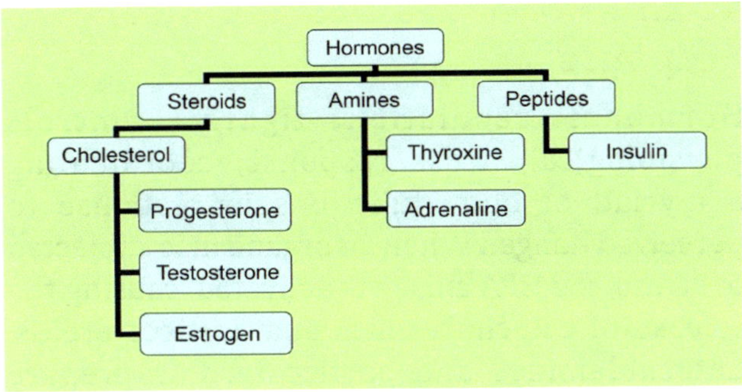

Figure 12.9. Hormones classification.

Source: https://external-content.duckduckgo.com/iu/?u=https%3A%2F%2Fimage.slideserve.com%2F545054%2Fhormone-classification-l.jpg&f=1&nofb=1&ipt=e2921b81e72ad6a5bec26e0ed4a0fb175de4f65133c4a74cf69d606560d6a4be.

12.2.2. Mechanisms of Hormone Action

Hormones exert their effects through a complex interplay of mechanisms that affect various physiological processes. Primarily, hormones bind to specific receptors, which initiate a cascade of intracellular events leading to a cellular response.

This binding has the potential to initiate or suppress gene expression, followed by modification of protein synthesis. For instance, in the scenario of endocrine-disrupting chemicals, such as PBDEs, their presence has the potential to induce alterations in hormone signaling pathways, which may lead to immune dysregulation. Hormonal evidence also indicates that this kind of exposure to such irritants may suppress pro-inflammatory cytokine release from activated macrophages, thereby implying that hormonal mechanisms are highly integrated into immune responses and respiratory health (Hennigar et al., 2010). Finally, the selectivity of hormone action is of special interest in that different hormones may respond differently depending on targeted tissues and receptor types. Thus, understanding such intricate mechanisms yields significant insights into the broader implications of hormonal regulation in the endocrine system.

12.2.3. Hormonal Regulation of Metabolism

The interaction of hormones with metabolic processes is crucial to maintaining homeostasis in the body. Hormonal regulation is a sophisticated control mechanism that impacts the storage, use, and transformation of energy. For instance, insulin released by the pancreas facilitates the uptake of glucose by cells, powering storage and inhibiting fat breakdown.

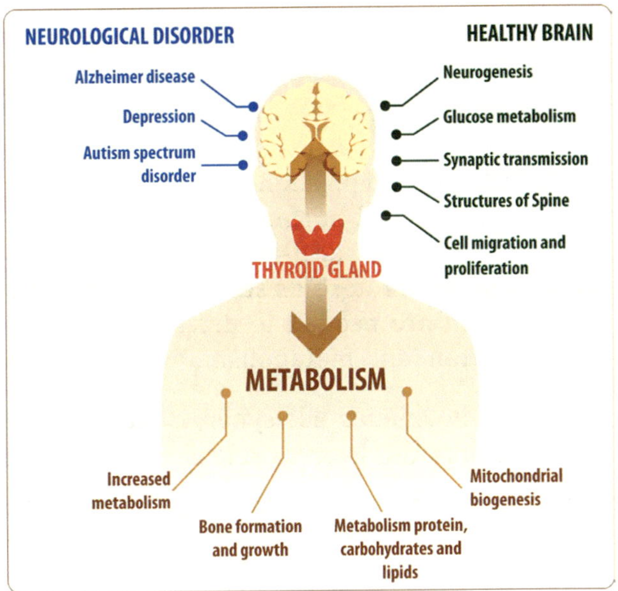

Figure 12.10. Hormones in control of metabolism.

Source: https://biyokimya.vet/wp-content/uploads/2023/05/image-1.png.

Conversely, hormones such as glucagon and cortisol mobilize energy reserves under fasting or stress conditions, illustrating dynamic equilibrium as required for metabolic homeostasis. The breakdown in this delicately balanced hormonal landscape can lead to metabolic disease, underscoring the importance of understanding the endocrine system's function in metabolism. Notably, hormonal therapy has a significant impact on such metabolic processes, as noted in assisted reproductive technologies (ART), such as in vitro fertilization (IVF). It is shown that hormonal treatments linked to IVF result in insulin resistance and inflammation, further complicating metabolic health (Barber et al., 2020). Also, circadian rhythm disturbances impact hormonal equilibrium, uncovering complex interactions between timekeeping and endocrine homeostasis with broad consequences for metabolic disorders (Bruscalupi et al., 2017) (Figure 12.10).

12.2.4. Hormones Involved in Growth and Development

Hormones are critical in the multifaceted processes of growth and development, coordinating varied physiological and metabolic processes. Principal hormones such as growth hormone (GH), insulin-like growth factors (IGFs), and sexual steroids such as testosterone and estrogen are needed to drive cell growth, differentiation, and metabolism.

These hormones act synergistically, since GH stimulates the liver to release IGFs, which stimulate bone and tissue development. In addition, sex steroids are pivotal in sexual development and the regulation of reproductive processes, guiding the body into puberty and regulating factors such as muscle composition and fat distribution. Notably, recent research highlights the sophistication of steroid hormones, particularly in their roles beyond growth, such as neuroprotection and metabolic programming, as seen in polycystic ovary syndrome (Gonzalez et al., 2016). It is crucial to understand these hormone interactions to fully grasp the larger context of the endocrine system's contribution to overall health and development (Arnold et al., 2001).

12.2.5. Hormones and the Stress Response

Hormonal regulation tightly controls physiological stress response, coordinating a myriad of body functions in response to perceived danger. When an organism is subjected to stress, the HPA axis gets activated, causing the release of catecholamines and corticosteroids. Catecholamines and corticosteroids prepare the body for rapid response, regulating heart rate and mobilization of energy and altering other functions such as digestion and immune function. An interesting stress response phenomenon can be seen in different species, i.e., in fish, in which environmental conditions significantly affect hormonal responses (Abdel-Tawwab et al., 2019). Also, in dairy cattle, pursuing greater milk yield has been linked with impaired fertility due to the disturbed regulation of hormones causing estrous activity (Beerda et al., 2010). The above examples also emphasize the important role that hormones play not only in acute stress responses but also in chronic physiological adjustments across a broad scope of species. This complex relationship yields useful insights in optimizing animal welfare as well as productivity in varied agricultural conditions (Figure 12.11).

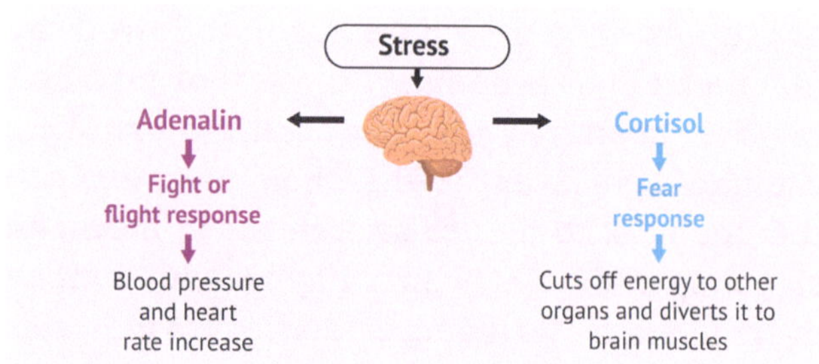

Figure 12.11. Stress hormones.

Source: https://external-content.duckduckgo.com/iu/?u=https%3A%2F%2Fwww.invitra.com%2Fen%2Fwp-content%2Fuploads%2F2022%2F01%2Fstress-hormones.png&f=1&nofb=1&ipt=b0d8e22b593e9d8894ec31dd0a7824ef7c1512413014fcd06eb3f9052a9d4206.

12.2.6. Reproductive Hormones and Their Effects

Reproductive hormones play a significant role in the regulation of various physiological processes, with effects not only on individual reproductive function but also on long-term health outcomes. The dynamic interaction between hormones such as estrogen, testosterone, and progesterone determines the development and maintenance of reproductive organs throughout the life course. Reproductive hormones are most sensitive during critical windows of development because prenatal exposure to hormonal as well as environmental factors can result in substantial neuroendocrine programming. For instance, it has been established that alterations in the gestational environment can affect the reproductive axis, hence leading to issues such as infertility or hormonal imbalance in adulthood (Bellingham et al., 2016). Secondly, plasticity in the gonadotropin-releasing hormone (GnRH) neurosecretory system defines the adaptive process of hormonal impact, demonstrating how early life exposures could define reproductive potential in future generations (Arnold et al., 2001). Not surprisingly, understanding these dynamics is required to comprehend the broader meanings of reproductive disease and health fully.

12.2.7. Hormones and Fluid Balance

The delicate equilibrium of body fluid balance is managed to a significant degree by hormones that regulate the manner in which kidneys manage fluid and electrolyte loss. Primary hormones involved in this regulation are renin, angiotensin, aldosterone, and antidiuretic hormone (ADH), all critical for maintaining homeostasis. For instance, the renin-angiotensin-aldosterone system responds to changes in blood pressure and blood volume by promoting sodium and water reabsorption in the kidneys to preserve dehydration and blood pressure (Leonard et al., 2020). In addition, endocrine changes can drastically influence body fluid composition, as seen in the study of oviduct fluid, demonstrating how hormones and environmental parameters can control the microenvironment required for reproduction (Arnold et al., 2016). Understanding these hormonal interactions not only clarifies fluid dynamics but highlights their crucial importance in overall health and physiologic homeostasis.

12.2.8. Feedback Mechanisms in Hormonal Regulation

Hormonal regulation relies to a great degree on feedback systems to maintain homeostasis in the body. Feedback systems are divided as negative and positive feedback systems. Negative feedback is the primary mechanism where an increase in the amount of a hormone initiates physiological activities that hinder further hormone production to stabilize the system. For instance, the hypothalamic-pituitary axis demonstrates this because changes in the body trigger the release of hormones, and once equilibrium has been restored, further secretion is inhibited. Positive feedback, on the other hand, builds the concentration of hormones, as seen with oxytocin release during parturition, which augments contractions. Understanding these feedback mechanisms is significant because not only do they regulate the release of hormones, but also influence other physiological processes, including reproductive and metabolic systems. This data sets the stage for understanding why the disruption of these feedback loops leads to pathologies, highlighting the importance of regulatory balance in health and disease (Gonzalez et al., 2016; Bruscalupi et al., 2017).

12.2.9. Disorders Related to Hormonal Imbalance

The endocrine system regulates most of the body's functions through the production and secretion of hormones; therefore, it is essential to be aware of the diseases resulting from hormonal imbalance. They lead to severe health issues like diabetes, obesity, and thyroid problems. For instance, populations impacted by industrial pollution, like in the Dokkarat region of Fez, have been discovered to suffer from a correlation between toxic environmental factors and the onset of some endocrine disorders, including hormonal imbalance and diabetes (Merzouki et al., 2018). Furthermore, traumatic brain injury can disrupt neuroendocrine regulation, manifesting as hypopituitarism and cognitive loss. The connection between endocrine diseases and external factors sheds light on the importance of early diagnosis and treatment, which can guarantee a decrease in long-term health effects. It is necessary to have an absolute understanding of these diseases to improve patient management and avoid adverse outcomes in patients with hormonal disorder (Quldashev et al.., 2023).

Test Your Knowledge

1. Which hormones regulate metabolism, and how do they maintain energy balance in the body?
2. What are the key hormones involved in growth, development, stress response, and reproduction, and what are their primary effects?

12.3. Endocrine System Disorders

Learning Outcome

1. Provide an overview of common endocrine disorders
2. Differentiate between types of diabetes mellitus
3. Explain the causes, symptoms, and effects of hyperthyroidism and hypothyroidism on metabolism
4. Describe the causes and symptoms of Cushing's syndrome
5. Explain the pathophysiology of Addison's disease
6. Identify the symptoms and hormonal imbalances associated with polycystic ovary syndrome (PCOS).
7. Describe disorders related to growth hormone
8. Explain what thyroid nodules and thyroid cancer are, and describe how they are detected and evaluated
9. Discuss various treatment options for endocrine disorders

The multifaceted operation of the endocrine system can become disordered, leading to a multitude of disorders that greatly influence overall health. Endocrine balance is produced by a variety of factors, including gene forms, autoimmune diseases, and environmental states. Endocrine disorders exist in various forms, such as diabetes, thyroid diseases, and adrenal insufficiencies, each with its unique symptoms and treatment procedures.

For instance, chronic stress exacerbates these conditions through its impact on the hypothalamic-pituitary-adrenal axis and induces dysregulation in hormone secretion and release (Daryl B. O'Connor et al., 2020). The effects of prolonged exposure to endocrine-disrupting chemicals also add complexity to these diseases, with devastating health effects. Early intervention and management are critical to avert the long-term effects of these disorders. With growing recognition of the crucial relationship between the outside stressors and endocrine health, active research seeks to reveal these intricate relationships for more effective therapy (Figure 12.12).

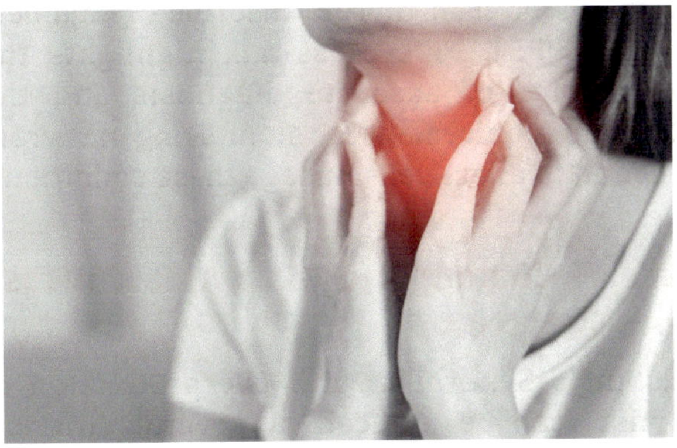

Figure 12.12. Woman experiencing discomfort in the neck area, indicating a possible thyroid or endocrine disorder.

Source: https://gvhcol.com/wp-content/uploads/sites/29/2024/06/Endocrine.jpg.

12.3.1. Overview of Common Endocrine Disorders

Hormonal imbalance can lead to a variety of endocrine disorders, which affect various body systems and the overall functioning of these systems. Hypothyroidism or an underactive thyroid leads to tiredness, weight gain, and depression, while hyperthyroidism produces hypermetabolism, leading to weight loss and nervousness. A critical concern is androgen-related disorders such as polycystic ovary syndrome (PCOS), which is linked to insulin resistance and endocrine disturbances that can impair reproductive function and lead to a susceptibility to diabetes. Furthermore, exposure to endocrine-disrupting chemicals such as PBDEs has been detected to suppress the release of pro-inflammatory cytokines from alveolar macrophages, potentially detracting from immune function and susceptibility to respiratory disease (Hennigar et al., 2010). Equally, the long-term side effects of such drugs as finasteride bear testament to the intricate interplay between endocrine and psychological health and make it a cautious area of treatment to enter (Banu et al., 2016) (Figure 12.13).

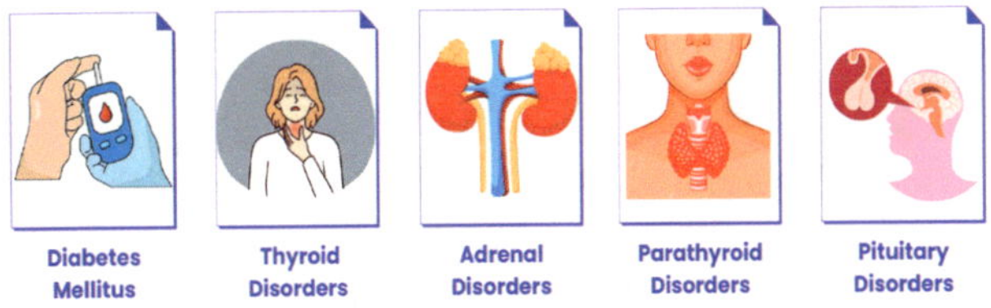

Figure 12.13. Common endocrine disorders.

Source: https://external-content.duckduckgo.com/iu/?u=https%3A%2F%2Fimages.examples.com%2Fwp-content%2Fuploads%2F2024%2F11%2FCommon-Endocrine-Disorders-1.png&f=1&nofb=1&ipt=f4a5457b9458d705dcaed73851f4272f3db9f4a3852b6f7934f82db4afd53cc3.

12.3.2. Diabetes Mellitus: Types and Management

Understanding diabetes mellitus involves recognizing its various forms and the management strategies essential for each. Type 1 and Type 2 diabetes, the two primary forms, have unique challenges and require disparate management. Type 1, by nature, is diagnosed in children and results from autoimmune destruction of the beta cells that produce insulin. In contrast, Type 2 is primarily associated with insulin resistance and is more likely to occur in adults. Effective control of either type is dependent upon monitoring blood glucose, dietary modification, and compliance with medications. More importantly, advancement in communication technology has been promising towards enhancing control. A systematic review attributed the advancement in electronic devices to facilitate more patient and healthcare provider interactions that resulted in better health outcomes in certain patients (Bandura et al., 2011). Specifically, conditions such as fibrocalculous pancreatic diabetes, related to chronic pancreatitis, illustrate the multifaceted nature of diabetes and its treatment, emphasizing the need for a multidimensional approach tailored to individual circumstances (Chowdhury et al., 1994) (Figure 12.14).

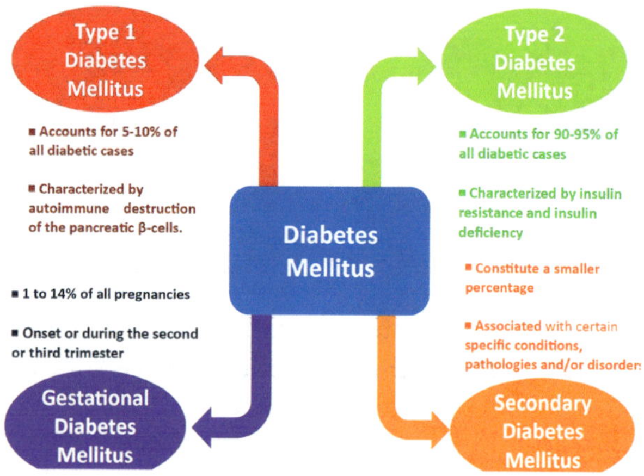

Figure 12.14. Types of diabetes mellitus.

Source: https://external-content.duckduckgo.com/iu/?u=https%3A%2F%2Fwww.researchgate.net%2Fpublication%2F365051474%2Ffigure%2Ffig1%2FAS%3A11431281095025936%401667696871709%2FClassification-of-Diabetes-Mellitus-Source-Banday-et-al-2020.png&f=1&nofb=1&ipt=1180a8265b0c0f4c96953a4ababbbeb84fc2fd7bd30a8438906a0a77f3cc6b0f.

12.3.3. Hyperthyroidism and Hypothyroidism

Endocrine disorders in the thyroid gland lead to two prominent conditions: hyperthyroidism and hypothyroidism. Overproduction of thyroid hormones in hyperthyroidism tends to manifest in loss of weight, tachycardia, and nervousness due to enhanced metabolic functions. Hypothyroidism leads to the underproduction of hormones and manifests itself through fatigue, weight gain, and depression as metabolic functions slow down. Its impact is not restricted to metabolic manifestations; subclinical thyroid disease (SCTD) is becoming a cause of growing alarm. SCTD can progress to overt disease, with implications for cardiovascular fitness and bone density (Biondi et al., 2008). It is also crucial to research the dynamics of TSH because the response of the hormone to thyrotropin-releasing hormone (TRH) is central to the diagnosis of such thyroid disorders (Enjalbert et al., 1985). This cross-talk highlights the importance of accurate diagnosis and the potential requirement for monitoring of thyroid function to effectively manage these conditions.

12.3.4. Cushing's Syndrome: Causes and Symptoms

Cushing's Syndrome with overproduction of cortisol can be induced by several different etiologies, resulting in a range of characteristic signs. These include the chief causes of adrenal tumors, such as adenomas or carcinomas, and pituitary adenomas that can lead to excess adrenocorticotropic hormone (ACTH) production, which stimulates hyperfunction of the adrenal cortex.

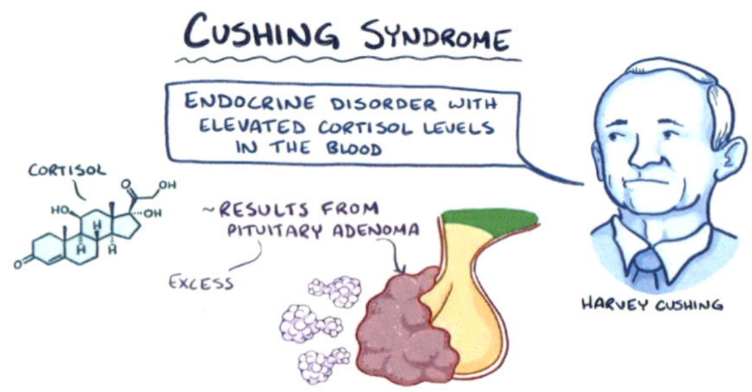

Figure 12.15. Cushing syndrome.

Source: https://www.osmosis.org/_next/image?url=https%3A%2F%2Fd16qt3wv6xm098.cloudfront.net%2Ft1w4xoMFQ8ys9JoZSoaWhn-iT8O_N7k3%2F_.jpg&w=3840&q=75.

Additionally, ectopic ACTH syndrome due to non-pituitary tumors secreting ACTH can induce related signs. Clinically, these patients have Cushing's Syndrome with features of weight gain, typically central obesity, rounding of the face, and cutaneous changes, including easy bruising and purple striae. Other frequent presentations include hypertension, diabetes, and mood disorders, showing the systemic impact of excess cortisol on various organ systems (Frantzcess et al., 2024). The interdependent nature of these symptoms illustrates the pervasive effect of hormonal dysregulation on overall well-being, emphasizing the significance of identifying and treating this syndrome within the broader context of the endocrine system (Yutaka, 2023) (Figure 12.15).

12.3.5. Addison's Disease: Adrenal Insufficiency

Addison's disease refers to adrenal insufficiency, characterized by the inability to generate hormones needed to maintain various processes in the body. The condition typically arises as a consequence of autoimmune destruction of the adrenal glands that leads to an insufficiency of critical hormones such as cortisol and aldosterone (Wolff et al., 2023). Symptoms may be extremely severe, including fatigue and weight loss as well as electrolyte disturbances, which result in adrenal crisis if left untreated. Clinical evidence has also previously been reported in recent times that survivors of COVID-19 develop adrenal insufficiency due to autoimmunity rather than hemorrhage, as seen in a case report of a young female patient with acute adrenal insufficiency diagnosed some months after her COVID-19 illness (Özge et al., 2023). Understanding these diverse pathways to adrenal insufficiency is crucial for prompt diagnosis and effective treatment, revealing the importance of the endocrine system for overall well-being.

12.3.6. Polycystic Ovary Syndrome (PCOS)

Of the various endocrine disorders that afflict women, Polycystic Ovary Syndrome (PCOS) stands out for its complex set of signs and causes. With signs and features such as hyperandrogenemia, disordered ovulation, and cystic ovaries, PCOS has a drastic impact on childbearing age females, affecting up to 5-10% of this population (Bernier et al., 2012). Pathophysiology in PCOS suggests a strong neuroendocrine etiology, not just involving endocrine imbalance but with potential alterations of the hypothalamic axis governing reproductive functions. The proof is that elevated levels of luteinizing hormone (LH) and increased frequency of gonadotropin-releasing hormone (GnRH) may be primarily responsible for exacerbating the symptoms of the conditions (Coutinho et al., 2019). Complementing this issue, insulin resistance in PCOS is associated with several related health issues, including metabolic syndrome and type II diabetes, necessitating parallel focus on pharmacologic and lifestyle intervention to attain effective control.

12.3.7. Growth Hormone Disorders

The reason for the complexity of growth hormone disorders is the complex developmental events in the pituitary gland, where numerous transcription factors and signaling molecules are essential for proper function. Maldevelopment in such events can lead to diseases such as congenital hypopituitarism, which often manifests in terms of growth hormone deficiency, the most common form of isolated hormone deficiency (Aarskog et al., 2009).

Changes in anterior pituitary development and differentiation can be induced through mutations in genes, which underscores the importance of heredity in such conditions. Furthermore, endocrine regulation by the skin also raises the broader implications of hormonal balance, for the cutaneous hypothalamus-pituitary-adrenal axis suggests that growth hormone disease might not occur in a vacuum but in conjunction with overall dysfunction of the entire endocrine system (Clark et al., 2020). Appreciation of these interconnections is crucial for the creation of focused interventions and treatments for patients afflicted with such disorders.

12.3.8. Thyroid Nodules and Cancer

Thyroid nodules, incidentally found on imaging studies, can present complex diagnostic issues due to their wide range in nature and their potential malignancy. While most are benign, the rising incidence of thyroid cancer necessitates meticulous evaluation.

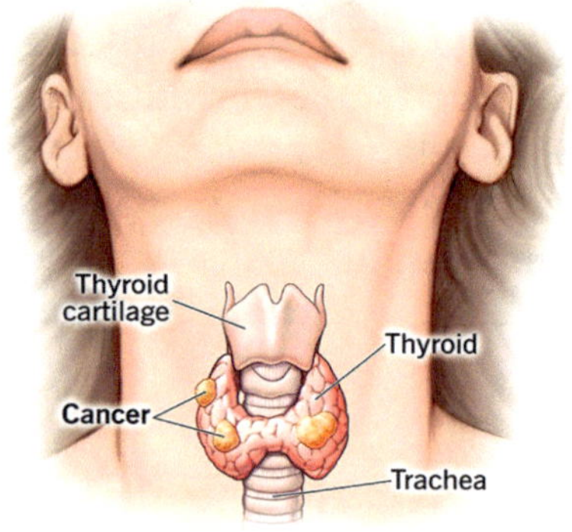

Figure 12.16. Thyroid cancer.

Source: https://my.clevelandclinic.org/-/scassets/images/org/health/articles/12210-thryoid-cancer.

Molecular genetic analysis is now an essential tool in the assessment of nodules, allowing the clinician to risk-stratify and determine surgery versus conservative management (Richmond et al., 2023). Nuclear imaging modalities such as radioiodine scanning and FDG PET/CT also become necessary in further defining thyroid cancer behavior. These modalities not only enable diagnosis and staging of thyroid cancer but also assist with monitoring response to treatment and detecting recurrences (Singh et al., 2023). Therefore, an all-encompassing approach that encompasses genetic and imaging studies is essential in the effective management of thyroid nodules as well as broader implications for patient outcomes in endocrine health (Figure 12.16).

12.3.9. Treatment Options for Endocrine Disorders

Endocrine disorders, affecting hormonal activity and equilibrium, require a multidisciplinary approach to treatment. Patients are managed in most instances by means of lifestyle modifications, pharmacotherapy, and, in a few cases, surgery. For example, diabetic patients can be managed by insulin therapy or oral hypoglycemic agents for glycemic control, together with dietary modifications favoring metabolic health. Further, emerging research highlights the overlap between COVID-19 and metabolic disease, given that infection has been theorized to worsen existing conditions like diabetes or even induce new-onset disease (Charlotte et al., 2021). Second, the intricate interaction between endocrine and gut function has been a point of interest, with emerging therapies in the form of probiotics and prebiotics promising to modulate the gut-brain axis, a mechanism whereby endocrine function is preserved (Hannibal et al., 2020). Collectively, an individualized treatment strategy, aligning with these diverse interventions, is essential for managing endocrine disorders effectively and improving patient outcomes.

Test Your Knowledge

1. How do the symptoms of hyperthyroidism differ from those of hypothyroidism, and what are their common causes?
2. What are the causes and significant symptoms of Cushing's syndrome and Addison's disease?

12.4. The Role of the Endocrine System in Homeostasis

Learning Outcome

1. Define homeostasis
2. Describe how the nervous system interacts with homeostatic mechanisms
3. Explain the regulation of blood glucose levels
4. Describe the mechanisms controlling blood pressure
5. Explain how the body maintains temperature homeostasis through various physiological responses
6. Describe the regulation of water and electrolyte balance
7. Explain the impact of homeostasis on immune function
8. Describe how hormones influence behavior through homeostatic regulation
9. Explain how the body adapts to environmental changes to maintain homeostasis

The endocrine system plays a vital role in maintaining homeostasis in the body by regulating a vast range of physiological processes. Endocrine glands secrete hormones into the blood, which act as chemical messengers and coordinate functions such as metabolism, growth, and mood. Hormone release of the gastrointestinal tract, for instance, not only participates in digestion but also in the balance of energy and appetite, demonstrating its neuroendocrine functions, which are involved in the overall metabolism (Calderón et al., 2023). Moreover, hormone response to target cells orchestrates complex pathways which are significant to the body's adaptive responses to internal as well as to external stimuli. In diseases like obesity, the alteration of these endocrine signals can lead to metabolic disorders, highlighting just how sensitive the endocrine system is in terms of ensuring homeostasis (Baldari et al., 2016). Learning about the intricate relationships and functions of the endocrine system is thus vital for overcoming some of these health problems and maximizing treatment regimens.

12.4.1. Definition of Homeostasis

Homeostasis, or the creation of a steady state internal environment, is essential for survival and effective operation in biological organisms. This encompasses the regulation of various physiological values, such as temperature, pH, and energy balance, to maintain conditions optimal even under adverse external changes.

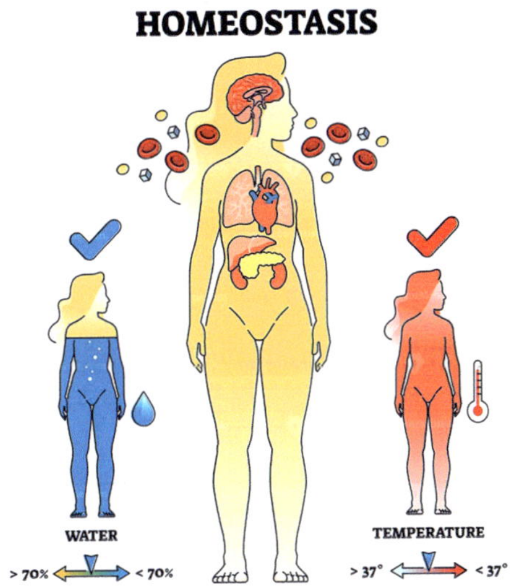

Figure 12.17. Homeostasis state with body temperature and water regulation.

Source: https://i.pinimg.com/originals/fa/f2/73/faf273ea4c417fb3c84fa8bde2e5f9ff.jpg.

For instance, during disturbances, such as illness or climatic change, the organism employs feedback mechanisms to restore balance. These homeostatic reactions are necessary, since a failure to maintain homeostasis may result in disease or death. As shown in the literature, the understanding of homeostasis is particularly pertinent to the application of physiological findings in medicine; it allows for the creation of more effective treatments and interventions (Ivan et al., 2011). Moreover, homeostatic processes also give insight into aging, where changes in body composition, such as sarcopenia and lipotoxicity, can also disturb the homeostatic balance (Carter et al., 2019). Thus, the understanding of homeostasis stands at the center of physiology as well as clinical aspects (Figure 12.17).

12.4.2. Interaction with the Nervous System

The intricate interaction between the endocrine and nervous systems illustrates the intricacy of the body processes and mechanisms of health regulation. The nervous system interacts with numerous endocrine glands in a highly complex manner, regulating the discharge of hormones and having a significant impact on physiological and psychological states. For instance, stress can potentially activate the HPA axis to release cortisol, hence impacting immune response and general homeostasis. In addition, the association of the central nervous system with adipose tissue further illustrates this dynamic relationship; adipocytes release adipokines, which communicate information about metabolic status and energy homeostasis to the brain, as illustrated by the leptin-kisspeptin axis (Bruno et al., 2021). Such interaction provokes the likelihood of disruption of endocrine signaling as an expression of psychological disorder, substantiating the crucial role played by the nervous system in endocrine well-being (Alaín et al., 2017). Knowledge of these interactions is essential in understanding health problems that result from hormonal imbalances.

12.4.3. Regulation of Blood Glucose Levels

Stable blood glucose levels are necessary for both good health and regular metabolic processes. Insulin, glucagon, and adrenaline are the three hormones that the body employs in a delicate balance to control glucose levels within a specific range. This system is carefully regulated to avoid both hyperglycemia and hypoglycemia. Insulin is secreted in response to elevated blood sugar, allowing glucose to be taken into cells and thus lowering blood sugar. In contrast, when blood glucose is reduced, glucagon stimulates the liver to release stored glucose to give a sufficient supply of energy. The autonomic nervous system also plays its part in glucose regulation, as shown by rat overfeeding experiments, which demonstrate impaired sympathetic and parasympathetic activity, which can increase obesity and insulin resistance diseases (Alingh et al., 1996). Therefore, the nervous system and endocrine system play an essential role in controlling blood glucose levels, highlighting the significance of such feedback control mechanisms to maintain physiological homeostasis (Mujtahid et al., 2020) (Figure 12.18).

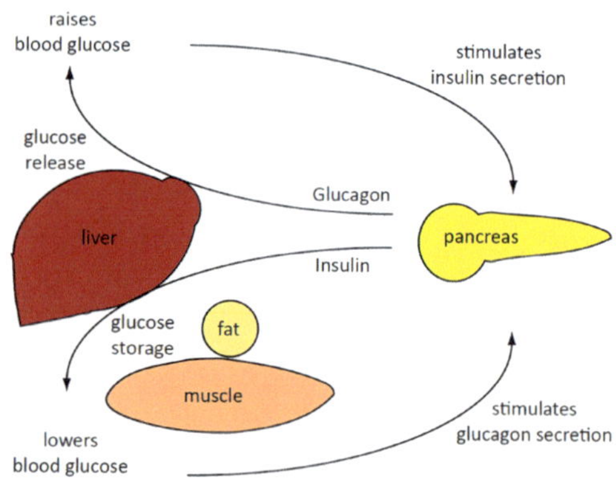

Figure 12.18. Regulation of blood glucose levels by insulin and glucagon.

Source: https://www.researchgate.net/figure/Regulation-of-blood-glucose-levels-by-insulin-and-glucagon-When-blood-glucose-tends-When_fig3_51451430.

12.4.4. Control of Blood Pressure

Control of blood pressure is a complex interaction among various physiological mechanisms, primarily the neural and hormonal systems. A specific critical regulatory pathway involves the renin-angiotensin system (RAS), which plays a central role in vascular homeostasis. As blood pressure drops, the kidneys release renin, leading to the production of angiotensin II. This potent vasoconstrictor not only increases blood pressure but also leads to the release of aldosterone, which enhances sodium and water reabsorption. Notably, it has been found just recently that cholinergic stimulation can also control these processes. For instance, intravenous infusion of carbachol in fetal sheep influenced heart rate and blood pressure as well as expressed an over-activated fetal RAS, indicating a direct relationship between cholinergic stimulation and control of blood pressure (Chen et al., 2009). Moreover, lifestyle factors, most notably dietary patterns like adherence to the Mediterranean diet, have also been reported to confer cardiovascular protection, avoiding the development of diseases such as myocardial infarction and stroke, which underscores the importance of combined interventions in blood pressure control (Cammisotto et al., 2017).

12.4.5. Maintenance of Body Temperature

Regulation of body temperature is part of homeostasis, a closely associated process with the endocrine system. Regulation is largely focused on the hypothalamus, which acts as the body's thermostat, responding to both internal and external temperature variations. When temperatures fluctuate, the hypothalamus releases hormones, which induce physiological responses, such as altering metabolic rate and stimulating sweat glands or blood vessel dilation for heat loss. In addition, dysregulation in this system can lead to circadian dysregulations impacting overall endocrine and metabolic function, as has been emphasized in recent work identifying the interface between circadian rhythms and physiological regulation (Bruscalupi et al., 2017). Furthermore, issues such as caloric restriction and hypothalamic estrogen signaling can significantly impact energy balance and temperature control, illustrating how precise the interfaces are between thermoregulation and metabolic health (Barakat et al., 2017). The value of these interrelationships emphasizes the endocrine system's key role in sustaining optimal body temperature.

12.4.6. Regulation of Water and Electrolyte Balance

Homeostasis in the body is essential, with respect to water and electrolyte balance, which is controlled mainly by the kidneys. The kidneys filter different substances, allowing the selective reabsorption of water and electrolytes to maintain equilibrium, thereby playing a central role in the regulation of blood pressure and the total fluid content in the body.

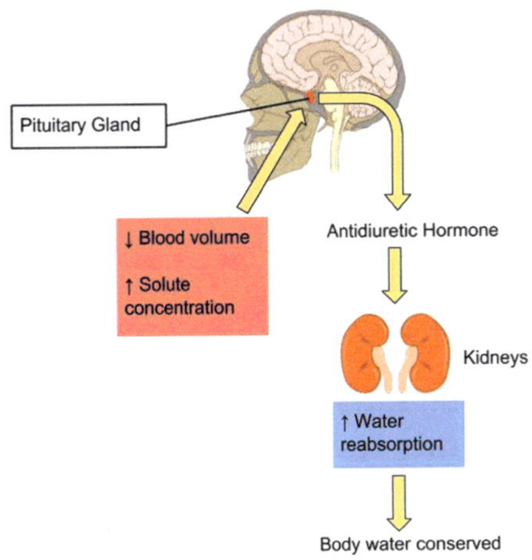

Figure 12.19. Regulation of water balance.

Source: https://pressbooks.bccampus.ca/nutr1100/wp-content/uploads/sites/774/2019/06/Regulating-water-output.jpg.

There are various hormones, such as renin and erythropoietin, which play roles in this process, showing the endocrine contribution to renal activity. Besides, breaks in this balance can lead to serious diseases. For instance, in end-stage renal disease (ESRD), the kidneys no longer have a functioning capacity, leading to uremic syndrome, manifested in dehydration and electrolyte imbalance (Petra, 2017). These conditions indicate the importance of the kidneys to not only control metabolic wastes but also essential fluids and electrolytes for sustaining life, marking the interdependence of the excretory and endocrine systems (Petra, 2017) (Figure 12.19).

12.4.7. Impact on Immune Function

The interrelation between endocrine and immunity is complex and important to the organism's well-being. Among the significant impacts on immunity is the role that Krebs cycle intermediaries have in being directly engaged in immune reactions by modifying cellular activation and energy metabolism. These intermediates play a central role in the production of many biosynthetic pathways that enhance immune cell functions, thereby enhancing the ability of the body to respond to infection (Arneth, 2023). Furthermore, quality sleep significantly affects immune function, particularly in professional athletes, who predominantly have reduced sleep duration and quality.

The restorative effect of adequate sleep maintains the endocrine system's ability to regulate physiological processes, a need for effective immune responses (Hadi et al., 2023). Thus, understanding how these interconnected systems function can provide valuable insights into potential therapeutic methods, underscoring the importance of maintaining endocrine balance and immune resilience.

12.4.8. Hormonal Influence on Behavior

The intricate interdependence of behavior and hormones emphasizes the remarkable influence endocrine systems play in regulating social interactions and physiological responses. Male meerkats, for instance, have a strong link between androgens such as testosterone and dominance rank and aggression. One discovers that subordinate helpers do not possess rank-related variation in testosterone levels, but that androgen receptors block varying behaviors among them.

Specifically, flutamide-treated meerkats were less aggressive but more prosocial, which refers to the way androgens influence behavioral trade-offs in a social setting (Albers et al., 2016). Additionally, hormone regulation is essential during situations of severe stress, e.g., space flight, when fluid and electrolyte status is the most important. In this regard, hormones like renin-angiotensin and ADH work together to control renal excretion, essentially exhibiting hormonal influence on behavior and adaptation to physical environment changes (Leonard et al., 2020). Thus, not only do hormones regulate individual behaviors, but they also work together to influence the social dynamics of groups.

12.4.9. Adaptation to Environmental Changes

The ability to adapt to environmental change is most important for the maintenance of homeostatic balance and the assurance of survival.

The endocrine system has a crucial role to play in doing this in its primary mechanism, the hypothalamic-pituitary-adrenal (HPA) axis, which reacts to stressors by regulating hormone secretion. For instance, during stress in the body, there is a cascade of hormonal reactions that stimulate the sympathetic nervous system while simultaneously suppressing reproductive hormones such as TSH, LH, and FSH. This highlights the sensitive communication between the endocrine and immune system, essential in adjusting effectively to varied conditions, as reported in (Baran et al., 2008). In addition, consideration of how these adaptive responses can manifest themselves in many different ways, particularly in endocrine diseases, is also required. Therefore, understanding the adaptation mechanisms not only contributes value to the knowledge of the endocrine system but also emphasizes its applicability in clinical settings, particularly patient care with different endocrine diseases, as depicted in (Carlos et al., 2010).

Test Your Knowledge

1. What is the definition of homeostasis, and why is it essential for the body?
2. How does the nervous system contribute to maintaining homeostasis?

SUMMARY

Briefly, it is necessary to know the intricate functions and impacts of the endocrine system to comprehend human health and disease. The interaction between endocrine disruptors, such as those present in cosmetics, provokes essential concerns about chemical exposure daily and their lasting implications for hormonal balance. As charted, the extensive research of such compounds illustrates the necessity to continue more investigation into their topical effect and cumulative risk of various ingredients (Chantelouve et al., 2022). The causal role of endocrine therapies in treating diseases like breast cancer also illustrates the effectiveness of targeted agents and how complex endocrine interactions are. As established by the efficacy of treatment interventions, such as aromatase inhibitors and selective estrogen receptor modulators, continued expansion of our understanding of the endocrine system can lead to improved health and new forms of treatment (Basso et al., 2015). Awareness of these factors in conjunction underscores the importance of continued research and understanding within the field of endocrinology.

The intricate relationship between environmental pollutants and endocrine well-being is evoked by the revelation of vast amounts of research studies conducted on fish populations, primarily sticklebacks. The results from the EDCAT project indicate that endocrine-disrupting chemicals (EDCs) significantly impact aquatic life, leading to alterations in reproductive physiology as well as metabolic processes (Abel et al., 2009). Notably, the absence of demonstrable estrogenic effects in men and increased reproductive endocrine indicators in women following remediation interventions signifies the complex dynamics present within ecosystems (Abel et al., 2009). Additionally, the significance of continued investment in medical research is accentuated by the Office of Health Economics through the recognition of the dependency of public and charitable funding in addressing health outcomes. Together, these studies illustrate the necessity for further research and intervention to address the multileveled difficulties that EDCs pose toward ultimately safeguarding both environmental and human health.

KEY TERMS FROM THIS CHAPTER

- Pituitary Gland
- Pineal Gland
- Parathyroid Glands
- Pancreas
- Testes
- Growth Hormone
- Insulin
- Cortisol
- Hypothalamus
- Thyroid Gland
- Adrenal Glands
- Ovaries
- Hormones
- Thyroxine
- Glucagon
- Adrenaline

CRITICAL THINKING QUESTIONS

1. **Which gland is known as the "master gland" of the endocrine system?**
   a. Thyroid gland
   b. Adrenal gland
   c. Pituitary gland
   d. Pineal gland
2. **Which hormone regulates blood sugar levels?**
   a. Insulin
   b. Thyroxine
   c. Estrogen
   d. Cortisol
3. **The adrenal glands are located:**
   a. In the brain
   b. On top of the kidneys
   c. In the neck
   d. Behind the stomach
4. **Which hormone is produced by the thyroid gland?**
   a. Insulin
   b. Thyroxine (T4)
   c. Glucagon
   d. Cortisone
5. **What is the primary function of parathyroid hormone (PTH)?**
   a. Regulate metabolism
   b. Increase blood calcium levels
   c. Stimulate milk production
   d. Control circadian rhythms

Short Answer Questions

1. What are the major glands of the endocrine system and where are they located?
2. What hormone is produced by the thyroid gland and what is its primary function?
3. How does the pituitary gland influence other endocrine glands?
4. What role does insulin play in regulating blood glucose levels?
5. What are the symptoms and causes of hypothyroidism?
6. How does adrenal gland dysfunction affect the body?
7. What is the role of the endocrine system in maintaining homeostasis?
8. How do feedback mechanisms regulate hormone levels in the body?

Answer to Critical Thinking Questions

1.(c) 2. (a) 3. (b) 4.(b) 5.(b)

REFERENCES

1. Abel, D., Cook, A., Juergens, M. D., Katsiadaki, I., Pottinger, T. G., Rhodes, G., & Sanders, M. (2009). A catchment-based study of endocrine disruption in surface waters: Multivariate evaluation of the health of a sentinel fish species exposed to sewage treatment works effluent. *EDCAT Consortium*. https://core.ac.uk/download/60806.pdf (accessed on 14th June 2025).
2. Farokhnia, M., McDiarmid, G. R., Newmeyer, M. N., Munjal, V., Abulseoud, O. A., Huestis, M. A., & Leggio, L. (2020). Effects of oral, smoked, and vaporized cannabis on endocrine pathways related to appetite and metabolism: a randomized, double-blind, placebo-controlled, human laboratory study. *Translational Psychiatry*, *10*(1). https://doi.org/10.1038/s41398-020-0756-3Ahnert-Hilger, G., Bader, M. F., Baumert, M., Bittner, M. A., Blasi, J., Elferink, L. A., Fischer, G., Geppert, M., Halpern, J. L., Hess, S. D., Jahn, R., Gratzl, M., Marqueze-Pouey, B., McMahon, H. T., Schiavo, G., Schmidle, T., Shirataki, H., Shoji-Kasai, Y., Stecher, B., Thomas, L., Trimble, W. S., Walch-Solimena, C., Wright, J. F., & Yoshida, A. (1994). Molecular aspects of secretory granule exocytosis by neurons and endocrine cells. *Wiley*. https://core.ac.uk/download/12168168.pdf (accessed on 14th June 2025).
3. Alonso Remedios, A., López González, E. J., López Cabrera, E., & Cabrera Macias, Y. (2017). Do we get worried sick? An answer from the Psiconeuroinmunoendocrinology. *Centro Provincial de Información de Ciencias Médicas, Cienfuegos*. https://core.ac.uk/download/201107423.pdf (accessed on 14th June 2025).
4. Appetecchia, M., Lauretta, R., Romanelli, F., Sansone, A., & Sansone, M. (2018). Gender in endocrine diseases: Role of sex gonadal hormones. *Hindawi Limited*. https://core.ac.uk/download/188826984.pdf (accessed on 14th June 2025).
5. Arneth, B. (2023). The impact of Krebs cycle intermediates on the endocrine system and immune system: A comparison. https://www.semanticscholar.org/paper/bfdbcbfa34420f85468af86e81a9d69780b77fda (accessed on 14th June 2025).
6. Arnold, B. S., Gross, T. S., McDonald, K., & Spulveda, M. S. (2001). Relations of environmental contaminants, algal toxins, and diet with the reproductive success of American alligators on Florida lakes. *Florida Cooperative Fish and Wildlife Research Unit, University of Florida*. https://core.ac.uk/download/11016994.pdf (accessed on 14th June 2025).
7. Arnold, G., Froehlich, T., Leese, H. J., Sathyapalan, T., Simintiras, C. A., & Ulbrich, S. E. (2016). Modelling aspects of oviduct fluid formation *in vitro*. *Bioscientific*. https://core.ac.uk/download/151161500.pdf (accessed on 14th June 2025).
8. Baan, C. C., van den Berg-Garrelds, I. M., Bindels, E. M. J., van den Bosch, T. P. P., Clahsen-van Groningen, M. C., Danser, A. H. J., Du, Z., Gribnau, J. H., Hoogduijn, M. J., Hoorn, E. J., Korevaar, S. S., Lopez-Iglesias, C., Mora, H. T., & Shankar, A. S. (2020). Human kidney organoids produce functional renin. *Elsevier BV*. https://core.ac.uk/download/373092792.pdf (accessed on 14th June 2025).
9. Balali-Mood, M., Naseri, K., Tahergorabi, Z., Khazdair, M. R., & Sadeghi, M. (2021). Toxic mechanisms of five heavy metals: Mercury, lead, chromium, cadmium, and arsenic. *12*. https://doi.org/10.3389/fphar.2021.643972 (accessed on 14th June 2025).
10. Baldari, C., Bimonte, V. M., Di Luigi, L., Donini, L. M., Emerenziani, G. P., Fittipaldi, S., Fornari, R., Greco, E. A., Guidetti, L., Lenzi, A., Marocco, C., Migliaccio, S., Nicolai, E., & Poggiogalle,

E. (2016). Physical activity and hypocaloric diet recover osteoblasts homeostasis in women affected by abdominal obesity. *Springer Science and Business Media LLC.* https://core.ac.uk/download/80310762.pdf (accessed on 14th June 2025).

11. Banu, P., Bălălău, C., Constantin, V. D., Motofei, I. G., Popa, F., Păunică, G. P., Păunică, I., Păunică, S., Rowland, D. L., & Vasilache, A. (2016). The post finasteride syndrome: An overview. *ValpoScholar.* https://core.ac.uk/download/144552981.pdf (accessed on 14th June 2025).
12. Barakat, R., Brooks, G. A., Efe, G., Garan, S. A., Gouw, A. M., Mehdizadeh, M., & Preecha, A. (2017). Roles of estrogen receptor-alpha in mediating life span: The hypothalamic deregulation hypothesis. *eScholarship, University of California.* https://core.ac.uk/download/305124015.pdf (accessed on 14th June 2025).
13. Baran, A., Jakiel, G., & Wójcik, G. (2008). The utilization of the climatic chamber to evaluate the influence of ambient conditions on endocrine, nervous and immune systems of rats. *Walter de Gruyter GmbH.* https://core.ac.uk/download/268436790.pdf (accessed on 14th June 2025).
14. Barber, T. M., Coussa, A., & Hassan, H. (2020). Impact of contraception and IVF hormones on metabolic, endocrine, and inflammatory status. *Springer Science and Business Media LLC.* https://core.ac.uk/download/293755293.pdf (accessed on 14th June 2025).
15. Basso, S. M. M., Lumachi, F., & Santeufemia, D. A. (2015). Current medical treatment of estrogen receptor-positive breast cancer. *Baishideng Publishing Group Inc.* https://core.ac.uk/download/53525256.pdf (accessed on 14th June 2025).
16. Beerda, B., Boer, H. M. T., Veerkamp, R. F., & Woelders, H. (2010). Estrous behavior in dairy cows: Identification of underlying mechanisms and gene functions. https://core.ac.uk/download/pdf/29246031.pdf (accessed on 14th June 2025).
17. Bellingham, M., Cotinot, C., Evans, N. P., Fowler, P. A., MacDonald, E. S., Mandon-Pepin, B., Rhind, S., & Sharpe, R. M. (2016). Timing of maternal exposure and fetal sex determine the effects of low-level chemical mixture exposure on the fetal neuroendocrine system in sheep. *Wiley.* https://core.ac.uk/download/74230048.pdf (accessed on 14th June 2025).
18. Bellingham, M., Evans, N. P., & Robinson, J. E. (2016). Prenatal programming of neuroendocrine reproductive function. *Elsevier BV.* https://core.ac.uk/download/42371121.pdf (accessed on 14th June 2025).
19. Bernier, D. (2012). *Polycystic Ovary Syndrome: Pathogenesis, Health Consequences, and Treatment of PCOS in Relation to Insulin Resistance.* University of New Hampshire Scholars' Repository. https://core.ac.uk/download/72048051.pdf (accessed on 14th June 2025).
20. Bich, L., Mossio, M., & Soto, A. M. (2020). Glycemia regulation: From feedback loops to organizational closure. https://core.ac.uk/download/287611700.pdf (accessed on 14th June 2025).
21. Biondi, B., & Cooper, D. S. (2008). The clinical significance of subclinical thyroid dysfunction. *The Endocrine Society.* https://core.ac.uk/download/54955329.pdf (accessed on 14th June 2025).
22. Boehm, O., Bornstein, S. R., Grotemeyer, D., Hamann, L., Koch, A., Kurt, M., Schott, M., Schumann, R. R., Schwenke, C., & Zacharowski, K. (2011). Genetic variation of TLR4 influences immunoendocrine stress response: An observational study in cardiac surgical patients. https://core.ac.uk/download/14521219.pdf (accessed on 14th June 2025).

23. Brucker, C., Downing, J. E. G., Head, G. M., Kendall, M. D., & Mentlein, R. (1999). Rapid progesterone actions on thymosin-secreting epithelial cells cultured from rat thymus. *S. Karger AG*. https://core.ac.uk/download/16432465.pdf (accessed on 14th June 2025).

24. Bruno, C., Cipolla, C., Giusti, M., Mancini, A., Oliva, A., Pitocco, D., & Vergani, E. (2021). The "adipo-cerebral" dialogue in childhood obesity: Focus on growth and puberty. Physio pathological and nutritional aspects. *MDPI AG*. https://core.ac.uk/download/551387441.pdf (accessed on 14th June 2025).

25. Bruscalupi, G., & Gnocchi, D. (2017). Circadian rhythms and hormonal homeostasis: Pathophysiological implications. *MDPI AG*. https://core.ac.uk/download/98342817.pdf (accessed on 14th June 2025).

26. Calderón Cornejo, H. W., Gorozabel Alman, A. E., Intriago Freire, M. N., Reyes Vélez, J. J., & Romero Suárez, T. L. (2023). Rol neuroendocrine del Sistema gastrointestinal. *Editorial Ciencia Digital*. https://core.ac.uk/download/588276083.pdf (accessed on 14th June 2025).

27. Cammisotto, V., Carnevale, R., Castellani, V., D'Amico, A., Fianchini, L., Nocella, C., Novo, M., Stefanini, L., & Violi, F. (2017). Extra virgin olive oil and cardiovascular diseases: Benefits for human health. *Bentham Science Publishers Ltd*. https://core.ac.uk/download/141695177.pdf (accessed on 14th June 2025).

28. Cardon, S. Z., & Iberall, A. S. (n.d.). A study on dynamic systems response of the performance characteristics of some major biophysical systems. https://core.ac.uk/download/pdf/80680406.pdf (accessed on 14th June 2025).

29. Carter, C. S., Justice, J. N., & Thompson, L. (2019). Lipotoxicity, aging, and muscle contractility: Does fiber type matter? *Springer Science and Business Media LLC*. https://open.bu.edu/bitstream/2144/40625/7/carter_justice_thompson_Lipotoxicity_paper_04302019.pdf (accessed on 14th June 2025).

30. Chantelouve, M., & Ripoll, L. (2022). Endocrine disruptors in cosmetics: A review. https://core.ac.uk/download/541080721.pdf (accessed on 14th June 2025).

31. Chen, B., Chen, L., Cheng, Y., Geng, C., Liu, R., Mao, C., Wu, L., Xu, Z., & Zhang, L. (2009). Cholinergic signal activated renin angiotensin system associated with cardiovascular changes in the ovine fetus. *Walter de Gruyter GmbH*. https://core.ac.uk/download/127603817.pdf (accessed on 14th June 2025).

32. Clark, A. K., Saric-Bosanac, S., Shi, V. Y., & Sivamani, R. K. (2020). The role of hypothalamus–pituitary–adrenal (HPA)-like axis in inflammatory pilosebaceous disorders. *eScholarship, University of California*. https://core.ac.uk/download/288432496.pdf (accessed on 14th June 2025).

33. Clavijo, R., & Hsiao, W. (2018). Update on male reproductive endocrinology. *eScholarship, University of California*. https://core.ac.uk/download/323070097.pdf (accessed on 14th June 2025).

34. Colombetti, G., & Zavala, E. (2019). Are emotional states based in the brain? A critique of affective brain centrism from a physiological perspective. *Springer Science and Business Media LLC*. https://core.ac.uk/download/226955103.pdf (accessed on 14th June 2025).

35. Compas, F., Desai, N. S., Moalem, J., & Harbuz-Miller, I. (2024). 8793 bilateral pheochromocytoma related to multiple endocrine neoplasia syndrome 2. *Semantics Scholar, 8*. https://www.

semanticscholar.org/paper/e327140f85effc27c74f2426659f5f037c2491c5 (accessed on 14th June 2025).

36. Costa, R. M., Lobato, N. S., Neves, K. B., & Tostes, R. C. (2018). Perivascular adipose tissue as a relevant fat depot for cardiovascular risk in obesity. *Frontiers Media SA*. https://core.ac.uk/download/153572426.pdf (accessed on 14th June 2025).

37. Coutinho, E. A., & Kauffman, A. S. (2019). The role of the brain in the pathogenesis and physiology of polycystic ovary syndrome (PCOS). *eScholarship, University of California*. https://core.ac.uk/download/323065551.pdf (accessed on 14th June 2025).

38. Crane, P., Farrell, C., Garau, M., Grassano, N., Hernandez-Villafuerte, K., Hopkins, M. M., Hutton, J., Lang, F., Mawer, A., Pateman, C., Rotolo, D., Shah, K., Sharp, T., & Sussex, J. (2014). Exploring the interdependencies of research funders in the UK. *Cancer Research UK*. https://core.ac.uk/download/30608686.pdf (accessed on 14th June 2025).

39. Czarnywojtek, A., Borowska, M., Dyrka, K., Moskal, J., Kościński, J., Krela-Kaźmierczak, I., Lewandowska, A. M., Abou Hjeily, B., Gut, P., Hoffmann, K., Van Gool, S., Sawicka-Gutaj, N., & Ruchała, M. (2023). The influence of various endocrine disruptors on the reproductive system. *74*(3), 221–233. https://www.semanticscholar.org/paper/f246c9a5e61e7888efa2b6b2adaf0beafa66e905 (accessed on 14th June 2025).

40. Dalile, B., Van Oudenhove, L., Vervliet, B., & Verbeke, K. (2019). The role of short-chain fatty acids in microbiota–gut–brain communication. *16*, 461–478. https://doi.org/10.1038/s41575-019-0157-3 (accessed on 14th June 2025).

41. Demas, G., Klein, S., Kriegsfeld, L., & Nelson, R. (1995). The influence of season, photoperiod, and pineal melatonin on immune function. *eScholarship, University of California*. https://core.ac.uk/download/323081880.pdf (accessed on 14th June 2025).

42. Desesquelles, A., Meslé, F., Frova, L., Pappagallo, M., Salvatore, M. A., Pace, M., & Egidi, V. (n.d.). Revisiting the mortality of France and Italy with the multiple-cause-of-death approach. https://core.ac.uk/download/pdf/6544416.pdf (accessed on 14th June 2025).

43. Dominguez-Chicas, A., Asano, T., Bannerman, R., Casani, S., Crook, J., Davison, A., Defra, A., Del Pino, S., Dyck, E. C., Environment Agency, Gurr, G., Hamilton, A., Kasprzyk-Hordern, B., Scrimshaw, M. D., Metcalf, L., NRC, NRMMC, Rodriguez, C., Singapore Public Utilities Board (PUB), WHO, & Yuan, Z. (2010). Hazard and risk assessment for indirect potable reuse schemes: An approach for use in developing Water Safety Plans. *Elsevier BV*. https://core.ac.uk/download/20665858.pdf (accessed on 14th June 2025).

44. Duston, S., & Reiter, B. (2010). Definition of disability under the ADA: A practical overview and update. *DigitalCommons@ILR*. https://core.ac.uk/download/19958974.pdf (accessed on 14th June 2025).

45. Engert, V., Grant, J., & Linz, R. (2018). Embodied stress: The physiological resonance of psychosocial stress. *Elsevier BV*. https://core.ac.uk/download/210979585.pdf (accessed on 14th June 2025).

46. Estrine, J., & DeLisle, L. (2006). Stress: Putting the brain back into medicine. *International Longevity Center–USA*. https://core.ac.uk/download/71356692.pdf (accessed on 14th June 2025).

47. Evans, P. C. (1979). *The Effect of Ethanol on Cortisol Metabolism in Man: A Thesis Presented in Partial Fulfilment of The Requirements for The Degree of Master of Science in Biochemistry at Massey University*. Massey University. https://core.ac.uk/download/148645529.pdf (accessed on 14th June 2025).

48. Fabiani, M., Askenfelt, A., Granqvist, S., Jansson, E., Ternström, S., Sundberg, J., et al. (2011). Interactive computer-aided expressive music performance. https://www.semanticscholar.org/paper/1c97da8b4b2fd5e9b826e0becd5b27dbcd81ee33 (accessed on 14th June 2025).

49. Fabuel, C., Jiménez Soriano, L., & Sarrión Pérez, M. G. (2010). Dental management of patients with endocrine disorders. https://core.ac.uk/download/71059943.pdf (accessed on 14th June 2025).

50. Gonzalez Deniselle, M. C., Lara, H. E., Recabarren, S. E., Roselli, C. E., & Zubeldia Brenner, L. (2016). Developmental and functional effects of steroid hormones on the neuroendocrine axis and spinal cord. *Wiley*. https://core.ac.uk/download/159294623.pdf (accessed on 14th June 2025).

51. Green, E., Khakshooy, S., Pieters, H. C., Sleven, M., & Stanton, A. L. (2019). A qualitative comparison of how older breast cancer survivors process treatment information regarding endocrine therapy. *eScholarship, University of California*. https://core.ac.uk/download/323079874.pdf (accessed on 14th June 2025).

52. Hada, D. S., Thakur, S., Hada, P., & Chaudhary, A. (2016). Proforma for salivary sample and candidal carriage collection (Figs 1 to 5): Saliva sample collection. https://www.semanticscholar.org/paper/ef6034d64bfea8c4bdfa09c45e4bcc1b1df296c1 (accessed on 14th June 2025).

53. Hennigar, S. R. (2010). Exposure to polybrominated diphenyl ethers (PBDEs) suppresses the release of pro-inflammatory products by alveolar macrophages *in vitro*. *University of New Hampshire Scholars' Repository*. https://core.ac.uk/download/215515896.pdf (accessed on 14th June 2025).

54. Javakhishvili, I., Sanikidze, T., Mardaleishvili, K., Momtselidze, N., Urdulashvili, T., Mantskava, M., Prantl, L., & Jung, F. (2024). Finding possible diagnostic markers for differentiating benign and malignant thyroid tumors on example investigate of rheological properties. https://www.semanticscholar.org/paper/c71e18a0a2dad5c83c3ef64255d66f1cf508befc (accessed on 14th June 2025).

55. Karin, O., Swisa, A., Gläser, B., Dor, Y., & Alon, U. (2016). Dynamical compensation in physiological circuits. *12*. https://doi.org/10.15252/msb.20167216 (accessed on 14th June 2025).

56. Kling, I. H. (1939). *The Hormones of Invertebrates*. Boston University. https://open.bu.edu/bitstream/2144/4470/1/Kling_1939_web.pdf (accessed on 14th June 2025).

57. Leonard, J. I. (n.d.). *The Behavior of Renal-Regulating Hormones During Hypogravic Stress*. https://core.ac.uk/download/pdf/42845534.pdf (accessed on 14th June 2025).

58. Merzouki, M., Chetouani, A., Taleb, M., Rais, Z., Omor, A., Ben Abbou, M., El Rhazi, K., Mtarfi, N., Elhajjaji, F., Metarfi, Y., Elmadani, F., Idrissi, N., & Elallaoui, N. (2018). The impact of chronic exposure on the Dokkarat district population of Fez city to endocrine disrupting chemicals. *Moroccan Journal of Chemistry*. https://core.ac.uk/download/492978291.pdf (accessed on 14th June 2025).

59. Mujtahid, M. (2020). Blood glucose regulating hormones and their physiological and biochemical roles. *TathQeef Scientific Publishing*. https://core.ac.uk/download/356679375.pdf (accessed on 14th June 2025).

60. Nagami, G. T., & Kraut, J. A. (2024). The role of the endocrine system in the regulation of acid–base balance by the kidney and the progression of chronic kidney disease. *Semantics Scholar, 25*. https://www.semanticscholar.org/paper/71f946e7dbef8bd1d6e91bc25334242 0414ed105 (accessed on 14th June 2025).

61. Nobari, H., Banihashemi, M., Saedmocheshi, S., Prieto-González, P., & Oliveira, R. (2023). Overview of the impact of sleep monitoring on optimal performance, immune system function and injury risk reduction in athletes: A narrative review. *106*. https://www.semanticscholar.org/paper/f12da0d5532b3a01f441d552821b9bfaba615c1a (accessed on 14th June 2025).

62. O'Connor, D. B., Thayer, J. F., & Vedhara, K. (2020). Stress and health: A review of psychobiological processes. *72*, 663–688. https://doi.org/10.1146/annurev-psych-062520-122331 (accessed on 14th June 2025).

63. Olauson, H. (2013). The role of FGF23/Klotho in mineral metabolism and chronic kidney disease. *Springer Science and Business Media LLC*. https://core.ac.uk/download/70340681.pdf (accessed on 14th June 2025).

64. Özer, Ö., Yorulmaz, G., & Şahin Tekin, M. (2023). A newly developing case of adrenal insufficiency developing after coronavirus disease. *1*. https://www.semanticscholar.org/paper/91bb0f85 d72f6767aa34d5b7e1e47b3dbc771171 (accessed on 14th June 2025).

65. Parker, K. (1972). A consideration of the hormone calcitonin and its possible mode of action. https://core.ac.uk/download/616454993.pdf (accessed on 14th June 2025).

66. Person, H., & Keefer, L. (2020). Psychological comorbidity in gastrointestinal diseases: Update on the brain–gut–microbiome axis. *107*, 110209. https://doi.org/10.1016/j.pnpbp.2020.110209 (accessed on 14th June 2025).

67. Plant, J., Stanley, E., & Voulvoulis, N. (2016). Environmental chemical exposures and breast cancer. *American Institute of Mathematical Sciences (AIMS)*. https://core.ac.uk/download/77011572.pdf (accessed on 14th June 2025).

68. Pocar, P., Grieco, V., Aidos, L., & Borromeo, V. (2023). Endocrine-disrupting chemicals and their effects in pet dogs and cats: An overview. *13*. https://www.semanticscholar.org/paper/f697d21d478bd660f85058bec92344b0e4b1fa50 (accessed on 14th June 2025).

69. Prangley, J. R. (1993). Radioimmunoassay and immunocytochemical studies on the recovery of pineal innervation and function following unilateral denervation: A thesis presented in partial fulfilment of the requirements for the degree of Master of Science in Physiology at Massey University. *Massey University*. https://core.ac.uk/download/159449358.pdf (accessed on 14th June 2025).

70. Quignon, C., Backer, A., & Wray, S. (2023). SAT591 Abnormal levels of thyroid hormones during development alters the migration and activity of GnRH reproductive neurons. *7*. https://www.semanticscholar.org/paper/15e4f5574fc148c7e72c0d437b571759a40d953a (accessed on 14th June 2025).

71. Quldashev, Q. A., Rasulov, J. M., Akbarov, I. N., Mamadaminova, M. A., & Quldasheva, Ya. M. (2023). Complex diagnostics and prognostic aspects of neuro-endocrinological parameters

in acute combined traumatic brain injuries. *Assoc Advancement Zoology, Azadanagar Colony, Rustampur, Gorakhpur, India, 273001*. https://core.ac.uk/download/603896901.pdf (accessed on 14th June 2025).

72. Richmond, B., & Gallimore, J. (2023). Genetic considerations in the tumorigenesis, diagnosis, and treatment of differentiated thyroid cancer: Current state of the science. *89*, 4853–4859. https://www.semanticscholar.org/paper/f198d875db68aef19c75621f9d794ea882fef4f4 (accessed on 14th June 2025).
73. Russell, G., & Lightman, S. L. (2019). The human stress response. *Nature Reviews Endocrinology, 15*, 525–534. https://doi.org/10.1038/s41574-019-0228-0 (accessed on 14th June 2025).
74. Singh, N. K., Hage, N., Ramamourthy, B., Nagaraju, S., & Kappagantu, K. M. (2023). Nuclear imaging modalities in the diagnosis and management of thyroid cancer. https://www.semanticscholar.org/paper/c74a0d424cd2052fefb4f2f14b3b916bd6864920 (accessed on 14th June 2025).
75. Soukup, A. (2012). The mind-body narrative: The evolution of psychoneuroimmunology and its implications for nursing research and practice. *Sophia Centre Press*. https://core.ac.uk/download/200292926.pdf (accessed on 14th June 2025).
76. Spasojevic, I. (2011). Integrative concept of homeostasis: Translating physiology into medicine. https://core.ac.uk/download/pdf/290549.pdf (accessed on 14th June 2025).
77. Steinhart, E. (2001). Persons versus brains: Biological intelligence in human organisms. https://core.ac.uk/download/287611886.pdf (accessed on 14th June 2025).
78. Strajhar, P. (2017). The effects of xenobiotics on steroidogenesis in human: "*In vitro*" and "*in vivo*" investigations. https://www.semanticscholar.org/paper/f1616ccb5a0041f80e88c745618e9e9218cecfed (accessed on 14th June 2025).
79. Takahashi, Y. (2023). Paraneoplastic autoimmune hypophysis's: A novel form of paraneoplastic endocrine syndrome. https://www.semanticscholar.org/paper/3ca07604893ae59670e6a7ae1082da3f507fe38b (accessed on 14th June 2025).
80. Technology Information and Communication Technology. (2018). Real-time Cloudlet PaaS for GreenIoT: Design of a scalable server PaaS and a GreenIoT application. https://www.semanticscholar.org/paper/04f6b0dee037112871e891c747704eb2ae9058de (accessed on 14th June 2025).
81. Walker, W. H., Walton, J. C., DeVries, A. C., & Nelson, R. J. (2020). Circadian rhythm disruption and mental health. *10*. https://doi.org/10.1038/s41398-020-0694-0 (accessed on 14th June 2025).
82. Wolff, A. S., Kucuka, I., & Oftedal, B. (2023). Autoimmune primary adrenal insufficiency–Current diagnostic approaches and future perspectives. *14*. https://www.semanticscholar.org/paper/b5355dab80f9e8da832e84aa397359f84354376a (accessed on 14th June 2025).

SPECIAL SENSES

13

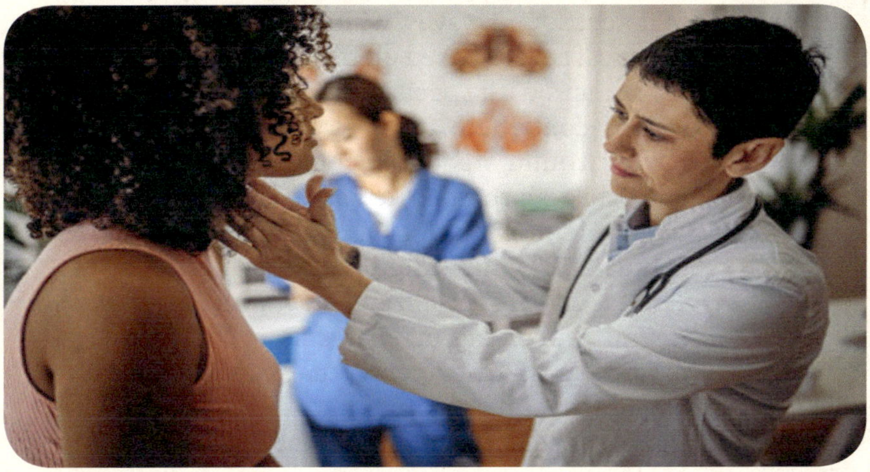

LEARNING OBJECTIVES

After studying this chapter, you will be able to:

1. Explain the anatomy and physiology of the sense of vision
2. Describe the structure and functioning of the auditory system
3. Describe the mechanisms of the senses of touch, smell, and taste
4. Explain how the special senses are integrated

Introduction

The human sensory system is crucial to information reception and processing about our world, and the special senses form the foundation for our perception and interaction with the world. Of the five traditional senses—vision, hearing, taste, touch, and smell—each of the special senses has evolved intricate anatomical and neurological systems for the processing of sensory information. The intricate brain structure, as illustrated in detailed works, emphasizes the significance of the sensory modalities, their interconnectedness, and their singular contribution to human experience. Understanding the physiological and psychological processes underlying these senses is essential not only for comprehending normal sensory function but also for predicting the outcomes of sensory dysfunction in deviant contexts, thereby pointing to the pivotal position of these systems in promoting overall human well-being and health (Gaiseanu et al., 2020). In delving deeper into the mechanisms of special senses, one finds a rich tapestry of neural networks and biological systems responsible for enabling sensory processing. Research indicates that sensory receptor signals are transmitted to some areas of the brain where they are interpreted, which leads to perceptual consciousness and informed responses. Evolution of brain hierarchical organization, as posited by the Informational Model of Consciousness, illustrates how senses evolve and change to fit incoming stimuli from the outside environment. By this model, sensory input gets integrated and encoded within neurophysiological entities, with the anterior cingulate cortex playing a significant role in modulating affective response and choice-making (Gaiseanu et al., 2020).

Thus, an extended investigation of these mechanisms illustrates the intersection of sensory experience and cognitive activity, reminding us of the necessity for special senses in negotiating life's complexities. The cognition of special senses moves beyond physiological fact and into cognitive and affective realms, with implications far-reaching for psychological as well as physical health. Sensory impairments affecting any of the special senses have the potential to result in significant disruption to perception, communication, and interaction with the world, with significant social consequences. The process of working through developing new technologies to facilitate individuals with sensory impairments is a good example of the interactive nature of sensory perception and adaptive function. Continuing our exploration of the complexity of special senses, we understand that not only are they biological processes, but an inherent part of human nature that demarcates our reality. This understanding highlights the importance of maintaining and enhancing sensory proficiency to reach peak functioning in various environmental conditions, paving the way for future investigation and innovative solutions in sensory rehabilitation.

Definition of Special Senses

Special senses refer to a specialized group of sensory modalities that provide human perception of the environment in a more sophisticated way. The primary senses are vision, hearing, taste, smell, and touch, each of which has corresponding special sensory organs and neural pathways. Vision has special sensory organs in the form of eyes, which assist in sensing light and interpreting visual information. Similarly, hearing employs the auditory system to detect sound waves, while taste and smell are chemical senses based on the binding of external substances with specialized receptors. All these senses contribute to an organism's ability to move around its world, build up memories, and establish complicated social interactions. So their role in evolution in a complex biosphere is crucial. The intricate processes of the special senses rely on specialized sensory receptors and neural processing mechanisms, which convert external stimuli to perceptual experience. For example, photoreceptors in the retina translate light into electric signals that are processed by the brain to create visual representations. For hearing, hair cells in the cochlea convert sound waves into neural impulses, allowing the perception of sound. In addition, sensory integration occurs in specific regions of the brain where higher-order processing takes place. This complex interplay between anatomy and physiology is a demonstration of how special senses not only play a role in better survival through immediate feedback from the environment but also impact cognitive processes such as memory and decision-making. Of specific note are the developments in cognitive neuroscience, as they illustrate the interdependence of sensory perception and cognitive function, thus pointing out their relative significance in human functioning (Georgiev et al., 2025). In addition, special senses are not only responsible for detecting stimuli; they are central to the formation of experiences and the direction of behavior. For example, the capacity to access food flavor by smell and taste strongly determines food selection and nutrient consumption, thus impacting health. Further, sensory modalities as a group contribute to learning and accommodation through informative feedback in relation to individual settings and experiences. With ongoing technological progress, it increasingly supports overcoming the human perception-computer interaction delay. For instance, the concept of transparent telepresence illustrates how sensory data can be technology-mediated to offer rich and immersive interactions with enhanced perception of and control over remote environments (Mair et al., 2007). Such associations between sensory modalities and technology illustrate the far-reaching impacts and applications of special senses, transcending their traditional bounds and indicating their significance in modern society (Figure 13.1).

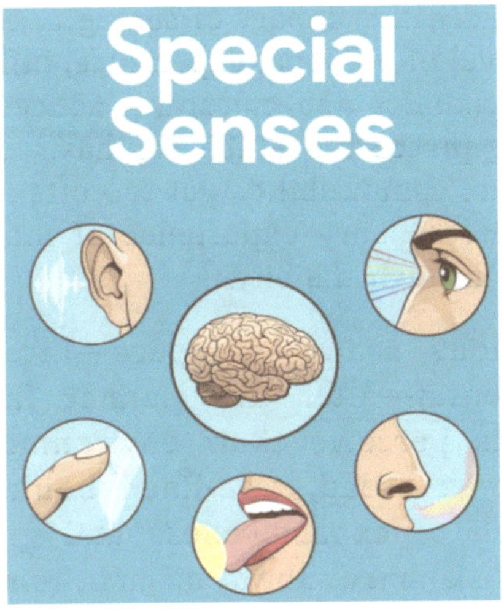

Figure 13.1. Illustration of the five special senses.

Source: https://i.pinimg.com/736x/a4/a2/e3/a4a2e372d921a2d20fd4678c442c4265.jpg.

Importance of Special Senses in Human Perception

One of the oldest understandings of human perception is dependent upon the contribution of the special senses, namely vision, hearing, taste, touch, and smell. All sensory modalities make independent contributions toward how individuals live and structure their experience of the world. Vision, as a case in point, typically dominates in circumstances where quick judgments and evaluations are required, such as product selection or navigation through environments. Evidence indicates that sensory dominance could switch at different stages of product use; what could begin with visual appraisal could go on to include other senses such as touch or smell, especially as users gain familiarity with the product (Fenko et al., 2009). This suggests a multi-layered complexity to sensory experience, with early reliance upon sight giving way to a more integrated multisensory experience, highlighting once more the importance of designers and marketers understanding these dynamics within their strategy. In addition, the integration of different senses is fundamental to creating meaningful experiences, which in turn profoundly impacts the human percept. Telepresence, in turn, describes how individuals are made to be present in a different setting by the use of virtual tools and not merely by visual engagement, but also auditory and bodily sense. An indication of it can be found in gamers' experiences, in which the combination of audio cues and haptic feedback brings about a state of presence that transcends physical location. These findings underscore the point that perception is not an independent phenomenon to single senses but an overall experience crafted through the interaction of them. The provision of various sensory inputs enriches the level of perception. It can even transform emotional and psychological responses fundamentally, which is essential in multiple applications, such as virtual reality and product design (Ozok et al., 2019). Furthermore, the significance of special senses extends beyond perception to cognitive and affective levels, influencing learning and memory. For example, sensory experience with particular emotions can result in more memories and retention of knowledge. This is observed in learning settings where multisensory instruction has been known to facilitate improved understanding and learner participation. When sensory phenomena become linked with emotive contexts, they engage on a more fundamental level and allow for memory and comprehension. Such understanding of special senses' operations is thus crucial to enhance teaching pedagogies, user experience design, and even therapy. The integration of the sensory modalities into so many aspects of human life speaks to the profound impact these senses have on the manner in which people look, interact with, and understand their worlds, and attests to their importance within the larger framework of human perception.

13.1. The Sense of Vision

Learning Outcome

1. Define the anatomy of the eye
2. Discuss the mechanism of vision
3. Identify the common vision disorders

The sense of vision is a central element in the set of human senses that profoundly impacts our experience of the world. Vision allows us to move about our world, identify faces, and decode intricate visual information. Seeing starts when light enters the eye and is brought into focus on the retina, where light is translated into neural signals by photoreceptor cells. This intricate process is further conditioned by observers prior experience and environmental knowledge, highlighting the value placed in a multisensory context in the study of perception. Vision thus operates not independently but alongside other senses, allowing us to interpret dynamic environments. As city spaces are designed with the visual modality in mind to begin with, it is critical to note how the variances of scale and spatial composition can influence our visual experiences to reveal the limitations of sight as a singular sense (Lucas et al., 2008). While investigating the sense of vision, it is crucial to have in mind its entanglement with other senses. Whereas vision is likely to be the most prepotent sense of human experience, smell and taste also contribute significantly to making our experience of the world rich and vivid. Studies indicate that these senses do not exist in a latent way; instead, they blend with visual sensation to generate rich, continuous experiences. For instance, food cannot be limited to its taste alone; the sight of food, along with the aroma, enhances the perception of taste as a whole. This integration of the senses contradicts the long-held argument that each occurrence of sensation is held within one modality alone and thus requires a general notion of perception (Smith et al., 2015). Feeling this interconnectedness is critical to fields based on sensory design, including architecture and urban planning. Additionally, the impact of seeing doesn't end at the level of personal experience, influencing social dynamics and cultural practices. Urban planning places too much emphasis on looks and visual compatibility, yet too often ignores the whole sensory experience of individuals passing through the city.

Various scales of space—interior to monumental—alter the manner in which residents perceive their environment. For example, a broad, tree-lined boulevard is evocative of expansiveness and grandeur, whereas a jammed subway might be reminiscent of discomfort or disorientation. If designers couple evidence from the study of seeing with an appreciation for the remaining sensory modalities, they can create spaces more available and beneficial to a diversity of populations. This hybrid strategy promotes multisensory urban experiences that accommodate the richness of human perception, leading to a more tangible engagement with our built environment (Lucas et al., 2008).

13.1.1. Anatomy of the Eye

The anatomy of the eye is the structural part of the special senses, where each component plays its role in the elaborate process of vision. The eye is broadly classified under structures such as the cornea, lens, retina, and optic nerve. The cornea, transparent outer covering of the eye, refracts light to help project it onto the retina, which is packed with photoreceptor cells to detect light and color. The lens further refines this focus to a higher level through accommodation by altering shape to focus at different distances. This intricate interaction among the optical components not only allows for registration of visual stimuli but also underscores the sophisticated nature of the sensory processing in the eye, proving that vision is far from being a mere optical phenomenon. Additionally, the arrangement of the retinas is awe-inspiring, being constituted by several layers that are responsible for light transduction into neural signals. The outer layer contains photoreceptors: rods, sensitive to light in dim light and required for night vision, and cones, which enable color perception and clear vision in brighter light. The photoreceptors are the ones that convert light into electrical impulses, which are relayed by bipolar and ganglion cells before reaching the optic nerve. The fovea, a minute depression in the retina, is another critical area, closely packed with cones, that provides the keenest visual acuity. This closely packed arrangement illustrates the special adaptations in the eye that not only allow human beings to perceive their world in fine detail but also illustrates the survival benefit of vision as a primary sensory mode in survival and interaction with the environment. The anatomy of the eye is crucial for enabling an engaging relationship between vision and overall sensory perception. In collaboration with other senses, the eye collaborates to provide an integrated perception of environmental stimuli.

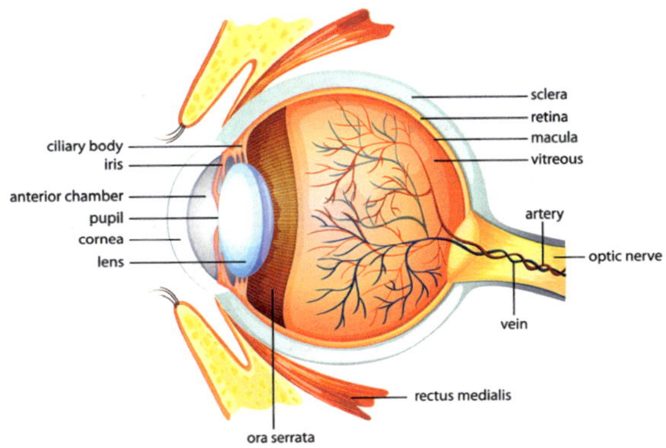

Figure 13.2. Anatomy of the human eye.

Source: https://www.exetereye.co.uk/wp-content/uploads/Exeter-Eye-Anatomy-of-the-human-eye-diagram.jpg.

The integration, for instance, of the visual information with the auditory and tactile feedback offers a richer cognitive interpretation of complex situations such as navigating the city environment full of mixed sensory inputs. This multi-layered encounter speaks to the conversations supplied through the UK AHRC/EPSRC research project that investigates our sensory experience of place. Through the investigation into how architecture and urban planning affect sensory modalities, attention is given to the manner in which visual forms shape our interaction with the world, highlighting the importance of the eyes anatomy within a broader sensory experience framework and its contribution to the formation of human perception and behavior (Azzolini et al., 2004; Lucas et al., 2008) (Figure 13.2).

13.1.2. Mechanism of Vision

The vision process is a sophisticated process that begins when light rays travel through the human eye. The process starts at the cornea, which bends the incoming light and directs it through the pupil, a changing aperture regulated by the iris. The lens further adjusts this light, changing the shape of the light to cause images to fall on the retina, the light-sensitive part of the eye. In the retina, there are photoreceptor cells known as rods and cones, which are essential. Rods function to detect low light levels and peripheral motion, while cones are used in color vision and sharp vision. This redundancy enables humans to see an astronomical number of visual stimuli under varying environmental conditions, contributing to overall sensory input in the special senses. Once the retina has absorbed the light, light is translated into electrical impulses through a series of processes referred to as phototransduction. The process begins when light photons strike photopigments of cone and rod cells, leading to a cascade of chemical reactions that modify the flow of ions across photoreceptor membranes. Rhodopsin pigment is involved in rods, undergoing a transformation that initiates the cascade of signals. In the case of cones, three different types of photopigments are responsible for the detection of red, green, and blue light, enabling the discrimination of colors. The optic nerve thus passes electrical signals to the different regions of the brain, specifically the visual cortex, where they are interpreted and integrated. This complex interaction not only makes visual perception a receptive representation of external stimuli but also an active cognitive process, building our conception of the world. The role of vision in special senses illustrates its flexibility and complexity. For instance, studies on other creatures, e.g., manatees, have explained different mechanisms of vision according to environmental demands. Manatees possess dichromatic vision, which allows them to perceive a diminished color spectrum, primarily to assist their foraging lifestyle in murky water. These contrasts are used to demonstrate that vision is not a fixed trait but a sensory modality strongly suited to the ecological stress exerted upon a species. Comparative studies of sensory modalities in animals have the ability to give insight into evolutionary processes and emphasize the subtle interplay between anatomy and interaction with the environment, and give a broader view of how vision functions in special sense contexts (N/A, 2025; Moore et al., 2020) (Figure 13.3).

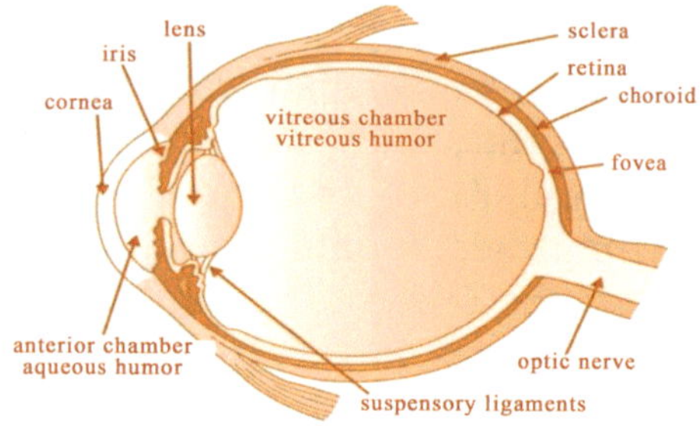

Figure 13.3. The mechanism of vision.

Source: https://i.ytimg.com/vi/KcNuQ09ngpY/maxresdefault.jpg.

13.1.3. Common Vision Disorders

Vision disorders are one of the most prevalent disorders among the special senses, with a profound effect on daily life and quality of life among individuals. Some examples of prevalent disorders include myopia, hyperopia, astigmatism, and presbyopia, showing the diversity of vision disorders among the population.

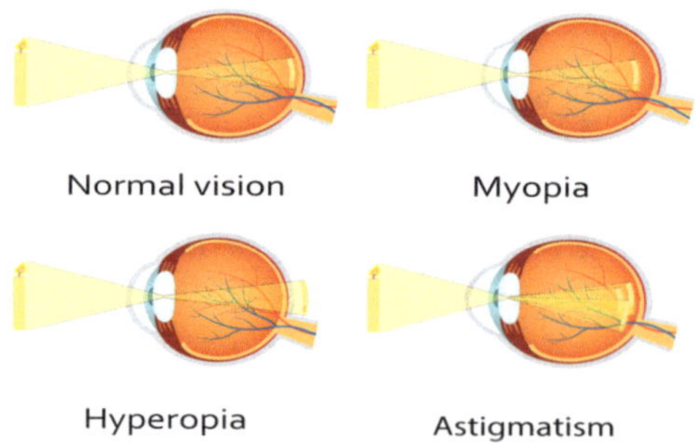

Figure 13.4. Vision disorders.

Source: https://www.greenbergeye.com/wp-content/uploads/2020/08/shutterstock_641320765-1-300x300.jpg.

Myopia, or nearsightedness, results in blurred vision at distance, and approximately

30% of the U.S. population is affected. On the other hand, hyperopia, or farsightedness, compromises near vision, and astigmatism results in blurred vision at all distances because of an irregular corneal curvature (Figure 13.4).

Presbyopia, a standard process with age, creates the gradual loss of focusing ability by the eye for near objects, typically becoming apparent in an individual in their 40s. Identification of these common disorders is necessary for the development of effective treatment regimens and for preserving visual health in all age categories. Other than the listed refractive errors, more complex vision disorders can be complicated. For instance, glaucoma and cataracts may result in severe impairment if left untreated. Cataracts, characterized by lens clouding, typically result from aging and eventually may lead to blurred vision and sensitivity to glare. Glaucoma, however, is primarily associated with increased intraocular pressure, which will be harmful to the optic nerve and cause permanent loss of vision. Early treatment is crucial in the management of these disorders; cataract surgical procedures and medication or surgery to control intraocular pressure in glaucoma can significantly improve visual outcomes. An understanding of these conditions and their symptoms is necessary to prevent late diagnosis and treatment, significant predictors that can avert long-term vision loss among affected individuals. Furthermore, certain neurological conditions may also impact visual processing, leading to special vision disorders. For example, patients with Parkinson's disease (PD) typically develop compromised visual perception as a significant nonmotor manifestation of the illness. As PD pathology advances over time, alterations in cognitive functioning and perception can make the visual experience more challenging, highlighting the interconnectedness of sensory systems under pathological brain conditions. Additionally, research on multi-sensory environments suggests potential ways to help patients with various visual and cognitive deficits (Atari et al., 2014). The observation of such relationships can enhance therapeutic interventions and determine the extent to which nonvisual factors play a role in the expression of vision disorders and their effect on the activity of daily living. Lastly, the treatment of the complex nature of vision disorders requires vast information on sensory and cognitive issues to maximize quality of life in infected individuals. (Cronin-Golomb et al., 2013).

Test Your Knowledge

1. What are the main anatomical structures of the eye involved in vision?
2. How does the eye convert light into visual signals through the mechanism of vision?

13.2. The Sense of Hearing

Learning Outcome

1. Describe the anatomy of the ear
2. Explain the process of sound perception
3. Identify common hearing impairments

Hearing is a sensitive and complex mechanism upon which human consciousness and interaction in the world depend. It concerns sound waves, which are vibrations transmitted in air and other media, perceived by the auditory system, and undergoing a highly developed process of transduction. The ear, made up of outer, middle, and inner structures, is organized to detect such sound waves, amplify them, and send them as electrical impulses to the brain. Through this intricate process, individuals cannot only appreciate the pitch and loudness of sounds but also the rich textures of sounds, which are crucial for communication, warning, and enjoyment in daily life. The multidimensionality of hearing gives a glimpse of the larger range of sensory experience, highlighting the value of hearing as a special sense that expands human connection and sensitivity to the world around us. The auditory system is also an excellent model to employ in studying the concept that senses do not exist in isolation but, rather, exist interwoven to bring richness to human experience. Philosophers resist a reductionist explanation of distinguishable senses, pointing out that various criteria—e.g., representation, phenomenal character, and sense organ—can be employed to achieve an enriched understanding of the way hearing belongs in a general taxonomy of sensory experiences (Macpherson et al., 2010). This perspective allows one to realize that the experience of hearing does not exist in its own independent sensory modality, but is entwined with other senses such as vision and touch, providing a total sensory experience of reality. The synergy of the senses can greatly augment cognitive processes, emotional reactions, and even social behaviors, implying that the very richness of hearing cannot be fully experienced if its contextual compatibility with other sensory modalities is not recognized. Also, the cultural and historical aspects of hearing serve to underscore its status as a special sense further. From the earliest rhythmic patterns of tribal communication to classical music's symphonic masterpieces, sound experiences have informed and structured human societies in profound and far-reaching ways. An illustration of this is the importance of an organ audition, as experienced by the individual with regard to sound, as it encapsulates the combination of risk, creativity, and professional assessment constitutive of the auditory performance (Foley et al., 1996). Such contexts help to emphasize the way that hearing experiences connect on an emotional and cognitive plane, reaffirming the idea that hearing is a matter of more than mere physiology but also of personal and communal identity. Grasping the sense of hearing, as a result, involves both appreciation for its biological underpinnings and a recognition of its profound influence on culture, creativity, and human relationships.

13.2.1. Anatomy of the Ear

The anatomy of the ear is a very complex and advanced system that enables us to hear and is one of the key components of the special senses. It is composed of three main divisions: the outer ear, middle ear, and inner ear. Each division has specific functions that assist in hearing and balance. The pinna and ear canal constitute the outer ear and are used to direct sound onto the eardrum, or tympanic membrane. The vibrations of the sound waves cause the eardrum to oscillate and transmit the vibrations onto the ossicles within the middle ear. The ossicles, made up of the stapes, incus, and malleus, amplify the sound waves before they reach the inner ear. This multi-step process not only emphasizes the precision of the hearing system but also directs to the requirement of anatomical integrity to maintain effective auditory perception. When the vibrations reach the inner ear, they pass through the cochlea, where neural impulses are created from sound signals. The spiral-shaped fluid-filled organ, the cochlea, contains hair cells that respond to the mechanical motion caused by sound waves. When the fluid in the cochlea moves, these hair cells bend, which triggers an electrochemical cascade of signals passed on to the auditory nerve, to the brain (Figure 13.5).

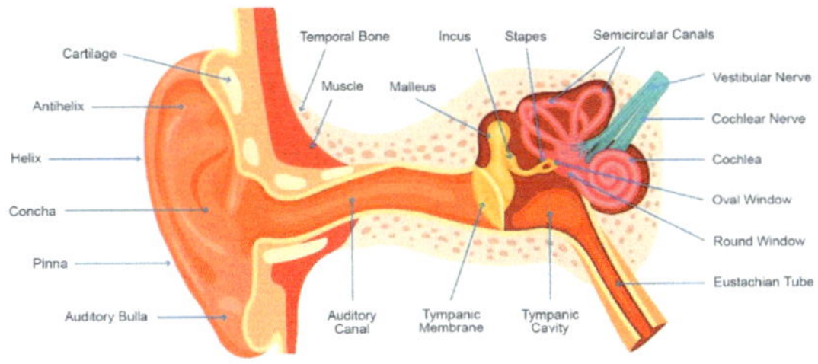

Figure 13.5. Anatomy of the ear.

Source: https://cdn-bihkj.nitrocdn.com/DhBThIwDIXwRSTyDepOvPddhGGndQQIo/assets/images/optimized/rev-f79c4a5/www.hearingsolutions.ca/wp-content/uploads/2023/11/Anatomy-of-the-Ear.jpg.

The brain interprets these signals, enabling us to experience sounds as pitch, volume, and direction, enhancing our auditory experience. The inner ear contains the vestibular system, which is important for equilibrium, in addition to hearing. Interconnectedness of these functions is a testimony to the ear as a versatile organ, essential in the interaction with our environment and rooted in our senses. Understanding the anatomy of the ear extends past physical details; it encompasses the larger significance of sound perception in our lives. The ability of the ears to perceive and understand sound not just dictates how we communicate but also our emotional and social lives. As research has discussed, our experience of sound can bring about memory and emotion, making ear anatomy even more vital in the larger human experience and interaction with the world. This is similar to the discussion of the sensory experience of urban places, where multiple modalities blend to produce a complete sense of place (Lucas et al., 2008). In addition, the active relationship between sound experience and our self can be compared to the manner in which taste contributes to our knowledge of "elsewhere," intertwining sensory experience to deepen our sense of self and the world around us (Sinha et al., 2016).

13.2.2. Process of Sound Perception

The process of sound perception entails intricate interactions among sound signals, physiological processes, and cognitive meanings. First, sound waves enter the ear and are transduced into neural signals by the organs of the auditory system. This process is critical, as the ear is not a passive receiver but rather an active component of the process of sound perception. The cochlea, for example, contains hair cells that convert mechanical movement into electrochemical signals, which are then sent to the brain to be processed. The brain interprets these signals, enabling individuals to perceive a variety of sounds, including speech, music, and external noises. Recognition of this change highlights the sophistication of sound processing. It highlights the fact that the hearing of sound is an active interaction between cognition and biology that holds power over our interaction with the world. Beyond physiology, the perception of sound also strongly relies on personal experience and culture. Each person's entry into the world of sound is shaped by their unique experiences with sounds throughout life, which significantly contribute to creating meanings and associations. Sounds are not simply signals; they tend to call out images and feelings that have to do with specific events or experiences. A case in point is listening to the voice of someone who is loved, which can evoke powerful feelings due to the emotional connection the person has. This link between sound and memory highlights the importance of considering personal histories in sound perception. By recognizing the strong bonds created through listening experiences, we can begin to appreciate the subjective space in which sound is felt and the rich manner in which it enriches our sensory experience of the world (Makhlouf et al., 2017) (Figure 13.6).

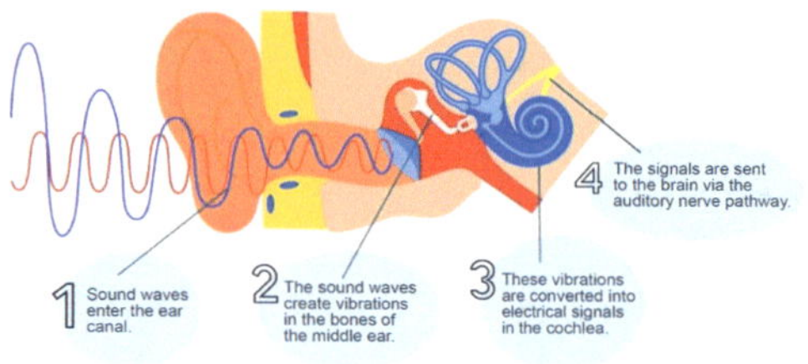

Figure 13.6. Human hearing works.

Source: https://www.healthyhearing.com/report/53241-How-we-hear-explainer-hearing.

In addition, the multi-sensory nature of cityscapes underscores the need for a more comprehensive understanding of sound perception in design and architecture. As has been evidenced in recent research, the sensory experience of location encompasses far more than visual data; sound is an essential dimension in understanding how spaces are perceived and moved through (Lucas et al., 2008). Urban designers can potentially create environments that engage multiple senses, building more interactive experiences with these environments. The inclusion of sound in urban design not only improves the atmosphere but also encourages an appreciation of the acoustic qualities that may influence mood and social interaction. As cities themselves are formed, it is increasingly critical to speak to how the experience of sound can enhance the lived and deepen more integrated and inclusive conceptions of city planning. In these efforts, the value of sound in our understanding of space can be established and embraced as an integral component of our sensorial connection to the world.

13.2.3. Hearing Impairments and Their Impact

Hearing impairments are a significant public health issue, and increasing age in the population only adds to it. Evidence indicates that almost 15% of people aged 70 years and older have dementia, and sensory impairment often occurs concomitantly with cognitive impairment. This implies that the neural mechanisms governing sensory processing could be affected by overlapping mechanisms producing hearing impairment and cognitive dysfunction. The implications of these findings emphasize the value of rigorous sensory function measurements in older adults, as the alleviation of hearing impairment could potentially improve cognitive outcomes. With the population aging, the prevalence of hearing impairments demands intervention that not only addresses sensory loss but also considers the resultant cascading effect upon cognitive functioning and quality of life (Cronin-Golomb et al., 2018). The quality of life of the hearing-impaired is greatly influenced by the degree of their impairment. The ability to conduct social life, be confronted with information, and communicate effectively can be severely compromised, which results in a state of isolation and frustration. A recent study suggests that measures of health status, such as self-assessed health, are directly correlated with the subjective experience of hearing loss. Since these disabilities control daily living and emotional function, it is crucial to utilize holistic approaches that quantify the impact of these disabilities on individuals' lives. Utilizing sophisticated measures that account for the dynamic experience of hearing-impaired individuals, medical specialists can design more effective systems of support and interventions to enhance overall life satisfaction and functional capacity in this group (Allison et al., 2025). In addition, the co-existence of hearing loss and psychological impact should not be downplayed. The patients with hearing loss also experience problems with mental illness in terms of depression and anxiety that may be attributable to extensive withdrawal from social activities and communication problems. The domino effect illustrates the compelling necessity for intervention that, apart from addressing the physical loss, intervenes in the concomitant psychological load. Conference studies on sensory disabilities in the elderly prove that interventions with comprehensive teamwork, like new treatments and local resources, play an essential part in improving the quality of life of the affected. Focusing on research and intervention strategies that address sensory as well as mental health issues will allow us to treat people with hearing disabilities more effectively, ultimately allowing them to contribute to and become part of society (Cronin-Golomb et al., 2018) (Figure 13.7).

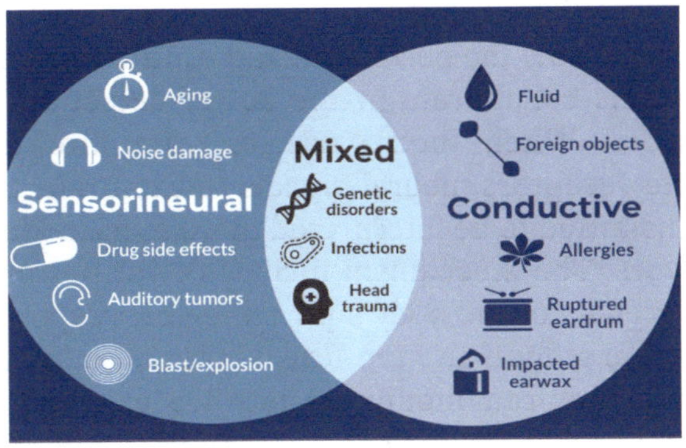

Figure 13.7. Types of hearing loss.

Source: https://static.wixstatic.com/media/0ebae5_8db3711a2b1f4cbd9f2d00a549d35ec6~mv2.png/v1/fill/w_568,h_438,al_c,q_85,usm_0.66_1.00_0.01,enc_avif,quality_auto/0ebae5_8db3711a2b1f4cbd9f2d00a549d35ec6~mv2.png.

Test Your Knowledge

1. How does the ear process sound waves to enable sound perception?
2. What are common types of hearing impairments, and how do they affect hearing ability?

13.3. The Sense of Taste

Learning Outcome

1. Discuss the anatomy of the taste buds
2. Understand the five basic tastes
3. Describe the factors influencing taste perception

The perception of taste, or gustation, is critical to human existence, not only guiding the selection of food but social experience and cultural heritage as well. It relies on the sensing of chemicals in food through taste receptors on the tongue. Taste receptors most fundamentally react to five elemental tastes: sweet, sour, salty, bitter, and umami, which trigger appropriate bodily and affective responses. The interaction between taste and emotion highlights the importance of gustation beyond mere survival; it constrains our pleasure and displeasure and therefore food preference. Emotional reactions to taste may range from pleasure at the sweetness of spoiled fruit to displeasure at the bitterness of decayed food. This intricate relationship illustrates how the sense of taste is linked to various aspects of human consciousness and experience, and thereby forms a part of our diet and emotional well-being as well. In order to appreciate the biological foundation of taste, one needs to observe how the peripheral and central nervous systems collaborate in the act of detection of flavors. When food particles stimulate the taste receptors, neural signals to the brain are transmitted to be interpreted there as individual flavors. The mechanism includes both bottom-up signals of the body's physiological response to taste stimuli and top-down influences by the brain that can modulate how we experience flavor based on context or memory. Under the cover of modern affective neuroscience, taste is a manifestation of the dynamic integration of physiological change and conscious perception. This can unveil mechanisms responsible for the subjective nature of taste and related emotional experience, consistent with recent theories regarding how taste informs feelings toward food and the world (Edward F Pace-Schott et al., 2019). Further, the sense of taste is not just the tongue's receptors but also the complex relationship between taste and smell, flavor being the term for this interaction. This mixture heightens our distinction among foods, along with emotional and sensory richness in our cuisine. Studies indicate that flavor perception is built through memory and experience, again repeating how deeply taste has penetrated human and cultural life. The role of culture in shaping taste is not to be denied, in that cultural convention and practice determine what will be viewed as acceptable or pleasant. The sense of taste, then, becomes a multifaceted domain in the interplay of biology, affect, and culture, and as a development of a more encompassing system of human sensory perception and experience (Elizabeth et al., 2019).

13.3.1. Anatomy of the Taste Buds

The organization of taste buds plays an essential role in the human sensory system, which is crucial in food assessment, transmission of safety, and enjoyment of meals. Taste buds, which are located predominantly on the rear of the tongue, are complex organs comprising specialized sensory cells that are referred to as taste receptor cells. There are between 50 to 150 taste cells in a taste bud. Microvilli extend into a taste pore that links these cells to the oral cavity, giving them an onion-like arrangement. The coordination of several types of epithelium allows taste buds to sense the five fundamental taste modalities: sweet, salty, sour, bitter, and umami. This intricate organization is a testament to the remarkable versatility of human physiology in accommodating diverse chemical stimuli in foods and beverages to maximize survival via correct ingestion response. The role of the taste buds is closely associated with the respective gustatory pathways, which transmit taste information from the mouth to the brain. Upon stimulation by food molecules, a series of biochemical events is initiated in the taste receptor cells to generate action potentials which are transmitted through cranial nerves VII (facial), IX (glossopharyngeal), and X (vagus) (Figure 13.8).

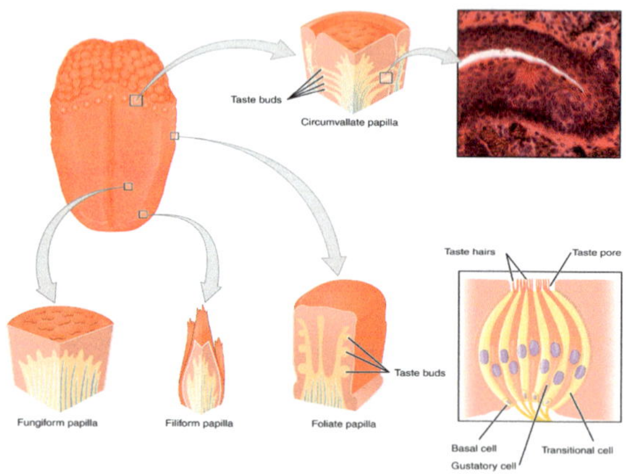

Figure 13.8. Taste buds are small structures present within the papillae of the tongue.

Source: https://en.wikipedia.org/wiki/Taste_bud#/media/File:1402_The_Tongue.jpg.

This information is then sent to the nucleus of the solitary tract and subsequently to the thalamus, where it is further processed and then sent to the gustatory cortex. This route not only facilitates the experience of taste but also combines other sensory modalities, such as smell and texture, to generate an integrated flavor experience. The integration of taste buds with these pathways is essential for effective behavioral reactions to food and possible toxins, illustrating the intricacy of our sensory machinery. Furthermore, the anatomy of taste buds is under the control of many physiological variables, including aging, wellness, and experience with different stimuli. As one ages, the quantity and sensitivity of taste buds may decline, causing differences in taste perception and influencing dietary absorption. Also, diseases like smoking or certain medical interventions can impair the function of taste receptor cells, leading to taste disturbances. Studies have demonstrated that tastes can trigger intense emotional and physiological responses, which only serve further to underline the importance of taste in human existence. Exploring the nuances of taste bud anatomy and associated functions gives critical information regarding the subtleties of human sensory processing, in keeping with broader themes of special senses and emphasizing the complexity of relationships within our sensory systems, corroborated by follow-up research into sensory modalities in equivalent species, which shows how organisms adapt their sensory mechanisms (Rao et al., 1967; Moore et al., 2020).

13.3.2. The Five Basic Tastes

The study of the five basic tastes—sweet, sour, salty, bitter, and umami—is insightful about how our sensory experiences drive food preference and nutrient intake. All the tastes serve an evolutionary purpose, guiding individuals to beneficial substances while away from potentially toxic ones. Sweetness, for instance, is most commonly associated with foods containing high levels of energy, signaling the presence of the sugar molecules that are essential for survival. At the same time, bitterness serves as an alert to toxic chemicals, inducing a rapid distaste. The slight interface between chemical senses and human survival underscores the importance of taste in human existence and its role in food choice decisions, highlighting the significance of sensory perception on behavior and health status in Special Senses (Smith et al., 2015) (Figure 13.9).

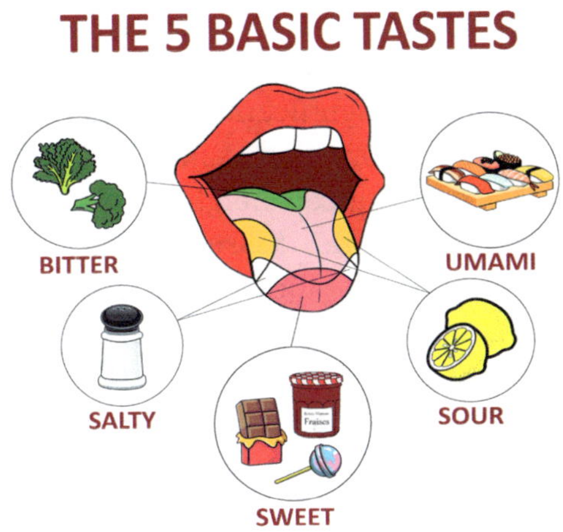

Figure 13.9. The five basic tastes.

Source: https://blogger.googleusercontent.com/img/b/R29vZ2xl/AVvXsEjF13SXAYTPmOOOPMyTu3ymL PxaErFu1Anak3oA7VSSTBvLRB0XyMlKB22U3_1DAt2247wg8mTcVOumKV7rcefsBiyKykL_IiigHISLbhrfeN2fEzZhGKt194SV6njNxYKUj0aa4PPOLQD8u8-wscBgP6R5aQL4hXeUSiA3Yfx4fJ21kYeNZzLZDSTi/s2600/20220421%20-%20The%205%20Basic%20Tastes%20by%20%C2%A9LeDomduvin%202022.png.

The chemical process of taste is the activation of specialized taste receptors on the tongue, which respond to various modalities of taste. Each taste bud contains cells that transmit signals to the nervous system when activated by chemical molecules in food. For example, sodium ion activation of taste receptors produces salty taste, a necessary message for electrolyte equilibrium. Umami, or as it has been described as savory, is a consequence of the detection of glutamate and specific nucleotides, linking it with protein-containing food to support growth and development. The meeting of chemical signal and sensory processing indicates a complex system that not only enhances flavor but also impacts our physiological responses, ultimately determining our overall sensory experience (Smith et al., 2015). In addition, the combination of taste with the other senses—primarily smell and texture—enriches flavor experience. Mastication is rarely a process of tasting food per se; odor is a significant contributor to the perception of flavors. For example, the aromas emitted by cooking can heighten the intrinsic tastes of ingredients. Moreover, the texture of food also tells us about taste, and crunchy textures as opposed to smooth textures evoke different levels of flavor intensity. Considering this multisensory experience, it is evident that taste cannot be appropriately described as a solo entity, but rather emerges from an integrative sensory context that prepares our understanding of food and the world at large. This unified approach to taste highlights the interdependence of sensory modalities and the broader ramifications for research into Special Senses.

13.3.3. Factors Influencing Taste Perception

Perception of flavor is a complex interaction of various factors that are more than the perception of basic taste qualities such as sweetness and bitterness. Color and appearance of food also contribute a lot in generating our perceptions and expectations regarding flavor. Research and observation have shown that color influences person-to-person judgments of taste, as different colors are associated with distinct flavors or food types. For example, a red plate can add sweetness to a dish because of the symbolic properties accorded to the color, hence its importance in fine dining where looks matter most (Mercês et al., 2025). The consumptive sensory enjoyment is thus not just a function of taste. Still, it includes visual beauty and emotional and memory aspects of different colors that highlight the multimodal nature of flavor perception. The sense of smell is also a factor in the perception of taste, since how we perceive smells is intricately related to how we perceive flavors. While we are consuming food, the volatiles given off by food come into contact with taste receptors on the tongue and enhance the sensory input further. This is demonstrated quite clearly in individuals with constricted nasal passages, as sinus disorders essentially impair the sense of taste. It has been demonstrated that food preference and aversion are largely a function of the combination of taste and smell because they influence dietary intake and nutritional behavior. Also, varying sensitivities to smell in individuals can result in varying taste experiences, acknowledging that each person's distinctive sensory pattern influences how they detect and enjoy flavors (Dietsch et al., 2024) (Figure 13.10).

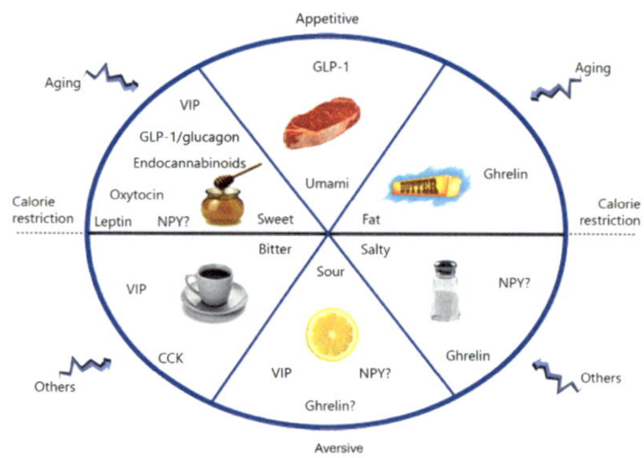

Figure 13.10. Overview of the modulation of different taste modalities by metabolically-related hormones. Six taste modalities are shown: umami, sweet, bitter, sour, salty, and fat.

Source: https://www.researchgate.net/figure/Overview-of-the-modulation-of-different-taste-modalities-by-metabolically-related_fig1_261735858.

Thus, the olfactory component is a vital element in taste perception, which affirms the interconnectedness of the special senses. Beyond sensory modalities, personal variation such as genetics, age, and culture play a considerable role in the perception of taste. Genetically determined inclinations can regulate an individual's sensitivity towards specific tastes, to a greater extent bitterness, and influence food choice early in life. For instance, individuals carrying specific genetic markers might experience cruciferous vegetables as extremely bitter, which serves as an avoidance cue. Age also comes into play, as sensitivity to taste tends to decrease with increasing years and affects food choices and overall nutrition. Cultural factors also influence taste preferences through exposure to diverse cuisine and traditional flavors, thus shaping the taste profile of a person over time. Understanding these persons and sociocultural factors is imperative in contexts such as clinical nutrition and food counseling because they inform focused approaches to enhancing meal experiences and successfully managing dietary problems (Dietsch et al., 2024).

Test Your Knowledge

1. What are the five basic tastes recognized by the human tongue?
2. What factors can influence or alter taste perception?

13.4. The Sense of Smell

Learning Outcome

1. Discuss the anatomy of the olfactory system
2. Understand the mechanism of smell detection
3. Describe the role of smell in memory and emotion

The use of the sense of smell, overshadowed by the dominance of vision and hearing in the hierarchy of the senses, is a vital part of our perception of the world. As opposed to visual stimuli, broadly characterized as immediate and objective, olfactory stimuli are inherently subjective and personal. This unique property of scent affects our emotional responses as well as our memory, typically inducing vivid memories linked to particular smells. For instance, the aroma of freshly baked cookies could transport someone to their childhood years, highlighting the powerful connection between smell and emotional memory. The exclusion of this sense in perception philosophy stems from a broader lack of understanding of its relevance; nonetheless, empirical research highlights that the chemical senses, including odor, provide valuable insights into our perception of environmental features and human experiences in general (Smith et al., 2015). In addition, the complexity of olfactory perception is demystified once examined alongside other chemical senses, like taste. Together, these senses braid one experience of flavor that captures the multisensory dynamic of human perception. In gastronomical contexts, for instance, smell and taste work in tandem to regulate our whole gastronomical experience. This synergy is the key to understanding how the chemical senses operate in presenting a more complex conception of perception beyond the historical bifurcation of the five senses. When one is enjoying a meal, flavors do not come solely from taste—smell must contribute to extending and cueing the broad sensory experience, allowing individuals to savor and engage with food more fully. This cross-modal integration challenges the perspective that chemical senses are subordinate or simply derivative of stronger senses like vision and necessitates them to be revisited in light of holistic sensory perception (Lucas et al., 2008). Besides, the importance of smell extends beyond simple perception to having a bearing on urban design and on contact with the environment. As environments are designed, the sensory properties offered by an environment—smell, sound, and texture—must all be tempered along with visual attractiveness. The urban landscape is replete with sensory images of odor, from the natural odors of parkland to the odors of food in thick markets. These sensory interactions build our place experience, illustrating the fact that our experiences of spaces are more than visual stimulation. Highlighted in recent research in urban design is the importance of an emphasis on the coordinated sensory experience to inform more successful architectural practice, and ultimately make urban environments more navigable and understood. By gaining a better insight into the interdependence of the chemical senses, planners can develop more sensitive, interactive, and inclusive spaces that take into account the diversity of human sensory experience (Lucas et al., 2008).

13.4.1. Anatomy of the Olfactory System

The anatomy of the olfactory system is paramount in the perception of smells and, therefore, makes significant input into the general system of special senses. The olfactory epithelium and its specialized olfactory sensory neurons are located in the nasal cavity and form the core of the system. These sensory neurons have cilia that bear olfactory receptors, which are each tuned to identify specific odorant molecules. When the odorant is bound to its receptor, it triggers a signal transduction cascade that will ultimately excite the olfactory bulb. This olfactory bulb, an extremely critical relay center, works on the odor information before transmitting it to higher centers of the brain, including the olfactory cortex. This complexity in layers enables not only the perception of diverse odors but also the intricate conjunction of the olfactory stimuli with memory and affective response, highlighting the olfactory system's critical impact on human behavior. Understanding the functional architecture of the olfactory system also includes examination of the unique organizational features of the olfactory bulbs themselves.

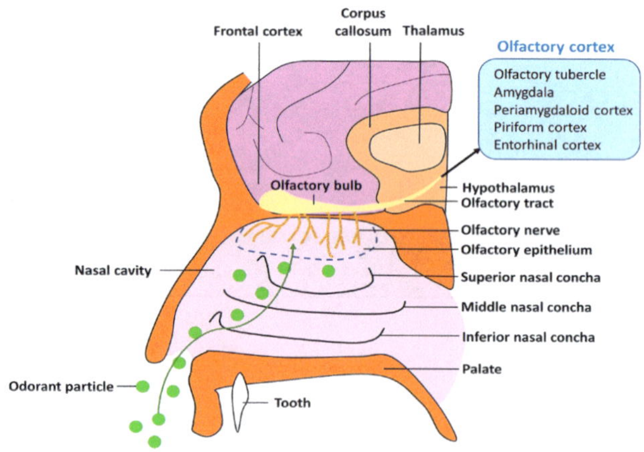

Figure 13.11. The human olfactory system.

Source: https://www.researchgate.net/figure/The-human-olfactory-system-The-diagram-shows-the-intricate-anatomy-of-the-human_fig1_384008447.

They consist of individual glomeruli that receive input from the olfactory sensory neurons and are initial centers for processing the odor. Specific sets of odors selectively activate single glomeruli, so a pattern of neural activity that results in perceived odor is feasible. This is in agreement with findings in other animals, such as sharks, which show an interesting evolutionary perspective on olfactory form. As suggested in recent research, the smooth dogfish shark possesses bilateral paired olfactory bulbs that might be adapted to specific odor processing, a significant deviation from the olfactory organization of bony fish. Such a functional divergence is a sign that different organisms have adjusted their olfactory apparatuses to adapt to some selective ecological demands, a pointer to the evolutionary pressures that govern sensory systems in species (Lohe et al., 2017) (Figure 13.11).

Further research reveals that the olfactory system is not only responsible for passive detection of smell but is also closely linked with behavioral response and adaptation. The existence of double pathways in the olfactory system, particularly in higher olfactory animals, suggests a comprehensive interaction between fundamental sensory experience and behavior. For instance, anatomical specialization of the olfactory bulbs in the smooth dogfish shark is thought to support diffcrential behavioral responses for food and social odors in favor of principal survival functions. Selective transection experiments demonstrate that impairment in the lateral olfactory tract weakens tracking of food without compromising social behavior, delineating a multifunctional organization. This tetrapod dualism is exemplified in their special olfactory and vomeronasal systems. It highlights the functional and adaptive significance of olfaction as a sense that bridges anatomical traits to ecological interactions (Lohe et al., 2017).

13.4.2. Mechanism of Smell Detection

The Smell detection begins with the interaction of volatile chemical substances with the olfactory receptors of the olfactory epithelium, a specialized mucous membrane lining the nasal cavity. As odor molecules are breathed in, they bind to their corresponding receptors, which are all specifically tuned to detect distinct chemical shapes. The binding action triggers a cascade of biochemical pathways, leading to depolarization of olfactory sensory neurons. Upon stimulation, these neurons transmit action potentials through the olfactory nerve to the olfactory bulb, an important processing center in the brain. There, the first information regarding the odor characteristics is classified, sorted out, and relayed to higher cortical areas for further processing.

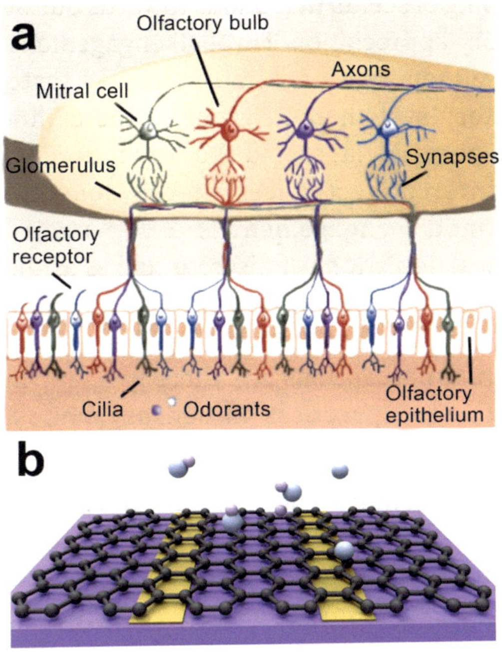

Figure 13.12. (a) The schematic illustration of the mechanism of smell. Reproduced with permission; and (b) The adsorption of the gas molecules on the surface of graphene serving as gas sensor.

Source: https://www.researchgate.net/figure/a-The-schematic-illustration-of-the-mechanism-of-smell-Reproduced-with-permission_fig9_303955702.

The intricate network that exists between neurons and receptors is a mirror of the intricacy of the olfactory system and demonstrates how the perception of odor comprises more than just bodily sensations, possibly illuminating fuller perceptual experiences (Smith et al., 2015). The convergence of olfactory sensory neurons further augments the precision and efficiency of the odor detection system onto tufted cells in the olfactory bulb. This synaptic arrangement enables the integration of signals from more than one receptor type, and in so doing, allows the brain to take account of a vast variety of smells simultaneously. Olfactory processing is not linear but rather a richer, multidimensional mapping of scents that builds towards our overall sensory appreciation. Through engagement with several sensory modalities, such as taste, the olfactory system contributes to the compound perception of flavor and the way it accentuates the interconnectedness of the senses. This multimodal engagement is a departure from classical depictions of discrete senses as distinct faculties, demonstrating the integration of smell, taste, and chemical irritations into presenting coherent perceptions and thereby undermining reductionist practices in sensory philosophy (Macpherson et al., 2010) (Figure 13.12).

Furthermore, the interaction between the sense of smell and feelings accounts for the broader significance of detecting smells in human life. The early connection between smell stimuli and the limbic system highlights the primacy of smell in releasing memory and emotional responses. The connection accounts for the way smells evoke visceral response and associations, again confirming that chemical senses give us an in-depth knowledge of our surroundings. Therefore, the mechanism of smell detection must not simply be addressed in the limited context of sensory experience but as an intricate component of an overarching epistemological process by which perception operates. As the philosophical debate unfolds, recognizing the importance of the chemical senses can provide much insight into the nature of perception and the variability of human sensory life (Smith et al., 2015).

13.4.3. The Role of Smell in Memory and Emotion

The intricate interdependence of smell, memory, and emotion contains profound truths about the human experience, remarkably illuminating the ability of olfactory stimuli to evoke vivid memories and emotions. Unlike the other senses, the sense of smell is uniquely associated with the limbic system, the region of the brain responsible for emotions and memory. This neurologic connection is the basis for how scents can transport individuals back to specific times in their lives, allowing immediate recall of associated feelings.

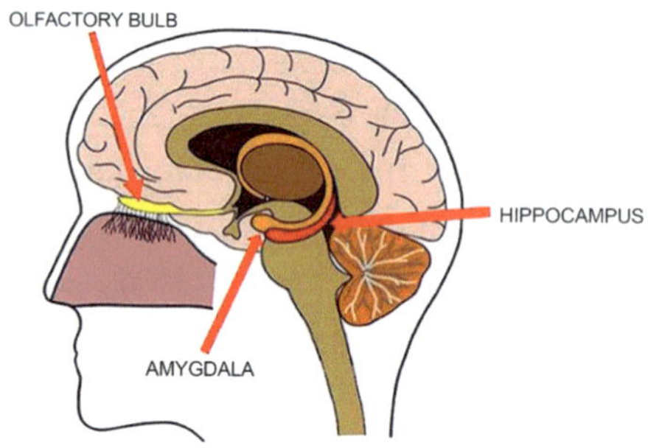

Figure 13.13. Smell is sent through the olfactory bulb (yellow) to the amygdala and hippocampus areas (orange).

Source: https://kids.frontiersin.org/articles/10.3389/frym.2022.667792.

The potency of this sense is often exemplified by the ability of a particular smell to trigger remembrances of childhood, along with an onslaught of sentimentality. This intense recall emphasizes the place of smell in forming emotional connections, ultimately shaping individual lives and experiences. Research has consistently shown that olfactory stimulation can significantly influence emotional states.

For instance, favorable odors such as lavender or vanilla often stimulate feelings of comfort and relaxation, while foul smells evoke feelings of disgust or fear. This dual-mode function of odors to enhance or decay emotional states defines their application range in therapy. Aromatherapy, for instance, uses specific scents to induce relaxation, stress relief, and mental focus (Figure 13.13).

Secondly, the ability of odor to evoke emotional bonds suggests its role in social and cultural contexts, where shared odors can promote group solidarity and facilitate bonding activities. An understanding of such processes offers valuable knowledge regarding the role of smell in not only personal emotional regulation but also group interaction. The integration of odor experience with more general sensory research has the potential to illuminate the complex ways human beings experience and engage with their environment. As described in recent dialogue regarding the promise of next-generation technologies, sensory experiences can be enhanced in virtual environments that simulate real-world experience. The metaverse, for example, is being explored for its potential to shape human interaction, including multisensory properties such as smell (Yogesh et al., 2022). The association of smells with specific places or activities can increase the sense of presence, thereby eliciting responses that might resonate from actual experiences. Further, since the concept of a reality augmented by technology gains momentum, the role of smell signals looms large in establishing true emotional connections within virtual spaces. Thus, the combination of odor with emotion and memory remains a rich subject for exploration, being a reason for more research as well as development of psychological and technological applications (Park et al., 2022).

Test Your Knowledge

1. How does the olfactory system detect and process smells?
2. What is the role of the sense of smell in memory and emotional responses?

13.5. The Sense of Touch

Learning Outcome

1. Discuss types of tactile receptors
2. Describe the role of touch in human interaction
3. Explain the disorders affecting the sense of touch

The sense of touch is a fundamental aspect of human experience, closely related to our interaction with the world. Touch encompasses a range of pressure, temperature, and texture sensations, detected by a range of specialized receptors distributed over the whole of the skin. The receptors convert mechanical stimuli into neural impulses that are interpreted by the brain to convey a direct and intimate connection with the world. In contrast to the sense of vision, which relies predominantly upon light, the sense of touch is a more intimate and instant experience that allows subtle understanding. Not only is this sense informative regarding potential dangers, such as heat or sharpness, but it also adds depth to our emotional lives as a means of communication and reassurance, especially in interpersonal relationships. Moreover, our environment is also a crucial determinant of our tactile senses. Urban environments, for instance, present a rich set of varied textures and sensations that are directly relevant to our comprehension of place. According to studies examining multimodal perceptions of urban space, the haptic interaction in these environments shapes our experience of space and atmosphere. Widespread tree-lined avenues provide a certain haptic feeling compared to the cold, smooth texture of subway tile or the jarring cobblestones of city square (Lucas et al., 2008) (Figure 13.14).

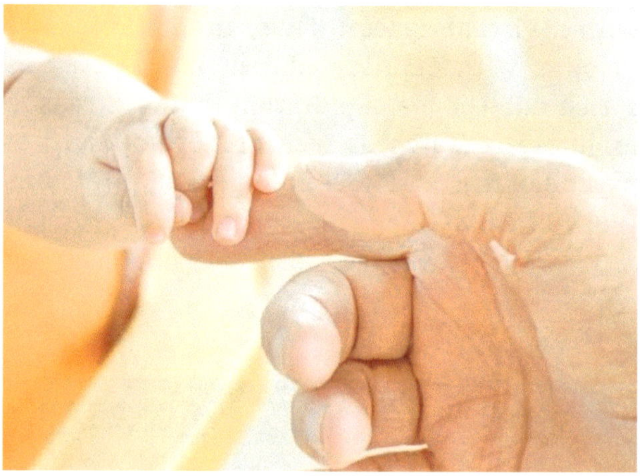

Figure 13.14. A child holding a parent's finger, symbolizing touch as a fundamental sense and form of connection.

Source: https://www.griffinot.com/wp-content/uploads/child-holding-parent-hand-600x441.jpg.

The variability of tactile input not only informs us about the physical character of our world but also enriches our sensory experience, stressing the interdependence of the senses in sensing city space. Finally, the sense of touch is integrated with the other sensory modalities, creating an intricate tapestry of perceptions. Philosophical discourse tends to underemphasize the richness of the chemical senses—taste and smell—and their integration with touch. These senses all come together to create synthesized perceptions, such as the combination of flavors upon consumption, which are not simply derived from taste and smell but also from food texture and temperature (Smith et al., 2015). This synthesis of several senses points out that touch is not an isolated sense; it is part of an extensive network affecting our experiences and interactions. Through the understanding of the intricateness of the sense of touch and the relationships of the senses, we can understand perception more holistically, something essential for interpreting and appreciating the intricateness of our worlds.

13.5.1. Types of Tactile Receptors

The human body harbors a variety of tactile receptors that are required to sense touch, pressure, temperature, and pain. Such receptors provide vital sensory information, enabling individuals to respond effectively to their environment. Among the most studied tactile receptors are Meissner's corpuscles, which contribute towards detecting light touch and changes in texture.

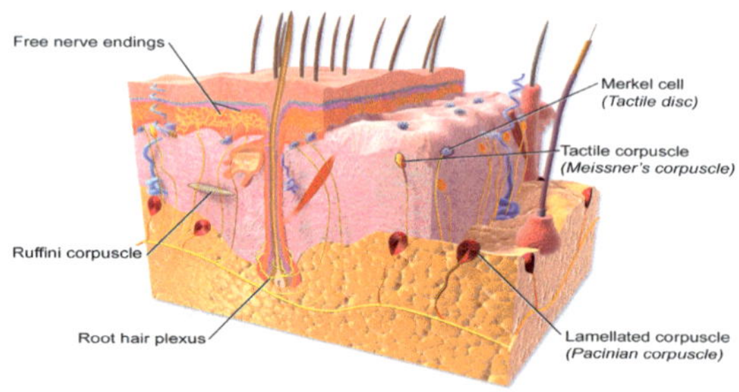

Figure 13.15. Tactile receptors in the skin include free nerve endings, Merkel cells, Meissner's corpuscles, Pacinian corpuscles, root hair plexuses, and Ruffini corpuscles.

Source: https://bio.libretexts.org/Courses/Cosumnes_River_College/Introductory_Anatomy_and_Physiology_%28Aptekar%29/07%3A_Senses/7.05%3A_Touch.

Present predominantly in the dermal papillae of glabrous skin, these receptors are sensitive to low-frequency vibration. In addition, Merkel cells play a critical role in the perception of light touch and provide spatial resolution that allows individuals to discern fine detail and form. Additionally, Pacinian corpuscles respond to deep pressure as well as high-frequency vibration, thus providing the ability to perceive intense tactile stimuli. This functional diversity illuminates the importance of touch receptors in building our sensory experience and understanding of our surroundings, lending credence to discussions about the multidimensional classification of the senses being argued within the literature (Macpherson et al., 2010) (Figure 13.15).

An understanding of the various types of tactile receptors and their role can help one appreciate the richness of sensory experience in a variety of contexts. The city context, for example, engages multiple sensory modalities beyond the dominance of sight. Tactile receptors play a role in perceiving the texture of surfaces, which influences the way individuals navigate spaces considerably. From asphalt's roughness to glass's smoothness, information relayed by sense receptors informs the direction of our movement and interaction. Furthermore, the psychological and emotional responses evoked by such tactile stimuli emphasize the nature of human sensory perception as complex. Evidence indicates that the urban sensory experience creates a more complicated, richer experience of space, and thus the value of urban design that can embrace diversity of the senses (Lucas et al., 2008). Such a multi-faceted process is consistent with thinking through the application of multiple criteria in the definition of our sensory experience more inclusively, as suggested in the debate about sensory classification. The interactions among different types of tactile receptors not only add to our understanding of sensory processing but also direct beneficial applications for rehabilitation and robotics. For instance, knowledge of the sensitivity of different receptors can lead to better techniques for sensory substitution in patients with sensory impairment. Prosthetic limbs, for example, can be created to mimic the work of cutaneous receptors to allow users to obtain feedback that can enhance their reaction to the environment. Furthermore, the development of technology enables the creation of haptic feedback systems in virtual reality that simulate tactile sensations, thereby creating immersive reactions from users through interaction with the depth of human sense perception. The complexity of the operation of tactile receptors underlines the necessity for a more global strategy to sensory modalities, in keeping with broad-scope models of comprehension of our sensory experience and its implications (Macpherson et al., 2010).

13.5.2. The Role of Touch in Human Interaction

Touch in human interaction is the primordial element of our sensory existence, which leads us to the way we connect and with the world. Whereas visual or auditory cues are more processed and less reactive, touch is instantaneous and creates emotional intimacy and social connection. Physical contact, a handshake, a hug, or a pat on the back, is a powerful nonverbal indicator of trust and compassion. Research indicates that contact induces the physiological response, i.e., the release of oxytocin, the so-called "bonding hormone," which stimulates inter-human interactions. Besides, touch can transmit delicate messages about love, warmth, or support, enriching interpersonal contacts in personal and public life. As our society progresses towards online communication, the declining emphasis on physical contact can lead to a lack of emotional expression, and the most crucial use of touch becomes apparent: maintaining human connection. In addition to facilitating emotional bonds, touch also plays a significant role in how we perceive and interact with the world. Contrary to the traditional view of visual dominance, tactile perception is vital in determining our understanding of the physical world. The chemical senses, like touch, provide rich feedback about texture, temperature, and pressure, thus providing us with a multisensory experience that optimizes environmental awareness. Such experiences involve objective features and subjective sensations, as indicated by the co-action of taste, touch, and smell in the perception of flavor. This multisensory approach dispels the myth that all perceptual episodes are confined to a single sense, emphasizing touch's interconnected role in our reasoning, thinking, and decision-making. The richness of touch, not just our sensory experience, but also our emotional experience and social interactions, promotes its wholesome contribution to human interaction (Smith et al., 2015) (Figure 13.16).

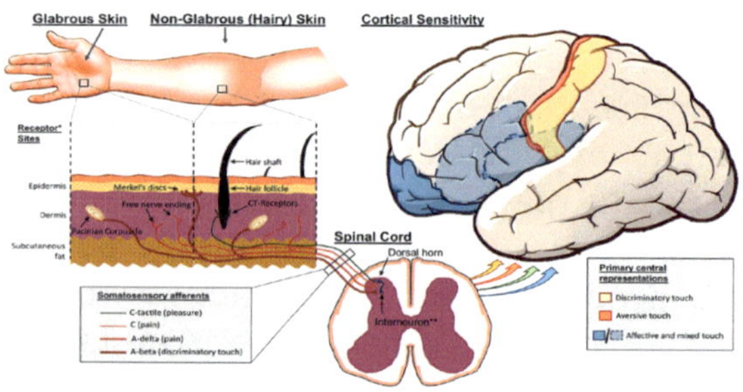

Figure 13.16. Schematic of parallel somatosensory pathways. Somatosensory information is received at the tactile receptors embedded within skin.

Source: https://nyaspubs.onlinelibrary.wiley.com/doi/full/10.1111/nyas.15056.

In addition, the role of touch is also mirrored in many aspects, including product design and user experience. Designers today increasingly recognize that a general awareness of user-product interaction involves sensitivity to the haptic quality of products over time, which can significantly influence user satisfaction. While vision will be the dominant driver in consumer choice at the point of sale, a product's haptic qualities increase in importance as it is used, leading to a rich experience that shapes consumer opinion. As examined in research on sensory dominance, haptic feedback may change user interaction direction based on the duration of interaction with a product, finally shaping long-term attitudes and satisfaction. This intersection of touch within the realm of design illuminates its broader significance for establishing human meanings and connections, reminding us of the sensory modality's central role in shaping individual relationships and consumer behavior (Fenko et al., 2009).

13.5.3. Disorders Affecting the Sense of Touch

Sensory disorders affecting the sense of touch can have far-reaching impacts on a person's perception of the environment and their interactions with the world around them. Conditions such as neuropathy, which is notorious for peripheral nerve damage, can lead to decreased sensitivity and result in loss of sensation in multiple parts of the body. This has severe consequences, including unnoticed infection or injury, especially in cases where immediate response by touch is necessary, e.g., exercise or body cleanliness.

The difficulty of treating these disorders lies not only in the physiology of nerve damage but also in the psychological aspect, where patients get anxious or depressed due to the altered sensory inputs. It is essential to understand the underlying mechanisms and implications of such disorders in an attempt to provide more effective treatment interventions and enhance the quality of life for individuals suffering from these afflictions. Tactile defensiveness, a disorder that often accompanies sensory processing disorders, is another critical disorder of touch sensation. Individuals with tactile defensiveness may be susceptible to some textures or sensations and feel uncomfortable or disgusted by ordinary sensations such as clothing tags or fabrics. Hypersensitivity for such individuals interferes with social relationships and causes problems in the classroom and the workplace. The neurologic bases of tactile defensiveness are abnormal brain responses in the sensory pathways, which provide difficulties in sensory integration of tactile information. Therapy for this disorder is typically a multidisciplinary approach that includes occupational therapy using the methods of desensitization. These techniques are aimed at slowly moving individuals forward toward the formerly aversive stimuli, toward more flexible and relaxed interaction with their own body space. The role of early interpersonal relations in the development of touch-related disorders cannot be overlooked. Developmental psychology research identifies the importance of early social experience, the foundations for tactility, and self-other relatedness. In particular, the concept of kinaesthetic intersubjectivity highlights the mechanisms by which shared movement and embodiment during early relational life influence sensory integration and the formation of personal identity. For instance, in non-verbal autism disorder therapies, mutual body contact and movement can build experiences of understanding and being in touch that need not involve words. This mode suggests that embodied interaction's therapeutic potential should not be downplayed, and it needs further exploration to help foster effective interventions that capitalize on these dynamics. By adopting the multi-sensory nature of touch in treatment settings, practitioners are able to heighten emotional and physiological care for those affected by touch-related disorders.

Test Your Knowledge

1. How does the sense of touch contribute to human interaction and communication?
2. What are some disorders that can affect the sense of touch, and how do they impact sensation?

13.6. Integration of Special Senses

Learning Outcome

1. Understand the brain's role in sensory integration
2. Define multisensory perception
3. Identify the impact of sensory integration on daily life

Special sense integration is a complex process that showcases human capacity to perceive and interpret the world through a blanket sensory system. The five primary senses—vision, hearing, taste, touch, and smell—each convey unique information that is consolidated by the brain to create a coherent representation of our environment. This interconnection of senses is required to live day-to-day life because it enables individuals to respond appropriately to stimulation. Interconnection between the senses can be illustrated in instances where, say, food is tasted not only through taste but also through smell and texture, showing that the modalities are interconnected in producing a whole sensory experience. For overall health and to increase the richness of human experience, this system must operate smoothly. Research has indicated that there are special populations, including those with autism spectrum disorder (ASD) or special health care needs, who may be faced with unusual challenges in sensory integration. For instance, a study on the effect of a multi-sensory environment (MSE) on children with ASD found the therapeutic potential of individualized sensory interventions to modulate physiological responses, including anxiety. This finding points to the role of adaptive sensory environments in coping with developmental challenges, as they have the potential to reactivate otherwise dormant sensory pathways. By tailoring sensory experience, for instance, through highly structured therapy environments, therapists can enhance participation and children's affective status, with the implication that sensory integration might be applied in a focused manner to improve therapy outcomes for groups of children with sensory processing disorders (Atari et al., 2014).

Beyond influencing individual perception, integration of special senses influences more general human communication and social functioning. The European 'Measuring the Impossible' Network (MINET) focuses on human perception being understood across various contexts, ranging from measuring product quality to measuring social well-being. The project shows a growing recognition of the need for metrological strategies involving not just the traditional physiological measurements but also human subjective experience across sensory modalities. MINET's research focus is aimed towards the development of consensus on measurement concepts and techniques that can be extended to human perception, and through that, improve decision-making processes in critical areas such as health and safety. Understanding the integration of multiple senses in measurement aids us in triggering innovations based on improved understanding of human integration of the senses and, thereby, better individual and collective results (Berglund et al., 2010).

13.6.1. The Brain's Role in Sensory Integration

The human brain plays a pivotal role in sensory integration, which ensures coordination of a smooth blend of information from multiple senses to create an integrated perceptual experience. Rather than processing individual sense modalities, the brain integrates inputs from the visual, auditory, and chemical senses and demonstrates a superior ability to enhance our understanding of the environment. For example, the experience of flavor—a smell and taste construct—illustrates the way in which the brain integrates information from multiple senses to create a complex experience. The complexity of these multimodal interactions contradicts the long-standing assumption that perception is a function of one of the five senses only, to suggest that chemical senses, long held in lower esteem, are central to the appreciation of the holistic nature of perception itself (Smith et al., 2015). Through the conjunction of stimuli, the brain allows for a more subtle and amplified interaction with the world around us, and the importance of sensory integration becomes evident in day-to-day life. While describing the intricacies of sensory integration, the concept of the brain being a prediction machine is a significant paradigm. As Clark has hinted, this framework encompasses a range of cognitive processes like perception, action, and cognition. It suggests that the brain is continuously engaged in estimating the consequences from sensor data. By generating predictions of the arriving stimuli, not only does the brain facilitate information processing, but it also reduces uncertainty in our experience of perception. As an example, during food tasting, the brain anticipates expectations of flavors through experience, facilitating effective identification and emotional responses to an array of stimuli. Predictive coding of sensory stimuli enhances our ability to interact with the environment, supporting the intimate link between sensory integration and intellectual processes such as attention and imagination (Muckli et al., 2013) (Figure 13.17).

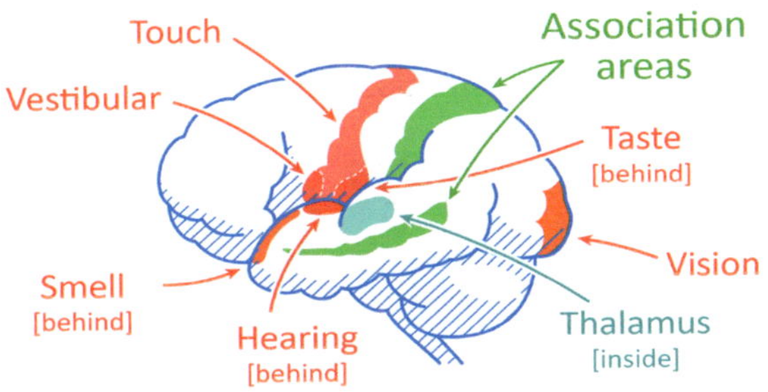

Figure 13.17. Multimodal association areas process information from multiple sensory areas in the brain.

Source: https://learn.genetics.utah.edu/content/senses/worktogether/.

Thus, the brain function transcends mere response to stimulus, asserting that it actually builds our perceptual world. In addition, sensory integration calls attention to the interconnectedness of mind and feelings present in perceptual experience. The conflict of different senses allows us to have a more subtle appreciation of what's present around us and lays the foundation of our decision-making processes. For instance, the combination of taste and smell not only informs us of the palatability of food but also evokes memories and emotions associated with a given taste. The brain's ability to form robust associational networks that facilitate learning and adaptation is a result of this multimodal data. Hence, the combination of sensorial inputs emphasizes the importance of sensory learning in comprehending how such processes are vital to the cognitive domain. The richness of our sensory experience is constructed to a significant degree by the capacity of the brain to bring information from diverse domains together, and this underscores the significance of sensory integration in research on the special senses (Smith et al., 2015). It is through such compounding that the brain navigates the world's complexities and provides us with an entire framework for comprehending our sensory experience.

13.6.2. Multisensory Perception

Multisensory perception fundamentally enlarges our understanding of how information from separate sensory modalities is processed in the brain to form a single perceptual experience. Traditional perception models are prone to individual sensory channels, therefore relegating some senses, particularly chemical senses such as smell and taste, to a subordinate role. However, recent theoretical advancements question this premise on the basis that chemical senses are essential to determining our relationship with the environment. Scientists have identified that these senses do not merely provide discrete sensory input; instead, they are part of a unified perception that possesses the properties of flavor and scent, influencing emotional and cognitive responses. Through the reevaluation of the role played by the chemical senses, philosophers and researchers both challenge the assertion that these modalities are essential to the comprehension of the complexity of multisensory perception, providing necessary hints regarding how various senses blend into our perception of the real world (Smith et al., 2015). In food consumption contexts, multisensory perception is even more elevated since it is an activity that implies the application of all five senses—taste, smell, sight, touch, and hearing—to eating. The combination of these senses has a striking effect on people's perception of taste and pleasure, reflecting the intricate process of multisensory integration. For instance, research has determined that visual information, such as food color and appearance, can enhance or suppress perceived taste. In contrast, olfactory information significantly influences flavor profiles. This complex interaction is well explained in novel systems like LeviSense, which systematically explore the effect of different sensory inputs during the tasting process. These experiments illuminate how multisensory integration creates immersive experiences that flavor our ordinary lives and are an important area of research in the study of human experience (Ablart et al., 2020). Furthermore, the implications of multisensory perception extend far beyond the culinary domain into such diverse fields as advertising, education, and therapy. By leveraging the findings from multisensory integration, professionals can create more sensory-rich, stimulating environments that better engage a wide range of sensory modalities, leading to improved learning and retention. For example, educators can use multisensory teaching methods to support different learning modalities, thereby enhancing student motivation and knowledge attainment. Alternatively, multisensory interventions in therapeutic settings can inspire emotional insight and improve intervention effectiveness. As science continues to advance, the comprehension of multisensory perception can provide innovative applications for the enhancement of human experience in various settings, challenging traditional assumptions of sensory order and emphasizing the richness of human perception (Smith et al., 2015).

13.6.3. Impact of Sensory Integration on Daily Life

Sensory integration is essential in developing the way individuals move and perceive their everyday lives, particularly in relation to special senses such as sight, hearing, and the sense of touch. Sensory processing ability is what allows individuals to perform simple activities, respond to the environment, and engage in social interactions. When sensory integration is properly functioning, individuals are not even aware of the complexities involved; nevertheless, challenges in this aspect can lead to tremendous disruptions. For instance, an individual with heightened sound sensitivity can struggle to attend social gatherings, which impacts their ability to form and maintain interpersonal relationships. Therefore, it is essential to study how sensory integration affects daily functioning for individuals and communities since it informs approaches on how to improve the quality of life and facilitate inclusion (Figure 13.18).

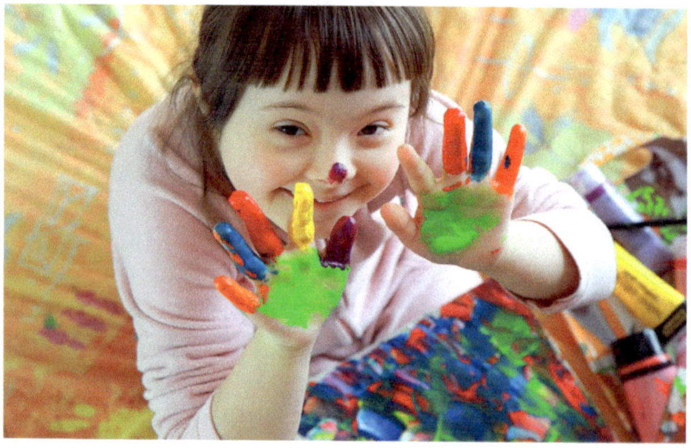

Figure 13.18. Finger painting activity promoting sensory integration and creativity in children.

Source: https://growinghealthyseasons.com/wp-content/uploads/2024/05/sensory-integration.jpg.

Also, the impacts of sensory integration extend beyond individual experience to affect greater societal interests. In school settings, effective sensory processing enhances learning outcomes for students, particularly students with sensory processing disorders. Organizations that incorporate multisensory teaching in education not only provide a more inclusive environment but also enhance involvement and comprehension for students with varying backgrounds. An integrated teaching strategy that stimulates multiple senses can significantly improve cognitive and affective development, offering students a more substantial learning experience. As attested through studies that provide evidence of self-directed learning strategies allowing vocabulary to be acquired by older adults through multisensory interaction, it is clear that auditory sensory integration has the potential to make learning environments richer and more supportive of diverse learning styles (Gonz et al., 2019; López Gómez et al., 2019). Outside of academic and social settings, sensory integration also significantly affects health and well-being, particularly with aging. The aging population is also likely to experience sensory perception changes that impact daily life, with increased risks of isolation and diminished quality of life. For example, decreased hearing and visual acuity may interfere with elderly engagement in social interaction or access to significant services, making the sensation of loneliness worse. Therefore, enhancing sensory integration by using therapies among older adults, such as multisensory stimulation methods, can reverse such challenges. By understanding the importance of sensory input and processing, societies can implement enabling strategies that augment the active participation of older adults and achieve their empowerment as well as reintegration into society. Addressing sensory integration in daily life provides an opportunity to create a more interactive and inclusive environment for people of all ages.

Test Your Knowledge

1. What is the brain's role in integrating sensory information from different modalities?
2. How does multisensory perception enhance our understanding of the environment?

SUMMARY

In summarizing the multifaceted roles of the special senses, one must acknowledge their profound influence on human experience and knowledge. Senses of vision, hearing, taste, touch, and olfaction are not separate abilities but integrated systems that operate to account for the world around us. These sensory modes operate collectively to provide a general comprehension of our world, allowing individuals to create meaningful relationships with the world around us. Therefore, sound perception, at times considered to be secondary to visual input, is integral to the conveyance of emotion and memory. The intricate interrelationship of auditory perception, emotional response, and memory serves to underscore the necessity of considering all senses in any examination of human cognition (Makhlouf et al., 2017). Therefore, by determining how these modalities interact, we gain insight into the nuances of human perception. Examination of the significance of sensory perception reveals its fundamental role in shaping the way individuals navigate their world and engage with others. By mixing sensory inputs, individuals can accommodate various surroundings, organize interpersonal interactions, and construct themselves. This perceptual level of experience is most visible with regard to auditory perception, which generates memory recall and emotional resonance. Cognitive science studies confirm that human knowers are epistemically open in the sense of cross-modal integration of sensory intuitions beyond visual experience. The interplay between the senses not only enriches our self-knowledge but also reveals the richness of our epistemic relations to the world (Anderson et al., 2005). Thus, each sense is worthy of close study in scientific and philosophical research. Finally, to learn the special senses, one can only approach them in an interdisciplinary way, which is commensurate with their complicatedness. The study of sensory modalities gives rise to other questions about how we know and make sense through lived experience. When individuals become more aware of each sense's subtlety of functioning, there is promise for more appreciation of the sense's role in existence. Moreover, recognizing the variation of sensory perception can highlight the subjective nature of human experience; different histories and cultures determine how individuals are engaged with the world. By cultivating a rich understanding of the special senses, we reinforce their significance in human cognition and affective life, leading the way to innovation in psychology, neuroscience, and design that focuses on the complete sensory experience.

To adequately appreciate the workings of special senses, one has to examine their primary mechanisms and significance in daily existence. Special senses—vision, hearing, taste, smell, and touch—are employed for explaining the world and guiding action. Each sense operates based on distinct physiological mechanisms responsible for detecting sensory stimuli, which are further elaborated upon by the nervous system. The neuroscientific findings provide significant insights into such processes, lighting the way sensory inputs are transformed into perceptions. For instance, research on visual imagery highlights how imagination and sensory perception are interconnected, with the potential that an understanding of the brain's mechanisms will further scientific and philosophical debates regarding these senses (Agamben et al., 2016). These findings reiterate the inseparability of perception, cognition, and imagination in the building of our sensory perceptions, an area that requires investigation. Importantly, the philosophic roots of sensory perceptions must be acknowledged. From the records of the past, it is apparent that issues relating to perception predate centuries, with important contributions from philosophers and psychologists. Their insight supports the intricacies of interpretation regarding how each sense is not only a passive receptive surface to stimuli but also positively constructs experience and cognition. The concept of "affordance" in media technologies, for instance, highlights how sensory engagements can contribute to our understanding of technology and its use and how the environment influences behavior by means of sensory interaction (Scarlett et al., 2019). This synthesis of science and philosophy shows the persisting relevance of studying special senses in empirical and theoretical contexts, reinforcing the necessity of multiplicity of discourse in interpreting the senses. Also, the synthesis of contemporary scientific inquiry with previous philosophy allows for a greater understanding of the special senses. By reviewing the manner in which recent advancements in neuroscience inform traditional philosophical debates, one can ascertain where empirical evidence refutes prevailing beliefs or reinforces assumptions already held. The dialogue between disciplines promotes the scientific community's understanding of sensory processing while easing problems with conceptual understanding derived from each school of thought. Emphasizing the importance of visualization, as suggested by recent neuroscience research, showcases how empirical findings can illuminate age-old philosophical queries concerning imagination and perception (Agamben et al., 2016). As our understanding of special senses continues to evolve, it is clear that such interdisciplinary exchanges are vital for addressing the intricacies and significance of sensory experience in the context of human cognition and interaction.

KEY TERMS FROM THIS CHAPTER

- Vision
- Taste
- Smell
- Hyperopia
- presbyopia
- External noises
- Human perception
- Chemical senses
- Hearing
- Touch
- Myopia
- Astigmatism
- Speech
- Special senses
- Neural pathways
- Taste buds

CRITICAL THINKING QUESTIONS

1. **Which part of the eye is responsible for controlling the amount of light entering the eye?**
   a. Retina
   b. Cornea
   c. Iris
   d. Lens
2. **The receptors for hearing are located in which part of the ear?**
   a. Outer ear
   b. Cochlea
   c. Tympanic membrane
   d. Eustachian tube
3. **Which of the following is NOT one of the five traditional special senses?**
   a. Taste
   b. Balance
   c. Smell
   d. Touch
4. **The sense of smell is primarily detected by receptors in the:**
   a. Nasal cavity
   b. Tongue
   c. Inner ear
   d. Cornea
5. **Which type of receptor is responsible for detecting color in vision?**
   a. Rod cells
   b. Cone cells
   c. Hair cells
   d. Olfactory receptors

Short Answer Questions

1. What are the main anatomical structures involved in the sense of vision?
2. How does the eye convert light into neural signals?
3. What are the key components of the ear responsible for hearing?
4. How is sound transmitted and processed within the auditory system?
5. What are the primary receptors involved in the sense of taste?
6. How do olfactory receptors contribute to the sense of smell?
7. What types of receptors are involved in the sense of touch, and what stimuli do they detect?
8. How does the nervous system integrate information from multiple special senses to create a cohesive perception?

Answer to Critical Thinking Questions

1.(c) 2.(b) 3.(d) 4.(a) 5.(b)

REFERENCES

1. Vi, C. T., Marzo, A., Memoli, G., Maggioni, E., Ablart, D., Yeomans, M., & Obrist, M. (2020). LeviSense: A platform for the multisensory integration in levitating food and insights into its effect on flavour perception. *International Journal of Human-Computer Studies, 139*, 102428. https://doi.org/10.1016/j.ijhcs.2020.102428Agamben, G., Amedi, A., Anderson, M., Aquinas, T., Aristotle, B., Belardinelli, M., et al. (2016). On picturing a candle: The prehistory of imagery science. https://core.ac.uk/download/41995105.pdf (accessed on 14th June 2025).
2. Anderson, M. L. (2005). Cognitive science and epistemic openness. https://core.ac.uk/download/pdf/86098.pdf (accessed on 14th June 2025).
3. Anonymous, A., Barrough, H., et al. (2014). Female barrenness, bodily access and aromatic treatments in seventeenth-century England. https://core.ac.uk/download/29841905.pdf (accessed on 14th June 2025).
4. Atari, R. (2014). The influence of multi-sensory environment on physiological response in children with autism spectrum disorders and children with special health care needs. https://core.ac.uk/download/67757154.pdf (accessed on 14th June 2025).
5. Azzolini, M. (2004). Anatomy of a dispute: Leonardo, Pacioli, and scientific entertainment in Renaissance Milan. https://core.ac.uk/download/28963208.pdf (accessed on 14th June 2025).
6. Berglund, B., Cancedda, A., Crenna, F., Drnovek, G., et al. (2010). Measurement with persons: A European network. https://core.ac.uk/download/pdf/29239442.pdf (accessed on 14th June 2025).
7. Cronin-Golomb, A. (2013). Emergence of nonmotor symptoms as the focus of research and treatment of Parkinson's disease: Introduction to the special section on nonmotor dysfunctions in Parkinson's disease. https://open.bu.edu/bitstream/2144/34944/3/nihms503527.pdf (accessed on 14th June 2025).
8. Cronin-Golomb, A., Cruickshanks, K. J., Gilmore, G. C., Lin, F., et al. (2018). American Geriatrics Society and National Institute on Aging Bench-to-Bedside Conference: Sensory impairment and cognitive decline in older adults. https://open.bu.edu/bitstream/2144/34380/1/JAGS%20paper%20in%20press%202018.pdf (accessed on 14th June 2025).
9. Dietsch, A. M., Mulheren, R. W., & Westemeyer, R. M. (2024). Applying the evidence: Taste manipulation as a dysphagia management strategy. https://core.ac.uk/download/620961190.pdf (accessed on 14th June 2025).
10. Dwivedi, Y. K., Hughes, L., Baabdullah, A. M., Ribeiro-Navarrete, S., Giannakis, M., Al-Debei, M. M., Dennehy, D., et al. (2022). Metaverse beyond the hype: Multidisciplinary perspectives on emerging challenges, opportunities, and agenda for research, practice and policy. *International Journal of Information Management, 66*, 102542. https://doi.org/10.1016/j.ijinfomgt.2022.102542 (accessed on 14th June 2025).
11. Fenko, A., Hekkert, P., & Schifferstein, H. N. J. (2009). Which senses dominate at different stages of product experience? https://core.ac.uk/download/99979.pdf (accessed on 14th June 2025).
12. Foley, E. (1996). Sound theology: The risk of audition. https://core.ac.uk/download/144550701.pdf (accessed on 14th June 2025).

13. Gaiseanu, F. (2020). Information-based hierarchical brain organization/evolution from the perspective of the informational model of consciousness. https://core.ac.uk/download/322492692.pdf (accessed on 14th June 2025).

14. Georgiev, D., Gregoric-Kramberger, M., & Pirtosek, Z. (2025). Decision making and the brain: Neurologists' view. https://core.ac.uk/download/pdf/6481489.pdf (accessed on 14th June 2025).

15. Gong, Z., Hartel, P. H., Law, Y. W., Moniava, R., et al. (2008). KALwEN: A new practical and interoperable key management scheme for body sensor networks. https://core.ac.uk/download/pdf/11468866.pdf (accessed on 14th June 2025).

16. Largo Gonzáles, J. C., Rojas Rodríguez, L. M., & Valencia Parra, A. (2019). The teaching of vocabulary through the multisensory approach to EFL third age adults in a public nursing home in Pereira, Colombia. https://core.ac.uk/download/288157870.pdf (accessed on 14th June 2025).

17. Lohe, A. (2017). The role of two anatomically separate olfactory bulbs in shark food odor tracking. https://open.bu.edu/bitstream/2144/20706/1/Lohe_bu_0017N_12581.pdf (accessed on 14th June 2025).

18. López Gómez, L. F., Montes Osorio, B., & Rodríguez Ramírez, Y. E. (2019). The teaching of English vocabulary through the multisensory approach to older adults in a private nursing home in Pereira, Colombia. https://core.ac.uk/download/288157871.pdf (accessed on 14th June 2025).

19. Lucas, R., Mair, G., & Romice, O. (2008). The scale of sense: Spatial extent and multimodal urban design. https://core.ac.uk/download/9023652.pdf (accessed on 14th June 2025).

20. Macpherson, F. (2010). Taxonomizing the senses. https://core.ac.uk/download/80155.pdf (accessed on 14th June 2025).

21. Mair, G. M. (2007). Towards transparent telepresence. https://core.ac.uk/download/9030453.pdf (accessed on 14th June 2025).

22. Makhlouf, M. M. (2017). Sound perception: Encapsulating intangible voice memories in a physical memento. https://core.ac.uk/download/84402596.pdf (accessed on 14th June 2025).

23. Mercês, M. J. (2025). Color in the food, color on the ceramic plate–Symbolic perception of the whole. https://core.ac.uk/download/654359772.pdf (accessed on 14th June 2025).

24. Moore, A. M. (2020). The use of multiple sensory modalities by the Antillean manatee (*Trichechus manatus manatus*) to locate food in their natural environments. https://core.ac.uk/download/346468486.pdf (accessed on 14th June 2025).

25. Muckli, L., Petro, L. S., & Smith, F. W. (2013). Backwards is the way forward: Feedback in the cortical hierarchy predicts the expected future. https://core.ac.uk/download/16459952.pdf (accessed on 14th June 2025).

26. N/A. (2025). *Aerospace Medicine and Biology: A Continuing Bibliography with Indexes, Supplement 144*. https://core.ac.uk/download/pdf/42887122.pdf (accessed on 14th June 2025).

27. Ozok, A. A., Tripathi, A. K., Turing, A. M., Nanay, B., Witmer, B. G., Street, C. N., Ihde, D., et al. (2019). Telepresence and the role of the senses. https://core.ac.uk/download/186332565.pdf (accessed on 14th June 2025).

28. Pace-Schott, E. F., Amole, M. C., Aue, T., Balconi, M., Bylsma, L. M., Critchley, H., Demaree, H. A., et al. (2019). Physiological feelings. *Neuroscience & Biobehavioral Reviews, 103*, 267–304. https://doi.org/10.1016/j.neubiorev.2019.05.002 (accessed on 14th June 2025).

29. Park, S., & Kim, Y. G. (2022). A metaverse: Taxonomy, components, applications, and open challenges. *IEEE Access, 10*, 4209–4251. https://doi.org/10.1109/access.2021.3140175 (accessed on 14th June 2025).

30. Paul, E. S., Sher, S., Tamietto, M., Winkielman, P., & Mendl, M. (2019). Towards a comparative science of emotion: Affect and consciousness in humans and animals. *Neuroscience & Biobehavioral Reviews, 108*, 749–770. https://doi.org/10.1016/j.neubiorev.2019.11.014 (accessed on 14th June 2025).

31. Payne, H., & Samaritter, R. (2012). Kinesthetic intersubjectivity: A dance-informed contribution to self-other relatedness and shared experience in nonverbal psychotherapy with an example from autism. https://core.ac.uk/download/9840405.pdf (accessed on 14th June 2025).

32. Rao, H. R. M. N. (1967). A comparative study of the distribution of *gemma gustatoria* in the dog, cat, sheep, and chicken. https://core.ac.uk/download/33362968.pdf (accessed on 14th June 2025).

33. Rosen, A. B., Cutler, D. M., Woodward, R. M., & Stewart, S. T. (2025). A proposed method for monitoring U.S. population health: Linking symptoms, impairments, and health ratings. https://core.ac.uk/download/pdf/6786188.pdf (accessed on 14th June 2025).

34. Scarlett, A., & Zeilinger, M. (2019). Rethinking affordance. https://core.ac.uk/download/250590491.pdf (accessed on 14th June 2025).

35. Sinha, S. R. (2016). From *sapore* to *sapere*: The gustatory perception of elsewhere in Calvino's 'Under the Jaguar Sun.' https://core.ac.uk/download/46604413.pdf (accessed on 14th June 2025).

36. Smith, B. C. (2015). The chemical senses. https://core.ac.uk/download/186332187.pdf (accessed on 14th June 2025).

INDEX

C

D

E

F

G

H

I

K

L

M

N